D1302131

Understanding

Health Care

Financial

Management

Second Edition

Understanding

Health Care

Financial

Management

Text, Cases, and Models
Second Edition

Louis C. Gapenski

AUPHA Press/Health Administration Press
Chicago, Illinois 1996

00 99 98 97 96   5 4 3 2 1

Library of Congress Cataloging-in-Publication Data

Gapenski, Louis C.
    Understanding health care financial management : text, cases, and models / Louis C. Gapenski. — 2nd ed.
        p.   cm.
    Includes bibliographical references and index.
    ISBN 1-56793-041-7 (hardcover : alk. paper)
    1. Health facilities—Business management.   2. Health facilities—United States—Business management.   3. Medical care—United States—Finance.
4. Health services administration—Economic aspects—United States.   I. Title.
RA971.3.G37   1996
362.1'068'1—dc20   96-2139
                                                                            CIP

The paper used in this publication meets the minimum requirements of American National Standard for Information Sciences—Permanence of Paper for Printed Library Materials, ANSI Z39.48-1984. ∞ ™

Health Administration Press
A division of the Foundation
   of the American College of
   Healthcare Executives
One North Franklin Street
Suite 1700
Chicago, Illinois 60606
312/424-2800

Association of University Programs
   in Health Administration
1911 North Fort Myer Drive
Suite 503
Arlington, VA 22209
703/524-5500

Contents

Part VII Working Capital Management

Part VIII Other Topics

Preface

After years of teaching corporate finance and writing related textbooks and casebooks, I began teaching the health care financial management course in the University of Florida's joint MBA/MHA program. The first thing that struck me was that no textbook was available that truly focused on health care financial management. To me, financial management primarily involves analysis and decision making, yet the books available at the time mostly covered accounting and institutional detail, with only a very limited number of pages devoted to financial management.

Thus, I set about creating a health care financial management text that emphasized analysis and decision making. In creating this book, I adopted a very broad definition of the health care industry that included suppliers, such as drug and medical equipment manufacturers, in addition to traditional health care providers such as hospitals and nursing homes. More and more health care administration students are electing careers outside of the hospital industry, and it is important that a health care financial management text presents a broad range of settings. Also, I identified those environmental factors unique to the health care industry that made health care financial management different from corporate financial management, and created a text that focused on these factors.

Concept of the Book

My goals in writing *Health Care Financial Management: Text, Cases, and Models* were to create a text that provided health administration students with (1) an operational knowledge of financial management theory, principles, and concepts; (2) the opportunity to apply these ideas to "real world" health care industry settings; and (3) the opportunity to use spreadsheet analyses to help make better financial decisions. Additionally, I wanted to create a book that could be used as a reference during residencies and after graduation. Finally, I wanted a text that students would find "user-friendly," meaning one that they would enjoy reading and could learn from on their own. If students don't find a text interesting, understandable, and useful, they won't read it.

This book begins with basic concepts about both the health care industry and financial management. It then progresses to show how financial management theory, principles, and concepts can be applied to the health care industry to help managers make better financial decisions, where "better" is defined as decisions that promote the financial well-being of the organization.

Beginning with Chapter 4, each chapter has one or more accompanying cases. The 20 cases give students the opportunity to apply the material covered in the chapters to real-world decision making. The cases are relatively short, about three to five pages each, and focus on a single health care financial management decision. Students typically will be required to either present their case analyses in class or to write up their results, conclusions, and recommendations. In the old days, I thought that it wasn't the job of health care administration faculty to teach communications skills. Now that I am older (and maybe wiser), I have concluded that students need all the communications skills exposure they can get, and the cases serve this purpose.

Most cases have an accompanying spreadsheet model created in both Lotus1-2-3 and Excel. The models are provided to instructors, who can then distribute them to students. Although the cases can be worked by hand, without using the spreadsheet models, this would be very time-consuming. Furthermore, the models allow students to (1) spend more time on decision making, rather than number crunching, and (2) conduct an analysis in much greater depth than otherwise would be possible. To be successful in today's rough-and-tumble health care world, managers need to be proficient in computer modeling. Using spreadsheet models with the cases allows students to gain insights into financial management principles and concepts that they would have simply missed in the old days of pencil and calculator.

Intended Market and Use

The text is targeted for the health care financial management course required in graduate programs in health administration. Students will typically have some background in basic business topics such as financial and managerial accounting, probability and statistics, spreadsheet analysis, and perhaps even corporate finance. However, the text contains a great deal of background information in these areas, and it can be used in programs where students have not had prior exposure to business topics if the instructor takes additional time to ensure that students have an adequate knowledge of fundamental business concepts. The book should also be useful to health care professionals, including both those holding general management positions, and those working as members of financial staffs.

Changes in the Second Edition

Since the first edition of the text was published, I have used the book several times and have received many comments from users at other universities. Furthermore, Health Administration Press has solicited and received a number of thoughtful reviews. The reaction of students, other professors, and the market in general has been overwhelmingly positive—everything indicates that the basic concept of the book is sound. Even so, nothing is perfect, and the health care industry is evolving at a dizzying pace. These circumstances have led to a number of changes to the book, with the most important listed here:

1. All aspects of text discussion, cases, and references were updated and clarified. Particular care was taken to include the latest tax law and reimbursement changes and to update the real-world examples. Also, case data were updated both to improve the cases and to make sure that solutions to the new cases were not identical to the old solutions.

2. The organization of the text was changed slightly to conform to reviewers' suggestions:

   a. A separate chapter was created that deals with financial risk. Although much of the material in the new chapter had been included in the first edition, placing it in a separate chapter consolidated the material so that it could be presented in a more logical manner, as well as allowing for somewhat greater coverage.

   b. The chapter on lease financing was moved from the Capital Acquisition section to the Other Topics section. Although leasing is clearly an alternative form of financing, and hence part of capital acquisition, it is sufficiently specialized to be treated as an "other" topic that may be omitted if time pressures dictate.

    c. A new chapter was added on mergers and acquisitions. Over the past several years, such activity in the health care industry has been extensive, and a chapter devoted to the topic seemed appropriate.

    d. Finally, a new chapter titled "Capitation and Risk Sharing" has been added to the second edition. Health care providers are integrating at breakneck speed, and managed care plans are using capitation payment for provider reimbursement with ever-increasing frequency. The result is that health administration students need to be better prepared to deal with capitation and risk sharing.

3. There are three basic types of cases: (1) directed (which contain questions); (2) semidirected (which contain a guidance paragraph or other forms of guidance, but no questions); and (3) nondirected (which tend to be very long and contain almost no guidance). The cases in the first edition were all directed, which forced all students along the same solution path, and hence kept them from straying too far afield. However, students did not have to develop their own solution strategies, which is, perhaps, the most important element of financial analysis. Furthermore, the directed cases inhibited student discussion, because students believed that all worthy issues were addressed by the case questions.

    Most of the cases in the second edition have been changed to the semidirected type. Now students have to develop their own solution strategies, and the case discussions are less structured and more stimulating. However, if an instructor prefers to use directed cases, case questions for the semidirected cases are included in the Instructor's Manual, and can be copied and provided to students.

4. Finally, one or more "Self-Test Questions" have been added to the end of each major section. These questions allow students to "test" their understanding of the material in that section. (No answers are provided; if a student cannot answer the self-test questions, he or she should reread the section.)

Ancillary Materials

Two important teaching aids were developed to accompany the text:

    Instructor's Manual. A comprehensive manual is available to instructors who adopt the book. The manual includes a sample course outline, suggestions for using the cases, and extensive solutions to all cases. Finally, the Instructor's Manual includes case questions for the semidirected cases that can be distributed to students if more focus is desired.

Model Diskette. The model diskette, which is also available to adopters, contains spreadsheet models that match 15 of the 20 cases. These models can be distributed by instructors to their students as required.

Acknowledgments

This book reflects the efforts of many people. First, I would like to thank the following individuals, who reviewed the first edition of the text and provided many valuable comments and suggestions for improving the book:

Doug Conrad	University of Washington
Tom Getzen	Temple University
Mike McCue	Virginia Commonwealth University
Dean Smith	University of Michigan
Jack Wheeler	University of Michigan

Special thanks are due to Barbara Langland-Orban of the University of Florida, Deborah S. Kolb and J. Bruce Ryan of Jennings Ryan & Kolb, and Peter F. Straley of Baycare Health Partners, who coauthored text chapters; and to Mike McCue and Jack Wheeler, who coauthored text sections.

Colleagues, students, and staff at the University of Florida provided inspirational support, as well as more tangible support, during the development and class testing of the first and second editions of the text. Also, the Health Administration Press staff was instrumental in ensuring the quality and usefulness of the test. Members of the team at the Press showed dedication, skill, and a sense of humor that helped greatly with all phases of text development and production.

Errors in the Text

In spite of the significant effort that has been expended on this edition, it is safe to say that some errors exist. In an attempt to create the most error-free and useful text possible, I strongly encourage both instructors and students to write me at the address below with comments and suggestions for improving the text. I welcome your input!

Conclusion

Good financial management is vital to the economic well-being of the health care industry. Because of its importance, financial management theory, principles, and concepts should be thoroughly understood; but this is easier said than done. I hope that *Understanding Health Care Financial Management: Text, Cases, and Models* will help you understand the financial management problems faced by the health care industry today, and that it will provide guidance on how best to solve them.

Louis C. Gapenski, Ph.D.
Box 100195
Health Science Center
University of Florida
Gainesville, Florida 32610-0195

February 1996

Part I

The Health Care Environment

1

Introduction

$\mathbf{T}$his chapter presents the philosophy and organization of the text and provides a brief overview of the health care industry. In Chapters 2 and 3, we discuss in more detail those features that make the health care industry unique. An appreciation of the motivation for the book, and of the nature of the industry, will make it easier for students to understand the intricacies of health care financial management.

Philosophy of the Text

First and foremost, financial management is a *decision science*. Whereas accounting provides decision makers with rational means by which to measure a business's financial performance, financial management provides the theory, principles, concepts, and tools necessary to make better decisions. Thus, the primary purpose of this text is to help health services administration students become better decision makers. The text is designed primarily for general managers rather than for financial management specialists, although such specialists, especially those with accounting rather than finance backgrounds, or those who are moving into the health care industry from other industries, will find the text useful.

The major difference between this book and corporate finance texts is that this book focuses on those factors that are unique to the health care industry. For example, the provision of health care services is dominated by *not-for-profit* organizations, both private and governmental, and such entities are inherently different from *investor-owned* firms.[1]

This chapter was coauthored by Barbara Langland-Orban of the University of Florida.

Also, the majority of the payments for services provided by the health care industry are not made by the consumers of the service, but rather by some *third party payer* (for example, a commercial insurance company or a government program). Indeed, even the purchase of health insurance is dominated by employers rather than the individuals who will receive the services. Throughout the text, we emphasize ways in which the unique features of the health care industry affect financial management decisions.

Although this book contains some theory, and a great number of financial management concepts and principles, its primary emphasis is on how managers can apply the theory, concepts, and principles. Thus, rather than end-of-chapter problems, the book contains cases, most of which are based on "real life" decisions faced by practicing health care managers. The cases are designed to enable students to apply the skills learned in the chapters in a realistic context, where judgment is just as critical to good decision making as numerical analysis. Furthermore, the cases are semidirected, meaning that students receive some guidance, but must formulate their own approach to the analyses just as real-world decision makers must do.[2]

Also, personal computers are changing the way managers think about structuring and performing financial analyses. Managers, and students, must recognize that computers are capable of providing answers to questions that were not even asked a few years ago. Thus, the cases are oriented toward using spreadsheets to help make better decisions, and instructors are furnished with spreadsheet models that can be distributed to students to make the case numerical analyses both easier and more complete.

Note, however, that it is impossible to create a text that includes everything that a manager needs to know about health care financial management. Indeed, it would be foolish even to try, because the industry is so vast and is changing so rapidly that many of the details needed to become completely knowledgeable in the field can only be learned through contemporary experience. Thus, we do not expect students to fully understand every nuance of every financial management theory and practice that pertains to the industry. Nor do we expect students to become experts in quantitative analysis. Nevertheless, this book will provide students with a sufficient knowledge of health care financial management so that they will be able to (1) judge the competency of analyses performed by others, usually financial staff specialists or consultants, and (2) incorporate sound financial management concepts and principles in their own managerial and personal decision making.

Self-Test Questions:

How does financial management differ from accounting?

The Role of Financial Management
in the Health Care Industry

Until the 1950s, financial management in all industries was generally viewed as descriptive in nature, with its primary role being to secure the financing needed to meet a business's operating objectives. A firm's marketing (or planning) department would project demand for the firm's goods or services, operating personnel would estimate the assets needed to meet the projected demand, and the finance department was responsible for raising the money needed to purchase the required plant, equipment, and supplies. The study of financial management concentrated on financial securities and markets, and on how businesses could interact with the markets to raise funds. Consequently, financial management textbooks of that era were almost totally descriptive in nature.

Today, financial management plays a much larger role in the overall management of a business. Now its primary role is to plan for, acquire, and utilize funds in order to maximize the efficiency and value of the enterprise. The specific goals of financial management depend on the nature of the firm, so we must postpone that discussion until Chapter 2. We also should emphasize that financial management and accounting are separate functions, although the accounting function is often carried out under the direction of the organization's chief financial officer (CFO), and hence falls under the overall category of "finance." The role of accounting is to provide the quantitative information needed to make financial and operating decisions, while the role of financial management is to provide the decision methodologies.

In general, financial management activities include the following:

Evaluation, forecasting, and planning. The financial staff must interact with the firm's other managers as they jointly assess the current situation, and then look ahead and lay the plans that will shape the firm's future.

Long-term investment decisions. It is essential that a firm's financial staff be involved in capital investment decisions, for such decisions (1) dictate the financing needs of the firm, and (2) are the primary determinants of the firm's strategic direction, and hence financial condition.

Financing decisions. The financial staff must raise the funds necessary to support the operating plans of the firm. Such decisions involve the choice between internal and external funds, the use of debt versus equity capital, and the use of long-term versus short-term debt.

Short-term asset management. The financial staff must manage the firm's current, or short-term, assets such as cash, marketable securities, receivables, and inventories. Included here is the management of contracts with third-party payers.

Certainly, no business can prosper unless all functions—accounting, financial management, operations, marketing, personnel, and so on—are performed in a competent manner. Of course, in times of high profitability and abundant financial resources, the role of financial management tends to decline in importance. Thus, when most health care providers were reimbursed on the basis of costs incurred, the role of financial management in the health services industry was minimal—the most critical functional area at that time was accounting, because the most important function was to account for costs, not to manage them. Today, however, the health care industry is facing an increasingly hostile environment, and any firm that ignores the financial management function runs the risk of financial decline, which can lead to bankruptcy and closure. As one prominent Catholic sister put it when discussing the necessity of maintaining hospital profitability, "No margin, no mission."

In recent years, providers have been redesigning their finance functions to recognize the changes that have been occurring in the industry. For the most part, the function of financial management had been driven by the Medicare program, which demanded that hospitals churn out a multitude of reports to help maximize reimbursement and comply with government regulations. Third-party reimbursement complexities meant that a large percentage of the financial staff's time was spent on cumbersome accounting, billing, and collection procedures. Thus, instead of focusing on value-adding activities, the financial staff spent most of its time on bureaucratic functions. Today, to be of maximum value to the enterprise, the financial staff must be able to provide analyses to support managed care contract negotiations, joint venture decisions, and integrated delivery system participation. In essence, financial staffs must help lead organizations into the future, rather than account for what has happened in the past.

We have been emphasizing the financial management function, but we hasten to note that there are no unimportant functions in a business. Also, all business decisions have financial implications, so nonfinancial executives must know enough about financial management to incorporate these implications into their own specialized areas. It is important for general managers, as well as functional managers in marketing, accounting, operations, facilities, and personnel, to understand the principles and concepts of financial management, because this knowledge will make them even better at their own jobs.

Self-Test Questions:

What is the role of financial management in today's health care organization?

How has this role changed over time?

Organization of the Text

Lewis Carroll wrote, in *Alice in Wonderland*, "Any road will do if you don't know where you are going." Therefore, we have carefully charted our destination—the readers of this text need to learn those financial management theories, principles, concepts, and techniques that are most important to managers in the health care industry—and the organization of the book paves the road to this destination.

Part I contains fundamental background materials on the health care environment upon which the remainder of the book builds. Chapter 1 introduces the text, while Chapters 2 and 3 provide additional insights into the uniqueness of the health care industry. Health care financial management cannot be studied in a vacuum—financial decisions are profoundly influenced by the economic and social environment of the industry in which they are made.

Part II contains two concepts fundamental to virtually all financial management decisions. Chapter 4 discusses discounted cash flow (DCF) analysis, which provides techniques for valuing cash flows that occur in the future, and Chapter 5 presents financial risk, one of the cornerstones of financial decision making.

Part III turns to the capital acquisition process. Businesses need capital, or funds, to purchase assets, and Chapters 6 and 7 cover the two primary types of long-term financing: long-term debt and equity. In Part III, we not only provide descriptive information about securities and the markets in which they are traded, but we also discuss security valuation and bond refunding decisions.

Part IV sets forth the framework for analyzing the appropriate mix of capital financing and assessing its cost to the business. In essence, firms use the particular mix of debt and equity financing that maximizes the value of the firm or, alternatively, minimizes the overall cost of funds to the firm. In turn, the cost of funds raised sets the firm's cost of capital, the return that investment opportunities must provide if they are to be financially profitable.

In Chapters 10 and 11 (Part V), we consider the vital subject of long-term investment decisions, or *capital budgeting*. Because major capital projects take years to plan and execute, and because these decisions are generally not easily reversed and will affect operations for many years, their impact on the financial condition of a firm is profound.

Part VI focuses on analysis and forecasting. It is important for a health care manager to be able to assess the current financial condition of his or her firm. Even more important, managers must be able to monitor and control current operations, and to assess ways in which alternative courses of action will affect the firm's future financial condition. The techniques used to analyze a firm's financial and operating strengths and weaknesses, as well as to forecast future financial condition, are discussed here.

Part VII examines current, ongoing operations, as opposed to long-term, strategic decisions. Assets that are expected to be converted into cash within one year, such as inventories and receivables, are called current, or short-term, assets. The management of current assets and current liabilities, such as payables and short-term debt, is discussed in Chapters 14 and 15.

Finally, in Part VIII, we examine some other topics of relevance to health care financial management. Chapter 16 discusses leasing, an alternative way of obtaining the use of fixed assets. In Chapter 17, we focus on mergers and acquisitions, an area of current importance as firms combine to help position themselves better for the health care environment of the future. To close the book, Chapter 18 focuses on capitation and risk sharing. The trend toward integrated delivery systems is creating new challenges for managers, and some of the unique issues associated with such systems are covered in this chapter.

Self-Test Question:

Briefly explain the organization of the book.

Health Care Expenditures

The U.S. health care industry is a diverse collection of subindustries that involve, either directly or indirectly, the provision of *health care services.*

The major players in the industry are: (1) the *providers* of health care services, such as medical (physician) practices, hospitals, and nursing homes; (2) the *suppliers* of drugs and equipment, such as pharmaceutical and medical equipment manufacturers; (3) the *traditional third party payers*, including both government programs and commercial insurers; (4) *managed care plans*, such as health maintenance and preferred provider organizations; and (5) a diverse collection of other entities, ranging from consulting firms to educational institutions to government and private research agencies. We will generally focus on providers, because they are the unique element of the industry, but one must never forget that the industry includes firms such as General Electric, which makes, markets, and leases medical diagnostic equipment, along with lightbulbs, appliances, and jet engines.

The health care industry is the second largest industry in the United States—only the real estate industry is bigger. As shown in Table 1.1, with total spending estimated at over $1 trillion in 1994, the health care industry consumed about 14 percent of the nation's gross national product. As measured by percentage of GNP, the resources devoted to health care in the United States have more than tripled since 1950.

Although it is impossible to effectively pinpoint the causes of rapidly escalating health care expenditures in the United States, some of the reasons that are most often cited are:

1. the rapid advance in the use of high technology to diagnose and treat disease, coupled with the high cost of new technology;

Table 1.1   Total Health Care Expenditures, Per Capita Expenditures, and Percent of Gross National Product, 1950–1994

Calendar Year	Total Health Care Expenditures (in Billions)	Per Capita	Percentage of GNP
1950	$ 12.7	$ 82	4.4%
1960	26.9	146	5.3%
1970	74.3	346	7.4%
1980	251.1	1,068	9.3%
1990	675.7	2,660	12.4%
1993	884.2	3,299	13.9%
1994	1,060.0	3,655	14.0%

Sources: Statistical Abstract of United States. 1990; *Health Care Financing Review.* 1994. (Fall); Department of Congress statistics.

2. the aging of the population;

3. Society's view of the value of life, and the resultant belief that good health is worth any price (it has been said that Americans are the only people on earth who believe that death is optional);

4. the fact that the third party payer system removes the economic responsibility from the consumers of health care goods and services, which results in overutilization;

5. the high cost of malpractice insurance;

6. operational inefficiencies, including duplication of services and excess capacity;

7. the willingness of the federal government to fund health care expenditures through its Medicare and Medicaid programs;

8. the high cost of physician education; and

9. the high cost of new facilities and equipment.

Table 1.2 provides a breakdown of expenditures by service type. Hospitals capture the largest percentage of the health care dollar, while physicians are the next largest beneficiary of health care expenditures. It is interesting to note that nursing home care now consumes over 8 percent of all health care expenditures, whereas nursing home care was almost nonexistent 40 years ago. Because hospitals and physicians

Table 1.2   Health Care Expenditures by Type of Service, 1993

Health Care Expenditure	Percentage of Total
Hospital care	39.3%
Physician services	20.6
Drugs and expendable supplies	9.0
Other direct care	8.5
Nursing home care	8.4
Administration	5.7
Dental services	4.5
Home health care	2.5
Medical equipment	1.5
Total	100.0%

Source: American College of Healthcare Executives. 1995. *Healthcare Executive Key Industry Facts* (March/April).

combined receive over half of the expenditures on health care, cost containment efforts have been directed first toward hospitals, and more recently toward physicians.

Self-Test Questions:

What has been the trend in health care expenditures over the past several decades?

How is the health care dollar split among the providers of goods and services?

Sources of Funding

Funding for health care services is provided by private as well as by federal, state, and local government sources. Although total spending by all sources has increased, the percentage of total expenditures covered by *private sources* decreased in the period from 1950 to 1993, while the percentage from the *federal government* increased. The percentage of expenditures covered by *state and local sources* remained about constant during this 40-year period. The trend of increasing participation by the federal government is a direct result of the Medicare and Medicaid programs.

In 1993, private sources covered 57 percent of health care expenditures, the federal government paid for 33 percent, and state and local government covered 10 percent. Table 1.3 summarizes the sources of national health expenditures.

Table 1.3   Health Care Funding Sources, 1993

Source	Percentage of Total Funding
Private health insurance	33.0%
Medicare	17.1
Medicaid	10.3
Other government programs	15.7
Out-of-pocket payments	20.1
Other private sources	3.8
Total	100.0%

Source: American College of Healthcare Executives. 1995. *Healthcare Executive Key Industry Facts* (March/April).

Self-Test Question:

What are the major sources of funding for health care services?

Trends in Health Care Financing

Numerous factors led to the development and growth of health insurance programs, particularly as health care services became more expensive and the provision of charity care became less practical. In this section, we provide a brief overview of the *third party payer system.* Since reimbursement is an essential element of health care financial management, we will discuss this subject in much more detail in Chapter 3.

During the 1920s, the science of medicine advanced and hospital care became more expensive. By the decade's end, the country faced the Great Depression. As a result, the financial condition of hospitals began to erode and the need for insurance protection became evident. Hospitals, through the American Hospital Association, encouraged the development of hospital insurance plans, primarily Blue Cross and Blue Shield. Private health insurance grew rapidly following World War II, increasing both the proportion of the population with insurance and the scope of coverage. In 1966, the Medicare and Medicaid programs—the two largest government programs financing health care services—were initiated to provide coverage to the elderly and poor.

Medicare is a federal insurance program designed to cover health care services for persons 65 years and older. In 1995, about 40 million persons were enrolled in Medicare. Medicare has two parts, and each has its own federal trust fund designed to ensure that adequate funds are available. The health insurance portion (Part A) pays for inpatient hospital care, posthospital skilled nursing care, home health services, and hospice care. The supplementary medical insurance portion (Part B) covers physician services, hospital outpatient services, and selected other services. Although Medicare is currently funded at adequate levels by payroll taxes and by Part B charges to enrollees, the rapid aging of the population, together with health care costs that are increasing faster than inflation, have caused many to predict that Medicare will be bankrupt by about 2005 unless substantial changes are made.

Medicaid is funded jointly by the federal and state governments. The federal government establishes the minimum requirements for eligibility and specifies the services that must be provided, and the states are allowed to design the scope of their programs within these guidelines.

States receive roughly one dollar from the federal government for each dollar they contribute to the program. This creates an incentive for the states, especially the more affluent, to expand Medicaid coverage, since they have to bear only half the costs. In 1995, over 30 million persons received some type of Medicaid benefit, with a majority of benefits directed toward the aged, blind, and disabled.

Private health insurance is offered by state and local *Blue Cross/Blue Shield* organizations, which are either not-for-profit or for-profit corporations established for the sole purpose of providing health insurance, and by *commercial insurers*, such as Aetna and Prudential, which are investor-owned insurance companies that offer a complete line of insurance services. Private health insurance varies widely in terms of hospital and outpatient physician benefits, depth of major medical coverage, and protection against large out-of-pocket expenses.

Traditional health insurance, or *indemnity plans*, typically use *deductibles* and *copayments* to curtail the demand for health services. Such out-of-pocket payments require beneficiaries to share some level of expense, thus avoiding first-dollar coverage. Despite the use of these financial incentives, indemnity plans, which provide almost unlimited access to services with relatively small out-of-pocket costs, encourage consumers to seek additional or higher-quality health care services, and thus place considerable pressure on overall costs.

Managed care plans, which reflect the current movement to control health care spending, strive to combine providers and insurers into a single entity. One type of managed care organization is the *health maintenance organization (HMO)*. HMOs are based on the premise that the current fee-for-service system creates perverse incentives that reward providers for treating patients' illnesses while offering few or no incentives for providing prevention and rehabilitation services. By combining the financing and delivery of comprehensive health care services into a single system, HMOs, at least theoretically, have as strong an incentive to prevent illnesses as to treat illnesses.

Due to the many different types of organizational structures, ownership, and financial incentives provided, HMOs vary widely in cost and quality. HMOs use a variety of methods to control costs. These include limiting patients to particular providers, including "gatekeeper" physicians who must authorize any specialized or referral services, utilization review to ensure that services rendered are appropriate and needed, discounted rate schedules for providers, and payment methods that transfer some risk to providers. In general, services are not covered if beneficiaries bypass their gatekeeper physician or use non-HMO providers. Today, about 65 percent of HMOs are investor-owned, while the remaining 35 percent are not-for-profit entities.

The federal Health Maintenance Act of 1973 encouraged the development of HMOs and created a great deal of interest in the concept by providing federal funds for HMO operating grants and loans. In addition, the Act required larger employers offering health care benefits to their employees to include a federally qualified HMO as one of the health care alternatives, if one was available, in addition to traditional insurance plans.

Another type of managed care plan, the *preferred provider organization (PPO)*, evolved during the early 1980s. PPOs are a hybrid of HMOs and traditional health care insurance. They use many of the cost-saving strategies developed by HMOs, such as specific provider panels, utilization review, and reduced rate schedules for providers. However, PPOs do not mandate that beneficiaries use specific providers, although financial incentives are created that encourage members to use those providers with which the PPO has discounted-fee contracts (the PPO panel). Unlike HMOs, PPOs do not require beneficiaries to use preselected gatekeeper physicians who serve as the initial contact and authorize all services received. PPOs are less likely than HMOs to provide preventive services, and they do not assume any responsibility for quality assurance since the enrollees are not constrained to use only the PPO panel of providers.

HMOs and PPOs grew rapidly in numbers and size during the 1980s and have continued to expand thus far in the 1990s. Further, hybrids of HMOs and PPOs continue to develop, such as *exclusive provider organizations*, which are PPO-like plans that require members to use only participating providers but do not designate a specific gatekeeper, and *point of service (POS) plans*, in which enrollees may choose either to obtain services from within the HMO or to bear higher out-of-pocket costs to obtain services from providers outside the HMO. HMOs now cover about 21 percent of all insured individuals, PPOs cover 36 percent, and POS plans cover 7 percent, while only 36 percent remain covered by free-choice indemnity plans. Just a few years ago, 61 percent of the insured population was covered by indemnity plans, so the movement to managed care has accelerated over time.

In an effort to achieve the potential cost savings of managed care plans, conventional insurance companies have started to apply managed care strategies to their own plans. Such plans, which are called managed fee-for-service plans, are using preadmission certification, utilization review, and second surgical opinions to control inappropriate utilization. Although the distinctions between managed care and conventional plans were once quite apparent, considerable overlap now exists in the strategies and incentives employed. Thus, the term "managed care" now describes a continuum of plans, which can vary significantly in their approaches to providing combined insurance and health care services. The common feature in managed care programs and plans is that the insurer has some mechanism by which it controls, or at least influences, patients' utilization of health care services.

In spite of the trend toward managed care plans, about 40 million Americans at any one time are without any type of health care insurance. This lack of insurance effectively denies them complete access to health care services, even though a large percentage of national expenditures is devoted to those services. Although the health system appears well funded, at least when compared with other industrialized nations, it clearly does not meet the complete health care needs of the entire population.

The rapidly increasing costs of health care services, coupled with the lack of universal access, have prompted policymakers to consider serious structural reform of the health care system. The federal government's highest priority is to reduce the budget deficit without creating new taxes, and state and local governments are also under significant budget constraints. Thus, government programs are unlikely to fund the ever increasing costs of health care services.

Whereas federal and state governments have made limited progress in changing the health care system, employers—the primary purchasers of health care insurance—are taking an ever more active role in attempting to rein in health care costs. Since for years the cost of insurance has steadily risen at two or more times the general inflation rate, employers are now finding it impossible to continue the old ways. Thus, employers are passing on to employees an increasing percentage of health insurance costs, as well as demanding that insurers be more aggressive in their efforts to reduce the rate of growth in health care costs.

If current trends continue, health care managers will be facing more and more pressure from all parties to offer quality services at the lowest possible costs. This means that the financial consequences of actions will become more and more important to the decision-making process, and that managers will have to become more and more sophisticated in their financial management skills.

Self-Test Questions:

Describe the recent trends in health care financing.

What are the implications of these trends for health care managers?

Delivery Settings and Trends

Health care services are provided in numerous settings including hospitals, ambulatory care facilities, long-term care facilities, and even at home. Prior to the 1980s, most health care organizations were free-standing and not formally linked with other organizations. Those that were linked tended to be part of horizontally-integrated systems that controlled a single type of health care facility, such as hospitals or nursing homes. Recently, however, many health care services organizations have diversified and become vertically integrated. The benefits of providing hospital care, ambulatory care, long-term care, and business support services through a multi-institutional entity can be considerable. Some of the more obvious benefits include the following:

1. Patients are kept in the corporate network of services (*patient capture*).
2. Providers have access to managerial and functional specialists (for example, reimbursement and marketing professionals).
3. Information systems that track all aspects of patient care, as well as insurance and other data, can be developed more easily.
4. Linked organizations have better access to capital.
5. The ability to recruit and retain management and professional staff is enhanced.
6. Integrated delivery systems are able to offer insurers a complete package of services ("one-stop shopping").
7. Incentives can be created that encourage all providers in the system to work in common for the good of the system; this has the potential to both improve quality and control costs.

Hospitals

Hospitals provide diagnostic and therapeutic services to persons who require more than several hours of care, although most hospitals are actively engaged in ambulatory services as well. To ensure a minimum standard of safety and quality, hospitals must be licensed by the state and undergo inspections for compliance with state regulations. In addition, most hospitals are accredited by the *Joint Commission on Accreditation of Healthcare Organizations (JCAHO)*. JCAHO accreditation is a voluntary process that is intended to promote high standards of care. Although the cost to achieve and maintain compliance with standards can be substantial, accreditation provides eligibility for participation in the Medicare program, and hence most general, acute care hospitals seek accreditation.

Recent environmental and operational changes have created significant challenges for hospital managers. For example, hospitals are experiencing decreasing admission rates and shorter average lengths of stay, resulting in excess capacity. At the same time, hospitals have been pressured to give discounts to managed care plans, to limit the growth in patient charges, and to assume greater risk in their contracts with third party payers. These trends are illustrated in Table 1.4, which contains selected community hospital statistics for 1979, 1989, and 1993. As can be seen, the number of hospitals is declining, and increasing cost-containment pressures are likely to accelerate the trend toward fewer, more efficient hospitals.

Hospitals differ in function, length of patient stay, size, and ownership. These factors affect the type and quantity of fixed assets, programs, and management requirements, and often determine the type and level of reimbursement available. Hospitals are classified as either general, acute care facilities or specialty facilities. Function not only dictates the type of patients who will be treated, but also the source of patients, capital intensity required (the amount of fixed assets such as buildings and equipment), staff mix, and reimbursement structure.

General, acute care hospitals provide general medical and surgical services and selected acute specialty services. General, acute care hospitals are short-stay facilities, and account for the majority of hospitals. *Specialty hospitals*, such as psychiatric, childrens, womens, rehabilitation,

Table 1.4   Selected General Acute Care Hospital Operating Measures

Measure	1979	1989	1993
Number of hospitals	5,842	5,533	5,261
Total number of beds	984,000	933,000	918,786
Average number of beds per hospital	168	171	175
Average length of stay (days)	7.6	7.2	7.0
Average occupancy rate	73.9%	65.5%	65.6%
Profit margin	5.6%	3.7%	5.2%

Sources: AHA Hospital Statistics. 1990–1991; American College of Healthcare Executives. Healthcare Executive Key Industry Facts, 1995. (March/April).

and cancer, limit admission of patients to specific ages, sexes, illnesses, or conditions. The number of psychiatric and rehabilitation hospitals has grown tremendously in the past decade due to the increased needs created by substance abuse, as well as increased government reimbursement for such services.

Hospitals vary in size from fewer than 25 beds to more than 1,000 beds, with general, acute care hospitals tending to be larger than specialty hospitals. Small hospitals, those with under 100 beds, tend to be located in rural areas. Many small hospitals have experienced financial difficulties under ever tighter reimbursement methods, since they are less able to reduce their cost structures than are the larger, urban hospitals. Larger hospitals tend to be academic health centers or teaching hospitals offering a wider range of services, including tertiary services.

Hospitals are organized as voluntary not-for-profit, investor-owned, public (nonfederal), and federal entities.[3] *Federal hospitals* serve special purposes, such as those run by the military services or the Department of Veterans Affairs. *Public hospitals* are funded wholly or in part by a city, county, tax district, or state. In general, federal and public hospitals provide substantial services to indigent patients. In recent years, many public hospitals have converted to other ownership categories— primarily private, not-for-profit—due to the financial burdens placed on governments, which limit the amount of public funds available for hospital care, and the inability of bureaucratic organizations to respond quickly to changes in the health care operating environment.

Private, not-for-profit hospitals are nongovernment entities organized for the sole purpose of providing health care. Due to the charitable origins of U.S. hospitals and a tradition of community service, roughly 87 percent of nonfederal community hospitals are not-for-profit entities, either public or private. In return for charitable service, these hospitals receive numerous benefits, including exemption from federal and state income taxes, exemption from property and sales taxes, eligibility to receive tax-deductible charitable contributions, favorable postal rates, favorable tax-exempt financing, and tax-favored annuities for employees.

The remaining 13 percent of nonfederal community hospitals are *investor owned*. This means that they have shareholders that benefit directly from any profits generated by the hospital and that they do not share the charitable mission of not-for-profit hospitals. Historically, most investor-owned hospitals have been owned by doctors, but now most are held by large corporations such as Columbia/HCA Healthcare, which owns over 300 hospitals across the United States. Unlike not-for-profit hospitals, investor-owned hospitals pay taxes, and they forgo the other benefits of not-for-profit ownership. Despite the expressed differences in mission between investor-owned and not-for-profit hospitals, not-for-profit hospitals are being forced to place greater emphasis on the financial implications of operating decisions than in the past. This trend has raised concerns in some quarters that many not-for-profit hospitals are now failing to meet their charitable mission, and hence should lose some, if not all, of the benefits associated with not-for-profit status.

Hospitals are labor-intensive due to the necessity of providing continuous nursing supervision to patients, in addition to the other services provided by professional and semiprofessional staffs. Physicians petition for privileges to practice in hospitals. While they admit and provide care to hospitalized patients, physicians are not hospital employees, and so are not directly accountable to hospital management. However, physicians retain a major responsibility for determining which hospital services will be provided to patients, so physicians play a critical role in determining a hospital's costs and revenues, and hence financial condition.

Ambulatory, or outpatient, care

Ambulatory care, also known as *outpatient care,* encompasses services provided to noninstitutionalized patients. Traditional outpatient settings include medical (physician) practices, hospital outpatient departments, and emergency rooms. In addition, the 1980s and early 1990s witnessed substantial growth in nontraditional ambulatory care settings such as home health care, ambulatory surgery centers, urgent care centers, diagnostic imaging centers, rehabilitation/sports medicine centers, and clinical laboratories. In general, the new settings offer patients increased amenities and convenience (atmosphere, parking, scheduling, waiting times, and privacy) compared to hospital-based services, and, in many situations, provide services at a lower cost than hospitals. For example, urgent care and ambulatory surgery centers are typically less expensive than their hospital counterparts, because hospitals have higher overhead costs that are factored into patient charges.

Many factors have contributed to the expansion of ambulatory services, but technology has been a leading one. Patients who once required hospitalization due to the complexity, intensity, invasiveness, or risk associated with certain procedures often can now be treated in outpatient settings. In addition, third party payers have encouraged providers to expand their outpatient services through mandatory authorization for inpatient services and by payment mechanisms that provide incentives to perform services on an outpatient basis. Finally, fewer entry barriers exist to developing outpatient services relative to institutional care. Ambulatory facilities ordinarily are less costly, less often subject to licensure and certificate-of-need regulations (exceptions are hospital outpatient units and ambulatory surgery centers), and generally are not accredited. (Licensure and certificate-of-need regulation are discussed in detail in a later section.)

As outpatient care consumes an increasing portion of the health care dollar, and efforts to control outpatient spending are enhanced, the traditional role of the ambulatory care manager is changing. Ambulatory care managers have typically met the needs of physician owners, specifically assuring adequate billing, collections, staffing, scheduling, and patient relations, while physicians have tended to make the more important business decisions. However, reimbursement changes, including managed care affiliations, are requiring a higher level of management expertise. Increasing competition as well as the increasing complexity of the environment are forcing managers of ambulatory care facilities to become more sophisticated in making business decisions, including financial management decisions.

Long-term care

Long-term care entails health care services as well as some personal services provided to individuals who lack some degree of functional ability. It usually covers an extended period of time, and long-term care includes both inpatient and outpatient services, many of which focus on mental health, rehabilitation, and nursing home care. Although the greatest use is among the elderly, long-term care services are used by individuals of all ages.

Long-term care is concerned with levels of independent functioning, specifically activities of daily living (ADLs), such as eating, bathing, and locomotion. Individuals become candidates for long-term care when they become too mentally or physically incapacitated to perform tasks necessary to their environment, and their family members are unable to provide the services needed. Long-term care is a hybrid of health services and social services, and *nursing homes* are a major source of such care.

Three levels of nursing home care exist: (1) skilled nursing facilities; (2) intermediate care facilities; and (3) residential care facilities. *Skilled nursing facilities (SNFs)* provide the level of care closest to hospital care. Services must be under the supervision of a physician and must include 24-hour daily nursing care. *Intermediate care facilities (ICFs)* are intended for persons who do not require hospital or SNF care, but whose mental or physical conditions require daily continuity of one or more medical services. *Residential care* facilities are sheltered environments that do not provide professional health care services, and thus for which most insurance programs, including Medicare and Medicaid, do not provide coverage.

It is interesting to note that the dominant payer for nursing home services, by far, is Medicaid. In the United States, most of the patients in nursing homes, at least those who stay for more than a year or two, exhaust their life savings, and then are forced to turn to the government to fund the care.[4] Nursing homes, with almost 20,000 facilities, are more abundant than hospitals and are also smaller, with average bed size of about 100 beds, compared with 175 beds for hospitals. About 75 percent of nursing homes are investor owned; their occupancy rate is a high 92 percent, and the average patient length of stay is 2.9 years. Nursing homes are licensed by states and nursing home administrators are licensed as well. Although the JCAHO accredits nursing homes, only a small percentage participate, since accreditation is not required for reimbursement and the standards to achieve accreditation are much higher than licensure requirements.

The long-term care industry has experienced tremendous growth in the past three decades. Long-term care accounted for only 1 percent of health care expenditures in 1960, but by 1993, it accounted for over 8 percent. Further demand increases are anticipated, as the percentage of the U.S. population 65 and older increases from less than 15 percent in 1993 to a forecasted 20 percent in 2030. The elderly are disproportionately high users of health care services, and they are major users of long-term care.

Although long-term care is often perceived as nursing home care, many new services are developing to meet society's needs in less institutional surroundings, such as adult day care, life care centers, and hospice programs. These services tend to offer a higher quality of life, although they are not necessarily less expensive than institutional care. Home health care, provided for an extended time period, could be an alternative to nursing home care for many people, but it is not as readily available as nursing home care in many areas. Furthermore, third party payers are just starting to view home health care as a cost-effective alternative to nursing home care.

Integrated delivery systems

Hospitals and physicians currently are developing new organizations that provide a coordinated continuum of health care services to a defined population. Although these organizations can be structured in many different ways, they all fall under the broad category of *integrated delivery systems*. The defining characteristic of an integrated delivery system is that the organization assumes full clinical and financial responsibility for the health care needs of the members of a managed care plan or the employees of a major company or government unit. Additionally, integrated delivery systems receive a fixed premium if contracting directly with an employer or government unit, or a fixed capitation payment if contracting with a managed care plan. Thus, integrated delivery systems assume all of the risks associated with providing health care services.

To be an effective competitor, integrated delivery systems must minimize the provision of unnecessary services, since additional services create added costs but do not result in additional revenues. The objective of integrated delivery systems is thus to provide all needed services to its member population in the lowest-cost setting. To achieve this goal, integrated delivery systems invest heavily in primary care services, especially prevention, early intervention, and wellness programs. The primary care gatekeeper concept is frequently used to control utilization, and hence costs. While hospitals continue to be centers of technology, the main focus of integrated delivery systems is to shift patients toward lower-cost outpatient settings, and clinical integration among the various providers and components of care is essential to achieving quality, efficiency, and patient satisfaction.

One of the most common types of integrated delivery system is the *physician-hospital organization (PHO)*, which is a separate organization formed by a hospital and a physician group to provide contracted health care services to managed care plans and employers. The PHO must provide utilization and quality management, physician credentialing, claims processing, marketing, and revenue distribution for the system. Another common type is the *management service organization (MSO)*, which is a hospital-based organization that provides physician billing and medical group management services.

Integrated delivery systems are in their formative years, so they will evolve over time. Perhaps one form will become dominant, but the provision of health care services may be sufficiently diverse to support a large range of integrated delivery system structures. In any event, they appear to be the future of health care delivery in the United States.

Self-Test Questions:

What are some different types of hospitals, and what trends are occurring in the hospital industry?

What trends are occurring in outpatient and long-term care?

What is an integrated delivery system?

Do you think that integrated delivery systems will be more or less prevalent in the future? Explain.

Health Care Services Manpower

More than 7.5 million individuals are employed in health care services, of which about 4 million full-time equivalents (FTEs) are employed in hospitals and 1.5 million are employed in long-term care facilities. The health care services industry is not only labor-intensive, but one whose labor force has moved toward extreme specialization. For example, hospitals have 200 to 300 different types of position descriptions, and the number is growing. Further, many of these positions require professional and paramedical staff who are licensed, registered, or certified.

Specialization of professionals creates a number of problem areas for managers. First, specialization reduces continuity of patient care. As providers deliver a more narrow scope of services, a greater number of providers must be involved in the overall management of an individual patient. In this environment, continuity of services can be achieved only at the cost of additional resources to coordinate services. Second, specialists demand higher incomes, and hence higher levels of reimbursement than generalists, thus increasing costs. Such cost increases are especially burdensome when specialists provide routine care along with specialized care.

When one thinks about health care professionals, the first profession to come to mind is the *physician*. Due to a perceived shortage of physicians during the 1960s and 1970s, federal assistance programs encouraged growth in the number of medical schools, as well as in the number of students enrolled in existing schools. Thus, the number of physicians per 100,000 population increased from 168 in 1970 to 241 in 1993. Today, most of the growth incentives have been eliminated, partly as a result of the forecasts that the United States currently has, or will soon have, a surplus of physicians. Although a national surplus is not readily apparent, due primarily to growth in specialization and increased opportunities in primary care, many communities are "over-doctored." (For a more detailed discussion of future needs for physicians and hospitals, see Chapter 18, which discusses the impact of *capitation* payment on the provision of health care services. Under capitation, providers receive a fixed payment per month for each patient covered, regardless of the amount or intensity of services provided.)

Physicians primarily control the quantity and mix of health care services utilized, and thus their role in health care expenditures receives much attention from health policymakers. It has been estimated that about 70 percent of all health care costs for services result directly from physician decisions. In addition, it has been argued that physicians even have some ability to create demand for health care services.[5] Optimizing physician numbers, mix, distribution, and practice patterns are key factors in controlling health care costs.

Many types of nonphysician professionals also provide direct health care services to patients. Some of these, such as dentists, podiatrists, psychologists, and chiropractors, are independent *health professionals* who do not practice under physician supervision. Numerous other *paramedical personnel* are university educated, for example pharmacists, dietitians, and physician assistants. Depending on the profession, paramedical personnel are either licensed by the state or registered or certified by a professional association. Their roles are more narrow in focus than those of physicians, independent health professionals, or nurses. The diversity of health care professionals and restrictions on their scope of practice make cost control strategies that attempt to utilize personnel across service areas impractical in many health care settings.

Nurses comprise the largest professional group in health care services. Active registered nurses total about 1.7 million, with hospitals the dominant employer. Unlike medical schools, the numbers of nursing schools and graduates have decreased since 1980. The decline in nursing education, together with the growing demand for health care services, resulted in nursing shortages in some geographic areas, especially in hospitals and nursing homes. However, this shortage has been somewhat offset in recent years by the reduction in demand for hospital services. The nursing profession is confronting many problems, including low levels of work satisfaction relative to that of other professional occupations. Satisfaction studies indicate that nurses perceive the need for more autonomy, higher salaries, and greater professional respect.

One dominant problem that must be overcome before the profession can enhance its image is the variety of educational programs that can lead to licensure. About 42 percent of hospital nurses have associate degrees in nursing, 32 percent have nursing diplomas, 23 percent have baccalaureate degrees in nursing, and 3 percent have masters degrees in nursing. The current system of licensure recognizes only one skill level, although nursing education produces professionals with very different levels of technical and professional expertise. With only one licensure level, nursing salaries are rarely adjusted to recognize the educational and skill differences among nurses.

Technicians and *technologists* (for example, radiology technicians and medical technologists) are usually trained in community colleges or hospital-based programs, although some baccalaureate programs exist for these paramedical personnel. Such personnel are essential to the provision of many types of health care service, although their scope of responsibility is quite narrow. Facilities often face problems in retaining technicians and technologists because their focused education and training generally limit advancement opportunities.

A major factor contributing to increasing health care costs is growing labor expenses. Labor costs now represent almost half of hospitals' total costs, and, in general, labor costs are rising more rapidly than nonlabor costs. Tight labor markets, minimum wage laws, the growth of unionization, and the "catching-up" process explain much of the increase in health care labor costs that has taken place. Historically, health care services employees have been underpaid relative to workers in other industries, and thus wage increases in excess of inflation have been necessary to achieve wage parity. Despite the prolonged upward trend in real wages, an equilibrium has not yet been reached, and wage inflation continues to be a major factor in increasing health care costs.[6]

Self-Test Questions:

What types of professionals work in the health care industry?

Which health care professional has the greatest impact on health care utilization, and hence costs?

Environmental Changes: Technology and Demographics

Changing technology and demographics alter the need for the delivery of health care services, and both ultimately affect health care costs. The advancement and proliferation of technology is a controversial area in health services, since cost-benefit assessments are difficult to perform and unnecessary duplication of expensive technologies is readily apparent. The rapid development of technology and demographic changes create opportunities and challenges for both providers and payers.

Technology

Technologies include drugs, equipment, devices, procedures, and application of specialized knowledge. New technologies are developed with the goal of improving patients' health, but their impact is often to shift delivery sites, stimulate reorganization of systems, and escalate costs.

Rapid and far-reaching technological improvements have occurred in the health care industry, in both diagnosing and treating patients. Major developments have resulted in improved patient care and outcomes, alternatives to invasive procedures, and enhanced patient comfort and convenience. Sophisticated diagnostic imaging devices, such as magnetic resonance imaging and digital subtraction angiography, provide examples of how technology can improve patient care. These technologies use enhanced computer capabilities to generate clinical information that was previously unavailable from diagnostic equipment. In addition, new drugs, devices, and surgical knowledge are facilitating highly complicated procedures, such as organ or tissue transplants and artificial implant surgeries. Prior to such developments, candidates for such procedures would not receive curative care, and instead would have poor prognoses or permanent disabilities.

Surgery is also experiencing rapid technological change. Less invasive procedures are being developed, including arthroscopic, endoscopic, percutaneous, laser, microsurgery, cryosurgery, and lithotripsy techniques. Such recently developed techniques are improving patient outcomes, reducing complication rates, and reducing risk of adverse outcomes. In addition, some techniques, such as balloon angioplasty, provide therapeutic interventions coincident with relatively noninvasive diagnostic equipment. Less invasive technologies also enhance patient satisfaction by reducing discomfort and recovery time.

Patient comfort and convenience are also improved by substituting ambulatory care for institutional care. New diagnostic imaging devices and less invasive surgical procedures permit more patients to be managed as outpatients. Also, improvements in anesthetics have permitted more procedures to be safely performed on an outpatient basis. In addition, new developments in clinical laboratory equipment allow an increased number of tests to be accurately performed in physicians' offices, so fewer patients must be referred to outside laboratories, while the development of mobile diagnostic and therapeutic units offers patients access to specialized services in more convenient locations. Finally, patient comfort and convenience have been improved by the development of comprehensive centers organized to manage particular diagnoses. For example, comprehensive cancer centers provide highly coordinated multidisciplinary services to patients, enhance communication among specialists, and improve patient education and information. Although cancer care is experiencing only incremental improvements in therapy (surgery, radiation therapy, and chemotherapy) and survival rates are not improving substantially, the art of providing cancer care is being improved through such centers.

Important new pharmaceuticals are discovered each year, and such developments have facilitated major improvements in health outcomes. For example, cyclosporin has permitted the development of organ transplant programs, and AZT has extended average longevity among patients with AIDS. In recent years, the four largest pharmaceutical companies (Bristol-Myers Squibb, Glaxo Wellcome, Merck, and SmithKline Beecham) have each developed individual drugs that generate annual sales of more than a billion dollars, thus generating the profits necessary to further develop new drugs. Despite significant advances in drug therapy, much of the research and development among pharmaceutical manufacturers has produced new drugs that contribute little to patient health because alternative medications already exist. Indeed, critics accuse pharmaceutical firms of price gouging because the industry profit margin has been a high 17–18 percent while the level of innovation has been relatively low.

As noted in an earlier section, technological advancements are responsible for at least some portion of recent health care cost increases. Some, such as imaging devices, require heavy capital investment, and many complement rather than substitute for existing services. Technological developments are also under fire for creating an imperative for use—regardless of their expense or whether patient benefit is incremental or substantial. Providers generally perceive new technologies as providing greater prestige, and therefore offering a competitive advantage. Thus, in the current competitive environment, providers are often compelled to purchase and use more expensive technologies to maintain a progressive, up-to-date image. There appears to be nothing in the near term that will reverse this trend in technological development, or that will minimize the impact of new technology on costs.

Demographics

Demographic changes have an impact on the demand for services and the type of services required. Major demographic changes include the increasing percentage of the population that is elderly, and the AIDS and chemical dependency epidemics. Such changes not only affect providers that deliver services, but also have a significant effect on payers that fund them, particularly since many services provided to these populations are funded through public sources.

The elderly

The aging of the population is expected to affect health care services more than any other environmental change. The number of older persons is increasing more rapidly than that of younger people, and the elderly population (65 years and over) is expected to represent 20 percent of the total U.S. population by the year 2030. This "graying of America" is a result of increased longevity coupled with the post-World War II baby boom. This trend is of major concern to policymakers, because the elderly are disproportionate users of health care services and a majority of their care is funded through public sources.

Although many elderly people are independent and active, they are likely to experience multiple chronic conditions that may become disabling. The elderly are admitted to hospitals three times more often than the general population, and their average length of stay is over three days longer than the general average. In addition, the elderly visit their physicians more often than younger persons, and comprise the majority of residents in nursing homes. Providers are concerned about the growth in elderly population because public funding sources (Medicare and Medicaid) have not been increasing their reimbursement rates sufficiently to cover inflation, and providers therefore earn a smaller real return on elderly patients each year.

The aging population also creates funding concerns because the percentage of employed individuals, who pay most of the income tax and all social security taxes, will decrease as the elderly population increases. Reform is needed to assure adequate delivery of health care services as the population ages. Suggestions for reform include increasing the age limits for Medicare eligibility, requiring beneficiaries to pay for a greater proportion of services provided, increasing the availability and coverage of long-term care insurance, increasing the incentives for prevention, and creating less expensive and more efficient delivery settings.

AIDS

Acquired immunodeficiency syndrome (AIDS) has been called the public health emergency of the 1990s. The first cases were diagnosed in the late 1970s and early 1980s. Fifteen years later there is no cure for AIDS, but treatments have been developed to prolong lives. By 1993, over 350,000 people had been diagnosed as having AIDS, and over 200,000 had died. It is estimated that another 1 to 1.5 million persons now carry the human immunodeficiency virus (HIV), which develops into AIDS after incubation.

The AIDS epidemic requires major health care expenditures in both research and personal health services. Over $15 billion has been spent on research and treatment thus far, and about 1.5 percent of health insurance claims are AIDS related. AIDS patients require care from infectious disease specialists, often require hospitalization, and are placing demands on an already burdened nursing home industry. A limited number of providers manage AIDS patients, and many of these are experiencing financial problems, which is not surprising since it costs a hospital about $60,000 to treat an AIDS patient for one year. In fact, AIDS has increased health care costs for all providers, because all health care workers must now handle any blood or body fluids as if they were AIDS contaminated. This results in higher costs to providers due to increased use of gowns, gloves, and goggles, as well as lower productivity.

Substance abuse

Alcohol, drug, and tobacco abuse are the source of numerous health and social problems. They often play a contributing role in accidents, homicides, suicides, cirrhosis, and cancer, all of which place demands on traditional health services. Substance abuse also places increased demands on mental health services and hospital emergency departments.

The costs associated with substance abuse programs have skyrocketed over the past few years. Inpatient and outpatient chemical dependency programs have been a growth area over the past decade because third party payers have been willing to fund such treatments. However, the trend cannot continue, and serious reforms are now occurring that will likely limit spending for such services in the future.

Self-Test Questions:

What are the costs and benefits associated with the relentless drive for technological innovation in health care?

What are some demographic factors that will affect the delivery of health care services in the future?

Regulatory and Legal Issues

The health care services industry is one in which entry traditionally has been heavily regulated. Examples of such regulation include licensure, certificate-of-need, rate-setting, and review programs. In addition, legal issues, specifically malpractice and antitrust, are prominent in discussions of health care cost control.

States require *licensure* of certain health care providers in an effort to protect the health, safety, and welfare of the public. Licensure regulations establish minimum standards that must be achieved in order to provide a service. Many types of providers are licensed, including whole facilities such as hospitals and nursing homes, as well as individuals such as physicians, dentists, and nurses. Facilities that are licensed must submit to periodic inspections and review activities. Such reviews have focused more on physical features and safety and less on patient care services and outcomes, although some progress has recently been made in outcomes research. Thus, licensure has not necessarily ensured that the public will receive quality services. Critics of licensure contend that it is designed to protect providers rather than consumers. For example, licensed paramedical professionals are required to work under the supervision of a physician or dentist, and thus it is impossible for the paramedical professions to compete with physicians or dentists. Despite the limitations of licensure, it is probably here to stay.

Certificate-of-need (CON) legislation was enacted by Congress in the early 1970s in an effort to control increasing health care costs. States were required to conduct health care planning, and a logical extension of this was to require that providers obtain approval based on community need for construction and renovation projects that either relate to specific services or exceed a defined cost threshold. This attempt to control capital expenditures by controlling expansion and preventing duplication of services lasted less than a decade before the Reagan administration began to downplay CON regulation and to promote cost controls through competition.

Criticisms of CON regulation include the following: (1) it does not provide as much control over capital expenditures as originally envisioned; (2) it increases health care costs by forcing providers to incur the administrative costs associated with applying for a CON; and (3) it creates a territorial franchise for services that it covers. That is, CON regulation makes it difficult for new entities to enter markets, even though those new entities may be able to provide services more efficiently than entrenched providers. Currently, CON regulation still exists in over half the states in order to regulate entry into very expensive new services, for example, creating new hospital or nursing home beds.

Additionally, *cost-containment programs* were enacted in many states at a time when most health care reimbursement was based on costs. By the late 1970s, nine states had mandatory cost-containment programs, and many other states had voluntary programs or programs that did not mandate compliance. The primary tool for cost-containment programs is the *rate review* system. Three types of systems have been used: (1) detailed budget reviews with approval or setting of rates; (2) formula methods, which use inflation formulas to set target rates; and (3) negotiated rates involving joint decision making between the provider and the rate setter. Some states using rate review systems have reduced the rate of increase in health care costs below the national average, while others have failed. However, rate review, as a sole means of cost containment, has been criticized because it does not address the issue of demand for health care services.

Health services are subject to many other forms of regulation. For example, pharmacy services are regulated by state and federal laws, and radiology services are highly regulated due to the handling and disposal of radioactive materials. The costs of complying with regulation are not trivial. The CEO of one 430-bed hospital estimated that the cost of dealing with regulatory agencies, including third party payers, is about $8 million annually, requiring a staff of 140 full-time workers to handle the process.

In addition, both federal and state agencies are involved in the regulation of *mergers* and *acquisitions*. In essence, *antitrust laws* prohibit businesses from combining in any way that would unduly limit future competition. Antitrust regulation will be considered further in Chapter 17, where we discuss mergers and acquisitions.

Finally, *professional liability* is yet another legal concern for health care providers. Malpractice suits are the oldest form of quality assurance in the U.S. health care system, and such suits now are used to an extreme extent. Many people believe that the United States is facing a malpractice insurance crisis. Total malpractice premiums, which have doubled in the last ten years, have been passed on to health care purchasers. Some specialists pay malpractice premiums of more than $100,000 per year, and each month U.S. courts manage approximately 20,000 new malpractice suits, with awards averaging $300,000 for those cases that go to trial. Although providers have been successful in achieving some tort reforms, malpractice litigation continues to be perceived as inefficient because it diverts resources to lawyers and courts and creates disincentives for physicians to practice high-risk specialties and for hospitals to offer high-risk services.

A major problem with the existing malpractice system is the lack of uniformity in compensating victims and protecting providers. Medical malpractice not only affects health care costs in terms of malpractice insurance premiums, but it also encourages the practice of defensive medicine, in which physicians overutilize diagnostic services in an effort to protect themselves. Although professional liability is the most visible legal concern in health care services, the health care industry is subject to many other legal issues, including those typical of other industries, such as general liability. Finally, health care providers are confronted with unique ethical issues, such as the right to die or to prolong life, which are often resolved through the legal system.

Self-Test Question:

What are some regulatory and legal issues facing health care providers today?

Summary

This chapter introduced the health care industry, discussed the role of financial management, and introduced the concept and organization of the book. Here are the key concepts:

- Financial management is a *decision science*, so the primary objective of this text is to provide students and practicing health care managers with the theory, principles, concepts, and tools necessary to make effective decisions. The book is structured to support this goal.

- The *primary role of financial management* is to plan for, acquire, and utilize funds in order to maximize the efficiency and value of the enterprise.

- Specific financial management functions include (1) *evaluation, forecasting, and planning*; (2) *long-term investment decisions*; (3) *financing decisions*; and (4) *short-term asset management.*

- The U.S. health care industry is a diverse collection of subindustries that are involved, directly or indirectly, in the provision of *health care services.*

- The major players in the industry are (1) the *providers* of health care services, such as hospitals and nursing homes; (2) the *suppliers* of drugs and equipment, such as pharmaceutical and medical equipment firms; (3) the *insurers*, including both governmental programs such as Medicare and private insurers; (4) *managed care plans*, such as health maintenance and preferred provider organizations; (5) *integrated delivery systems*, which combine multiple provider functions and often the insurance function into a single entity; and (6) a diverse collection of other entities ranging from consulting firms to educational institutions to research agencies.

- *Funding* for health care services is provided by private and federal, state, and local government sources. Although total spending by all sources has increased, the percentage of total expenditures covered by private sources decreased from 1950 to 1993, while the percentage derived from the federal government has increased.

- Most of the reimbursement for health care providers occurs through the *third party payer system*, which includes (1) *private insurers* such as Blue Cross/Blue Shield and Prudential; (2) *public insurance plans* such as Medicare and Medicaid; and (3) *managed care plans* such as health maintenance organizations (HMOs) and preferred provider organizations (PPOs).

- *Health care services* are provided in numerous settings, including hospital, ambulatory care, and long-term care facilities, and in the home.

- The health care services industry is not only *labor intensive,* but its labor force is extremely specialized. For example, hospitals have 200 to 300 different types of positions, and the number is growing. Further, many are professional and paramedical staff who are licensed, registered, or certified.

- *Changing technology* and *demographics* alter the needs and delivery of health services, and ultimately affect health care costs.

- Entry into the health care services industry has been heavily regulated. Examples of regulation include *licensure, certificate of need,* and *rate-setting and review* programs. In addition, legal issues, such as *malpractice* and *antitrust,* are prominent in discussions about controlling health care costs.

Notes

1. Not-for-profit organizations are also called *nonprofit,* but the former designation is becoming dominant within the health care services industry. Also, investor-owned firms are sometimes called *proprietary,* or *for-profit,* firms. We will discuss the differences in these forms of ownership in detail in Chapter 2.
2. There are questions for each case in the Instructor's Manual. Instructors who want to use directed cases in class can make these available to their students.
3. Here we briefly discuss hospital ownership. We will have much more to say about the impact of ownership on financial management goals in Chapter 2.

4. The cost to stay in a nursing home varies widely, but the average cost is close to $3,000 per month. At $36,000 a year, it does not take long for most people to exhaust their savings. Also, about one in five people in the United States will eventually require nursing home care. Considering all of this, it is not surprising that many elderly individuals with substantial savings are setting up trusts or other legal devices to try to protect their wealth from being spent on nursing home care. Additionally, long-term care insurance is beginning to become more widely available, but thus far has not achieved the same widespread acceptance as other forms of health insurance.

5. For example, a 1991 study by the Florida Health Care Cost Containment Board found that clinical laboratories owned by doctors performed almost twice as many tests per patient as similar laboratories with no physician investors. The average charge in a physician-owned lab was $43 per patient, as compared with $20 per patient in other labs.

6. *Real* wages are wages that are adjusted for inflation effects. Thus, for real wages to grow, the growth rate in wages must exceed inflation. In recent years, wages to health care workers, on average, have grown at about twice the inflation rate.

Selected Additional References

For more information on the health care industry, see
Raffel, M. W., and N. K. Raffel. 1989. *The U.S. Health System: Origins and Functions.* New York: Wiley.
For the latest information on events that affect the health care industry, see
Medical Benefits, published semimonthly by Kelly Communications Inc., Charlottesville, VA.
Modern Healthcare, published weekly by Crain Communications Inc., Chicago, IL.
For some ideas on where the health care industry is headed, see
Sullivan, J. M. 1992. "Health Care Reform: Towards a Healthier Society," *Hospital & Health Services Administration* (Winter 1992): 519–32.

2

Organization, Ownership, Goals, and Taxes

In this chapter, we discuss four important, and inter-related, topics. Unlike most industries, which tend to be dominated by one form of business organization and ownership, firms in the health care industry have diverse ownership and organizational structures. For example, health care is provided by both investor-owned and not-for-profit businesses that are organized as proprietorships, partnerships, corporations, joint ventures, and loose alliances. The diverse forms of organization and ownership create an industry in which the participants can have significantly different goals and tax structures. Since financial management decisions are greatly influenced by the goals and ownership of the organization, and the resulting tax consequences, it is necessary for managers to have a good understanding of the similarities and differences in ownership and organization that occur within the health care industry.

Alternative Forms of Business Organization

There are three primary forms of *business organization*: the sole proprietorship, the partnership, and the corporation. Because most health administration students go to work for corporations, and because not-for-profit businesses are organized as corporations, we will concentrate on this form of organization. However, many individual physician practices are organized as proprietorships, and partnerships are common in group practices and joint ventures, so it is important for students to be familiar with all forms of business organization.

35

Sole proprietorship

A *sole proprietorship* is a business owned by one individual. Going into business as a sole proprietor is easy—one merely begins business operations. However, most cities require even the smallest businesses to be licensed, and state licensure is required for most health care professionals.

The sole proprietorship form of organization has three important advantages: (1) It is easily and inexpensively formed. (2) It is subject to few governmental regulations. (3) The business pays no corporate income taxes—all earnings of the business, whether they are reinvested in the business or withdrawn by the owner, are taxed as personal income to the proprietor. In general, a sole proprietorship will pay lower total taxes than a comparable corporation because corporate profits are taxed twice: once at the corporate level, and again at the personal level when the profits are distributed as dividends. Taxation will be discussed in more detail later in the chapter.

Sole proprietorships have three important limitations: (1) Unless the proprietor is very wealthy, it is difficult for a proprietorship to obtain large sums of capital. (2) The proprietor has unlimited personal liability for the debts of the business, which can result in losses greater than the amount put into the business. (3) The life of the business is limited to the life of the proprietor. For these reasons, the sole proprietorship form of organization is restricted primarily to small businesses. However, many corporations start as sole proprietorships (or partnerships) and then are converted to corporations when their growth causes the disadvantages of being a proprietorship to outweigh the advantages.

Partnership

A *partnership* is formed whenever two or more persons associate to conduct a nonincorporated business. Partnerships may operate under different degrees of formality, ranging from informal, oral understandings to formal agreements filed with the state in which the partnership does business. Like a sole proprietorship, the major advantage of the partnership form of organization is its low cost and ease of formation. The disadvantages are also similar to those of a sole proprietorship: (1) unlimited liability; (2) limited life of the business entity; (3) difficulty of transferring ownership; and (4) difficulty in raising large sums of capital. In addition, the tax treatment of a partnership is similar to that of a sole proprietorship: the partnership's earnings are allocated to the partners and taxed as personal income, regardless of whether the earnings are actually paid out to the partners or retained in the business.

Regarding liability, the partners risk all of their personal assets, even those not invested in the business, because each partner is liable for all of the debts of the business. This means that if any partner is unable to meet his or her pro rata obligation in the event of bankruptcy, the remaining partners are responsible for the unsatisfied claims and must draw on their personal assets if necessary.

The first three disadvantages—unlimited liability, impermanence of the business, and difficulty in transferring ownership—lead to the fourth, the difficulty that partnerships (and sole proprietorships) have in attracting substantial amounts of capital. This is no particular problem in a slow-growing business, but if a business needs to expand rapidly to capitalize on market opportunities, the difficulty of attracting capital becomes a real handicap. Thus, many growth companies start out as sole proprietorships or partnerships, but then ultimately convert to the corporate form of organization.

Note that some specialized types of partnerships have somewhat different characteristics than the "plain vanilla" kind. First, it is possible to limit the liabilities of some of the partners by establishing a *limited partnership*, wherein certain partners are designated *general partners* and others *limited partners*. In a limited partnership, the limited partners are liable only for the amount of their investment in the partnership, while the general partners have unlimited liability. However, the limited partners typically have no control, which rests solely with the general partners. Limited partnerships are quite common in real estate and mineral investments, but they are not widely used in the health care industry because one partner is usually unwilling to accept the majority of the business's risk, while the other is unwilling to forgo control.

The *limited liability partnership (LLP)*, sometimes called a *limited liability company (LLC)* (although it is not a corporation) is a relatively new type of partnership that is now available in many states. In a regular or limited partnership, at least one partner is liable for the debts of the partnership. However, in an LLP, all partners enjoy limited liability, just as if they were shareholders in a corporation. In effect, as we discuss in the next section, the LLP form of organization combines the limited liability advantage of a corporation with the tax advantages of a partnership.

Corporation

A *corporation* is a legal entity that is separate and distinct from its owners and managers. The creation of a separate business entity gives the corporation three main advantages: (1) a corporation has unlimited life—it can continue in existence after its original owners and managers have died or left the company; (2) it is easy to transfer ownership in a corporation because ownership is divided into shares of stock that can be easily sold; and (3) owners of a corporation have limited liability. To illustrate, suppose that you invested $10,000 in a partnership that subsequently went bankrupt, owing $100,000. Since the partners are liable for the debts of the partnership, you could be assessed for a share of the partnership's debt in addition to your $10,000 contribution. In fact, if your partners are unable to pay their shares of the indebtedness, you could be held liable for the entire $100,000. However, had your $10,000 been invested in a corporation that went bankrupt, your potential loss would be limited to your $10,000 investment. (Note, though, that in the case of small, financially weak corporations, the limited liability feature of ownership is often fictitious because bankers and other lenders will require personal guarantees from the stockholders.)

These three factors—unlimited life, ease of ownership transfer, and limited liability—make it much easier for corporations to raise money in the capital markets than it is for sole proprietorships or partnerships. Additionally, corporations have been able to provide more generous insurance and retirement plans to their managers than have sole proprietorships or partnerships, although this advantage has been reduced in recent years.

The corporate form of organization does have two primary disadvantages: (1) corporate earnings of taxable entities are subject to double taxation—once at the corporate level and then again at the personal level when dividends are paid to stockholders; and (2) setting up a corporation, and then filing the required periodic state and federal reports, is more costly and time-consuming than that required for establishing a sole proprietorship or partnership.

Although a sole proprietorship or partnership can begin operations without much legal paperwork, setting up a corporation requires that the incorporators prepare a charter and a set of bylaws, or, more typically, hire a lawyer to do it for them. Today, attorneys have standard forms for charters and bylaws on their personal computers, so they can set up a "no frills" corporation relatively easily. The *charter* is filed with the appropriate official of the state in which the firm will be incorporated, and, when approved, the corporation is officially in existence.[1] After the corporation has been officially formed, it must file quarterly and annual financial and tax reports with state and federal agencies.

The *bylaws* are a set of rules drawn up by a corporation's founders to provide guidance for the governing and internal management of the company. Bylaws include features such as the following: (1) how directors are to be elected; (2) whether the existing shareholders have the first right to buy any new shares that the firm issues; and (3) what procedures must be followed to change the charter or the bylaws.

As with partnerships, there are several different types of corporate forms. One type that is common among physicians and other individual and group practice health care professionals is the *professional corporation (PC)*, or in some states, the *professional association (PA)*. All 50 states have statutes that prescribe the requirements for such corporations, which provide the usual benefits of incorporation, but do not relieve the participants of professional liability. Indeed, the primary motivation behind the professional corporation originally was to provide a way for professionals to incorporate yet still be held liable in the courts for professional liability.

Note that if certain requirements are met, one (or more) individuals can establish a corporation but elect to be taxed as if the business were a proprietorship (or partnership). Such corporations, which differ only in how the owners are taxed, are called *S corporations*. Although S corporations are similar in many ways to limited liability partnerships, LLPs actually offer more flexibility and benefits to owners, so we expect to see many businesses, especially group practices, converting to this relatively new organizational form.

Self-Test Questions:

Describe the three major forms of business organization.

What are some different types of partnerships?

What are some different types of corporations?

Alternative Forms of Ownership

Unlike other industries, not-for-profit corporations play a major role in health care, especially among providers. For example, about 60 percent of the hospitals in the United States are private, not-for-profit, hospitals; 25 percent are governmental; and only 15 percent are investor-owned. Further, not-for-profit ownership is common in the nursing home, home health care, and managed care industries. Thus, it is essential for managers in the health care industry to understand the forms of ownership and how differences among the forms affect financial management decisions.

Investor-owned (for-profit) corporations

When the average person thinks of a corporation, he or she probably thinks of an *investor-owned*, or *for-profit, corporation.* The IBMs and General Motors of this world are investor-owned corporations. Investors become owners of such companies by buying the firms' common stock. Investors may buy the common stock of the firm when it first sells its shares to the public: this is called an *initial public offering (IPO)*. In this situation, the funds raised from the new shareholders generally go to the corporation.[2]

Once the shares have been initially sold, they are traded in the *secondary market*, either through exchanges such as the New York Stock Exchange (NYSE) and the American Stock Exchange (AMEX), or in the over-the-counter (OTC) market, which is composed of a large number of dealer/brokers connected by a sophisticated electronic trading system. When shares are bought and sold in the secondary market, the corporations whose stocks are traded receive no funds from the trades—corporations receive funds only when the shares are initially sold. An example of a *publicly held* investor-owned health care company is Columbia/HCA Healthcare, which owns and operates over 300 hospitals and has over 500 million shares outstanding, owned by some 50,000 individual and institutional stockholders. Another example is Beverly Enterprises, which owns and operates about 775 nursing homes and has over 80 million shares outstanding owned by about 8,000 stockholders. Of course, drug companies, such as Merck and Pfizer, and medical equipment manufacturers, such as St. Jude Medical (which makes heart valves) and U.S. Surgical (which makes surgical stapling instruments), are all investor-owned businesses.

The *stockholders*, or *shareholders*, are the owners of investor-owned companies. As owners, they have three basic rights:

1. The right of control. Common stockholders, and no one else, have the right to vote for the corporation's board of directors. Each year, a company's shareholders receive a *proxy* ballot, which they use to vote for directors and to vote on other issues that are proposed by management or shareholders. In this way, shareholders exercise control. In the voting process, shareholders cast one vote for each common share held.

2. A claim on the residual earnings, or net income, of the firm. A corporation sells products or services and realizes revenues from the sales. To produce these revenues, the corporation must incur expenses for materials, labor, insurance, debt capital, and so on.

Any excess (or loss) of revenues after expenses belongs to the owners (the shareholders) of the firm. Management may elect to retain some of the earnings in the firm rather than pay them out to the shareholders as dividends; if so, this is presumably done with the owners' blessing, since the funds belong to the shareholders.

3. In the event of bankruptcy and liquidation, entitlement to any proceeds that remain after all other claimants have been satisfied.

There are three key features of investor-owned corporations: (1) the owners of the firm are well defined, and they exercise control of the firm by the proxy process; (2) the residual earnings of the firm belong to the owners, so management is responsible to a single, well-defined group (the stockholders) for the profitability of the firm; and (3) investor-owned corporations are subject to taxation at the local, state, and federal levels.

Not-for-profit corporations

If a corporation meets a set of stringent requirements, it can qualify for *tax-exempt status*. Such businesses are called *not-for-profit corporations*.[3] Tax-exempt status is granted to organizations that meet the tax definition of a charitable organization, as defined by Internal Revenue Service (IRS) Tax Code Section 501(c)(3) or (4). Hence, such corporations are also known as *501(c)(3) or (4) corporations*.[4]

The tax code defines a charitable organization as any corporation, community chest, fund, or foundation that is organized and operated exclusively for religious, charitable, scientific, public safety, literary, or educational purposes. Since the promotion of health is commonly considered a charitable activity, a corporation that provides health care services can qualify for tax-exempt status, provided it meets other requirements. In addition to the charitable purpose, a not-for-profit corporation must be organized and operated so that (1) it operates exclusively for the public, rather than private, interest; (2) no profits are used for private inurement; (3) no political activity is conducted; and (4) if liquidation occurs, the assets will continue to be used for a charitable purpose. Note that *private inurement* means personal benefit from the profits (net income) of the corporation. Since individuals cannot benefit from the profits of not-for-profit corporations, such organizations cannot pay dividends. Note, though, that prohibition of private inurement does not prevent parties to not-for-profit corporations, such as managers and physicians, from benefiting through salaries, perquisites, contracts, and the like.

Hospital corporations that qualify for tax-exempt status tend to exhibit the following characteristics: (1) control rests in a board of trustees composed of community leaders who have no direct economic interest in the organization; (2) the organization maintains an open medical staff, with privileges available to all qualified physicians; (3) if the hospital leases office space to physicians, it can be leased by any member of the medical staff; (4) the hospital operates an emergency department accessible to the general public; (5) the hospital is engaged in medical research and education; and (6) the hospital undertakes various programs to improve the health of the community.

Conversely, any of the following activities may disqualify a hospital from tax-exempt status: (1) the hospital is controlled by members of the medical staff; (2) the hospital restricts staff privileges to controlling physicians; (3) the hospital leases office space to some physicians at less than fair market value; (4) the hospital limits the use of its facilities; (5) the hospital has contractual agreements that provide direct economic benefit to controlling physicians; or (6) the hospital provides a negligible amount of charity care.

Not-for-profit corporations differ significantly from investor-owned corporations. Since not-for-profit firms have no shareholders, there is no single body of individuals that has ownership rights to the firm's residual earnings and that exercises control of the firm. Rather, control is exercised by a *board of trustees* that is not constrained by outside oversight. Also, not-for-profit corporations are generally exempt from taxation, including both property and income taxes, and they have the right to issue tax-exempt debt. Finally, individual contributions to not-for-profit organizations can be deducted from taxable income by the donor, so not-for-profit firms have access to tax- subsidized contribution capital.

The financial problems facing most federal, state, and local governments have caused politicians to take a closer look at the tax subsidies provided to not-for-profit hospitals. For example, two bills recently introduced in Congress require hospitals to meet minimum standards for care to the indigent or lose federal tax-exempt status. Sponsors say the bills are needed because not-for-profit hospitals provide insufficient services to indigent patients despite generous tax breaks designed to promote charity care. "Under current law, hospitals which are exempt from federal income tax as charitable organizations are not required to provide charity care as a condition of exemption," said Congressman Brian J. Donnelly, who introduced one of the bills. "The need for hospitals to provide charity care is increasing, and many hospitals which enjoy the benefits of tax exemption have done little or nothing to fulfill the need," Donnelly added.

Officials in several states also have been fighting to restrict or strip tax exemptions to hospitals, or to specify mandatory levels of charity care. For example, Texas has established minimum requirements for charity care, which in effect hold not-for-profit hospitals accountable to the public for the tax exemptions they receive. The Texas law specifies four tests, and each hospital must meet at least one of them. The test that most hospitals are expected to use to comply with the law requires that 4 percent of net patient services revenue be spent for charity care.

In addition, money-starved municipalities in several states have levied property taxes on not-for-profit hospitals that have "neglected" their charitable missions. For example, local tax assessors are fighting to remove property tax exemptions from not-for-profit hospitals in several Pennsylvania cities after a recent appellate court ruling supported the Erie school district's authority to tax a local hospital that had strayed too far from its charitable purpose. Hospitals are prime targets because they reap millions of dollars of tax breaks each year. According to one estimate, if all not-for-profit hospitals had to pay taxes comparable to their investor-owned counterparts, local, state, and federal governments would garner an additional $3.5 billion in tax revenues. Obviously, more initiatives to restrict, or even abolish, tax-exempt status are bound to appear in the future.[5]

The inherent differences between investor-owned and not-for-profit organizations have profound implications for almost all elements of financial management, including organizational goals, financing decisions (the choice between debt and equity financing and the types of securities to issue), and capital investment decisions. Much of the remainder of this book will be devoted to such issues.

Self-Test Questions:

What are the major differences between investor-owned and not-for-profit corporations?

What pressures recently have been placed on not-for-profit hospitals to ensure that they meet their charitable missions?

Organizational Structures

Whether investor-owned or not-for-profit, the number of ways of organizing a health care delivery organization is almost unlimited. At the
most basic level, a health care provider can be a single entity with
one operating unit. In this situation, all of the financial management
decisions are made by a single set of managers, since they must raise
the needed capital and decide how to allocate the capital within the
organization. Alternatively, corporations can be set up with separate
operating divisions or as holding companies with wholly or partially
owned subsidiary corporations, in which different management layers
have different financial management responsibilities.

Holding companies

Today many organizations, both investor-owned and not-for-profit, have
adopted *holding company* structures to take advantage of economies of
scale (or scope) in operations and financing, or to gain favorable legal
or tax treatment. Holding companies date from 1889, when New Jersey
became the first state to pass a law permitting corporations to be formed
for the sole purpose of owning the stocks of other companies. Many of
the advantages and disadvantages of holding companies are identical
to those inherent in a large company with several divisions. Whether
a company is organized on a divisional basis or as a holding company
with several subsidiary corporations does not affect the basic reasons
for conducting large-scale, multiproduct or multiservice, multifacility
operations. However, the holding company structure has some distinct
advantages and disadvantages over the divisional structure.

Advantages of holding companies

Control with fractional ownership. A holding company may buy 5, 10,
or 50 percent of the stock of another corporation. Such fractional
ownership may be sufficient to give the acquiring company effective
working control, or at least substantial influence, over the operations of
the company in which it has acquired stock ownership. Working control
is often considered to entail more than 25 percent of the common stock,
but it can be as low as 10 percent if the stock is widely held.

Isolation of risks. Because the various operating companies in a holding company system are separate legal entities, the obligations of one unit
are separate from those of the other units. Therefore, catastrophic losses
incurred by one unit of the system are not transferable into claims against

the other units. This can be especially beneficial when the operating units carry the potential for large losses from malpractice or other liability lawsuits. Note, though, that the parent company often steps in voluntarily to aid a subsidiary with large losses either to protect the good name of the company or to protect its investment in the subsidiary.

Separation of for-profit and not-for-profit subsidiaries. Holding company organization facilitates expansion into both tax-exempt and taxable activities well beyond patient care. However, a tax-exempt holding company must ensure that all transactions with the taxable subsidiaries are conducted at arm's length; otherwise, the tax-exempt status of the parent holding company could be challenged. Investor-owned multihospital systems are organized similarly, except that all of the entities are taxable, for-profit organizations.

Disadvantages of holding companies

Partial multiple taxation. Investor-owned holding companies that own at least 80 percent of a subsidiary's common stock can file a consolidated return for federal income tax purposes. In effect, the holding company and the subsidiary are treated as a single entity, with all of the revenues and costs aggregated. However, when less than 80 percent of the stock is owned, the only way that the subsidiary can transfer funds to the holding company is by paying dividends, and such dividends face partial multiple taxation. For example, holding companies that own over 20 percent but less than 80 percent of the stock of another corporation must pay tax on 20 percent of the dividends received (80 percent are nontaxable), and companies that own less than 20 percent must pay tax on 30 percent of the dividends (70 percent are nontaxable). Since the subsidiary must pay taxes on the earnings prior to making the dividend payment, the funds transferred to the parent are taxed twice.

Ease of forced divestiture. In the event of antitrust action, it is relatively easy for a holding company to relinquish ownership in a subsidiary by selling the stock to another party. This is considered a disadvantage because it increases the likelihood that government agencies will demand divestiture if antitrust concerns arise.

Multihospital systems

Multihospital systems, including both tax-exempt and for-profit organizations, have grown much faster than free-standing hospitals over the past 30 years. Several advantages of multihospital systems have been hypothesized, for instance:

1. better access to capital markets, resulting in lower capital costs;
2. elimination of duplicated services, which increases the volume of services at the remaining sites, resulting in lower unit costs and increased quality;
3. economies of scale or scope, or both;
4. access to specialized managerial skills within the system;
5. ability to recruit and retain better personnel because of superior training programs, advancement opportunities, and transfer opportunities; and
6. increased political power to deal with government issues such as property taxes, certificates of need, and government reimbursement systems.

Corporate alliances

Corporate alliances potentially can provide some of the benefits of multi-institutional systems without requiring common ownership. Perhaps the least binding alliances are industry trade groups, which tend to operate at both state and national levels. To illustrate, the American Hospital Association and its state organizations—for example, the Florida Hospital Association—constitute one major hospital trade association. Also, the American Association of Equipment Lessors is the trade group for companies that lease equipment to the health care industry.

Other types of alliances can be more binding, but provide more benefits to their members. For example, several hospital alliances exist primarily to provide purchasing clout for their members. One of the largest of such alliances is Voluntary Hospitals of America (VHA), which is a for-profit company whose shareholders are the member hospitals, all not-for-profit institutions. VHA's companies and subsidiaries provide members and affiliates with management services in such areas as procurement, data management, marketing, and even capital acquisition. VHA's members and affiliates retain local control and autonomy, yet gain many of the advantages of large systems.

In addition to alliances among similar organizations, alliances are also being formed among dissimilar providers in order to offer a more complete range of services. Such vertical alliances are discussed in the next section.

Integrated delivery systems

In recent years, the most dynamic changes in organizational structures in health care services have centered on the *integrated delivery system*.[6] In the

1970s, horizontal integration, such as the combining of hospitals, was the dominant trend in organization evolution. In the 1980s, and into today, the dominant organizational movement is toward vertically integrated systems. In an integrated delivery system, a single organization, or a closely aligned group of organizations, offers a broad range of patient care and support services operated in a unified manner. The range of services offered by an integrated delivery system may focus on a particular area, such as long-term care or mental health, or, more commonly, it may offer a full range of subacute, acute, and postacute services.

An integrated delivery system may have a single owner, or it may have multiple owners joined together by contracts and agreements. The driving force behind these systems is the motivation to offer a full line of coordinated services, and hence to increase the overall effectiveness and lower the overall cost of the services provided. Cost reduction is obtained by providing only those services that are necessary and ensuring that the services are provided at the most cost-effective clinical level. Integrated delivery systems may be formed by managed care plans or even directly by employers, but more often they are formed by providers to facilitate contracting with plans or employers.

Perhaps the key feature of integrated delivery systems is that, to be successful, the primary focus must be the clinical effectiveness and profitability of the system as a whole, as opposed to each individual element. This requires a much higher level of administrative and clinical integration than is seen in most organizations and, more importantly, it requires that managers of the individual elements of the system place their own interests second to that of the overall system.

Self-Test Questions:

What are the advantages and disadvantages of the holding company form of organization?

What is the difference between horizontal and vertical integration?

What are integrated delivery systems, and why are they such an important organizational structure today?

Firm Goals

Financial management decisions are made not in a vacuum, but with some objective in mind. It is clear that financial management goals must be consistent with and in support of the firm's goals. Thus, by discussing firm goals, we provide a framework for financial decision making within health care organizations.

Investor-owned firms

From a financial management perspective, the primary goal of investor-owned firms is generally assumed to be *shareholder wealth maximization*, which translates to stock price maximization. Investor-owned firms do, of course, have other objectives. Managers, who make the actual decisions, are interested in their own personal welfare, in their employees' welfare, and in the good of the community and of society at large. Still, as we shall see, the goal of stock price maximization is a reasonable operating objective upon which to build financial decision rules.

The primary obstacle to shareholder wealth maximization as the goal of investor-owned firms is the *agency problem*. An agency problem exists when one or more individuals (the *principals*) hire another individual or group of individuals (the *agents*) to perform some service on their behalf, and then delegate some decision-making authority to those agents. Within the financial management framework, the agency problem exists between stockholders and managers and between debtholders and stockholders. We will discuss the stockholder/manager problem now, but will defer our discussion of the debtholder/stockholder problem until Chapter 6.

The agency problem between stockholders and managers occurs because most managers own less than 100 percent of their firm's common stock. In general, the managers of large, investor-owned firms hold only a very small proportion of the firm's stock, so they benefit very little from stock price increases. On the other hand, managers benefit substantially from such actions as increasing the size of the firm to justify higher salaries and more fringe benefits, awarding themselves generous retirement plans, and spending too much on office space, personal staff, and travel, while these actions are often detrimental to shareholders' wealth. It is easy to visualize many situations in which managers are motivated to take actions that are in their best interests, rather than in the best interests of the firm's stockholders.

However, shareholders recognize the agency problem and counter it by creating incentives for managers to act in shareholders' interests. Additionally, some other factors are at work to keep managers focused on shareholder wealth maximization:

Structuring managerial incentives. More and more firms are creating *incentive compensation plans* that tie managers' compensation to the company's performance. One tool often used is *stock options*, which allow managers to purchase stock at some time in the future at a given price. Since the options are valuable only if the stock price climbs above the exercise price (the price that the managers must pay to buy the stock), managers are motivated to take actions to increase the stock price. However, since a firm's stock price is a function both of the actions taken by managers and the general state of the economy, a firm's managers could be doing a superlative job for shareholders and the options still prove to be worthless.

To overcome the inherent shortcoming of stock options, many firms today now use *performance shares* as the managerial incentive. Performance shares are given to managers on the basis of the firm's performance as indicated by objective measures such as earnings per share, return on equity, and so on. Performance shares have a value even if the firm's stock price remains constant because of general market conditions such as rising interest rates. Of course, the value of any shares received is dependent on stock price performance, because 1,000 shares are a lot more valuable if a stock sells for $50 than if it sells for only $10.

Finally, many firms are now using the concept of *economic value added (EVA)* to structure managerial compensation. (EVA is discussed in some detail in Chapter 12.) All incentive compensation plans—stock options, performance shares, profit-based bonuses, and so forth—are designed with two purposes in mind. First, they offer managers incentives to act on those factors under their control in a way that will contribute to stock price maximization. Second, the existence of such plans helps companies attract and retain top-quality managers.[7]

The threat of firing. Until recently, the probability of a large firm's management being ousted by its stockholders was so remote that it posed little threat. This situation existed because ownership of most firms was so widely held, and management's control over the proxy (voting) mechanism was so strong, that it was almost impossible for dissident stockholders to fire a firm's managers. Today, however, about 50 percent of the stock of an average large corporation is held by large institutions such as pension funds and mutual funds, rather than by individual investors. These institutional money managers have the clout, if they choose to use it, to exercise considerable influence over a firm's managers and, if necessary, to vote out the current management team.

The threat of takeover. Hostile takeovers, in which a firm is bought against its management's wishes, are most likely to occur when a firm's stock is undervalued relative to its potential because of poor management. In a hostile takeover, a potential acquirer makes a direct appeal to the shareholders of the target company to *tender*, or sell, their shares at some stated price. If 51 percent of the shareholders agree to tender their shares, the acquirer gains control. When a hostile takeover occurs, the managers of the acquired firm often lose their jobs, and any who are permitted to stay on generally lose the autonomy they had prior to the acquisition. Thus, managers have a strong incentive to take actions to maximize stock price. In the words of the president of a major drug manufacturing company, "If you want to keep control, don't let your company's stock sell at a bargain price."

In summary, it is clear that managers of investor-owned firms can have motivations that are inconsistent with shareholder wealth maximization. Still, sufficient mechanisms are at work to force managers to view shareholder wealth maximization as an important, if not primary, goal. Thus, shareholder wealth maximization is a reasonable goal for financial management decision making within investor-owned firms.

Not-for-profit firms

Because not-for-profit firms do not have shareholders, it is clear that shareholder wealth maximization is not an appropriate goal for such organizations. Indeed, not-for-profit firms consist of a number of classes of *stakeholders* who are directly affected by the organization. Stakeholders include all parties that have an interest (usually financial) in the organization. For example, a hospital's stakeholders include the board of trustees, managers, employees, physicians, creditors, suppliers, patients, and even potential patients, which might include the entire community. While managers of investor-owned companies have to please only one class of stakeholders—the shareholders—to keep their jobs, managers of not-for-profit firms face a different situation. They have to try to please all of the organizational stakeholders, because no single, well-defined group exercises control.

Many people argue that managers of not-for-profit firms do not have to please anyone at all, because they tend to dominate the board of trustees who are supposed to exercise oversight. Conversely, we would argue that managers of not-for-profit firms have to please all of the firm's stakeholders to a greater or lesser extent, because all are necessary to the continuance of the business. Also, even managers of investor-owned firms should not attempt to enhance shareholder wealth by treating any of their firm's other stakeholders unfairly, because such actions ultimately will be detrimental to shareholders.

Typically, the goal of not-for-profit firms is stated in terms of a mission. An example is the mission statement of Bayside Memorial Hospital, a 650-bed, not-for-profit, acute care hospital:

"Bayside Memorial Hospital, along with its medical staff, is a recognized, innovative health care leader dedicated to meeting the needs of the community. We strive to be the best comprehensive health care provider through our commitment to excellence."

Although this mission statement provides Bayside's managers and employees with a framework for developing specific goals and objectives, it does not provide much insight into the goal of financial management. For Bayside to accomplish its mission, the hospital's managers have identified five financial management goals.

1. The hospital must maintain its financial viability.

2. The hospital must generate sufficient profits to permit it to continue to provide the current range of health care services to the community. This means that current plant and equipment must be replaced as it becomes obsolete.

3. The hospital must generate sufficient profits to invest in new medical technologies and services as they are developed and needed.

4. Although the hospital has an aggressive philanthropy program in place, it does not want to rely upon this program, or government grants, to fund its operations.

5. The hospital will strive to provide services to the community as inexpensively as possible, given the above financial requirements.

In effect, Bayside's managers are saying that to achieve the "commitment to excellence" contained in its mission statement, the hospital must remain financially strong and profitable. Financially weak organizations cannot continue to accomplish their stated missions over the long run. It is interesting to note that Bayside's five goals for financial management are probably not much different from the financial management goals of Jefferson Regional Medical Center (JRMC), a for-profit competitor. Of course, JRMC has to worry about providing a return to its shareholders, and it receives only a very small amount of contributions and grants. But, to maximize shareholder wealth, it also must retain its financial viability and have the financial resources necessary to offer new services and technologies. Furthermore, competition in the market for hospital services will not permit JRMC to charge appreciably more for services than its not-for-profit competitors.

Self-Test Questions:

What is the difference in goals between investor-owned and not-for-profit firms?

What is the agency problem, and how does it apply to investor-owned firms?

What factors tend to reduce the agency problem?

Taxes

The value of any financial asset, such as a share of stock issued by Columbia/HCA Healthcare or a municipal bond issued by the Alachua County Healthcare Financing Authority, as well as the value of many real assets such as a medical office building or a hospital, depends on the stream of usable cash flows that the asset is expected to produce. Since taxes can reduce the cash flows that are usable to the business, financial management analyses must include the impact of local, state, and federal taxes. Local and state tax laws vary widely, so we will not attempt to cover them in this book. Rather, we will focus on the federal income tax system, since these taxes are normally much larger than the other taxes. Then, in our examples, we will typically increase the tax rate to approximate the effects of state and local taxes.

Tax laws can be changed by Congress, and major changes have occurred on average every three to four years since 1913 when the federal tax system was initiated. Further, certain aspects of the Tax Code are tied to inflation, so changes automatically occur each year based on the previous year's inflation rate. Therefore, although this section will give you an understanding of the basic nature of our federal tax system, **it is not intended to be a guide for actual use**. Tax laws are so complicated that many law schools offer a master's degree in taxation, and many of the lawyers who hold this degree also are CPAs. Managers and investors should and do, therefore, rely on tax experts rather than trust their own limited knowledge. Still, it is important to know the basic elements of the tax system as a starting point for discussions with tax specialists. In a field complicated enough to warrant such detailed study, we can cover only the highlights.

Current (1995) federal income tax rates on personal income go up to 39.6 percent, and when state and local income taxes are added, the marginal rate can approach or even exceed 50 percent. Business income is also taxed heavily. The income from partnerships and proprietorships is reported by the individual owners as personal income and, consequently, is taxed at rates going up to 50 percent. Corporate income is taxed by the federal government at marginal rates as high as 38 percent, in addition to state and local income taxes. Because of the magnitude of the tax bite, taxes play an important role in most financial management decisions made by individuals and by for-profit organizations.

Individual (personal) income taxes

Individuals pay personal taxes on wages and salaries; on investment income such as dividends, interest, and profits from the sale of securities; and on the profits of sole proprietorships, partnerships, and S corporations. Federal income taxes are *progressive*; that is, the higher one's income, the larger the *marginal tax rate*, which is the rate applied to the last dollar of earnings. Marginal rates on *ordinary income* begin at 15 percent, then rise to 28, 31, and 36 percent, and finally top out at 39.6 percent.

Taxes on dividend and interest income

Individuals can receive *dividend income* on stocks that they own and *interest income* on savings accounts, certificates of deposit, bonds, and the like. Such income from securities is taxed as ordinary income, and hence is taxed at federal rates going up to 39.6 percent, plus state and local income taxes if applicable. Because corporations pay dividends out of earnings that have already been taxed, there is double taxation on corporate income.

Note, however, that under federal tax laws, interest on most state and local government bonds, called *municipals* or "*munis*," is not subject to federal income taxes. Such bonds include those issued by municipal health care authorities on behalf of not-for-profit health care providers. Thus, investors get to keep all of the interest received from municipal bonds, but only a proportion of the interest received from bonds issued by the federal government or by corporations. This means that a lower interest rate muni bond could provide the same or higher after-tax return as a higher-yielding corporate or Treasury bond. For example, consider an individual in the 39.6 percent federal tax bracket who could buy a taxable corporate bond that yielded 10 percent interest. What yield would a similar-risk muni bond have to offer to make the investor indifferent between the muni and the corporate? Here is a way to think about this problem:

$$
\begin{aligned}
\text{After-tax yield on} \\
\text{corporate bond} \ &= \ \text{Pre-tax yield} \ - \ \text{Yield lost to taxes} \\
&= \ \text{Pre-tax yield} \ - \ \text{Pre-tax yield}(\text{Tax rate}) \\
&= \ \text{Pre-tax yield}(1 - T) \\
&= \ 10\%(1 - 0.396) = 10\%(0.604) = 6.04\%,
\end{aligned}
$$

where T is the investor's marginal tax rate. Thus, the investor would be indifferent between a corporate bond with a 10 percent yield and a municipal bond with a 6.04 percent yield.

If the investor wants to know what yield on a taxable bond is equivalent to, say, a 7.5 percent yield on a muni bond, then he or she would follow this procedure:

$$
\begin{aligned}
\text{Equivalent yield on taxable bond} \ &= \ \frac{\text{Yield on muni}}{1 - T} \\
&= \ \frac{7.5\%}{1 - 0.396} = \frac{7.5\%}{0.604} \\
&= \ 12.42\%.
\end{aligned}
$$

The exemption of municipal bonds from federal taxes stems from the separation of power between the federal government and state and local governments, and its primary effect is to allow state and local governments (and not-for-profit health care providers) to borrow at lower rates than otherwise would be possible.

Capital gains versus ordinary income

Assets such as stocks, bonds, real estate, and plant and equipment (land, buildings, x-ray machines, and the like) are defined as *capital assets*. If you buy a capital asset and later sell it at a profit—that is, you sell it for more than you paid for it—the profit is called a *capital gain*. If you sell it for less than you paid for it, the loss is called a *capital loss*. An asset sold within one year of the time it was purchased produces a *short-term capital gain or loss*, whereas an asset held for more than one year produces a *long-term capital gain or loss*. Thus, if you buy 100 shares of Beverly Enterprises, a nursing home company, for $10 per share, and sell the stock later for $15 per share, you will make a capital gain of $100(\$15 - \$10) = 100(\$5) = \$500$. However, if you sell the stock for $5 per share, you will incur a capital loss of $500. If you held the stock for one year or less, the gain or loss is short-term; otherwise, it is a long-term gain or loss. Note that if you sell the stock for $10 a share, you will make neither a capital gain nor a loss; you will simply get your $1,000 back and no taxes are due on the transaction.

Short-term capital gains are taxed as ordinary income—at the same rates as wages, interest, and dividends. However, long-term capital gains are taxed at slightly lower rates than ordinary income if an individual is in the highest (31 percent or higher) tax brackets, because the maximum tax on long-term capital gains is 28 percent. To illustrate the effect of this tax benefit on long-term capital gains, consider an investor in the top 39.6 percent tax bracket who makes a $500 long-term capital gain on the sale of her Beverly Enterprises stock. If the $500 were ordinary income, she would have to pay federal income taxes of 0.396($500) = $198. However, as a long-term capital gain, the tax would be only 0.28($500) = $140, for a savings of $58 in taxes.

Corporate income taxes

The corporate tax structure, shown in Table 2.1, has marginal rates as high as 38 percent, which brings the average rate up to 35 percent. To illustrate, if Midwest Home Health Services, Inc., an investor-owned home health care company headquartered in Chicago, had $80,000 of taxable income, its federal income tax bill would be $13,750:

$$\text{Taxes} = \$13,750 + 0.34(\$80,000 - \$75,000)$$
$$= \$13,750 + 0.34(\$5,000)$$
$$= \$13,750 + \$1,700 = \$15,450.$$

Midwest's marginal tax rate would be 34 percent, and its average tax rate would be $15,450/$80,000 = 19.3\%$. Note that the average federal corporate income tax rate is progressive to $18,333,333 of income, but is constant thereafter.

Unrelated business income earned by not-for-profit corporations

Even though tax-exempt holding companies can be created with both tax-exempt and taxable subsidiaries, it is also possible for tax-exempt corporations to have taxable income, which is usually referred to as *unrelated business income (UBI)*. UBI is created when a tax-exempt corporation has income from a trade or business that (1) is not substantially related to the charitable goal of the organization, and (2) is carried on

Table 2.1   1995 Corporate Tax Rates

Taxable Income	Tax	Average Tax Rate at Top of Bracket
Up to $50,000	15% of taxable income	15.0%
$50,000–$75,000	$7,500 + 25% of excess over $50,000	18.3
$75,000–$100,000	$13,750 + 34% of excess over $75,000	22.3
$100,000–$335,000	$22,250 + 39% of excess over $100,000	34.0
$335,000–$10,000,000	$113,900 + 34% of excess over $335,000	34.0
$10,000,000–$15,000,000	$3,400,000 + 35% of excess over $10,000,000	34.3
$15,000,000–$18,333,333	$5,150,000 + 38% of excess over $15,000,000	35.0
Over $18,333,333	$6,416,667 + 35% of excess over $18,333,333	35.0

with the frequency and regularity of comparable for-profit commercial businesses.

As an example of UBI, consider Bayside Memorial Hospital's pharmacy sales. In addition to its sales to the hospital's patients, the not-for-profit hospital's pharmacy has a second location adjacent to the parking garage that sells drugs and supplies to the general public. In general, the IRS views the charitable purpose of a hospital as providing health care services to its patients, so the income from Bayside's sale of drugs and supplies to nonpatients, which is done on a regular basis, is taxable. The fact that the profits from the sales are used for charitable purposes is immaterial. Note, however, that if the trade or business engaged in by a not-for-profit entity (1) is run by volunteers, or (2) is run for the convenience of employees, or (3) involves the sale of merchandise contributed to the organization, then the income generated remains tax-exempt. Thus, the profits on Bayside's sale of drugs and supplies to its employees, as well as the profits on the sale of items in its gift shop, which is run by volunteer "pink ladies," is exempt from taxation.

UBI tax returns must be filed with the IRS by not-for-profit organizations annually if the gross income from unrelated business activity exceeds $1,000. In determining taxable income, expenses related to UBI income production are deducted from gross income. Then, taxes are calculated as if the income were earned by a taxable corporation.

Interest and dividend income received by an investor-owned corporation

Interest income received by a taxable corporation is taxed as ordinary income at the regular tax rates contained in Table 2.1. However, some portion of the dividends received by one corporation from another is excluded from taxable income. As we mentioned earlier in our discussion of holding companies, the size of the dividend exclusion actually depends on the degree of ownership. In general, we will assume that corporations receiving dividends have only nominal ownership in the dividend-paying corporations, so 30 percent of the dividends received are taxable. The purpose of the dividend exclusion is to lessen the impact of triple taxation, which occurs when the earnings of Company A are taxed, then dividends are paid to Company B, which must pay partial taxes on the income, and then Company B pays out dividends to Individual C, who must pay personal taxes on the income.

To illustrate the effect of the dividend exclusion, a corporation earning $500,000 and paying a 34 percent marginal tax rate would have an *effective tax rate* of only $0.30(0.34) = 0.102 = 10.2\%$ on its dividend income. If this company had $10,000 in pre-tax dividend income, its after-tax dividend income would be $8,980:

$$
\begin{aligned}
\text{After-tax income} &= \text{Pre-tax income} - \text{Taxes} \\
&= \text{Pre-tax income} - \text{Pre-tax income (Effective tax rate)} \\
&= \text{Pre-tax income}(1 - \text{Effective tax rate}) \\
&= \$10,000[1 - 0.30(0.34)] \\
&= \$10,000(1 - 0.102) = \$10,000(0.898) \\
&= \$8,980.
\end{aligned}
$$

If a taxable corporation has surplus funds that can be temporarily invested in securities, the tax laws favor investment in stocks, which pay dividends, rather than in bonds, which pay interest. For example, suppose Midwest Home Health Services has $100,000 to invest temporarily, and it could buy either bonds that paid interest of $8,000 per year or preferred stock that paid dividends of $7,000 per year. Since Midwest is in the 34 percent tax bracket, its tax on the interest if it bought the bonds would be $0.34(\$8,000) = \$2,720$, and its after-tax income would be $\$7,000 - \$2,720 = \$5,280$. If it bought the preferred stock, its tax would be $0.34[0.30(\$7,000)] = \$714$, and its after-tax income would be $6,286. Other factors might lead Midwest to invest in the bonds, but the tax laws certainly favor stock investments when the investor is a corporation.

Interest and dividend income received by a not-for-profit corporation

Interest and dividend income received from securities purchased by not-for-profit corporations with **temporary surplus cash** is not taxable.

However, note that not-for-profit firms are prohibited from issuing tax-exempt bonds for the sole purpose of reinvesting the proceeds in other securities, although such firms can temporarily invest the proceeds from a tax-exempt issue in taxable securities while waiting for the planned expenditures to occur. If not-for-profit firms could engage in such *tax arbitrage* operations, they could, in theory, generate an unlimited amount of income by issuing tax-exempt bonds for the sole purpose of raising funds to invest in higher-yielding securities that are taxable to most investors. For example, a not-for-profit firm might sell tax-exempt bonds with an interest rate of 5 percent and use the proceeds to invest in U.S. Treasury bonds yielding 6 percent.

Interest and dividends paid by a corporation

A firm's assets can be financed either with debt or equity capital. If it uses debt financing, it must pay interest on that debt, whereas if an investor-owned firm uses equity financing, normally it will pay dividends to its stockholders. The interest paid by a taxable corporation is deducted from the corporation's operating income to obtain its taxable income, but dividends are not deductible. Put another way, dividends are paid from after-tax income. Therefore, Midwest Home Health Services, which is in the 34 percent tax bracket, needs only $1 of pre-tax earnings to pay $1 of interest expense, but it needs $1.52 of pre-tax earnings to pay $1 in dividends:

$$\text{Dollars of pre-tax income required} = \frac{\$1}{1 - \text{Tax rate}}$$
$$= \frac{\$1}{0.66} = \$1.52.$$

The fact that interest is a tax deductible expense while dividends are not has a profound impact on the way businesses are financed—the U.S. tax system favors debt financing over equity financing. This point will be discussed in detail in Chapter 9.

Corporate capital gains

At one time, corporate long-term capital gains were taxed at lower rates than ordinary income. However, under current law, corporate capital gains are taxed at the same rate as operating income.

Corporate loss carry-back and carry-forward

Corporate operating losses that occur in any year can be used to offset taxable income in other years. Such losses can be carried back to each of the preceding 3 years and forward for the next 15 years. For example, an operating loss in 1996 would first be applied to 1993. If the firm had taxable income in 1993, and hence paid taxes, the loss would be used to reduce 1993's taxable income, so the firm would receive a refund on taxes paid for 1993. If the 1996 loss exceeded the taxable income for 1993, the remainder would be applied to reduce taxable income for 1994, then 1995. If the firm had losses in the previous three years, the cumulative losses, including the loss for 1996, would be carried forward to 1997, then 1998, and so on up to year 2011. Note that losses that are carried back provide immediate tax benefits, but the tax benefits of losses that are carried forward are delayed until some time in the future. The tax benefits of losses that cannot be used to offset taxable income in 15 years or less are lost to the firm. The purpose of this provision in the tax laws is to avoid penalizing corporations whose incomes fluctuate substantially from year to year.

Consolidated tax returns

As we mentioned earlier, if a corporation owns 80 percent or more of another corporation's stock, it can aggregate income and expenses and file a single consolidated tax return. Thus, the losses of one company can be used to offset the profits of another. No business wants to incur losses (you can go broke losing 1 dollar to save 34 cents in taxes), but tax offsets do make it more feasible for large multicompany businesses to undertake risky new ventures that might suffer start-up losses.

Self-Test Questions:

Briefly explain the personal and corporate income tax systems.

What are capital gains and losses, and how are they differentiated from ordinary income?

What is unrelated business income?

How do federal income taxes treat dividends received by corporations as compared to dividends received by individuals? Why is this distinction made?

Do tax laws favor corporate financing by debt or by equity? Explain.

Depreciation

Suppose a medical group practice buys an x-ray machine for $100,000 and uses it for ten years, after which the machine is obsolete. The cost of the services provided by the machine must include a charge for the cost of the machine, and this charge is called *depreciation*. Because depreciation reduces profit as calculated by accountants, the higher a firm's depreciation charge, the lower its reported profit. However, depreciation is a noncash charge—it is an allocation of previous cash expenditures—so higher depreciation expense does not actually reduce cash flow. In fact, for taxable businesses, higher depreciation increases cash flow, because the greater a firm's depreciation expense in any year, the lower its tax bill.

To see more clearly how depreciation expense affects cash flow, consider Table 2.2. Here we examine the impact of depreciation on two investor-owned hospitals that are alike in all regards except for the amount of depreciation expense. Hospital A, with $100,000 of depreciation expense, has $200,000 of taxable income, pays $80,000 in taxes, and has $120,000 of after-tax income. Hospital B, with $200,000 of depreciation expense, has only $100,000 of taxable income, pays $40,000 in taxes, and has an after-tax income of $60,000.

However, depreciation is a noncash expense, whereas we assume that all other entries in Table 2.2 represent actual cash flows. To determine each hospital's cash flow, depreciation must be added back to after-tax income. When this is done, Hospital B, with the larger depreciation expense, has the larger cash flow. In fact, Hospital B's cash flow is larger by $260,000 − $220,000 = $40,000, which represents the tax savings on its additional $100,000 in depreciation expense:

Table 2.2   The Effect of Depreciation on Cash Flow

	Hospital A	*Hospital B*
Revenue	$1,000,000	$1,000,000
Costs except depreciation	700,000	700,000
Depreciation	100,000	200,000
Taxable income	$ 200,000	$ 100,000
Federal plus state taxes (assumed to be 40%)	80,000	40,000
After-tax income	$ 120,000	$ 60,000
Add back depreciation	100,000	200,000
Net cash flow	$ 220,000	$ 260,000

$$\text{Tax savings} = \text{Tax rate(Depreciation expense)}$$
$$= 0.40(\$100,000) = \$40,000.$$

Because a firm's financial condition depends on the actual amount of cash that it earns, as opposed to some arbitrarily determined accounting profit, a firm's managers should be more concerned with cash flow than reported profit. Note that if the hospitals in Table 2.2 were not-for-profit hospitals, taxes would be zero for both hospitals, and both hospitals would have $300,000 in net cash flow. However, Hospital A would report $200,000 in earnings, while Hospital B would report only $100,000 in earnings.

Companies generally calculate depreciation one way for tax returns and another way when reporting income to other parties such as investors, Medicare administrators, and state health care boards. For *tax depreciation*, businesses must follow the depreciation guidelines laid down by tax laws, but for other purposes, firms usually use *accounting*, or *book*, *depreciation* guidelines.

To determine book depreciation, the most common method is the *straight line* method. To apply the straight line method, start with the capitalized cost of the asset (price plus shipping plus installation), then subtract the asset's *salvage value*, which, for book purposes, is the estimated value of the asset at the end of its useful life, and finally divide the net amount by the asset's useful life. For example, consider the x-ray machine that costs $100,000 and has a ten-year useful life. Further, assume that it costs $10,000 to deliver and install the machine, and that its estimated salvage value after ten years of use is $5,000. In this case, the capitalized cost of the machine is $100,000 + $10,000 = $110,000, and the annual depreciation is ($110,000 − $5,000)/10 = $10,500. Thus, the depreciation expense reported to the hospital's investors would include a $10,500 charge for "wear and tear" on the x-ray machine. The name "straight line" comes from the fact that the annual depreciation under this method is constant; the book value of the asset, which is the cost minus the accumulated depreciation to date, declines evenly (follows a straight line) over time.

For tax purposes, depreciation is calculated according to the *Modified Accelerated Cost Recovery System (MACRS)*, which was established by the Tax Reform Act of 1986. MACRS actually spells out two procedures for calculating depreciation: (1) The *standard (accelerated) method*, which allows firms to depreciate assets on an accelerated basis, which is faster than the straight line method; and (2) an *alternative straight line method*, which is optional for some assets but mandatory for others. Since taxable firms want to gain the tax savings, or *tax shields*, associated with depreciation as early as possible, they will normally use the standard MACRS method whenever possible.

The standard method has two important features: a set of recovery periods that defines the length of time over which the asset is depreciated, and a set of allowance percentages for each recovery period.

MACRS recovery periods

Table 2.3 describes the general types of property that fit into each *recovery period*. Property in the 27.5- and 39-year classes (real estate) must be depreciated using the alternative straight line method, but 3-, 5-, 7-, and 10-year property (personal property) can be depreciated either by the accelerated method or by the alternative straight line method.

MACRS recovery allowances

Once the property is placed in the correct recovery period, the yearly recovery allowance, or depreciation expense, is determined by multiplying the asset's depreciable basis by the appropriate recovery percentage shown in Table 2.4. The specific calculation is discussed in the following sections.

Depreciable basis

The *depreciable basis* is a critical element of the depreciation calculation because each year's recovery allowance depends jointly on the asset's

Table 2.3   MACRS Recovery Periods

Period	Type of Property
3-year	Tractor units and certain equipment used in research
5-year	Automobiles, trucks, computers, and certain special manufacturing tools
7-year	Most equipment, office furniture, and fixtures
10-year	Certain longer-lived types of equipment
27.5-year	Residential rental property such as apartment buildings
39-year	All nonresidential property such as commercial and industrial buildings

Note: Land cannot be depreciated.

depreciable basis and its MACRS recovery period. The depreciable basis under MACRS is equal to the purchase price of the asset plus any transportation and installation costs. The basis is **not** adjusted for salvage value under MACRS regardless of whether the standard accelerated or alternative straight line method is used.

Half-year convention

Under MACRS, the assumption is generally made that an asset is placed in service in the middle of the first year. Thus, for three-year recovery period property, depreciation begins in the middle of the year the asset in placed in service and ends three years later. The effect of the *half-year convention* is to extend the recovery period out one more year, so three-year property is depreciated over four calendar years, five-year property is depreciated over six calendar years, and so on. This convention is incorporated in Table 2.4.

MACRS depreciation illustration

Assume that the $100,000 x-ray machine is purchased by the physician's group practice and placed in service in 1996. Further, assume that the group paid another $10,000 to ship and install the machine, and that the machine falls into the MACRS five-year class. Since salvage value does

Table 2.4   MACRS Recovery Allowances

Ownership Year	Recovery Period			
	3-Year	*5-Year*	*7-Year*	*10-Year*
1	33%	20%	14%	10%
2	45	32	25	18
3	15	19	17	14
4	7	12	13	12
5		11	9	9
6		6	9	7
7			9	7
8			4	7
9				7
10				6
11				3
	100%	100%	100%	100%

Note: The tax tables carry the recovery allowances out to two decimal places, but for ease of illustration, we will use the rounded allowances shown in this table throughout this book.

not play a part in tax depreciation, and since delivery and installation charges are included in the basis (are capitalized) rather than expensed in the year incurred, the machine's depreciable basis is $110,000. Each year's recovery allowance (tax depreciation expense) is determined by multiplying the depreciable basis by the applicable recovery percentage. Thus, the depreciation expense for 1996 is 0.20($110,000) = $22,000, and for 1997 it is 0.32($110,000) = $35,200. Similarly, the depreciation expense is $20,900 for 1998, $13,200 for 1999, $12,100 for 2000, and $6,600 for 2001. The total depreciation expense over the six-year recovery period is $110,000, which equals the depreciable basis of the x-ray machine. Note that the depreciation expense reported for tax purposes each year is different from the book depreciation calculated earlier.

Book value

The *book value* of an asset at any point in time is its depreciable basis minus the depreciation accumulated to date. Thus, at the end of 1996, the x-ray machine's tax book value is $110,000 − $22,000 = $88,000; at the end of 1997 the machine's tax book value is $110,000 − $22,000 − $35,200 = $52,800 (or $88,000 − $35,200 = $52,800), and so on. Again, note that the book value for accounting purposes is different from the book value for tax purposes.

Sale of a depreciable asset

According to the IRS, the value of a depreciable asset at any point in time is its tax book value. If a firm sells an asset for more than its tax book value, the implication is that the firm took too much depreciation, and the IRS will want to recover the excess tax benefit. Similarly, if an asset is sold for less than its book value, the implication is that the firm did not take sufficient depreciation, and it can take additional depreciation upon the sale of the asset. For example, suppose the medical group practice sells the x-ray machine in early 1998 for $60,000. Since the machine's tax book value is $52,800 at the time, $60,000 − $52,800 = $7,200 is added to the group's operating income and taxed. Conversely, if the group received only $40,000 for the machine, it would be able to deduct $52,800 − $40,000 = $12,800 from taxable income, and hence reduce taxes in 1998.

Self-Test Questions:

Briefly describe the MACRS tax depreciation system.

What is the effect of the sale of a depreciable asset on the firm's taxes?

Summary

This chapter presented some background information on organization, ownership, goals, and taxes. The key concepts are listed next:

- The three main forms of business organization are the *sole proprietorship*, the *partnership*, and the *corporation.*

- Although each form of organization has its own unique advantages and disadvantages, most large organizations, and all not-for-profit entities, are organized as *corporations.*

- *Investor-owned corporations* have *shareholders* who are the owners of the firm. Shareholders exercise control through the *proxy* process, in which they elect the firm's board of directors and vote on matters of major consequence to the firm. As owners, the shareholders have claim on the residual earnings of the firm. Investor-owned firms are fully taxable.

- Charitable organizations that meet certain criteria can be organized as *not-for-profit corporations.* Rather than having a well-defined set of owners, such organizations have a large number of *stakeholders* who have an interest in the organization. Not-for-profit firms do not pay taxes, they can accept tax-deductible contributions, and they can issue tax-exempt debt.

- From a financial management perspective, the goal of investor-owned firms is *shareholder wealth maximization*, which translates to stock price maximization. For not-for-profit firms, a reasonable goal for financial management is to *ensure the organization can fulfill its mission*, which translates to maintaining the firm's financial viability.

- An *agency problem* is a potential conflict of interests that can arise between principals and agents. One type of agency problem in financial management is the conflict between the owners of a firm and its managers.

- The value of any income stream depends on the amount of *usable*, or *after-tax, income.* Thus, tax laws play an important role in financial management decisions.

- Separate tax laws apply to *personal* income and *corporate* income.

- Fixed assets are *depreciated* over time to reflect the decline in their values. Depreciation is a deductible, but noncash, expense. Thus, for a taxable entity, the higher its depreciation, the lower its taxes, and hence the higher its cash flow, other things held constant.

- Current laws specify that the *Modified Accelerated Cost Recovery System (MACRS)* be used to depreciate assets for tax purposes.

Notes

1. Over 60 percent of corporations in the United States are chartered in Delaware, a state that, over the years, has provided a favorable governmental and legal environment for corporations. It is not necessary for a firm to be headquartered, or even to conduct business operations, in its state of incorporation.
2. In some situations, shares can be sold to the public for the first time by the company's original owners rather than by the company itself. In this case, the proceeds from the sale go the original owners, and not to the company. We will discuss stock sales in much more detail in Chapter 7, when we discuss equity financing.
3. Tax-exempt corporations are sometimes called *non-profit corporations.* Since non-profit businesses need profits to sustain operations, and since it is hard to explain to a layman why non-profit corporations should earn profits, we prefer to call such businesses not-for-profit corporations.
4. We could easily fill up the entire chapter with the details of obtaining and maintaining tax-exempt status. However, that is not the purpose of this book. Therefore, we will provide you with enough information to see the ways in which not-for-profit status has an impact on financial management decisions, but we will leave the myriad of details concerning tax-exempt status to outside readings or other courses. For additional information, see the Summer 1988 issue of *Topics in Health Care Financing,* titled "Tax Management for Exempt Providers."
5. For more information on the challenges to tax exemption, see the January 1991 issue of *Healthcare Financial Management.*
6. For a more thorough discussion of integrated delivery systems, see D. A. Conrad and W. L. Dowling, "Vertical Integration in Health Services: Theory and Managerial Implications," *Health Care Management Review* (Fall 1990).
7. Incentive compensation plans are also used by not-for-profit organizations. For more information, see the Winter 1989 issue of *Topics in Health Care Financing,* entitled "Incentive Compensation"; and W. O. Cleverley and R. K. Harvey, "Economic Value Added—A Framework for Health Care Executive Compensation." *Hospital and Health Services Administration* (Summer 1993).

Selected Additional References

Blair, J. D., G. T. Savage, and C. J. Whitehead. 1989. "A Strategic Approach for Negotiating with Hospital Stakeholders." *Health Care Management Review* (Winter): 13–23.

Clement, J. P., D. G. Smith, and J. R. C. Wheeler. 1994. "What Do We Want and What Do We Get from Not-for-Profit Hospitals?" *Hospital and Health Services Administration* (Summer): 159–78.

Fallon, R. P. 1991. "Not-For-Profit ≠ No Profit: Profitability Planning in Not-For-Profit Organizations." *Health Care Management Review* (Summer): 47–59.

Fottler, M. D., J. D. Blair, C. J. Whitehead, M. D. Laus, and G. T. Savage. 1989. "Assessing Key Stakeholders: Who Matters to Hospitals and Why?" *Hospital and Health Services Administration* (Winter): 525–46.

Herzlinger, R. E., and W. S. Krasker. 1987. "Who Profits From Nonprofits." *Harvard Business Review* (January-February): 93–105.

McLean, R. A. 1989. "Agency Costs and Complex Contracts in Health Care Organizations," *Health Care Management Review* (Winter): 65–71.

Nauert, R. C., A. B. Sanborn, II, C. F. MacKelvie, and J. L. Harvitt. 1988. "Hospitals Face Loss of Federal Tax-Exempt Status." *Healthcare Financial Management* (September): 48–60.

Pink, G. H., and P. Leatt. 1991. "Are Managers Compensated for Hospital Financial Performance?" *Health Care Management Review* (Summer): 37–45.

Umbdenstock, R. J., W. M. Hageman, and B. Amundson. 1990. "The Five Critical Areas for Effective Governance of Not-for-Profit Hospitals." *Hospital and Health Services Administration* (Winter): 481–92.

Walker, C. L., and L. W. Humphreys. 1993. "Hospital Control and Decision Making: A Financial Perspective." *Healthcare Financial Management* (June): 90–96.

Wolfson, J., and S. L. Hopes. 1994. "What Makes Tax-Exempt Hospitals Special?" *Healthcare Financial Management* (July): 57–60.

3

The Third Party Payer System

In general, companies in the health care industry that do not provide products or services directly to the public have the same operating environment as companies in any other industry. For example, Cincinnati Milicron, a machine tool manufacturer, and General Electric's Medical Equipment Division sell their products in roughly the same way. Cincinnati sells its machines directly to manufacturers that use the machines to produce other goods, and GE Medical sells its diagnostic equipment directly to hospitals, medical practices, and other organizations that use the equipment for diagnostic testing. The prices that the two companies charge for their products are set in the competitive marketplace, and it is relatively easy for buyers to distinguish among competing products. In general, the more expensive the product, the better the performance, where performance can be judged on the basis of a set of more or less objective measures. Thus, in some segments of the health care industry, and in most other industries, the consumer of the product or service (1) has a choice among many suppliers, (2) can distinguish the quality of competing goods or services, (3) makes a (presumably) rational decision regarding the purchase on the basis of quality and price, and (4) pays for the full cost of the purchase.

However, for the most part, the provision of health care services takes place in a unique way. First, often there are few providers of a particular service at hand. Next, it is very difficult, if not impossible, to judge the quality of competing goods or services. Then, the decision about which goods or services to purchase is usually not made by the consumer of those goods or services, but rather by a physician or some other clinician. Also, payment to the provider is not normally made by the user of the goods or services, but by a *third party payer*. Finally, for most individuals, the purchase of health insurance from third party payers is totally paid for or heavily subsidized by employers, so patients are insulated from the costs of health care. This highly unusual marketplace for health care has a profound effect on the supply of, and demand for, such services. We will leave most of the discussion concerning the market for health care services for health care economics courses, but, to get a better understanding of the unique payment mechanisms involved, we must examine the third party payment system in more detail. In the remainder of this chapter, we discuss those elements of the payer system that directly affect financial management decisions.

Insurance Concepts

To begin, note that the third party payer system is really an insurance system with a wide variety of insurance "companies" that come in all types and sizes. Some are investor-owned, while others are not-for-profit or government sponsored. Further, some "companies" require their policyholders, who may or may not be the beneficiaries of the insurance, to make the policy payments, while other "companies" collect partially or totally from society at large. Since insurance is the cornerstone of the third party payment system, an appreciation of the nature of insurance will help you better understand the marketplace for health care services.[1]

A simple illustration

To better understand insurance concepts, consider a simple example. Assume that no health insurance exists, and that you face only two medical outcomes in the coming year:

Outcome State	Probability	Medical Status	Cost
1	0.99	Stay healthy	$ 0
2	0.01	Get sick	20,000
	1.00		

Furthermore, assume that every other person faces the same medical outcomes, and hence "sees" the same odds and costs associated with health care.

Now, what is your expected health care cost for the coming year? To find the answer, we must multiply the cost of each outcome by its probability of occurrence, and then sum the products:

$$\text{Expected} $$

$$
\begin{aligned}
\text{health care cost} &= \text{(Probability of State 1)(Cost of State 1)} \\
&\quad + \text{(Probability of State 2)(Cost of State 2)} \\
&= 0.99(\$0) + 0.01(\$20{,}000) \\
&= \$0 + \$200 = \$200.
\end{aligned}
$$

Since you, and everyone else, makes $20,000 a year, you can easily afford the $200 "expected" health care cost. The problem is that no one's actual bill will be $200. If you stay healthy, your bill will be zero. But if you are unlucky and get sick, your bill will be $20,000, and this would force you, and most others who get sick, into personal bankruptcy, a ruinous event.

Now suppose a health insurer offered you an insurance policy for $250 that would pay all of your health care costs for the coming year. Would you take the policy, even though it cost $50 more than your "expected" health care costs? Most people would, because they are risk averse; they would be willing to pay a $50 premium over their expected benefit to eliminate the risk of financial ruin. In effect, policyholders are passing the costs associated with the risk of getting sick to the insurer.

Would the insurer be willing to offer the policy for $250? If the insurer could sell enough policies, it could take advantage of the *law of large numbers*. That is, it is impossible to predict the health care costs for any one individual for the coming year with any certainty, since the cost will either be $0 or $20,000, and you will not know for sure until the year is over. However, if the insurance company sells a million policies, it can predict its total policy payout with some accuracy—it is one million times the expected payout for each policy, or 1,000,000($200) = $200 million.[2] Since it will collect 1,000,000($250) = $250 million in health insurance premiums, the insurance company will have $50 million dollars to cover the administrative costs of the insurance operation, provide a reserve in case realized claims are greater than predicted by its actuaries, and make a profit.

Basic characteristics of insurance

The simple example of health insurance described above illustrates why individuals would seek health insurance, and why insurance companies would be formed to provide such insurance. Needless to say, the concept of insurance becomes much more complicated in the real world. Insurance is typically defined as having four distinct characteristics.

Pooling of losses

The pooling, or sharing, of losses is the heart of insurance. *Pooling* means that losses are spread over a large group of individuals, so that each individual realizes the average loss of the pool rather than the actual loss incurred. In addition, pooling involves the grouping of a large number of homogeneous *exposure units* (people or things having the same risk characteristics) so that the law of large numbers can apply. Thus, pooling implies (1) the sharing of losses by the entire group, and (2) the prediction of future losses with some accuracy based on the law of large numbers.

Payment only for random losses

A *random loss* is one that is unforeseen and unexpected and occurs as a result of chance. Insurance is based on the premise that payments are made only for losses that are random. We will discuss the moral hazard problem, in which losses are not random, in a later section.

Risk transfer

An insurance plan almost always involves *risk transfer*. The sole exception to the element of risk transfer is *self-insurance*, which occurs when a business assumes a risk itself rather than insuring the risk through an insurance company. (Self-insurance is discussed in a later section.) Risk transfer means that the risk is transferred from the insured to the insurer, which because of the premiums collected typically is in a better financial position to pay the loss than the insured.

Indemnification

The final characteristic of insurance is *indemnification* for losses; that is, the insured is reimbursed if a loss occurs. Within the context of health insurance, indemnification occurs when the insurer pays the insured (or the provider), in whole or in part, for the expenses related to an insured illness or injury.

Adverse selection

One of the major problems facing insurers is that of *adverse selection*. Adverse selection means that those individuals and companies that are most likely to have claims purchase insurance, while those that are least likely to have claims do not. For example, an otherwise healthy individual with no insurance who needs a costly surgical procedure will likely seek health insurance if he or she can afford it, whereas an identical individual without the threat of surgery is much less likely to purchase insurance. If this tendency toward adverse selection goes unchecked, a disproportionate number of sick people will seek health insurance, and the insurer will experience higher-than-expected claims. This will trigger a premium increase, which only worsens the problem, since the healthier members of the plan will seek insurance from other companies at a lower cost or totally forgo insurance. The adverse selection problem exists because of *asymmetric information*—individual buyers of health insurance know more about their health status than do insurers.

Insurance companies attempt to control the adverse selection problem by underwriting provisions. *Underwriting* refers to the selection and classification of candidates for insurance. From a health insurance perspective, there are two extreme positions that can be taken by insurers regarding underwriting. First, assuming that insurers offer insurance in all 50 states, but not elsewhere, insurers can base premiums on national average statistics without regard to individual characteristics. Thus, each individual (or each individual's employer, if the firm provides the insurance) would pay the same health insurance premium regardless of age, sex, geographic location, line of work, smoking habits, genetic disposition, and so on. The premium charged for each individual would be sufficient in the aggregate to cover all expected outlays, plus administrative expenses, plus earn a profit for the insurer. In this situation, *cross-subsidies* clearly exist, because young, healthy nonsmokers in relatively safe jobs would pay the same premiums as older, sickly smokers in relatively hazardous jobs. Thus, after taking administrative costs out of the insurance premium, healthy individuals would pay premiums that exceed their expected health care costs, while the sicker individuals would pay premiums that are less than their expected costs.

At the other extreme, if no information asymmetries existed and perfect information were available, insurance companies could charge a premium to each subscriber on the basis of that subscriber's expected health care costs over the coming year. Individuals who are expected to have high costs would be charged high premiums, and those with low expected costs would be charged low premiums. Of course, neither individuals nor insurers have perfect foresight, so the extreme of charging each person on the basis of his or her expected health care costs is not actually attainable. However, insurers could take into account all factors that are proven to affect health status (and hence costs), such as smoking habits, weight, cholesterol level, and hereditary factors, when fixing insurance rates.

What approach do health insurers take in practice? Initially, most health insurers used *community ratings*. Here, a single set of premiums, or rates, was offered to all members of a community without regard to age, sex, health status, and so on. Thus, rates reflected geographical differences, and potentially even ethnic and cultural differences if the community was dominated by a single ethnic or cultural group. However, within the community, rates represented an average of high- and low-cost individuals. Then, some insurers (particularly commercial insurers) started to offer *experience ratings*, whereby rates are set based on the claims experience of the specific group being insured.

For example, the Boeing Company might contract with a health insurer to insure all of Boeing's employees in the Seattle area. If Boeing's employees (who as a group tend to be younger and more educated) have lower health care costs than the community in general, then insurers competing for the contract that use experience ratings can offer Boeing lower rates than competitors that use community ratings. As more and more employers with low-risk employees seek health insurance based on experience ratings, the least costly groups are skimmed from the insurance pool, and those that remain have higher-than-average costs. Since the health care costs for those remaining are above the average for the community, insurers serving that population have no choice but to apply experience ratings, so higher premiums can be charged to the remaining groups. The trend, then, has been toward experience ratings and away from community ratings, although community ratings are still used.

Another way that health insurers protect themselves against adverse selection is by including *preexisting conditions* clauses in contracts. A preexisting condition is a physical or mental condition of the insured person that existed prior to the issuance of the policy. A typical clause states that preexisting conditions are not covered until the policy has been in force for some period of time, say, one or two years.

Health care reform as envisioned by the Clinton administration in 1993 and 1994 required all insurers to use community ratings and to offer coverage regardless of preexisting conditions. The purpose, of course, was to make health care coverage available and affordable to as many people as possible. Although a noble goal, political reform of the health care system faced many hurdles, some of which appeared to be insurmountable; so political reform has given way to industry-driven reforms, and experience ratings and preexisting condition clauses remain a fact of life.

Moral hazard

As we stated in the previous section, insurance is based on the premise that payments are made only for random losses. This basic characteristic of insurance highlights the *moral hazard* problem. The most common illustration of moral hazard in a casualty insurance setting is the owner who deliberately sets a failing business on fire to collect the insurance. Moral hazard is also present in health insurance, but its form typically is not so dramatic—not too many people are willing to voluntarily sustain injury or illness for the purpose of collecting health insurance. However, there undoubtedly are people who purposely use health care services that are not medically required. For example, some people who live alone might visit a physician or a walk-in clinic for the social value of human companionship rather than to address a medical necessity. Also, some hospital discharges might be delayed for the convenience of the patient rather than for medical purposes. Finally, when the full cost (or most of the cost) is covered by insurance, individuals often are quick to agree to a $1,000 MRI scan or other high-cost procedure that may not be necessary. If the same test required total out-of-pocket payment, individuals would think twice before agreeing to such an expensive procedure unless the medical necessity was clearly understood.

Even more insidious is the impact of insurance on individual behavior. Individuals are less likely to take preventive actions when the costs of not taking those actions will be borne by insurers. Why worry about getting a flu shot if the monetary costs associated with flu are borne by the insurance company, or why stop smoking if the likely adverse health consequences will be paid for by others? Clearly, the very fact that insurance exists causes individuals to forgo preventive actions and embrace unhealthy behaviors, both of which might be approached differently in the absence of insurance.

Insurers generally attempt to protect themselves from moral hazard claims by paying less than the full amount of health care costs borne by the insured. By making insured individuals bear some of the cost, there will be less of a tendency to consume unneeded services or engage in unhealthy behaviors. One way of doing this is to require a *deductible*. Medical policies usually contain some dollar amount that must be satisfied before benefits are paid. Although deductibles have some positive effect on the moral hazard problem, their primary purpose is to eliminate the payment of small claims, wherein the administrative cost of processing the claim may be larger than the claim itself. Although there are several types of deductibles, the most common form is the *calendar-year deductible.* Here, the first $100 (or $250 or more) of medical expenses incurred each year is paid by the individual insured. Once the deductible is met, the insurer will pay all eligible medical expenses (less any copayments) for the remainder of the year.

The primary weapon that insurers have against the moral hazard problem is the *copayment,* which requires insured individuals to pay a certain percentage of eligible medical expenses, say, 20 percent, in excess of the deductible amount. For example, assume that George Maynard, who has employer-provided medical insurance that pays 80 percent of eligible expenses after the $100 deductible is satisfied, incurs $10,000 in medical expenses during the year. The insurer will pay $0.80($10,000 - $100) = 0.80($9,900) = $7,920$, so Mr. Maynard's responsibility is $10,000 - $7,920 = $2,080$.

The purposes of copayments are to reduce premiums and to prevent overutilization of health care services, and hence insurance benefits. Since insured individuals pay part of the cost, premiums can be reduced. Additionally, by being forced to pay some of the costs, insured individuals will presumably seek fewer and more cost-effective treatments and embrace a more healthy lifestyle.

Some health insurance policies contain *stop-loss limits,* also called *out-of-pocket maximums,* whereby the insurer pays all covered costs, including the copayment, after the insured individual pays a certain amount of copayment costs, say, $2,000. Thus, if George Maynard had $50,000 of covered expenses above the deductible amount, his coinsurance share would be $10,000 if there were no stop-loss provision. If his policy contained a stop-loss amount of $2,000, George would only have to pay $2,000, and his insurer would pay the remaining $48,000 of costs. Of course, health insurance policies with stop-loss provisions are more costly than those without such features.

Finally, most insurance policies have *policy limits*—for example, $1,000,000 in total lifetime coverage, or $1,500 per year for mental health benefits, or $100 for eyeglasses. These limits are designed to control excessive use of certain services and to protect the insurer against catastrophic losses. Of course, a lifetime coverage limit means that subscribers must bear the risk of catastrophic losses.

Self-Test Questions:

Briefly explain the following characteristics of insurance:

1. Pooling of losses
2. Payment only for random losses

3. Risk transfer

4. Indemnification

What is adverse selection, and how do insurers deal with the problem?

What is the moral hazard problem?

Alternative Payment Methods

Regardless of the payer for a particular health care service, only a limited number of payment methods are used by payers to reimburse providers. In this section, we discuss alternative payment methods.

Charge-based reimbursement

When payers pay *charges,* they pay according to the schedule of charge rates established by the provider. Some insurers still reimburse providers according to billed charges, but the trend for payers is toward other, less generous reimbursement methods. If this trend continues, the only payers that will be expected to pay billed charges are self-pay, or private-pay, patients.

Negotiated, or *discounted, charges* are often used by insurers in conjunction with managed care plans such as health maintenance organizations (HMOs) and preferred provider organizations (PPOs). Because HMOs and PPOs, as well as some conventional insurers, have bargaining power due to the large number of enrollees who use a particular provider, they can negotiate discounts from billed charges. Such discounts generally range from 20 to 30 percent or even more of billed charges.

Cost-based reimbursement

Under a *retrospective cost* system, the payer agrees to pay the provider certain allowable costs that are incurred in providing services to the payer's enrollees. Typically, the payer makes *periodic interim payments (PIPs)* to the provider, and then a final reconciliation is made after the contract period expires and all costs have worked their way through the provider's accounting system.

The *prospective cost method* is another cost-based reimbursement method, but here costs are determined in advance. Thus, third-party payers know beforehand what the cost will be for services, but they do not know which services, in what amount, will be consumed. Note, however, that the prospective cost method usually includes provisions for retroactive adjustments when cost increases occur that exceed some preset limit.

Prospective payment reimbursement

In a *prospective payment system*, the rates paid by payers are determined in advance, but they are not directly related to either reimbursable costs or billed charges. Under prospective payment, there are four common payment units.

1. *Per diagnosis.* In the per diagnosis reimbursement method, the provider is paid a rate that depends on the patient's diagnosis—diagnoses that require higher resource utilization have higher reimbursement rates. This basis of payment is used in Medicare's diagnosis-related group (DRG) system, which we will discuss in some detail in a later section. When payment is made by this method, the provider bears the risk for costs incurred in excess of the fixed payment for each patient's diagnosis.

2. *Per day (per diem).* If reimbursement is based on a per diem rate, the provider is paid a fixed amount for each day that service is provided, regardless of the nature of the services. Because the nature of the services can vary widely, the provider bears the risk that costs associated with the services provided on any day will exceed the per diem rate. Since payment is not tied to diagnosis, the risk borne by providers under per diem reimbursement is higher than the risk under per diagnosis reimbursement. Note, however, that some per diem rates are *stratified.* For example, a hospital might be paid one rate for a medical/surgical day, a higher rate for a critical care unit day, and yet a different rate for an obstetrical day. Stratified per diems recognize that providers may incur widely different costs for providing different types of care.

3. *Per admission.* If reimbursement is made on a per admission basis, a single payment is made for each admission, regardless of the services provided or the length of stay. Here, the provider bears even more risk than under per diem reimbursement, because, in addition to diagnosis risk, the provider bears the risk associated with length of stay.

4. *Capitation.* Under capitated reimbursement, the provider is paid a fixed amount per enrollee per period (usually a month), regardless of whether any services are used. The reimbursement

risk to the provider under this system is generally regarded as being highest among the prospective payment systems. Chapter 18 discusses capitation payment in some detail.

All prospective payment methods involve a transfer of risk from insurers to providers, and this risk increases as the payment unit moves down the foregoing list. The added risk does not mean that providers should avoid such reimbursement methods—indeed, refusing to accept contracts with prospective payment provisions would be tantamount to organizational suicide for many providers. However, it is essential that providers understand the risks involved in prospective payment arrangements, especially the effect on profitability, and make every effort to negotiate a level of payment that is consistent with the risk incurred. One of the basic principles of finance is that investments with higher risk must have higher expected returns. Providers invest in assets, and when reimbursement provisions make the cash flows from these assets riskier, a higher return should be demanded. We will revisit this concept throughout the book in a myriad of situations.

Nonpayment

Before we close this section, we think it worthwhile to address briefly the issue of nonpayment. If a user of health care services does not have insurance, then the responsibility for payment of total billed charges falls on the patient or the patient's family. Since people without health insurance tend to be poor, many find it difficult, if not impossible, to pay for health care services that can quickly amount to tens of thousands of dollars. Nonpaying patients fall into two categories. First, those who have the capacity to pay, but are unwilling to pay. The lost revenues attributable to this class of nonpayer are called *bad debt losses*. The second group is made up of patients who are not able to pay. The revenues lost to these patients are called *charity*, or *indigent, care losses*.

Self-Test Questions:

Briefly describe the following payment methodologies:

1. Charges and discounted charges

2. Retrospective cost

3. Prospective cost

4. Per diagnosis

5. Per diem

6. Per admission

7. Capitation

Which of these payment methods carries the least risk for providers? The most risk?

Third Party Payers

Up to this point in the chapter we have discussed the basic concept of insurance, along with some key elements of health insurance. Now we move to the primary focus of this chapter, third party payers. We will provide here a brief background of the major third party payers and, more important, we will discuss the reimbursement methods that they use to pay health care providers. Health insurance originated in Europe in the early 1800s, when mutual benefit societies were formed to reduce the financial burden associated with illness or injury. Today, health insurers fall into two broad categories: private insurers and public programs.[3]

Private insurers

In the United States, the concept of public, or government, health insurance is relatively new, while private health insurance has been in existence since the turn of the century. In this section, we discuss the major private insurers, Blue Cross–Blue Shield, commercial insurers, and self-insurers.

Blue Cross–Blue Shield

Blue Cross–Blue Shield organizations trace their roots to the Great Depression, when both hospitals and physicians were concerned about their patients' abilities to pay health care bills.

Blue Cross originated as a number of separate insurance programs offered by individual hospitals. At the time, many patients were unable to pay their hospital bills, but most people, except the very poorest, could afford to purchase some type of hospitalization insurance. Thus, the programs were initially designed to benefit hospitals as well as patients. The programs were all similar in structure: hospitals agreed to provide a certain amount of services to program members who made periodic payments of fixed amounts to the hospitals whether services were used or not. In a short time, these programs were expanded from single hospital programs to community-wide, multihospital plans that were called *hospital service plans*. The American Hospital Association (AHA) recognized the benefits of such plans to hospitals, so a close relationship was formed between the AHA and the organizations that offered hospital service plans.

In the early years, several states ruled that the sale of hospital services by prepayment did not constitute insurance, so the plans were exempt from regulations governing insurance companies. However, it was clear that the legal status of hospital service plans would be subject to future scrutiny unless their status was formalized. So the states, one by one, passed enabling legislation that provided for the founding of not-for-profit hospital service corporations that were exempt both from taxes and from the capital requirements mandated for other insurers. However, state insurance departments had—and continue to have—oversight over most aspects of the plans' operations. The Blue Cross name was officially adopted by most of these plans in 1939.

Blue Shield plans developed in a manner similar to that of the Blue Cross plans, except that the providers were physicians instead of hospitals and the professional organization was the American Medical Association (AMA) instead of the AHA. Today, there are almost 70 Blue Cross–Blue Shield organizations; some offer only one of the two plans, but most offer both plans. For example, Blue Cross–Blue Shield of Virginia covers the entire state; the state of Washington has only one Blue Cross corporation, but eight Blue Shield organizations; and New York state has four Blue Cross and four Blue Shield organizations. The Blues are organized as local or statewide corporations, but all belong to a single national association that sets standards that must be met to use the Blue Cross–Blue Shield name.

Historically, the Blues have been not-for-profit corporations that enjoyed the full benefits accorded that status, including freedom from taxes. But in 1986, Congress eliminated the Blues' tax exemption on the grounds that they operated "commercial-type" insurance activities. However, the plans were given some special deductions, which resulted in taxes that are generally less than those paid by commercial insurance companies. In spite of the 1986 change in tax status, the national association continued to require all Blues to operate entirely as not-for-profit corporations, although they could establish for-profit subsidiaries. In 1994, however, the national association lifted its traditional ban on member plans becoming investor-owned companies.

The first state plan to announce conversion was Blue Cross of California, which at the time was embroiled in controversy over its WellPoint Health Networks, a for-profit subsidiary. Blue Cross sold 20 million shares of WellPoint to investors and retained 80 million shares of the business, which was valued at $2 billion. Critics at the time contended that Blue Cross used a loophole in state law to convert most of its assets from not-for-profit to investor-owned status without donating a like amount to a charitable foundation.[4] The final plan for conversion was predicated upon a merger between WellPoint and Health Systems International that would have created the nation's second-largest for-profit managed care company. The plan, which was approved by the California Department of Corporations, would have established charitable foundations worth $3 billion as part of Blue Cross's obligation to the state for converting to for-profit status. However, in late 1995 the proposed merger was abandoned, and a new plan for conversion must now be developed.

In spite of the action by Blue Cross of California, it is estimated that only a handful of state Blues will convert to for-profit status because of the legal problems inherent in conversion and because they already have the ability to create for-profit subsidiaries. At the time this chapter was written (early 1996), Blue Cross plans in Wisconsin, Indiana, California, and Missouri had established for-profit subsidiaries, while those in Georgia, Maryland, New Jersey, and Virginia were exploring options for conversion. The main rationale for converting or creating for-profit subsidiaries is access to investor-supplied equity capital, which many people believe is necessary to be competitive in today's health care market.

Since the Blue Cross–Blue Shield corporations operate independently, no one reimbursement method is universal to all of them. However, over the past few years the tendency has been to move away from cost-based and charge-based methods toward prospective payment systems. For example, some of the Blues use hospital reimbursement methods that are similar to Medicare's prospective payment system based on diagnosis-related groups, while others use a two-tier system in which a per diem rate is paid for routine hospitalizations while charge-based rates are paid for nonroutine services.

Virtually all of the Blues now offer managed care plans along with more traditional indemnity insurance, and many plans are contracting with integrated delivery systems. In these situations, capitation often is the method of payment to providers. We discuss capitation and risk sharing in detail in Chapter 18.

Commercial insurers

Commercial health insurance is issued by life insurance companies, by casualty insurance companies, and by companies that were formed exclusively to write health insurance. Commercial insurance companies can be organized either as stock or mutual companies. *Stock* companies are shareholder owned, and can raise equity capital just like any other for-profit company. Further, the stockholders assume the risks and responsibilities of ownership and management. A *mutual* company has no shareholders; its management is controlled by a board of directors elected by the company's policyholders. Regardless of the form of ownership, commercial insurance companies are taxable entities.

Commercial insurers moved strongly into health insurance following World War II. At that time, the United Auto Workers negotiated the first contract with employers where fringe benefits were a major part of the contract. Like the Blues, the majority of individuals with commercial health insurance are covered under *group policies* with employee groups, professional and other associations, and labor unions. Group health coverage has the following advantages over individual coverage:

1. Group coverage has low administrative costs because many individuals are insured under a single contract. This lowers the costs associated with sales and administration of the contract.

2. The group contract holder, say, the employer or labor union, usually pays a part of or all of the premium. Note, however, that employers that have costly employee health programs are usually forced by competitive pressures for their products and services to offset higher health care costs with lower wages or reductions in other fringe benefits. Also, the competitive market for labor forces firms to offer competitive aggregate benefits, although the benefit mix may differ.

3. Generally, eligibility for a group plan does not depend on the insured individual's health status. The insurance company bases premiums on the overall health status of the group. But note that the premiums charged group plans that involve small numbers of members can be adversely affected by the poor health of one individual.

4. In general, an individual's coverage cannot be canceled unless the individual leaves the group or the plan itself is terminated.

Commercial insurers have traditionally reimbursed health care providers on the basis of billed charges. However, with the dramatic increase in health care costs that has occurred over the past 20 years, the traditional providers of health insurance—employers and unions—have seen their health care costs grow to almost unbelievable amounts. For example, the Big Three automakers estimate that about $700 of the cost of each car and truck produced results from employee health care costs. Clearly, this trend cannot continue, so the major purchasers of group health insurance have put pressure on the insurance companies to trim costs. This, in turn, has forced commercial insurers to move toward other reimbursement methods and delivery systems, including managed care plans, that presumably have a better chance at controlling costs than does reimbursement on the basis of billed charges.

Self-insurers

The third major form of private insurance is *self-insurance*. One could argue that all individuals who do not have any other form of health insurance are self-insurers, but this is not technically correct. Self-insurers make a conscious decision to bear the risks associated with health care costs, and then set aside funds to pay future costs as they occur. Individuals are not good candidates for self-insurance because they face too much uncertainty concerning future health care expenses. On the other hand, large groups, especially employers, are good candidates for self-insurance. Indeed, today most large groups are self-insured. For example, employees of the State of Florida are covered by health insurance that is administered by Unisys, but the actual benefits to plan members are paid by the state. Unisys is paid for administering the plan, but the state bears all risks associated with cost and usage uncertainty.

Many firms today are even going one step further in their self-insurance programs by totally bypassing third party payers. For example, Digital Equipment Corporation, a major computer maker, negotiates discounts directly with hospitals and physicians. Others, such as Deere & Company, a farm implements manufacturer, have set up health services subsidiaries to provide health care services to their employees. For the most part, these companies use the same techniques as managed care organizations—they just count on doing them better and cheaper themselves by applying the kind of management attention to health care that they do to their core businesses.

Public insurers

Government is a major insurer and direct provider of health care services. For example, the government provides health care services directly to qualifying individuals through the Department of Veterans Affairs (VA), Department of Defense (DOD), and Public Health Service (PHS) medical facilities. In addition, the government either provides or mandates a variety of insurance programs such as workers compensation and CHAMPUS (Civilian Health and Medical Program of the Uniformed Services). However, in this section, we focus on the two major government insurance programs: Medicare and Medicaid.

Medicare

Medicare[5] was established by the federal government in 1966 to provide medical benefits to individuals age 65 and older. Medicare consists of two separate coverages: *Part A*, which provides hospital and some skilled nursing home coverage, and *Part B*, which covers physician services, ambulatory surgical services, outpatient services, and certain other miscellaneous services. Part A coverage is free to all persons eligible for social security benefits. Individuals who are not eligible for social security benefits can obtain Part A medical benefits by paying premiums of $289 per month (for 1996). Part B is optional to all individuals who have Part A coverage, and it requires a monthly premium of $42.50 (for 1996). About 97 percent of Part A participants purchase Part B coverage.

Administration of Medicare. The Medicare program falls under the *Department of Health and Human Services (DHHS)*, which creates the specific rules of the program on the basis of enabling legislation. Medicare is administered by an agency under DHHS called the *Health Care Financing Administration* (*HCFA*, pronounced "hicfah"). HCFA has eight regional offices that oversee the Medicare program and ensure that regulations are followed.

Medicare payments to health care providers are not made directly by HCFA, but rather by contractors at state or local level called *intermediaries* for Part A payments and *carriers* for Part B payments.[6] Part A intermediaries are all either Blue Cross associations or commercial insurers. For example, Blue Cross–Blue Shield of Florida is the HCFA fiscal intermediary for Florida, while Aetna is the fiscal intermediary for Oklahoma.

A short history of Part A reimbursement. From its inception in 1966 to 1983, hospital payments were based on a retrospective system that reimbursed hospitals for all reasonable costs. In general, reasonable costs were defined as (1) operating costs for labor and materials; (2) capital costs for depreciation, interest expense, lease payments, and return on equity for investor-owned hospitals; and (3) costs associated with medical educational programs. In effect, HCFA provided hospitals with blank checks that they could use to provide "gold-plated" services to Medicare beneficiaries.

For many providers, Medicare became the "goose that laid the golden egg." Per capita Medicare spending rose from $648 in 1967 to $4,472 in 1994, and total spending is expected to increase by 10 percent per year over the next decade. Unfortunately, in its early years, Medicare provided no incentives whatever for providers to offer cost-effective services. If anything, Medicare encouraged overbuilding, "gold plating," excessive services, and overly long hospital stays. However, Medicare did lead to many positive results, although at a high price. First, Medicare fueled a hospital boom that put a hospital nearby for most of the population. In addition, Medicare provided most elderly with access to health care that only a small proportion had had before. This access to health care is at least a partial reason why life expectancy has increased dramatically for the elderly—in 1966, a 65-year-old could expect to live to about 70; today he or she can expect to live to about 83. Finally, Medicare was a major factor in the desegregation of hospitals, since all providers had to desegregate to qualify for federal dollars.

Foundations of the prospective payment system. In an attempt to curb spending, on October 1, 1983, Congress established a new reimbursement system for Medicare Part A providers called the *prospective payment system (PPS)*. The intent of the PPS was (1) to reduce the growth in Medicare outlays, (2) to provide cost-containment incentives to providers, and yet (3) to maintain the quality of care achieved under the old cost-based system. The basic concept of the PPS is to reimburse hospitals with a fixed sum for each admission based on the patient's diagnosis. If the hospital is able to provide the services for less than the fixed reimbursement amount, it can keep the difference. Conversely, if a Medicare patient costs the hospital more than the reimbursement amount, the hospital must bear the loss.[7]

The PPS was phased in over several years, and the initial fixed reimbursement rates were based on hospital costs at that time. Thus, upon implementation of PPS, hospitals were able to embark on cost-cutting measures that allowed them to deliver services to Medicare beneficiaries for less than the fixed payments, and many hospitals were able to generate large profits. For example, operating margins on Medicare patients during the first two years of PPS averaged over 14 percent.[8]

Unfortunately for hospitals, from the system's inception PPS payments have not kept pace with hospital costs. For example, hospital operating costs rose 10 percent in 1987, but Medicare PPS rates were increased by only 3.8 percent. Furthermore, once the most obvious cost cutting took place, it was difficult for hospitals to generate additional efficiency gains. The result was that the average hospital's operating margin on Medicare patients fell steadily to a loss of 1.5 percent in 1992, but then rebounded to a plus 3.4 percent in 1994 as hospitals again were able to reign in costs while PPS payments rose 3.3 percent.

The PPS has had a direct influence on hospitals' lengths of stay. Prior to PPS, according to the AHA, the average hospital length of stay for Medicare patients was 10.3 days; now it is under 7 days. However, no evidence has been found to support the contention that Medicare patients are being discharged "quicker and sicker." Quicker yes, but probably not sicker. While the relationship between length of stay and quality is uncertain, shorter stays do often mean that ill Medicare patients or their families have to worry sooner about finding posthospital services when they are needed.

The PPS also has had a profound impact on the provision of outpatient care. Since outpatient care is paid by Medicare Part B, it continues to be reimbursed on a cost basis. This has provided an incentive for hospitals to shift health care services from inpatient to outpatient. For example, while the inpatient activity at community hospitals has fallen over the past decade, the number of outpatient visits has increased by about 75 percent. Furthermore, Medicare spending for outpatient services has been growing three times as fast as spending for inpatient services. In effect, some of the cost savings expected from PPS were lost because hospitals shifted inpatient services to outpatient services. In an effort to moderate this trend, HCFA has proposed a prospective payment system for outpatient care, but no implementation date has been set.

An overview of the prospective payment system.[9] Under PPS, a single payment for each patient covers the cost of routine inpatient care, special care, and ancillary services. The amount of the prospective payment is based on the patient's *diagnosis-related group (DRG)* as assigned at discharge. (Originally, the attending physician had to attest, in writing, to the principal diagnosis, secondary diagnosis, and procedures performed. However, the requirement for physician certification was dropped for 1996 and beyond.) The Medicare DRG payment generally covers all costs except medical education costs and bad debt costs, which we will discuss later along with capital costs.

The starting point in determining the amount of reimbursement is the DRG itself. HCFA has divided potential patient diagnoses into 23 *major diagnostic categories (MDCs)*, which correspond to the major organ systems. Within the 23 MDCs, there are almost 500 DRGs.[10] To illustrate the nature of DRGs, Table 3.1 contains Medicare's ten most frequently used DRGs.

The individual DRG *relative weights* represent the average resources consumed in treating that particular diagnosis relative to resources consumed in treating the average diagnosis. Thus, the costs associated with DRG 209, major joint and limb procedures, are over 2.2 times as much as the costs associated with the average diagnosis, while the costs associated with DRG 140, angina pectoris, are only 63 percent of the average diagnosis. To account for changes in resource consumption, treatment patterns, and technology, the DRG weights are *recalibrated* (updated) annually.

The Medicare *case-mix index* is a useful tool for judging the types of diagnoses that are being treated at a particular hospital. The index represents the average DRG weight for all Medicare patients treated in a specific period. Of course, the average DRG weight for an average hospital is 1.0. To illustrate the concept, the recent case-mix index for North Ridge Medical Center in Fort Lauderdale was 1.775, while that of

Table 3.1   Ten Most Frequently Used DRGs for Medicare Patients

DRG Name	DRG Number	MDC Number	1996 Relative Weight	Average Length of Stay
Heart failure and shock	127	5	1.0302	6.7 days
Angina pectoris	140	5	0.6312	3.8
Simple pneumonia, age > 17	89	4	1.1211	7.6
Specific cerebrovascular disorders	14	1	1.2065	8.2
Psychoses	430	19	0.8670	10.7
Esophagitis, age > 17	182	1	0.7794	5.4
Bronchitis and asthma with complications, age > 17	96	4	0.8390	5.9
Major joint and limb procedures	209	8	2.2707	7.6
Nutritional and metabolic disorders with complications, age > 17	296	10	0.9166	7.0
Cardiac arrhythmia with complications	138	5	0.8049	5.0

Source: Federal Register. 1995. (1 September): Vol. 60.

DeSoto Memorial Hospital in Arcadia, Florida, was 0.840. North Ridge is treating much more complex cases requiring greater services and longer lengths of stay than is DeSoto.

Hospitals are classified by HCFA as falling into one of two locational categories: (1) *large urban* and (2) *other areas,* where other areas is itself a combination of two formerly separate categories: (1) other urban and (2) rural. Forty-six urban areas across the country are classified as large urban, while the remainder of the country falls into the other area classification. Each year, HCFA publishes standardized national *labor-* and *nonlabor-related* costs per discharge for the two locational categories. For example, Table 3.2 contains the national average amounts for 1996. Most hospitals paid under PPS are reimbursed at the national rates; however, some hospitals, such as rural referral centers and hospitals with a disproportionate share of low-income patients, are subject to additional adjustments that effectively increase the reimbursement rates above those shown in Table 3.2.

The PPS rate computation is relatively simple given the standardized labor and nonlabor amounts, the local area wage index, and the DRG relative weight. To illustrate, consider Table 3.3, which displays the Medicare reimbursement computation for DRG 127 (heart failure and shock) for a hospital located in Miami, Florida (designated a large urban area). The national large urban labor amount, $2,741, is first adjusted by the local *area wage index,* which is published periodically by HCFA and reflects relative labor costs across the United States. This product, $2,618, which is the labor amount adjusted for area wage rates, is then added to the national nonlabor amount. The result is the adjusted hospital rate, $3,716, which is the base rate applied to all diagnoses. Finally, the adjusted hospital rate is multiplied by the DRG relative weight to obtain the reimbursement amount. In our illustration, the DRG relative weight is 1.0302, which produces a DRG payment of $3,828 for a patient discharged with a diagnosis of heart failure and shock.

Table 3.2   1995 National Average Standardized Amounts

Classification	Labor	Nonlabor
Large urban	$2,741	$1,098
Other areas	2,698	1,081

Source: Federal Register. 1995. (1 September): Vol. 60.

Table 3.3   Sample Medicare DRG Payment

Hospital location:	Large urban
Area wage index for Miami:	0.9552
DRG description:	127 (Heart failure and shock)
DRG relative weight:	1.0302

Large urban labor amount	$2,741
Multiplied by area wage index	× 0.9552
Adjusted labor amount	$2,618
Plus nonlabor amount	+ 1,098
Adjusted hospital rate	$3,716
Multiplied by DRG relative weight	× 1.0302
Hospital reimbursement for DRG 127	$3,828

Outlier payments. The PPS payment is based on the costs associated with an average patient for each diagnosis. Of course, for any given DRG in any given hospital, some patients will incur costs that are greater than average while some will be less costly than average. If the patients select hospitals randomly, that is, if all of the sicker patients in a given DRG do not go to a particular hospital, and if a large number of patients are treated in each DRG, then the high-cost and low-cost patients will offset one another, and the hospital will experience average costs for each DRG.

Reimbursement on an arithmetic mean, or average cost basis, works well if the distribution of patient costs within each DRG is symmetrical, but the distribution is actually skewed to the right—patients with a "mild" case of heart failure and shock may cost half of the average amount, but patients with a "severe" case might cost five times the average amount.

To provide some cushion for the high costs associated with severely ill patients within each diagnosis, PPS includes a provision for *outlier payments.* Outliers are classified into two categories: *length of stay (LOS) outliers* and *cost outliers.* Medicare will make additional payments when a patient's LOS or cost exceeds the established LOS or cost cutoff points. Hospitals are not required to request additional reimbursement for LOS outliers. For cost outliers, hospitals must file a form with Medicare's fiscal intermediary.

Capital-related costs. The major categories of *capital-related costs* are (1) depreciation expense; (2) interest expense; and (3) lease and rental expense. At one time, a return on equity payment was made to investor-owned hospitals, but these payments were discontinued some years ago. Prior to October 1, 1991, capital-related costs were excluded from Medicare's PPS. In lieu of folding these into DRG rates, capital-related costs were passed-through separately on the basis of costs incurred. Thus, such payments to hospitals are called *capital pass-through payments.* Medicare has eliminated the capital pass-through system for PPS hospitals and instead now includes capital payments as add-ons to prospective payments. However, Medicare does not use the PPS system for all hospitals, and some third party payers continue to use capital pass-through systems, so it is important for health care managers, especially those in hospitals, to have some understanding of capital pass-through.

To get a rough idea of the capital pass-through system, consider Manhattan Psychiatric Hospital. For 1996, Manhattan's interest expense was $1,542,000, its book depreciation was $4,130,000, and lease and rental expense was $3,360,000, for total capital-related costs of $9,032,000.[11] Thirty-four percent of Manhattan's patients were Medicare patients, and since Manhattan is a non-PPS hospital that qualifies for capital pass-through, Medicare traditionally would pay 34 percent of Manhattan's capital-related costs, or 0.34($9,032,000) = $3,070,880. However, because of recent fiscal constraints, pass-through reimbursement has been reduced to 85 percent of capital-related costs, so Manhattan's actual capital pass-through from Medicare in 1996 was 0.85($3,070,880) = $2,610,248.

For PPS hospitals, the basis for the prospective capital payment is the federal capital payment rate, which was set at $462 for 1996. In theory, each hospital under PPS would receive a capital payment of $376.83 for each Medicare discharge during the year. However, the new rules are quite complex, and adjustments are made to the federal rate to account for geographic and cost differentials, as well as medical education costs. Further, the new system is being phased in over a ten-year period that ends in 2001, so capital PPS calculations are quite involved.

The intent of the prospective capital payment system is to take away incentives for hospitals to purchase or lease too much plant and equipment or to use too much debt financing. Under capital pass-through, Medicare reimburses hospitals for a percentage of capital-related costs whether the capital expenditures are to promote efficient care, to build an emergency room, to build a luxury wing, or to build unneeded capacity. With prospective capital payments, hospitals are encouraged to be as prudent in making capital expenditure decisions as they are in making operating cost decisions.

Other Medicare payments to hospitals. In addition to the payments for operating and capital-related expenses just discussed, Medicare reimburses
hospitals for a variety of other costs related to inpatient services. For
example, Medicare reimburses hospitals for direct and indirect costs
associated with medical education programs. *Direct medical education costs*
include salaries for interns and residents, as well as salaries for teaching
personnel, net of tuition revenues, in approved training programs for
physicians, nurses, and certain allied health professionals. Direct medical education payments are based on costs and are paid in addition to
prospective payments. *Indirect medical education costs* are those operating
costs, in addition to direct costs, that arise from medical education
programs. Medicare reimburses hospitals for indirect medical education
costs by adjusting PPS payments.

Another example of Medicare's other payments is reimbursement
for bad debt losses by Medicare patients. Medicare reimburses hospitals
for unpaid deductible and copayment amounts from Medicare beneficiaries. However, Medicare does not reimburse hospitals for bad debt
losses from non-Medicare patients. There are several other types of
Medicare payments, such as payments for hospitals that have a disproportionate share of poor Medicare patients, who are typically in ill health and
hence cost more to treat than average Medicare patients. However, we
will leave additional details on Medicare reimbursement to your outside
readings.

Peer review organizations. An integral part of the Medicare reimbursement system is the *peer review organization (PRO)*. PROs are independent
organizations contracted by HCFA at the state level to monitor the
care, and the resulting reimbursement, provided by hospitals and other
providers that treat Medicare patients. Basically, PROs review hospital
admissions patterns, lengths of stay, transfers, outlier cases, and quality
of services. If a PRO determines that a hospital has misrepresented
admission, discharge, or billing data, payment for the services related
to that discharge may be denied. Patterns of behavior designed to cir-
cumvent PPS payment procedures could result in termination of the
provider agreement. As with most oversight of this nature, a process is
available by which hospitals and other Medicare providers can appeal
PRO rulings.

Part B reimbursement. Through 1991, Part B reimbursement to physicians
and suppliers was based on the concept of *reasonable charges*. In essence,
Medicare defined a reasonable charge as the lowest of (1) the actual

charge for the service performed, (2) the physician's customary charge, or (3) the prevailing charge for that service in the community. Medicare then paid providers 80 percent of the reasonable charge after the Medicare patient had satisfied his or her deductible amount. The patient was responsible for the 20 percent copayment.

However, Medicare changed its physician payment system beginning in 1992 to a *resource-based relative value scale (RBRVS)*. Under RBRVS, reimbursement is based on three resource components: (1) physician work; (2) practice expenses; and (3) malpractice insurance. Each of about 4,000 HCFA common procedure codes (HCPCs) have assigned relative value units for the three resource components, which are summed to get the total number of units per code. The total units for each code are then multiplied by a conversion factor that equals the dollar value of one unit to get the dollar reimbursement amount.[12] The 1996 conversion factors—the dollar amounts that services' "relative values" are multiplied by to determine the fee—are $35.42 for primary care, $40.80 for surgery, $34.63 for nonsurgical services, and $15.28 for anesthesiology. When the RBRVS payment system was first put into place, it appeared that Medicare payments for surgical and diagnostic procedures would be cut significantly, while payments for office visits would increase substantially. However, the system has not shifted payments to primary care physicians to the extent that was anticipated.

Medicaid

Medicaid was begun in 1966 as a modest program to be jointly funded and run by the states and the federal government to provide a medical safety net for low-income mothers and children, and for elderly, blind, and disabled individuals receiving benefits from the Supplemental Security Income program. Congress mandated that Medicaid cover hospital and physician care, but states were encouraged to expand on the basic package of benefits by either increasing the range of benefits or extending the program to the near-poor through optional eligibility. A mandatory nursing home benefit was added in 1972.

States with large tax bases were quick to expand coverage to many of the optional groups, while states with limited abilities to raise funds for Medicaid were forced to construct limited programs. In 1994, total Medicaid expenditures topped $100 billion, with the federal government picking up 55 percent of the tab and the states the rest. The program covered more than 28 million people, or about one in every ten Americans. Still, about 35–40 million people in the United States are uninsured and do not qualify for Medicaid benefits.

Because Medicaid is administered by the states, each state establishes its own reimbursement system for providers. Although in the past Medicaid has reimbursed providers on a cost basis, more and more states are moving to per diem and fixed-fee prospective rates. As Medicaid expenditures continue to rise, policymakers are struggling to find cost-effective ways to improve the program's access, quality, and reimbursement rates.

Hospitals recently have been very vocal in their claims that Medicaid reimbursement does not cover the costs of service, and some have even sued their state governments for increased payments on the grounds that Medicaid laws call for "fair market" rate reimbursement. Physicians historically have also fared badly under Medicaid because states have tried to cut Medicaid costs by freezing physicians' fees. Citing excess paperwork, high risks, and low fees, many physicians— particularly obstetricians and pediatricians—have either quit taking Medicaid patients or are limiting the numbers served.

Medicaid has been a major payer fueling growth in the nursing home industry. Medicaid pays about 44 percent of total nursing home income, but Medicaid patients consume about 65 percent of nursing homes' total patient days. Nursing homes cover the losses on Medicaid patients by shifting the costs to private-pay patients. Medicaid was not originally intended as a payment vehicle for long-term care, but the high per capita cost of care for the aged and disabled is taking up a big share of overall expenditures. Nearly 75 percent of Medicaid payments go for the aged, blind, and disabled, who represent about 28 percent of Medicaid's recipients.

Self-Test Questions:

Briefly describe some different types of private insurers.

What reimbursement methods are commonly used by private insurers?

Briefly describe the origins and purpose of Medicare.

What is the prospective payment system (PPS), and how does it work?

What is Medicaid, and how is it administered?

Other Issues

Two other issues that relate to reimbursement and the third party payer system merit discussion: cost shifting and case-mix management.

Cost shifting

Providers of most services, from fast-food restaurants to carpet cleaners, charge all customers the same rate for similar services. Furthermore, the rates charged are set by supply and demand conditions in a competitive marketplace. However, in the provision of health care services, there is typically a wide range of reimbursement amounts for a single treatment protocol. For example, assume a hospital treats six different patients for heart failure and shock (DRG 127) in a single week. Table 3.4 contains a hypothesized reimbursement pattern for those six patients.

Reimbursement for this single DRG ranges from a high of $5,575 for private-pay, or self-pay, patients to a low of $0 for indigent patients. On average, the hospital is reimbursed $3,860, which is only 1.6 percent above costs. Thus, a hospital with this payer mix is barely breaking even on this DRG. Now assume that this hospital's payer mix changes so that it now has one more Medicare patient and it loses its commercial insurance patient: its average reimbursement for this DRG now is only $3,682, which is $188 below costs.

Clearly, the hospital cannot allow this situation to persist, so it engages in *cost shifting*. That is, it increases its billed charges applicable to this DRG so that private-pay, commercially insured, and HMO/PPO patients pay even more than is indicated in Table 3.4. Thus, costs associated with patients whose reimbursement does not cover those costs are

Table 3.4   Typical Reimbursement Pattern

Payer	Reimbursement Method	Reimbursement Amount
Private pay	Billed charges	$ 5,575
Commerical insurance	Billed charges less 5%	5,296
HMO/PPO	Billed charges less 15%	4,739
Medicare	Prospective payment	4,128*
Medicaid	Cost less 10%	3,420†
Indigent patient	No payment	0
Total reimbursement		$23,158
Average reimbursement		$ 3,860

* Includes capital-related costs.

† Assumes $3,800 cost of treatment.

shifted to other payers who, at least temporarily, are willing to absorb, or pass on, the higher billings.

Cost shifting has been the remedy that many health care providers have used to maintain profitability in the face of higher indigent care loads and less generous government reimbursement amounts. However, as the burden of cost shifting falls more and more heavily on just a few classes of payers, it is becoming more and more difficult to continue the practice. As private-pay rates increase and insurance rates increase for group health insurance (especially for medium and small businesses) these parties are finding it very difficult, if not impossible, to carry the burden of payers that are paying less than costs. Indeed, cost shifting has contributed to the movement to managed care plans, which in turn have adopted reimbursement methodologies—such as discounted fee-for-service and capitation—that make further cost shifting difficult if not impossible.

Case-mix management

In addition to cost shifting, which is not sustainable in the long run, providers have been using *case-mix management* to try to control costs and enhance profitability. Case-mix management can be exercised at two levels. First, at the lowest level, it is used to lower the costs associated with a particular diagnosis by changing the mix of procedures applied to the diagnosis.[13] The provider, say, a hospital, examines the costs associated with treating a large number of patients with the same diagnosis. Typically, these costs will vary substantially on the basis of severity of illness and the particular treatments prescribed by attending physicians.

Although a complicated and challenging job, it is possible in many situations to identify lower-cost treatment regimens that result in outcomes that are just as good as those from higher-cost regimens. When these are identified, hospital managers and physicians can work together to adopt the lower-cost treatment patterns. Although this might lower revenues from third party payers that continue to reimburse on a cost basis, more and more payers are moving to prospective payment or capitation, so lower costs translate directly into higher profits.

The second type of case-mix management involves changing the provider's overall patient mix by lowering the number of patients with diagnoses that typically result in losses and increasing the number with diagnoses that are highly profitable. For example, many services associated with heart disease have been, and continue to be, highly profitable.

Thus, many hospitals have been very aggressive in their advertising campaigns to promote themselves as "your cardiac care center" or "leaders in the fight against heart disease." Conversely, hospitals are not promoting, and even attempt to discontinue, those services that are money losers. By doing this, hospitals are attempting to increase the percentage of high-profit treatments and decrease the percentage of treatments that result in losses.

Self-Test Questions:

What is cost shifting?

Will providers be able to continue to cost shift in the future?

What is case-mix management?

Summary

- Health insurance is widely used in the United States because individuals are *risk averse* and insurance companies can take advantage of the *law of large numbers.*

- Insurance is based on four key characteristics: (1) *pooling of losses*; (2) *payment for random losses*; (3) *risk transfer*; and (4) *indemnification.*

- *Adverse selection* occurs when those individuals most likely to have claims purchase insurance while those least likely to have claims do not.

- *Moral hazard* occurs when an insured individual purposely sustains a loss, as opposed to a random loss.

- When payers pay *billed charges*, they pay according to the schedule of charge rates established by the provider.

- *Negotiated charges*, which are discounted from billed charges, are often used by insurers in conjunction with managed care plans such as HMOs and PPOs.

- Under a *retrospective cost* system, the payer agrees to pay the provider certain allowable costs that are incurred in providing services to the payer's enrollees.

- In a *prospective payment system*, the rates paid by payers are determined in advance and are not tied directly to either reimbursable costs or billed charges.

- The major private insurers are *Blue Cross–Blue Shield, commercial insurers,* and *self-insurers.*

- Government is a major insurer, and direct provider, of health care services. The two major forms of government health insurance are *Medicare* and *Medicaid.*

- In 1983, the federal government adopted the *prospective payment system (PPS)* for Medicare hospital reimbursement. The intent of the PPS was (1) to reduce the growth in Medicare outlays; (2) to provide cost-containment incentives to providers; and yet (3) to maintain quality of care.

- Under PPS, the amount of the payment is based on the patient's *diagnosis-related group (DRG)* as determined by the attending physician.

- To attempt to provide some cushion for the high costs associated with severely ill patients within each diagnosis, PPS includes a provision for *outlier payments.*

- The major categories of capital-related costs are *depreciation expense, interest expense,* and *lease* and *rental* expense.

- Until recently, *capital-related costs* were excluded from Medicare's PPS. In lieu of folding capital-related costs into the DRG rate, such costs were passed-through separately on the basis of costs incurred. Thus, such payments to hospitals are called *capital pass-through payments.*

- Now, hospitals receive a *fixed amount* for each Medicare discharge to cover capital-related costs directly related to inpatient care.

- *Peer Review Organizations (PROs)* are independent organizations contracted by HCFA at the state level to monitor the care, and the resulting reimbursement, provided by hospitals and other health care providers that treat Medicare patients.

- *Cost shifting* results when a provider increases its billed charges to one set of payers to compensate for insufficient reimbursement from another set of payers.

- Providers employ *case-mix management* to try to control costs and enhance profitability. First, case-mix management is used to lower the costs associated with a particular diagnosis by changing the mix of procedures applied to the diagnosis. Second, case-mix management involves changing the diagnosis mix by lowering the number of patients with diagnoses that typically result in losses and increasing the number with diagnoses that are highly profitable.

Notes

1. For more information on the basics of insurance, see one of the many excellent insurance textbooks, for example, G. E. Rejda, *Principles of Insurance* (Glenview, IL.: Scott, Foresman, 1993), or E. J. Vaughan, *Fundamentals of Risk and Insurance* (New York: Wiley, 1993).

2. For any one individual, the standard deviation of health care costs is $1,990 per expected cost of $200, so there is significant uncertainty about the required expenditure. However, the law of large numbers tells us that the standard deviation of costs to an insurance company with a large number of policyholders is $\sigma/\sqrt{n}$, where σ is the standard deviation for one individual and n is the number of individuals insured. Thus, the expected payout for the insurance company with 1 million policyholders is $200 million, but payout uncertainty, as measured by the standard deviation, is only $1,990/\sqrt{1,000,000} = \$1.99$ per subscriber, or $1.99 million in total. Thus, if there were no uncertainty in the $20,000 estimated medical cost per claim, the insurance company could forecast its claims quite precisely. The problem for real world insurers is their inability to forecast the cost of each claim.

3. In the following sections, we provide only a brief introduction to the major third party payers. For more information, see Section E, entitled "Payment," in *Handbook of Health Care Accounting and Finance*, Volume II, edited by W. O. Cleverley (Rockville, MD: Aspen, 1989) or H. J. Berman, S. F. Kukla, and L. E. Weeks, *The Financial Management of Hospitals* (Ann Arbor, MI: Health Administration Press, 1993).

4. State laws typically require the assets of not-for-profit corporations to be used for charitable purposes in perpetuity, so conversion of ownership is a relatively complex endeavor. We discuss the issues involved in conversion in Chapter 17.

5. This section was coauthored by Michael J. McCue of Virginia Commonwealth University.

6. HCFA plans to consolidate the processing of Medicare claims at regional processing centers beginning in the fall of 1997. The new system, called the Medicare Transaction System, is designed to standardize claims processing by creating one national system. When completed, the system will allow hospitals to file Medicare claims—mostly in electronic format—directly to HCFA. Other functions such as audits, customer service, and medical reviews will continue to be performed by intermediaries.

7. The prospective payment system does not apply to all hospitals. For example, psychiatric and childrens hospitals are still reimbursed on a retrospective cost basis.

8. An operating margin of 14 percent means that for each dollar of Medicare revenue, operating costs amounted to 86 cents, so the hospital made a 14 cent operating profit. In most industries, operating margins run less than 10 percent, so most managers would view a 14 percent margin as highly profitable.

9. Our purpose here is not to make you an expert in Medicare's PPS. Indeed, most hospitals other than the very smallest have one or more specialists on the financial staff whose sole responsibility is to keep track of changes in Medicare reimbursement practices. However, some type of DRG-based prospective payment system is being used by many payers with many different types of providers, so some knowledge of the system is necessary for all health care managers.

10. The number of DRGs in Medicare's PPS changes frequently as diagnoses are refined. Originally, there were only 383 DRGs. Also, note that the prospective payment system proposed for outpatient services will be based on about 300 *ambulatory patient groups (APGs)*, which are designed to measure the type and amount of resources used in an ambulatory care visit.

11. As we discussed in Chapter 2, for tax purposes, investor-owned hospitals calculate depreciation expense using the accelerated method of the Modified Accelerated Cost Recovery System (MACRS). However, for Medicare reporting purposes, and hence for recovery of capital-related costs, both investor-owned and not-for-profit hospitals must use accounting, or book, depreciation methods.

12. Of course, the system is not quite that simple because payments are adjusted by cost indexes that reflect geographical differences in costs. For more details, see P. L. Grimaldi, "RBRVS: How New Physician Fee Schedule Will Work." *Healthcare Financial Management* (September 1991), 58–76.

13. For a more detailed discussion of case-mix management at the treatment level, see D. A. Tong and P. L. Jones, "Physicians, Financial Managers Join Forces to Control Costs." *Healthcare Financial Management* (January 1990), 21–30.

Selected Additional References

Coddington, D. C., D. J. Keene, K. D. Moore, and R. L. Clarke. 1991. "Factors Driving Costs Must Figure into Reform." *Healthcare Financial Management* (July): 44–62.

Grimaldi, P. L. 1993. "Capital Update Factor: A New Era Approaches." *Healthcare Financial Management* (February): 32–37.

Grimaldi, P. L. 1992. "Changes in Medicare Capital PPS Rates and Rules." *Healthcare Financial Management* (December): 40–47.

Guterman, S. P., W. Eggers, G. Riley, T. F. Greene, and S. A. Terrell. 1988. "The First 3 Years of Medicare Prospective Payment: An Overview." *Health Care Financing Review* (Spring): 67–77.

Healthcare Financial Management Association. 1988. *Medicare Prospective Price Setting.* Westchester, IL: Healthcare Financial Management Association.

Herr, W. W. 1991. "Taking a Deep Breath over Medicare Capital Payments." *Healthcare Financial Management* (April): 19–32.

Hottinger, M., C. L. Polich, and M. Parker. 1991. "At Risk: A Look at Managing Medicare Losses." *Healthcare Financial Management* (May): 23–32.

Hughes, K. E. 1993. "Medicare Physician Payment Reform: A View from the Field." *Healthcare Financial Management* (November): 48–54.

Lamm, R. D. 1990. "High-Tech Health Care and Society's Ability to Pay." *Healthcare Financial Management* (September): 20–30.

Micheletti, J. A., T. J. Shlala, and C. E. Greenfield. 1993. "Optimizing Medicare Reimbursement in Skilled Nursing Facilities." *Healthcare Financial Management* (February): 38–42.

Ryan, J. B., and S. B. Clay. 1995. "Understanding the Law of Large Numbers." *Healthcare Financial Management* (October): 22–24.

Smith, D. G. 1992. "Provider Involvement in Managed Care Underwriting." *Topics in Health Care Financing* (Winter): 33–39.

Part II

Basic Financial Management Concepts

4

Discounted Cash Flow Analysis

$\mathbf{O}$ne of the concepts that you will use frequently within health care financial management is asset valuation. The value of any asset, whether a *financial asset*, such as stocks and bonds, or a *real asset*, such as lithotripters and ambulatory surgery centers, is based on the cash flows that the asset is expected to produce in the future. But a dollar to be received in the future is worth less than a dollar in the hand today because current consumption is preferred to future consumption. (Or as one famous economist put it, a Big Mac today is better than a Big Mac tomorrow.) To think about it in another way, if you have a dollar today, you can invest it, say, in a bank savings account, earn interest, and end up with more than one dollar in the future. Thus, future dollars are worth less than current dollars.

The process of accounting for timing value differences is called *discounted cash flow analysis*, or *time value of money analysis*. It is an important part of many financial decisions, including bond and stock valuation, capital budgeting analysis, and lease analysis. In fact, of all of the techniques used in financial management, none is more important than discounted cash flow analysis. Discounted cash flow concepts will be used throughout the remainder of the book, so it is vital that you understand the material in this chapter thoroughly before going on to other topics.

Time Lines

One of the most important tools in discounted cash flow analysis is the *time line*. Time lines make it easier to visualize when the cash flows in a particular analysis occur. To illustrate the time line concept, consider the following five-period time line:

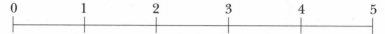

Time 0 is today (or, really, any starting point); Time 1 is one period from today, or the end of Period 1; Time 2 is two periods from today, or the end of Period 2; and so on. Thus, the numbers on top of the tick marks represent end-of-period values. Often, the periods are years, but other time intervals such as semiannual (six-month) periods, quarters, months, or even days are also used when needed to fit the timing of the cash flows being evaluated. If the time periods are years, the interval from 0 to 1 would be Year 1, and Time 1 would represent both the end of Year 1 and the beginning of Year 2.

Cash flows are shown on a time line directly below the tick marks, and interest rates are sometimes shown directly above the time line. Additionally, unknown cash flows—the ones you are trying to determine in the analysis—are sometimes indicated by question marks. To illustrate, consider the following time line:

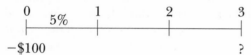

Here, the interest rate for each of the three periods is 5 percent, a *lump sum* investment of $100 is made at Time 0, and the Time 3 value is unknown. We know the $100 is an *outflow*, because it is shown as a negative cash flow. (Note that outflows are often designated by parentheses rather than a minus sign.)

Now consider the following situation, where an unknown lump sum investment must be made today to receive $100 at the end of Period 2:

The interest rate is 5 percent during the first period, but 10 percent during the second period. Generally, the interest rate is constant over all periods, in which case we show it in the first period only to avoid cluttering the time line.

Time lines are essential when first learning discounted cash flow analysis, but even experienced analysts use time lines when dealing with complex problems. The time line may be an actual line, as illustrated, or it may be a series of columns (or sometimes rows) on a spreadsheet. We will be using time lines throughout the book, and you should get into the habit of creating your own time lines when conducting analyses that involve future cash flows.

Self-Test Question:

Draw a three-year time line that illustrates the following situation:

    1. An investment of $10,000 at Time 0;

    2. Inflows of $5,000 at the end of Years 1, 2, and 3; and

    3. An interest rate during the entire three years of 10 percent.

Future Value of a Lump Sum (Compounding)

The process of going from today's values, or *present values*, to future values is called *compounding*. To illustrate *lump sum* compounding, suppose the cash manager of Meridian Clinics deposited $100 in a bank account that pays 5 percent interest each year. How much would be in the account at the end of one year? To begin, we define the following terms:

PV = $100 = present value, or beginning amount, of the account.

i = 5% = interest rate the bank pays on the account per year. The interest is based on the balance at the beginning of each year, and it is paid at the end of the year. Expressed as a decimal, i = 0.05.

I = dollars of interest earned during the year = Beginning amount $\times$ i.

FV_n = future value, or ending amount, of the account at the end of n years. Whereas PV is the value now, or *present value*, FV_n is the value n years into the *future*, after the interest earned has been added to the account.

n = number of years involved in the analysis.

In our example, n = 1, so FV_n can be calculated as follows:

$$FV_n = FV_1 = PV + I$$
$$= PV + PV(i)$$
$$= PV(1 + i).$$

Thus, the future value at the end of one year, FV_1, equals the present value multiplied by 1.0 plus the interest rate. We can now use these concepts to find how much $100 will be worth at the end of one year if it is invested in an account that pays 5 percent interest:

$$FV_1 = PV(1 + i) = \$100(1 + 0.05) = \$100(1.05) = \$105.$$

What would be the value of the $100 if Meridian Clinics left its money in the account for five years? Here is a time line set up to show the amount at the end of each year:

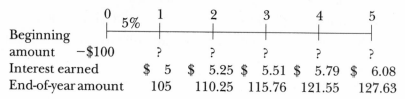

Note the following points:

1. The account is opened with a deposit of $100. This is shown as an outflow at $t = 0$.

2. Meridian earns $100(0.05) = \$5$ of interest during the first year, so the amount in the account at the end of Year 1 is $100 + \$5 = \$105$.

3. At the start of the second year, the account balance is $105. Interest of $5.25 is earned on the now larger amount, and the account balance at the end of the second year is $110.25. The Year 2 interest, $5.25, is higher than the first year's interest, $5, because $5(0.05) = \$0.25$ in interest was earned on the first year's interest.

4. This process continues, and because the beginning balance is higher in each succeeding year, the interest earned increases.

5. The total interest earned, $27.63, is reflected in the final balance at $t = 5$, $127.63.

Note that the Year 2 value, $110.25, is equal to

$$FV_2 = FV_1(1 + i)$$
$$= PV(1 + i)(1 + i)$$
$$= PV(1 + i)^2$$
$$= \$100(1.05)^2 = \$110.25.$$

Continuing, the balance at the end of Year 3 is

$$FV_3 = FV_2(1 + i)$$
$$= PV(1 + i)^3$$
$$= \$100(1.05)^3 = \$115.76,$$

and

$$FV_5 = \$100(1.05)^5 = \$127.63.$$

In general, the future value of a lump sum at the end of n years can be found by applying Equation 4.1:

$$FV_n = PV(1 + i)^n. \tag{4.1}$$

Future values, as well as most other discounted cash flow problems, can be solved in three ways:

1. *Use a regular calculator.* You can simply use a regular calculator, either by multiplying $(1 + i)$ by itself $n - 1$ times or by using the exponential function to raise $(1 + i)$ to the nth power. For most calculators, you would enter $1 + i = 1.05$ and multiply it by itself four times, or else enter 1.05, then press the y^x (exponential) function key, then enter 5. In either case, you would get 1.2763 (if you set your calculator to display four decimal places) as the answer, which you would then multiply by \$100 to get the final answer, \$127.63.

2. *Use a financial calculator.* Financial calculators have been programmed to solve many types of time value of money problems. In effect, Equation 4.1 is programmed directly into a financial calculator, and the future value is found using the time value of money input keys pictured below:

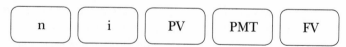

Note that there are five calculator keys that correspond to the five time value of money variables that are commonly used:

n (or N) = number of periods.

i (or I) = interest rate per period.

PV = present value.

PMT = payment. This key is used only if the cash flows involve a series of equal payments (an annuity).

FV = future value.

In this chapter, we will deal with equations that involve only four of the variables at any one time—three of the variables will be known, and the calculator will solve for the fourth (unknown) variable. In Chapter 5, when we deal with bond valuation, all five of the variables will be included in the analysis.[1]

To find the future value of $100 after 5 years at 5 percent interest using a financial calculator, just enter PV = 100, i = 5, and n = 5, and then press the FV key. The answer, 127.63 (rounded to two decimal places), will appear. Many financial calculators require that cash flows be designated as either inflows or outflows (shown as positive or negative values). Applying this logic to our illustration, Meridian deposits, or puts in, the initial amount (which is an outflow to the firm) and takes out, or receives, the ending amount (which is an inflow to the firm). If your calculator requires that you follow this sign convention, the PV would be entered as −100.

Also, on some calculators you are required to press a *Compute* key before pressing the FV key. Finally, financial calculators permit you to specify the number of decimal places that are displayed, even though 12 or more significant digits are actually used in the calculations. We generally use two places for answers in dollars or percentages, and four places for decimal answers, but the final answer should be rounded to reflect the accuracy of the input values—it makes no sense to say that the return on a particular investment is 14.63827 percent when the cash flows are highly uncertain. The nature of the analysis dictates how many decimal places should be displayed.

3. *Use a computer.* Computers, along with spreadsheet programs such as Lotus 1-2-3, Excel, and Quattro Pro, can also be used to solve many types of discounted cash flow problems.[2] Furthermore, spreadsheet users can create their own formulas to perform tasks that have not been preprogrammed. The discounted cash flow formulas that are provided in spreadsheet programs are part of a series of functions called *@functions* (pronounced "at functions"). Like any formula, @functions consist of a number of arithmetic calculations combined into one statement. By using @functions, spreadsheet users can save the time and tedium of building formulas from scratch.

Each @function begins with a unique function name that identifies the calculation to be performed, and contains one or more *arguments*, which are the input values for the calculation, enclosed in parentheses. There is no @function for finding the future value of a lump sum, since it can be quickly calculated by formula. For example, the spreadsheet formula for solving the Meridian Clinic example is:

$$100 * (1.05)^\wedge 5,$$

where $*$ is the spreadsheet multiplication sign and $\wedge$ is the spreadsheet exponential (or power) sign. When this formula is entered into a spreadsheet cell, the value 127.63 appears in the cell.[3]

The most efficient way to solve most problems involving time value of money is to use a financial calculator or a spreadsheet. However, you must understand the basic mathematics behind the calculations to set up complex problems before solving them. In addition, you need to understand the underlying logic in order to comprehend stock and bond valuation, lease analysis, capital budgeting analysis, and other important health care financial management topics.

To help you better understand the various types of time value analyses, we will use a more or less constant format in this chapter:

1. We lay out the situation on a time line and show the equation that must be solved.

2. We then present the regular calculator solution, if applicable.

3. Next, we show how the equation can be solved with a financial calculator.

4. Finally, we present the spreadsheet formula or @function.

Graphic view of the compounding, or growth, process

Figure 4.1 shows how $1 (or any other lump sum) grows over time at various rates of interest. The data used to plot the curves could be obtained by using any of the solution techniques described above. Note that the greater the rate of interest, the faster the growth rate. Thus, $100 on deposit for ten years at a 5 percent interest rate will grow to $162.89, but the same amount invested at 10 percent interest will grow to $259.37. The interest rate is, in fact, a growth rate: if a sum is deposited and earns 5 percent interest, the funds on deposit will grow at a rate of 5 percent per period. Note also that future value concepts are not

Figure 4.1   Relationships among Future Value, Interest Rates, and Time

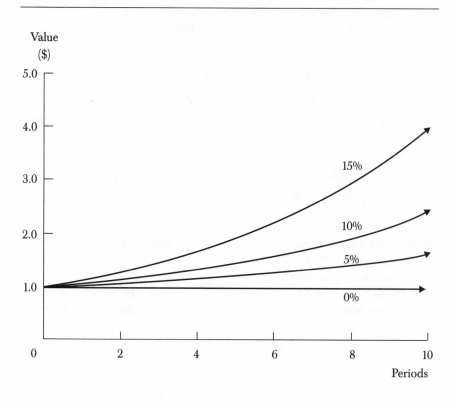

	Interest Rate Plot Points		
Period	*5%*	*10%*	*15%*
1	1.0500	1.1000	1.1500
2	1.1025	1.2100	1.3225
3	1.1576	1.3310	1.5209
4	1.2155	1.4641	1.7490
5	1.2763	1.6105	2.0114
6	1.3401	1.7716	2.3131
7	1.4071	1.9487	2.6600
8	1.4775	2.1436	3.0590
9	1.5513	2.3579	3.5179
10	1.6289	2.5937	4.0456

Source: E. F. Brigham and L. C. Gapenski. 1994. *Financial Management: Theory and Practice,* 7th ed. Fort Worth, TX: The Dryden Press.

restricted to deposits; they can be applied to any number that is growing (or declining)—sales, population, earnings per share, and so on.

Self-Test Questions:

Explain what is meant by the following statement: "A dollar in the hand today is worth more than a dollar to be received in the future."

What is compounding? What is interest on interest?

What are three solution techniques for solving lump sum compounding problems?

Present Value of a Lump Sum (Discounting)

Suppose Ridgewood Community Hospital, which currently has excess cash to invest, has been offered the chance to purchase a low-risk security from a local broker that will pay $127.63 at the end of five years. A local bank is currently offering 5 percent interest on a five-year certificate of deposit (CD), and the hospital's managers regard the security in question as being as safe as the bank CD. The 5 percent interest rate available on the bank CD is the hospital's opportunity cost rate, or the best rate of return it could earn on alternative investments of similar risk. (Opportunity costs will be discussed in detail in the next section.) How much would the hospital be willing to pay for a security that promises $127.63 after five years?

From the future value example presented in the previous section, we saw that an initial amount of $100 invested at 5 percent per year would be worth $127.63 at the end of five years. Thus, Ridgewood should be indifferent to the choice between $100 today and $127.63 at the end of five years. The $100 is defined as the *present value*, or *PV*, of $127.63 due in five years when the opportunity cost rate is 5 percent. If the price of the security is anything less than $100, the hospital should buy it; if the price is greater than $100, it should turn the offer down. If the price is exactly $100, the hospital could buy it or turn it down, because that is the security's "fair value."

In general, *the present value of a cash flow due n years in the future is the amount which, if it were on hand today, would grow to equal the future amount.* Since $100 would grow to $127.63 in five years at a 5 percent interest rate, $100 is the present value of $127.63 due five years in the future when the opportunity cost rate is 5 percent.

Finding present values is called *discounting*, and it is simply the reverse of compounding—if you know the PV, you compound to find the FV; if you know the FV, you discount to find the PV. Following are ways to solve the discounting problem.

Time line:

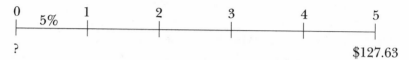

To develop the discounting equation, simply solve Equation 4.1 for *PV*:

$$FV_n = PV(1 + i)^n \qquad\qquad (4.1)$$

$$PV = \frac{FV_n}{(1 + i)^n} = FV_n \left(\frac{1}{1 + i}\right)^n$$

Regular calculator solution:

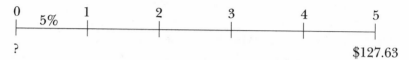

Financial calculator solution:

Inputs	5	5			127.63
	n	i	PV	PMT	FV
Output			=−100.00		

Spreadsheet solution:

Cell formula	127.63/(1.05)^5
Cell display	100.00

Graphic view of the discounting process

Figure 4.2 shows how the present value of $1 (or any other sum) to be received in the future diminishes as the years to receipt increase.

Figure 4.2   Relationships among Present Value, Interest Rates, and Time

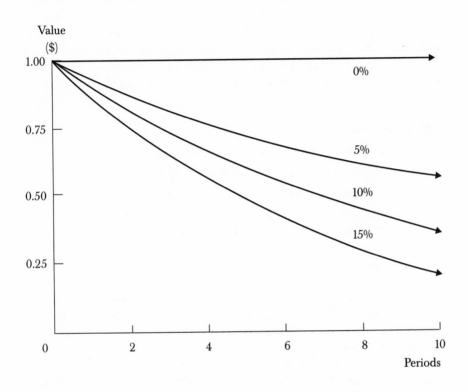

Period	Interest Rate Plot Points		
	5%	10%	15%
1	.9524	.9091	.8696
2	.9070	.8254	.7561
3	.8638	.7513	.6575
4	.8227	.6830	.5718
5	.7835	.6209	.4972
6	.7462	.5634	.4323
7	.7107	.5132	.3759
8	.6768	.4665	.3269
9	.6446	.4241	.2843
10	.6139	.3855	.2472

Source: E. F. Brigham and L. C. Gapenski. 1994. *Financial Management: Theory and Practice,* 7th ed. Fort Worth, TX: The Dryden Press.

Again, the data used to plot the curves can be developed by using any of the solution techniques. The graphs show (1) that the present value decreases and approaches zero as the payment date is extended further into the future, and (2) that the rate of decrease is greater the higher the interest (discount) rate. At relatively high interest rates, funds due in the future are worth very little today, and even at relatively low discount rates, the present value of a sum due in the distant future is quite small. For example, at a 10 percent discount rate, $100 due in 50 years is worth only 85 cents.

Self-Test Questions:

What does the term "opportunity cost rate" mean?

What is discounting? How is it related to compounding?

What are three techniques for solving lump sum discounting problems?

How does the present value of an amount to be received in the future change as the time is extended and as the interest rate increases?

Opportunity Costs

The *opportunity cost* concept plays a very important role in discounted cash flow analysis. To illustrate, suppose you found the winning Florida lottery ticket and now have $1 million to invest. Should you assign a cost to these funds? At first blush, it might appear that this money has zero cost to you since it cost you nothing. However, as soon as you think about what to do with the $1 million, you have to think in terms of the opportunity cost involved. By using the funds to invest in one alternative, say, Columbia/HCA stock, you forgo the opportunity to make some other investment, say, buying U.S. Treasury bonds. Thus, there is an opportunity cost associated with any investment planned for the $1 million even though your lottery winnings were "free."

Because one investment decision automatically negates all other possible investments with the same funds, the cash flows from any investment must be discounted at a rate that reflects the rate that could be earned on forgone opportunities, *regardless of the source of the funds.* The problem, of course, is that the number of forgone opportunities is virtually infinite, so which one should be chosen to establish the opportunity cost rate? The opportunity cost rate to be applied in discounted cash flow analysis is the *highest rate that could be earned on alternative investments of similar risk.* It would not be logical to assign a very low opportunity cost rate to a series of very risky cash flows, or vice versa.

Generally, opportunity cost rates are obtained by looking at rates that could be earned, or more precisely, the rates that are expected to be earned, on securities such as stocks and bonds. Securities are usually chosen to set opportunity cost rates because their expected returns are more easily estimated than rates of return on real assets such as group practices, hospital beds, MRI machines, and the like.

For example, assume that Green Valley Community Hospital is considering the purchase of a nursing home. The first step in the analysis is to forecast the cash flows that the nursing home is expected to generate if owned by Green Valley. Then, these cash flows must be discounted at some opportunity cost rate. Would the hospital's opportunity cost rate be (1) the expected rate of return on Treasury bonds, (2) the expected rate of return on the stock of Beverly Enterprises, which owns some 850 nursing homes, or (3) the expected rate of return on pork belly futures? (Pork belly futures are very risky investments that involve commodity contracts for delivery at some time in the future.) The answer is the expected rate of return on Beverly Enterprises' stock because that is the rate of return available to the hospital on alternative investments of similar risk. Treasury securities are low-risk investments, so they would understate the opportunity cost rate in owning a nursing home. Conversely, pork belly futures are very high-risk investments, so that rate of return is probably too high to apply to a nursing home investment.

Actually, owning a single nursing home is riskier than owning a chain that has geographical diversification, so the true opportunity cost is probably somewhat higher than the return expected on Beverly Enterprises' stock. Also, note that the source of the funds used for the nursing home investment is not relevant to the analysis. Green Valley may obtain the needed funds by issuing tax-exempt debt, or by soliciting contributions, or it may even have excess cash accumulated from retained earnings. The discount rate applied to the nursing home cash flows depends on the riskiness of those cash flows, not on the source of the investment funds.

The bottom line here is that some opportunity cost rate has to be applied to discount future cash flows. The proper rate is the rate that best reflects the riskiness inherent in the future cash flows, and this rate is normally established by looking at the expected returns available on securities of similar risk. (Chapter 8 presents a discussion of how baseline opportunity cost rates are established for capital investments, while Chapter 10 presents a detailed discussion on how the riskiness of a cash flow stream can be assessed.)

Self-Test Questions:

Why does an investment have an opportunity cost rate even when the funds employed have no explicit cost?

How are opportunity cost rates established?

Does the opportunity cost rate depend on the source of the investment funds?

Solving for Interest Rate and Time

At this point, it should be obvious that compounding and discounting are reciprocal processes. Furthermore, we have been working with four time-value-of-money variables: PV, FV, i, and n. If you know the values of three of the variables, you (perhaps with the help of your financial calculator or spreadsheet) can find the value of the fourth. Thus far we have always given you the interest rate, i, and the number of years, n, plus either the PV or the FV are known. In many situations, however, you will need to solve for either i or n.

Solving for the interest rate (i)

Suppose Ridgewood Community Hospital can buy a bank CD for $78.35 that will return $100 after five years. Here, we know PV, FV, and n, but we do not know i, the interest rate that the bank is paying. These types of problems are solved as follows.

Time line:

$$
\begin{array}{ccccccc}
0 & & 1 & 2 & 3 & 4 & 5 \\
\vdash & ? & & & & & \dashv \\
-\$78.35 & & & & & & \$100
\end{array}
$$

$$FV_n = PV(1 + i)^n \qquad\qquad (4.1)$$
$$\$100 = \$78.35(1 + i)^5$$

Financial calculator solution:

Inputs	5		-78.35		100
	n	i	PV	PMT	FV
Output		$= 5.0$			

Spreadsheet solution:

@Function	@RATE (FV,PV,n)
Cell formula	@RATE $(100,78.35,5)$
Cell display	0.050

Note that there is an @function, @RATE, which solves for interest rate in spreadsheet programs. Also, note that the answer is displayed in decimal form unless the cell is formatted to display in percent.

Solving for time (n)

Suppose the bank told Ridgewood Community Hospital that a certificate of deposit pays 5 percent interest each year, that it costs $78.35, and that at maturity the hospital would receive $100. How long must the funds be invested in the CD? Here, we know PV, FV, and i, but we do not know n, the number of periods. Following are ways to solve this type of problem.

Time line:

$$FV_n = PV(1 + i)^n \qquad\qquad (4.1)$$
$$\$100 = \$78.35(1.05)^n$$

Financial calculator solution:

Spreadsheet solution:

@Function	@CTERM (i,FV,PV)
Cell formula	@CTERM $(0.05,100,78.35)$
Cell display	5.00

Note that interest rates must be entered into @functions as decimals.

The Rule of 72

The *Rule of 72* is a simple and quick method for judging the effect of different interest rates on the growth of a lump sum deposit. It tells us that to find the number of years required to double the value of a lump sum, merely divide the number 72 by the interest rate paid. For example, if the interest rate is 10 percent, it would take $72/10 = 7.2$ years for the money in an account to double in value. The calculator solution is 7.27 years, so the Rule of 72 is relatively accurate, at least when reasonable interest rates are applied.

In a similar manner, the Rule of 72 can be used to determine the interest rate required to double the money in an account in a given number of years. To illustrate, an interest rate of $72/5 = 14.4\%$ is required to double the value of an account in five years. The calculator solution here is 14.9 percent, so the Rule of 72 again gives a reasonable approximation of the correct answer.

Self-Test Questions:

What are some real world situations that may require you to solve for interest rate or time?

What is the Rule of 72, and how is it used?

Future Value of an Annuity

Whereas lump sums are single values, an *annuity* is a series of equal payments at fixed intervals for a specified number of periods. Annuity payments, which are given the symbol PMT (for payment), can occur at the beginning or end of each period. If the payments occur at the end of each period, as they typically do, the annuity is an *ordinary*, or *deferred*, *annuity*. If payments are made at the beginning of each period, the annuity is an *annuity due*. Since ordinary annuities are far more common in finance, when the term "annuity" is used in this book you should assume that payments occur at the end of each period.

Ordinary annuities

A series of equal payments at the end of each period constitutes an ordinary annuity. If Meridian Clinics were to deposit $100 at the end of each year for three years in an account that paid 5 percent interest per year, how much would Meridian accumulate at the end of three years?

The answer to this question is the future value of the annuity, FVA_n, which occurs at the end of the final period, and hence coincides with the final payment.

Time line:

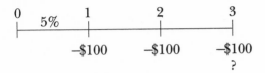

Regular calculator solution:

Of course, one approach to the problem is to compound each individual cash flow to Year 3.

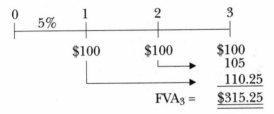

Financial calculator solution:

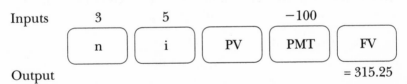

Note that in annuity problems, the PMT key is used in conjunction with either the PV or FV key.

Spreadsheet solution:

@Function	@FV(*PMT,i,n*)
Cell formula	@FV(100,0.05,3)
Cell display	315.25

Annuities due

Had the three $100 payments in the previous example been made at the beginning of each year, the annuity would have been an *annuity due*.

Note that the future value of an annuity is always defined as occurring at the end of the final period, so the future value of an annuity due occurs one period after the final payment.

Time line:

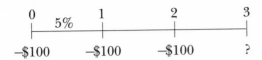

Regular calculator solution:

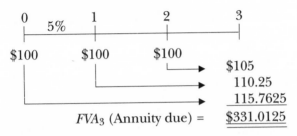

FVA_3 (Annuity due) = $\underline{\underline{\$331.0125}}$

In the case of an annuity due, as compared with an ordinary annuity, all of the cash flows are compounded for one additional period, and hence the future value of an annuity due is greater than the future value of a similar ordinary annuity by $(1 + i)$. Thus, the future value of an annuity due also can be found as follows:

$$FVA_n \text{ (Annuity due)} = FVA_n(1 + i)$$
$$= \$315.25(1.05) = \$331.01$$

Financial calculator solution:

Most financial calculators permit you to change the setting from end-of-period payments (ordinary annuity) to beginning-of-period payments (annuity due). When the beginning-of-period mode is activated, the display will normally indicate the changed mode with the word "BEGIN" or some other symbol. To deal with annuities due, merely change the mode to beginning of period and proceed as before.

			BEGIN	
Inputs	3	5		−100	
n	i	PV	PMT	FV
Output					= 331.01

Since most problems will deal with end-of-period cash flows, don't forget to switch your calculator back to the END mode.

Spreadsheet solution:

@Function	@FV(PMT,i,n)*(1 + i)
Cell formula	@FV(100,0.05,3)*(1.05)
Cell display	331.01

Self-Test Questions:

What is an annuity?

What is the difference between an ordinary annuity and an annuity due?

Which annuity has the greater future value: an ordinary annuity or an annuity due? Why?

Present Value of an Annuity

Suppose Vantage Health System was offered the following alternatives: (1) a three-year annuity with payments of $100 at the end of each year, or (2) a lump sum payment today. Vantage has no need for the money during the next three years, so if it accepts the annuity, it would simply deposit the payments in an account that pays 5 percent interest per year. Similarly, the lump sum payment would be deposited into the same account. How large must the lump sum payment today be to make it equivalent to the annuity?

Time line:

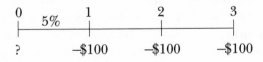

Regular calculator solution:

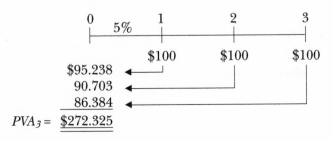

Financial calculator solution:

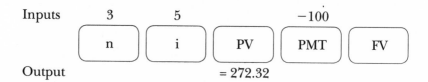

Inputs	3	5		−100	
	n	i	PV	PMT	FV
Output			= 272.32		

Spreadsheet solution:

@Function	@PV(*PMT,i,n*)
Cell formula	@PV(100,0.05,3)
Cell display	272.32

One especially important application of the annuity concept relates to loans with constant payments, such as mortgages and auto loans. With such loans, which are called *term,* or *amortized, loans,* the loan amount is the present value of an ordinary annuity, and the loan payments constitute the annuity stream. We will examine term loans in more depth in a later section on amortization.

Annuities due

If the three $100 payments in the previous example had been made at the beginning of each year, the annuity would have been an *annuity due.* Each payment would be shifted to the left one year, so each payment would be discounted for one less year. Since its payments come in faster, an annuity due is more valuable than an ordinary annuity. Note that the present value of an annuity is always defined as occurring at the beginning of the first period, so the present value of an annuity due coincides with the first payment.

Time line:

```
0       1        2       3
|  5%   |        |       |
-$100  -$100   -$100
  ?
```

Regular calculator solution:

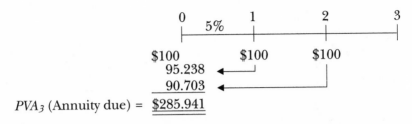

PVA_3 (Annuity due) = $\underline{\underline{\$285.941}}$

The present value of an annuity due can be thought of as the present value of an ordinary annuity that is compounded for one period, so it also can be found as follows:

$$PVA_n \text{ (Annuity due) } = PVA_n(1 + i)$$
$$= \$272.32(1.05) = \$285.94.$$

Financial calculator solution:

Activate the beginning of period mode (BEGIN), and then

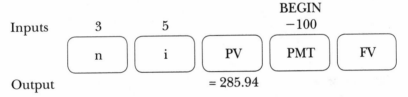

Again, since most problems will deal with end-of-period cash flows, don't forget to switch your calculator back to the END mode.

Spreadsheet solution:

@Function	@PV(PMT,i,n)*(1 + i)
Cell formula	@PV(100,0.05,3)*(1.05)
Cell display	285.94

Self-Test Questions:

Which annuity has the greater present value: an ordinary annuity or an annuity due? Why?

Perpetuities

Most annuities call for payments to be made over some finite period of time—for example, $100 per year for three years. However, some annuities go on indefinitely, or perpetually, and these annuities are called *perpetuities.* The present value of a perpetuity is found by applying Equation 4.3:

$$PV \text{ (Perpetuity)} = \frac{\text{Payment}}{\text{Interest rate}} = \frac{PMT}{i}. \tag{4.3}$$

Perpetuities can be illustrated by some securities issued by General Healthcare, Inc. Each security (actually, a preferred stock) promises to pay $100 every year in perpetuity. What would each security be worth if the opportunity cost rate, or discount rate, was 10 percent? The answer is $1,000:

$$PV \text{ (Perpetuity)} = \frac{\$100}{0.10} = \$1,000.$$

Suppose that interest rates, and hence the opportunity cost rate, rose to 15 percent; what would happen to the security's value? The interest rate increase would lower its value to $666.67:

$$PV \text{ (Perpetuity)} = \frac{\$100}{0.15} = \$666.67.$$

Now assume that interest rates fell to 5 percent. The rate decrease would increase the perpetuity's value to $2,000:

$$PV \text{ (Perpetuity)} = \frac{\$100}{0.05} = \$2,000.$$

We see that the value of a perpetuity changes dramatically when interest rates change. All securities' values are affected by interest rate changes, but some, like perpetuities, are more sensitive to interest rate changes than others, such as short-term government bonds. We will discuss the risks associated with interest rate changes in more detail in Chapter 6.

Self-Test Questions:

What is a perpetuity?

What happens to the value of a perpetuity when interest rates increase or decrease?

Uneven Cash Flow Streams

The definition of an annuity includes the words "constant amount," so annuities involve payments that are the same in every period. Although some financial decisions, such as bond valuation, do involve constant payments, most important financial management decisions involve uneven, or nonconstant, cash flows. For example, capital budgeting analyses, such as the evaluation of an outpatient clinic or MRI facility, rarely involve constant cash flows.

Throughout the book, we will follow convention and reserve the term *payment (PMT)* for annuity situations, where the cash flows are constant, and we will use the term *cash flow (CF)* to denote uneven cash flows. Financial calculators are set up to follow this convention, so if you are using one and dealing with uneven cash flows, you need to use the CF functions rather than the PMT key.

Present value of an uneven cash flow stream

The present value of an uneven cash flow stream (PVU_n) is found as the sum of the present values of the individual cash flows of the stream:

$$PVU_n = CF_1 \left(\frac{1}{1+i} \right)^1 + CF_2 \left(\frac{1}{1+i} \right)^2 + \ldots + CF_n \left(\frac{1}{1+i} \right)^n \quad (4.4)$$

$$= \sum_{t=1}^{n} CF_t \left(\frac{1}{1+i} \right)^t.$$

For example, suppose that Family Medical Practice of San Diego is considering opening a new office in a rapidly developing suburban area. The firm forecasts that the new office would produce the following stream of net cash flows (in thousands of dollars):

```
0      1       2       3       4       5       6       7
|------+-------+-------+-------+-------+-------+-------|
   $0     $100    $200    $200    $200    $300    $400
```

What is the present value of the new office investment if the appropriate discount (opportunity cost) rate is 10 percent?

Regular calculator solution:

We can simply find the PV of each individual cash flow using a regular calculator, and then sum these values to find the present value of the stream, $868.30[4]:

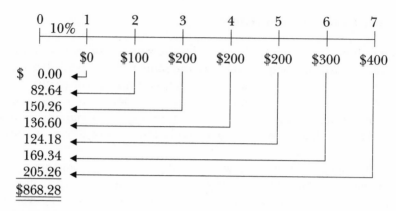

Also, in some situations, we may want to find the value of a cash flow stream at some point in time other than Year 0. In that situation, we proceed as above, but compound and discount the individual cash flows to some other point on the time line, say, Year 2.

Financial calculator solution:

Problems involving uneven cash flows can be solved in one step with most financial calculators. Here, you (1) input the individual cash flows, in chronological order, into the *cash flow registers*, usually designated as CF_0 and CF_j (CF_1, CF_2, CF_3, and so on) or just CF_j (CF_0, CF_1, CF_2, CF_3, and so on); (2) then enter the discount rate; and (3) finally push the NPV key. In effect, you have entered all the known values in Equation 4.4, and then the calculator finds and sums the present values. For this problem, enter 0, 0, 100, 200, 200, 200, 300, and 400 in that order into the calculator's cash flow registers, enter i = 10, and then push NPV to obtain the answer, 868.30. (A rounding difference occurs because the regular calculator method rounds the present value of each individual cash flow, while the financial calculator solution does not. Also, note that an implied cash flow of zero is entered for Year 0.)

Three points should be noted. First, when dealing with the cash flow registers, the term *NPV* is used to represent present value, rather than *PV*. The letter *N* in *NPV* stands for the word *net*, so *NPV* is the abbreviation for net present value. Net present value simply means the sum (or net) of the present values of a cash flow stream that generally contains both positive and negative cash flows (inflows and outflows)— in effect, the inflows and outflows are "netted out" on a present value basis. Our example has no negative cash flows, but if it did, we would simply input them into the cash flow registers as negative numbers.

Second, note that the annuity cash flows can be entered into the cash flow registers more efficiently on most calculators by using the n_j (or N_j) key. This key allows you to specify the number of times a constant payment occurs within an uneven cash flow stream. (On some calculators, you are prompted to enter the number of times the cash flow occurs.) In this illustration, you would enter $CF_0 = 0$, $CF_1 = 0$, $CF_2 = 100$, $CF_3 = 200$, $n_j = 3$, $CF_6 = 300$, and $CF_7 = 400$. Enter $i = 10$, press the NPV key, and 868.30 appears in the display.

Finally, note that amounts entered into the cash flow registers remain in those registers until they are cleared. Thus, if you had previously worked a problem with eight cash flows, and then moved to a problem with only four cash flows, the calculator would assume that the final four cash flows from the first calculation belonged to the second calculation. Be sure to clear the cash flow registers before starting a new problem!

Spreadsheet solution:

The *@NPV* function calculates the present value of a series (called a spreadsheet *range*) of cash flows. First, the cash flow values must be entered into consecutive cells in the spreadsheet. For example,

Cell Address:	A10	B10	C10	D10	E10	F10	G10
Value:	0	100	200	200	200	300	400

Then, the *@NPV* function is placed in an empty cell, say, A5:

@Function	@NPV($i, range$)
Cell formula	@NPV(0.10,A10.G10)
Cell display	868.30

Note that a spreadsheet's *@NPV* function assumes that cash flows occur at the end of each period, so the NPV is calculated as of the beginning of the period of the first cash flow specified in the range. Since we specified the Year 1 cash flow as the first flow in the range, the calculated NPV occurs at the beginning of Year 1 (or the end of Year 0), which is correct for this problem. However, many situations include a Year 0 cash flow, which means that the NPV would be calculated at the beginning of Year 0 (or the end of Year -1), which would be incorrect.

There are two solutions to the problem. One solution is to compound the calculated present value one period at 10 percent. The effect here is to move the PV one year to the right along the time line:

@Function   @NPV($i, range$ *including the Year 0 CF*)$*(1 + i)$

An alternative solution is to change the range in the @NPV function to force the first payment in the range to occur at Year 1, so the present value will be calculated at Year 0. However, since there is a Year 0 cash flow that must enter into the calculation, the Year 0 cash flow must be added to the spreadsheet-calculated NPV:

@Function   @NPV(*i, modified range without the Year 0 CF*) + *Year 0* Cell

Future value

The future value of an uneven cash flow stream (FVU_n, sometimes called the *terminal value*) is found by compounding each payment to the end of the stream and then summing the future values:

$$FVU_n = CF_1(1 + i)^{n-1} + C_2(1 + i)^{n-2} + \ldots + CF_n(1 - i)^{n-t}$$

$$= \sum_{t=1}^{n} CF_t(1 + i)^{n-t}. \tag{4.5}$$

Regular calculator solution:

We can simply find the future value of each individual cash flow using a regular calculator, and then sum these values to find the future value of the stream, $1,692.07:

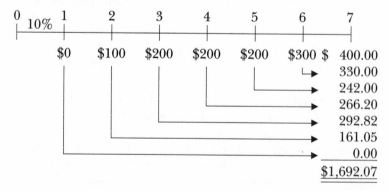

Financial calculator solution:

Some financial calculators have a net future value (NFV) key which, after the cash flows have been entered into the cash flow registers, can be used to obtain the future value of an uneven cash flow stream. However, we are generally more interested in the present value of a cash flow stream than in its future value, because the present value represents today's value, which can be compared to the cost of the asset, be it a stock, bond, or new group practice office.

Spreadsheet solution:

Most spreadsheet programs do not have a function that computes the future value of an uneven cash flow stream. However, future values can be found by building a formula in a cell that replicates the regular calculator solution.

Solving for the interest rate (i)

Although it is relatively easy to solve for i when the cash flows are lump sums or annuities, it is more difficult to solve for i when the present or future value is given and the cash flows are uneven. One can use a trial and error technique, in which various values of i are chosen until the correct one is found. Alternatively, a financial calculator's internal rate of return (IRR) function can be used when the present value is known. We will defer further discussion of this problem for now, but we will take it up later in Chapter 10, in our discussion of capital budgeting methods.

Self-Test Questions:

Give two examples of financial decisions that typically involve uneven cash flows.

What is meant by the term "net present value?"

What is meant by the term "terminal value?"

Semiannual and Other Compounding Periods

In all of our examples thus far, we have assumed that interest is compounded once a year, or annually. This is called *annual compounding.* Suppose, however, that Meridian Clinics puts $100 into a bank account that pays 6 percent annual interest, but compounded *semiannually.* How much would the clinic accumulate at the end of 1 year, 2 years, or some other period? Semiannual compounding means that interest is paid each six months, so interest is earned more often than under annual compounding.

To illustrate semiannual compounding, assume that the $100 is placed into the account for three years. The following situation occurs under annual compounding:

Time line:

$$FV_n = PV(1 + i)^n = \$100(1.06)^3.$$

Regular calculator solution:

Financial calculator solution:

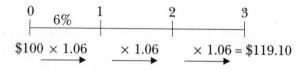

Inputs   3   6   −100

| n | i | PV | PMT | FV |

Output   = 119.10

Spreadsheet solution:

Cell formula   100*(1.06)^3
Cell display   119.10

Now consider what happens under *semiannual* compounding. Now, n = 2(3) = 6 semiannual periods, and i = 6/2 = 3% per semiannual period. Note that interest is always stated as an annual rate, for example, 6 percent (annual) interest, compounded semiannually. Here is the solution.

Time line:

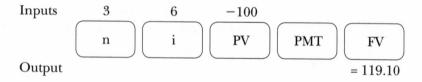

$$FV_n = PV(1 + i)^n = \$100(1.03)^6.$$

Regular calculator solution:

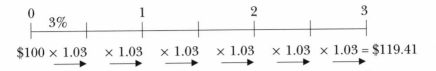

0   1   2   3

3%

$100 × 1.03   × 1.03   × 1.03   × 1.03   × 1.03   × 1.03 = $119.41

Financial calculator solution:

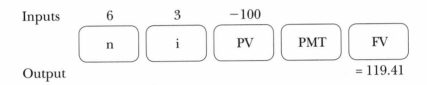

Inputs   6   3   −100

n   i   PV   PMT   FV

Output   = 119.41

Spreadsheet solution:

Cell formula   100*(1.03)^6
Cell display   119.41

We see that the $100 deposit grows to $119.41 under semiannual compounding, but only to $119.10 under annual compounding. This result occurs because interest on interest is being earned more frequently.

Throughout the economy, different compounding periods are used for different types of investments. For example, bank accounts often compound interest monthly or daily, most bonds pay interest semiannually, and stocks generally pay quarterly dividends.[5] Furthermore, the cash flows stemming from capital investments such as clinics and diagnostic equipment can be analyzed in monthly, quarterly, or annual periods, or even some other period. If we are to properly compare discounted cash flow analyses with different compounding periods, we need to put them on a common basis. This means that we must distinguish between the *stated* (sometimes called *nominal*) *interest rate* and the *effective annual rate.*

The stated interest rate in the Meridian Clinics semiannual compounding example is 6 percent. The effective annual rate is the rate that produces the same ending (future) value under annual compounding. In the example, the effective annual rate is the rate that would produce an account value of $119.41 at the end of Year 3 under annual compounding. The solution is 6.09 percent:

Inputs   3   −100   119.41

| n | i | PV | PMT | FV |

Output   = 6.09

Thus, if one bank offered to pay 6 percent interest with semiannual compounding on its savings accounts, while another offered 6.09 percent with annual compounding, they would both be paying the same effective annual rate because the ending value is the same under both sets of terms:

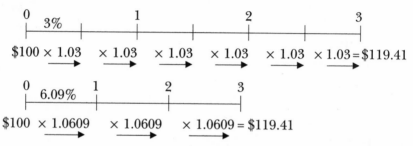

In general, we can determine the effective annual rate, given the stated rate and number of compounding periods per year, by solving Equation 4.6:

$$\text{Effective annual rate} = \left(1 + \frac{i_{Stated}}{m}\right)^m - 1.0. \tag{4.6}$$

Here i_{Stated} is the stated interest rate and m is the number of compounding periods per year. For example, the effective annual rate when the stated rate is 6 percent and semiannual compounding occurs is 6.09 percent:

$$\text{Effective annual rate} = \left(1 + \frac{0.06}{2}\right)^2 - 1.0.$$
$$= (1.03)^2 - 1.0$$
$$= 1.0609 - 1.0 = 0.0609 = 6.09\%.$$

We see that semiannual compounding, or for that matter, any compounding that occurs more than once a year, can be handled in two ways. First, the input variables can be expressed as periodic variables rather than annual variables. In the Meridian Clinics example, use n = 6 periods rather than n = 3 years and i = 3% per period rather than i = 6% per year. Second, find the effective annual rate by applying Equation 4.6, and then use this rate as an annual rate over the number of years. In the example, use i = 6.09% and n = 3 years.

The points made about semiannual compounding can be generalized as follows. When compounding periods are more frequent than once a year, we use a modified version of Equation 4.1 to find the future value of a lump sum:

$$\text{Annual compounding: } FV_n = PV(1 + i)^n. \tag{4.1}$$

$$\text{More frequent compounding: } FV_n = PV\left(1 + \frac{i_{Stated}}{m}\right)^{mn}. \tag{4.7}$$

Here m is the number of times per year compounding occurs, and n is the number of years. For example, when banks compute future values under daily interest, the value of m is set at 365 and Equation 4.7 is applied.

For another illustration, consider the interest rate charged on credit cards. Many banks charge 1.5 percent per month and, in their advertising, state that the annual percentage rate (APR) is 18.0 percent. However, the true cost rate to credit card users is the effective annual rate of 19.6 percent:[6]

$$\text{Effective annual rate } = (1.015)^{12} - 1.0 = 0.196 = 19.6\%.$$

Semiannual and other compounding periods can also be used for discounting, and for both lump sum cash flows and annuities. First, consider the case of an ordinary annuity of $100 per year for three years discounted at 8 percent compounded annually.

Time line:

```
0        1         2        3
|--8%----|---------|--------|
?      $100      $100     $100
```

Financial calculator solution:

Inputs	3	8		100	
	n	i	PV	PMT	FV
Output			= -257.71		

Spreadsheet solution:

@Function	@PV(PMT,i,n)
Cell formula	@PV(100,0.08,3)
Cell display	257.71

Now suppose the annuity calls for payments of $50 every six months for three years, and the interest rate is 8 percent compounded semiannually:

Time line:

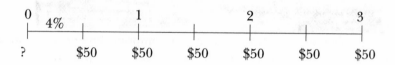

Financial calculator solution:

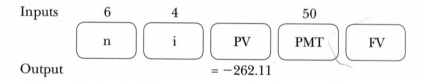

Spreadsheet solution:

Cell formula	@PV(PMT,i,n) = @PV(50,0.04,6)
Cell display	262.11

The semiannual payments come in a little earlier, so the $50 semiannual annuity is a little more valuable than the $100 annual annuity. Note, though, that an annuity with annual payments, but with semiannual compounding, cannot be treated in the same way. The discount rate period must match the annuity period, so if there are annual payments, then an annual discount rate must be used. Under semiannual compounding, the correct rate to apply to annual payments is not the stated rate, but rather the effective annual rate.

Self-Test Questions:

What changes must be made in your calculations to determine the future value of an amount being compounded at 8 percent semiannually versus one being compounded annually at 8 percent?

Why is semiannual compounding better than annual compounding from a saver's standpoint?

How does the effective annual rate differ from the stated rate?

Fractional Time Periods

In all of the examples used thus far in the chapter, we have assumed that payments occur at the beginning or the end of periods, but not *within* a period. However, we often encounter within-period situations. For example, Meridian Clinics might deposit $100 in a bank that pays 10 percent interest compounded annually, and leave it in the bank for nine months, or 0.75 years. How much would be in the account?

Time line:

```
0                    10%              1
├────────┼────────┼────────┼────────┤
-$100                                ?
```

$$FV_n = PV(1+k)^n.$$

Regular calculator solution:

$$FV_n = \$100(1.10)^{0.75} = \$100(1.0741) = \$107.41.$$

Financial calculator solution:

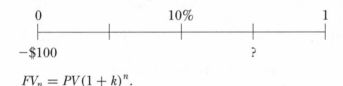

Inputs	0.75	10	−100		
	n	i	PV	PMT	FV
Output					= 107.41

Spreadsheet solution:

Cell formula	100*(1.10)^0.75
Cell display	107.41

Present values, annuities, and problems where you must find interest rates or numbers of periods with fractional time periods can all be handled with ease with a financial calculator or spreadsheet program.

Indeed, financial calculators and spreadsheet programs have calendar functions specifically designed to deal with fractional time periods. However, any further discussion is beyond the scope of this book.

Self-Test Question:

How are fractional time periods handled in discounted cash flow calculations?

Amortized, or Term, Loans

One important application of discounted cash flow analysis involves loans that are to be paid off in equal installments over time. Included are automobile loans, home mortgage loans, and most business debt other than very short-term loans and long-term bonds. If a loan is to be repaid in equal periodic amounts (monthly, quarterly, or annually), it is said to be an *amortized*, or *term, loan*. (The word *amortize* comes from the Latin *mors*, meaning *death*, so an amortized loan is one that is *killed off* over time.)

To illustrate, suppose Santa Fe Healthcare System borrows $1,000,000 from the Bank of New Mexico on a term loan to be repaid in three equal payments at the end of each of the next three years. The bank is to receive 6 percent interest on the loan balance that is outstanding at the beginning of each year. The first task is to determine the amount Santa Fe must repay each year, or the annual payment. To find this amount, recognize that the loan represents the present value of an annuity of PMT dollars per year for three years, discounted at 6 percent.

Time line:

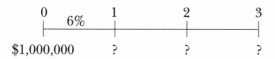

```
0        1        2        3
|  6%    |        |        |
$1,000,000    ?        ?        ?
```

Financial calculator solution:

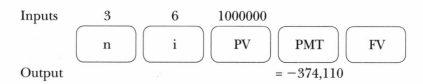

Inputs	3	6	1000000		
	n	i	PV	PMT	FV
Output				= −374,110	

Spreadsheet solution:

@Function	@PMT(PV,i,n)
Cell formula	@PMT(1000000,0.06,3)
Cell display	374,110

Therefore, if Santa Fe pays the bank $374,110 at the end of each of the next three years, then the percentage cost to the borrower, and the rate of return to the lender, will be 6 percent.

Each payment consists partly of interest and partly of repayment of principal. This breakdown is given in the *amortization schedule* shown in Table 4.1. The interest component is largest in the first year, and it declines as the outstanding balance of the loan is reduced over time. For tax purposes, a taxable business borrower reports as a deductible cost each year the interest payments in Column 3, while the lender reports these same amounts as taxable income.

Financial calculators are often programmed to calculate amortization schedules; you just key in the inputs, and then press one button to get each entry in Table 4.1.

Self-Test Questions:

When constructing an amortization schedule, how is the periodic payment amount calculated?

Do the principal and interest components stay at their initial levels over time? Explain.

Table 4.1 Loan Amortization Schedule at 6 Percent Rate

Year	Beginning Amount (1)	Payment (2)	Interest* (3)	Repayment of Principal† (2) − (3) = (4)	Remaining Balance (1) − (4) = (5)
1	$1,000,000	$ 374,110	$ 60,000	$ 314,110	$685,890
2	685,890	374,110	41,153	332,957	352,933
3	352,933	374,110	21,177	352,933	0
		$1,122,330	$122,330	$1,000,000	

* Interest is calculated by multiplying the loan balance at the beginning of the year by the interest rate. Therefore, interest in Year 1 is $1,000,000(0.06) = $60,000; in Year 2 it is $685,890(0.06) = $41,153; and in Year 3 it is $352,933(0.06) = $21,177.

† Repayment of principal is equal to the payment of $374,110 minus the interest charge for each year.

A Final Discussion of Interest Rate Types

Up to this point, we have covered many discounted cash flow concepts. Now it might be best to stop for a moment and review some points concerning the three types of interest rates.

Stated rate

This is the annual rate that is typically stated in financial contracts. Convention in the stock, bond, mortgage, commercial loan, consumer loan, and other markets calls for terms to be expressed in stated rates. So, if you talk with a banker, broker, or mortgage lender about rates, the stated rate will normally be quoted. However, to be meaningful, the stated rate must indicate the number of compounding periods per year. For example, a bank savings account might offer 10 percent interest compounded quarterly, or a money market mutual fund might offer a 12 percent rate, with interest paid monthly. You should *never* use the stated rate for calculations (that is, never use i_{Stated} on a time line or in your calculator) unless compounding occurs once a year ($m = 1$), in which case i_{Stated} = Periodic rate = Effective annual rate.

Periodic rate

This is the rate charged by a lender or paid by a borrower (or any other time value of money rate) expressed on a per period basis. It can be a rate per year, per six-month period, per quarter, per month, per day, or per any other time interval. For example, a bank might charge 1 percent per month on its credit card loans, or a finance company might charge 3 percent per quarter on consumer loans. Note that Periodic rate = i_{Stated}/m, which implies that i_{Stated} = (Periodic rate)(m), where m is the number of compounding periods per year. To illustrate, consider the finance company loan at 3 percent per quarter:

$$i_{Stated} = (\textit{Periodic rate})(m) = (3\%)(4) = 12\%,$$

and

$$\textit{Periodic rate} = i_{Stated}/m = 12\%/4 = 3\% \text{ per quarter.}$$

The periodic rate often is used when payments (or cash flows) occur more frequently than once a year, and the number of payments (or cash flows) per year corresponds to the number of compounding periods per year. Thus, if you are dealing with a retirement annuity that provides monthly payments, or with a semiannual payment bond, or with a consumer loan with quarterly payments, or with a credit card loan with monthly payments, then your calculations would use Periodic rate = i_{Stated}/m. Note that the implication in all of these examples is that the interest compounding period is the same as the payment (or cash flow) period. *The periodic rate can only be used directly in calculations when the cash flow period coincides with the interest rate compounding period—for example, quarterly payments and quarterly compounding.*

To illustrate use of the periodic rate, assume that you make eight quarterly payments of $100 into an account which pays 12 percent, compounded quarterly. What would you accumulate after two years?

Time line:

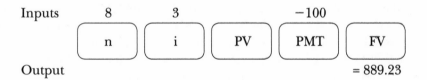

Financial calculator solution:

Inputs	8	3		−100	
	n	i	PV	PMT	FV
Output					= 889.23

Spreadsheet solution:

@Function	@FV(PMT,i,n)
Cell formula	@FV(100,0.03,8)
Cell display	889.23

Effective annual rate

This is the rate that, under annual compounding ($m = 1$), would produce the same results as a given stated rate with $m > 1$. The effective annual rate (*EAR*) is found as follows:

$$EAR = \left(1 + \frac{i_{Stated}}{m}\right)^m - 1.0.$$

In the *EAR* equation, i_{Stated}/m is the periodic rate and m is the number of periods per year. For example, suppose you could use either the 1 percent per month credit card loan or the 3 percent per quarter consumer loan to make a purchase. Which one should you choose? To answer this question, the cost rate of each alternative must be expressed as an *EAR*.

$$\text{Credit card loan: } EAR = (1+0.01)^{12} - 1.0 = (1.01)^{12} - 1.0$$
$$= 1.126825 - 1.0 = 0.126825 = 12.6825\%.$$

$$\text{Consumer loan: } EAR = (1+0.03)^{4} - 1.0 = (1.03)^{3} - 1.0$$
$$= 1.125509 - 1.0 = 0.125509 = 12.5509\%.$$

Thus, the consumer loan is slightly less costly than the credit card loan. This result should have been intuitive to you, because both loans have the same 12 percent stated rate, but you would have to make monthly payments on the credit card, while under the consumer loan terms you only would have to make quarterly payments.

The EAR is also used when the interest rate compounding period occurs more often than the period between payments or cash flows. For example, if payments occur semiannually, but interest is compounded quarterly, then the EAR must be used. Here, the EAR is really an "effective semiannual rate" calculated as $(1 + i_{Stated}/4)^2 - 1.0$, which is then applied to the semiannual payment stream. For example, assume that you make four semiannual payments of $100 into an account that pays 12 percent, compounded quarterly. What would you accumulate after two years?

Time line:

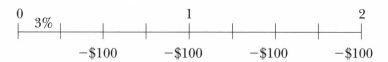

Now, you must calculate the *semiannual EAR* because, although the compounding is quarterly, the payments occur semiannually:

$$\text{Semiannual } EAR = (1 + 0.03)^{2} - 1.0 = (1.03)^{2} - 1.0$$
$$= 1.0609 - 1.0 = 0.0609 = 6.09\%.$$

Financial calculator solution:

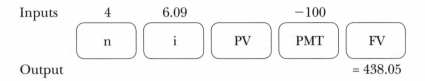

Inputs   4   6.09 -100

| n | i | PV | PMT | FV |

Output   = 438.05

Spreadsheet solution:

@Function	@FV(PMT,i,n)
Cell formula	@FV(100,0.0609,4)
Cell display	438.05

Note that the number of periods, n, must equal the number of payments when using the annuity formulas (and financial calculator PMT key). If the value for n that you are using in a calculation does not match the number of payments, then something is wrong!

Self-Test Questions:

Define the stated rate, the periodic rate, and the effective annual rate.

How are these three rates related?

Can you think of a situation where all three of these rates are the same?

Summary

Financial decisions often involve situations in which future cash flows must be valued. The process of valuing future cash flows is called *discounted cash flow analysis*, and the key concepts of this type of analysis are listed next:

- *Compounding* is the process of determining the *future value (FV)* of a lump sum cash flow or a series of payments.

- *Discounting* is the process of finding the *present value (PV)* of a future lump sum cash flow or series of payments.

- An *annuity* is a series of equal, periodic *payments (PMT)* for a specified number of periods.

- An annuity that has payments occurring at the end of each period is called an *ordinary* annuity.

- If each annuity payment occurs at the beginning of the period rather than at the end, the annuity is an *annuity due.*

- A *perpetuity* is an annuity that lasts forever.

- If the analysis involves more than one cash flow, but the cash flows do not constitute an annuity, the cash flows are called an *uneven cash flow stream.*

- The *stated rate* is the annual rate normally quoted in financial contracts.

- The *periodic rate* equals the stated rate divided by the number of compounding periods per year.

- If compounding occurs more frequently than once a year, it is often necessary to calculate the *effective annual rate*, which is that rate that produces the same results under annual compounding as compared with more frequent compounding.

- An *amortized* loan is one that is paid off in equal amounts over some specified number of periods. An *amortization schedule* shows how much of each payment represents interest, how much is used to reduce the principal, and the remaining balance on each payment date.

Notes

1. On some financial calculators, these keys are actually buttons on the face of the calculator; on others, they are shown on the display after accessing the time value of money menu. Also, some calculators use different symbols to represent the number of time periods and interest rate. For example, both lower and upper cases are used for n (N) and i (I), while other calculators use N/YR and I%/YR or similar variations. Finally, note that financial calculators today are quite powerful, in that they can directly solve relatively complex situations, such as when cash flows occur in between periods or when multiple cash flows occur in a single period. To focus on concepts rather than mechanics, all of the illustrations in this chapter and the remainder of the book assume that the cash flows occur at the end (or beginning) of a period, and that there is only one cash flow per period. Thus, to follow the illustrations, financial calculators must be set to one period per year, and it is not necessary to use the calendar function.
2. Since Lotus 1-2-3 created the early standard for spreadsheet programs, and since most other spreadsheet programs have the "look and feel" of Lotus, we will use Lotus conventions to illustrate spreadsheet discounted cash flow functions. We do not expect that most students will read this chapter in front of a personal computer and work our examples using a spreadsheet program. The primary purpose of including spreadsheet solutions in this chapter is to

acquaint you with the spreadsheet functions that you will be using in the future, either when working cases or on the job.

3. In constructing spreadsheets, you normally will want to create a formula that can accommodate changing inputs, so a more useful approach would be a formula like

$$+A1 * (1 + B1)^{\wedge}C1,$$

where the present value ($100) would be contained in Cell A1, the interest rate (5 percent) in Cell B1, and the number of periods (5) in Cell C1.

4. Since the cash flows in Years 3, 4, and 5 represent an annuity, the present value of the entire stream could be found by finding the PV of the ordinary annuity at Year 2 and then discounting this value, along with the lump sum values for Years 1, 2, 6, and 7, back to Year 0 and then summing. Indeed, there are numerous ways of organizing the cash flows to be discounted. These nuances, however, are of little real world value, because the actual present value calculation would be done with a calculator's cash flow registers or with a spreadsheet.

5. Some financial institutions even pay interest on accounts that is compounded *continuously*. However, continuous compounding generally is not relevant to health care financial management, so it will not be discussed here.

6. The *annual percentage rate (APR)* is the rate often used in bank loan advertisements, since it meets the minimum requirements contained in "truth in lending" laws. Typically, APR is defined as (Periodic rate) (Number of periods in one year). For example, the APR on a credit card with interest charges of 1.5 percent per month is 1.5%(12) = 18.0%. The APR understates the effective annual rate, so banks typically use APR when advertising loan rates. However, banks are quick to use the effective annual rate when advertising rates on savings accounts and certificates of deposit, because they want to make their rates look high.

Selected Additional References

Brigham, E. F., D. A. Aberwald, and L. C. Gapenski. 1992. *Finance with Lotus 1-2-3: Text and Models*. Fort Worth, TX: Dryden Press.

Gasteiger, D. 1988. *The Lotus Guide to @Functions* (Cambridge, MA: Lotus Publishing).

Owner's Manual for your calculator.

Reference Manual for your spreadsheet software.

Case 4

Empire State Clinics: Discounted Cash Flow Analysis

George Mitchell was born and raised in upstate New York. He obtained his bachelor's degree in business from Cornell University, where he enrolled in the NROTC program and, upon graduation, received a commission in the U.S. Marine Corps. After his release from active duty, George used his GI Bill benefits to obtain a master's degree in public administration from New York University with a concentration in health services management. His first job in health care was as a special projects coordinator/financial analyst at a large New York City hospital. He enjoyed his work there, but his ultimate goal was to become the manager of a smaller health care business, where he would have more responsibility and authority. After five years at the hospital, George became the chief operating officer of Empire State Clinics, an investor-owned chain of ambulatory surgery centers that has four locations in New York state's finger lakes region.

Immediately after assuming his new position, George faced several decisions. First, Empire State currently has $100,000 in its cash account, but the firm's target cash balance is only $50,000. Thus, George wants to temporarily invest the excess $50,000 in marketable securities, which typically consist of low-risk, short-term securities such as Treasury bills or money market mutual funds. One alternative that George is considering is to invest the $50,000 in a bank certificate of deposit (CD). CDs are generally available in maturities from six months to ten years, and interest can be handled in one of two ways: the investor (buyer) can receive interest payments every six months, or the interest can automatically be reinvested in the CD. In the latter case, the buyer receives no interest during the life of the CD, but receives the accumulated interest plus principal amount at maturity. Since George's goal is to accumulate funds for future use, all interest earned by Empire State would be reinvested in the CD.

Second, the firm recently bought a software package to handle its patient billings. However, it is obvious, even now, that the software will have to be replaced with a more sophisticated system in five years. After making some inquiries to software vendors, George estimates the future cost of the software to be $20,000. He does not want to count on the $50,000 current cash excess being available in five years, so to fund the future software purchase George is planning either to deposit a lump sum today in an interest-bearing account or to make annual payments of $2,000 into the same account.

Third, Empire State has some extra space in one of its clinics that it might lease out for five years. The initial renovation cost to add more electrical outlets and lighting to the space and to create an outside entrance is estimated to be $20,000. Because of some unusual terms in the proposed lease contract, and also due to the fact that Empire State promised to redecorate the office in three years, the net cash flows expected from the lease follow this uneven pattern:

End of Year	Net Cash Flow
1	$ 6,000
2	6,000
3	0
4	8,000
5	10,000

George's decisions all involve time value of money, or discounted cash flow (DCF) analysis. As a check on your skills, see if you can answer the following relevant questions.

Questions

1. Consider the $50,000 excess cash. Assume that George invests the funds in a one-year CD.

   a. What is the CD's value at maturity (future value) if it pays 10.0 percent (annual) interest?

   b. What would be its future value if the CD pays 5.0 percent interest? If it pays 15.0 percent interest?

c. The First National Bank of Rochester offers CDs with 10.0 percent nominal (stated) interest, but compounded semiannually. What is the effective annual rate on this CD? What would the future value be after one year if $50,000 is invested?

d. The Lakeside Branch of New York Trust Company offers a 10.0 percent CD with daily compounding. What is the CD's effective annual rate and its value at maturity one year from now if $50,000 is invested? (Assume a 365-day year.)

e. What nominal rate would the First National Bank have to offer to make its semiannually compounding CD competitive with New York Trust's daily compounding CD?

2. Rework Parts (a) through (d) of Question 1 assuming that each CD has a five-year maturity.

3. Now consider Empire State's goal of having $20,000 available in five years to buy new patient billing software.

a. What lump sum amount must be invested today in a CD paying 10.0 percent annual interest to accumulate the needed $20,000?

b. What annual interest rate is needed to produce $20,000 after five years if only $10,000 is invested?

c. What stated rate must the First National Bank, with semiannual compounding, offer in order to accumulate the required $20,000 when $10,000 is invested today?

4. Now consider the second alternative for accumulating funds to buy the new software—five annual payments of $2,000 each. Assume that the payments are made at the end of each year.

a. What type of annuity is this?

b. What is the present value of this annuity if the opportunity cost rate is 10.0 percent annually? Ten percent compounded semiannually?

c. What is the future value of this annuity if the payments are invested in an account paying 10.0 percent interest annually? Ten percent compounded semiannually?

d. What size annual payment would be needed to accumulate $20,000 under annual compounding at a 10.0 percent interest rate?

e. Suppose the payments are only $1,000 each, but they are made every six months, starting six months from now. What would be the future value if the ten payments were invested at 10.0 percent annual interest? If they were invested at the First National Bank at 10.0 percent, compounded semiannually?

5. Assume now that the payments are made at the beginning of each period. Repeat the analysis in Question 4.

6. Now consider the uneven cash flow stream stemming from the lease agreement that is given in the case.

   a. What is the present (Year 0) value of the lease payments if the opportunity cost rate is 10.0 percent annually?

   b. What is the value of this cash flow stream at the end of Year 5 if the cash flows are invested at 10.0 percent annually?

   c. Does the office renovation and subsequent lease agreement appear to be a good investment for Empire State? (Hint: Compare the cost of renovation with the present value of the lease payments. Use a 10 percent discount rate for the analysis.)

7. Now assume that it is five years later and Empire State was unable to accumulate the $20,000 needed to make the software purchase. Instead, the firm is forced to borrow the $20,000. The loan calls for repayment in equal annual installments over a four-year period, with the first payment due at the end of one year. Assuming that the firm can borrow the funds at a 10.0 percent rate, what amount of interest and principal will be repaid at the end of each year of the loan?

8. Throughout this case, you have been either discounting or compounding cash flows. Many financial analyses, such as bond refunding decisions, capital investment decisions, and lease decisions, involve discounting projected future cash flows. What factors must managers consider when choosing a discount rate to apply to forecasted cash flows?

5

Financial Risk

$\mathbf{O}$ne of the most important concepts in health care financial management is financial risk: what is it, how is it measured, and what impact does it have on managerial decisions? In all honesty, it would be great if we could just gloss over risk, and its related concept of return, and quickly move on to more applied topics such as capital budgeting and lease financing. Unfortunately, it is just not possible to gain a solid understanding of health care financial management without having a solid appreciation of financial risk, because risk assessment and incorporation are key elements in good decision making.

Introduction to Financial Risk

If investors—both individuals and businesses—viewed risk as a benign fact of life, there would be no problem. However, decision makers are, for the most part, averse to risk, believing that risk is to be avoided—and if it is to be taken on, that there must be some reward for doing so. Since risk is both dangerous and enticing because it usually promises higher returns, it is a basic part of financial decision making. Investments of higher risk, whether they be an individual investor's stock investment or an investment in diagnostic equipment by a radiology group, must offer higher returns to make the investment financially worthwhile. It is this characteristic of good financial decision making that makes financial risk such an important concept.

Two factors come into play that complicate any discussion of financial risk. First, financial risk is seen both by businesses and investors in those businesses. Some risk is inherent in the business itself depending on the nature of the business and its economic environment. For example, pharmaceutical firms face a great deal of risk, while hospitals are inherently less risky, because the research and development, production, and marketing of drugs is inherently more risky than the provision of health care services. The investors in any business (the stockholders and creditors) must bear the riskiness inherent in the business, but as modified by the nature of the securities they hold. For example, the stock of Beverly Enterprises is more risky than the debt of the firm, because contractual provisions place the claims of creditors above those of stockholders. Note, though, that the risk of both types of securities depends on the inherent risk of the nursing home business.

The second complicating factor results because the riskiness of any asset changes with the context in which the asset is held. For example, a stock held in isolation is riskier than a stock that is held as part of a large *portfolio* (collection) of stocks. Similarly, an MRI system that is operated independently is more risky than one that is operated by a large health care provider that operates numerous types of diagnostic equipment over a geographically dispersed area.

In this chapter, basic risk concepts are presented both from the standpoint of individual investors and that of businesses. It is necessary for managers to be familiar with both contexts because investors supply the capital that businesses need to function. But before beginning the discussion of financial risk, it is necessary to understand the concept of investment returns.

Self-Test Questions:

Why are risk concepts so important to financial decision making?

What factors complicate the discussion of financial risk?

Investment Returns

In most investments, an individual or a business spends money today with the expectation of receiving money in the future. To illustrate, suppose you buy ten shares of stock for $100. The stock pays no dividends, but at the end of one year, you sell the stock for $110. What is the return on your $100 investment? One way of expressing the return is in dollar terms. The *dollar return* is simply the total dollars received from the investment less the amount invested:

$$\text{Dollar return} = \text{Amount received} - \text{Amount invested}$$
$$= \$110 - \$100$$
$$= \$10.$$

If at the end of the year you sold the stock for only $90, your dollar return would be −$10.

Although expressing returns in dollars is simple to do, there are two problems. (1) To make a meaningful judgment about the adequacy of the return, you need to know the amount invested—a $10 return after one year on a $100 investment is a good return, while a $10 return on a $1,000 investment is a poor return. (2) You also need to know the timing of the return—a $10 return after one year on a $100 investment is a good return, while a $10 return after five years is a poor return.

The solution to the problem of interpreting dollar returns is to express investment returns as a *rate of return*, or *percentage return*. For example, the rate of return on the $100 stock investment, assuming the stock is sold for $110, is 10 percent:

$$\text{✳ Rate of return} = \frac{\text{Amount received} - \text{Amount invested}}{\text{Amount invested}}$$
$$= \frac{\$110 - \$100}{\$100} = \frac{\$10}{\$100}$$
$$= 0.10 = 10\%.$$

Rate of return "normalizes" the return by considering the return per unit of investment. In this example, the return of 0.10, or 10 percent, indicates that each dollar invested will earn 0.10($1.00) = $0.10, or ten cents on the dollar. A negative rate of return indicates that the original investment will not even be recovered. For example, selling the stock for only $90 results in a −10 percent rate of return, which means that only 90 cents of every dollar invested will be returned. Also, note that a $10 return on a $1,000 investment produces a rate of return of only 1 percent, so percentage rate of return takes into consideration the size of the investment.

Expressing rate of return on an annual basis also solves the timing (or holding period) problem. A $10 return after one year on a $100 investment produces a 10 percent annual rate of return, while a $10 return after five years only yields a 1.9 percent annual rate of return.

Self-Test Questions:

How are returns calculated?

Differentiate between dollar return and rate of return.

Why is rate of return superior to dollar return?

Introduction to Financial Risk

With the concept of financial return in mind, let us now turn our attention to financial risk. Risk is defined in most dictionaries as "a hazard; a peril; exposure to loss or injury." Thus, risk refers to the chance that some unfavorable event will occur. If you engage in skydiving, you are taking a chance with your life—skydiving is risky. If you gamble at roulette, you are not risking your life, but you are taking a financial risk. Even when you invest in stocks or bonds, you are taking a risk in the hope of earning a positive rate of return.

Consider your evaluation of two potential investments. The first investment consists of a $1,000 certificate of deposit (CD) offered by CitiBank that promises to pay $1,050 after one year. Your expected rate of return on the CD is ($1,050 − $1,000)/$1,000 = $50/$1,000 = 0.050 = 5.0%. Since the return is fixed by contract (the CD promises to pay this amount), and since CitiBank is certain to make the payment (the only exception would be a banking industry disaster, a very improbable event), there is virtually a 100 percent probability that your investment will actually earn the 5.0 percent return that you expect. In this situation, the investment is defined as being *riskless*, or *risk free*. (Note that the CD does have some purchasing power risk. Embedded in the 5.0 percent return is some inflation expectation, and if actual inflation exceeds expected inflation, the real, or inflation-adjusted, return will be less than expected. In many situations, however, purchasing power risk is not considered because it tends to affect all investments in a similar way.)

Now assume that your $1,000 is invested in a biotechnology partnership that will be terminated in one year. If the partnership develops a new commercially valuable drug, its rights will be sold and you will receive $2,100 from the partnership, for a rate of return of ($2,100 − $1,000)/$1,000 = $1,100/$1,000 = 1.100 = 110.0%. If nothing worthwhile is developed, the partnership will be worthless, so you will receive nothing, and your rate of return would be ($0 − $1,000)/$1,000 = −1.00 = −100%. Now assume that there is a 50 percent chance that a valuable product will be developed. In this admittedly unrealistic situation, your expected rate of return (in the statistical sense) is the same 5.0 percent as on the CD investment: 0.50(110.0%) + 0.50(−100.0%) = 5.0%. However, the biotechnology partnership is a far cry from being riskless. If things go poorly, your realized rate of return will be −100 percent—you will lose your entire $1,000 investment. Because there is a high probability of actually earning a return that is significantly less than you expect to earn, the partnership investment is described as being very risky.

Financial risk, then, is related to the probability of earning a return less than expected: the greater the chance of a return far less than expected (or even negative), the greater the amount of financial risk.

Self-Test Question:

Explain the concept of financial risk.

Risk Aversion

Why is it so important to define and measure financial risk? The reason is that both individual and business investors, for the most part, dislike risk. Suppose you were given the choice between a sure $1,000,000, and the flip of a coin for either $0 or $2,000,000. You, and just about everyone else, would "take the $1 million and run." Those people who take the sure $1,000,000 are said to be *risk averse*; a person who is indifferent between the two alternatives (views them as the same) is *risk neutral*; and an individual who prefers the gamble over the sure thing is a *risk seeker*.

Of course, people and businesses do gamble and take other chances, so all of us typically exhibit some risk-seeking behavior at one time or another. However, most individual investors would never put a sizable proportion of their net worth at risk, and most business executives would never "bet the business," because most people are risk averse when it really matters.

What are the implications of risk aversion for financial decision making? First, given two investments with similar returns but differing risk, most investors will favor the lower-risk alternative. Second, most investors will require higher returns to invest in higher-risk investments. These typical outcomes of risk-averse behavior have a significant impact on many facets of financial decision making, and hence these results will appear time and time again in later chapters.

Self-Test Questions:

What does the term "risk aversion" mean?

What are the implications of risk aversion for financial decision making?

Expected Rate of Return

We know now that financial risk is associated with returns less than those expected, but it is useful at this point to define the concept more precisely. Table 5.1 contains the estimated *returns distribution* developed by the financial staff of Crystal Beach Community Hospital for two proposed projects: an MRI system and a walk-in clinic. Here, the economic state reflects a combination of factors that affect each project's profitability. For example, for the MRI project, the very poor economic state signifies very low physician acceptance, and hence very low usage, very high discounts on reimbursements, very high operating costs, and so on. The economic states are defined in a similar fashion for the walk-in clinic project.

The *expected rate of return* on any investment, which we will designate as $\hat{k}$, is the weighted average of the return distribution, where the weights are the probabilities of occurrence. For example, the expected rate of return on the MRI system investment is 10.0 percent:

$$\hat{k}_{MRI} = \sum_{i=1}^{n} P_i k_i$$
$$= 0.10(-10\%) + 0.20(0\%) + 0.40(10\%)$$
$$+ 0.20(20\%) + 0.10(30\%)$$
$$= 10.0\%.$$

where P_i is the state's probability of occurrence, k_i is the return in that state, and n is the number of states. Calculated in a similar manner, the expected rate of return on the walk-in clinic investment is 15.0 percent.

The expected rate of return is the average return that would be realized if the situation were repeated many times. In our illustration, if 1,000 clinics were built in different areas, each of which faced the return distribution given in Table 5.1, the average return on the 1,000 investments would be 15.0 percent (assuming that the returns in each

Table 5.1   Estimated Returns for Two Proposed Investment Projects

Economic State	State's Probability of Occurrence	Rate of Return if State Occurs	
		MRI	*Clinic*
Very poor	0.10	−10%	−20%
Poor	0.20	0	0
Average	0.40	10	15
Good	0.20	20	30
Very good	0.10	30	50
	1.00		

area are independent). Of course, only one clinic would be built, and the realized rate of return may be less than the expected 15.0 percent, so the clinic investment (and the MRI investment) is risky.

Self-Test Questions:

How is the expected rate of return calculated?

What is the economic interpretation of expected rate of return?

Stand-Alone Risk

We can look at the two distributions in Table 5.1 and intuitively conclude that the clinic is more risky than the MRI system, because the clinic has a chance of a 20 percent loss while the worst possible loss on the MRI system is 10 percent. This intuitive risk assessment is based on the *stand-alone risk* of the two investments. That is, we are focusing on the riskiness of each investment under the assumption that the MRI system or the walk-in clinic would be the business's only asset (operated in isolation). In the next section, portfolio effects will be introduced, but for now, let us continue our discussion of stand-alone risk.

Stand-alone risk depends on the "tightness" of an investment's return distribution. If an investment has a tight return distribution, with returns falling close to the expected return, it has relatively low stand-alone risk. Conversely, an investment with a return distribution that is "loose," and hence has values well below the expected return, is relatively risky in the stand-alone sense. It is especially important to recognize that risk and return are two separate attributes of an investment. We might have a very tight distribution of returns, and hence a very low risk investment, but that investment might have an expected rate of return of only 2 percent. In this situation, the investment probably would not be financially attractive, in spite of its low risk. Conversely, a high-risk investment with a sufficiently high expected rate of return might be attractive.

To be truly useful, any definition of risk must have some measure, or numerical value, so we need some way to specify the "degree of tightness" of an investment's return distribution. One such measure is the *standard deviation*, which is often given the symbol "σ" (Greek lowercase sigma). Standard deviation is a common statistical measure of the dispersion of a distribution about its mean—the smaller the standard deviation, the tighter the distribution, and hence the lower the riskiness of the investment. To illustrate the calculation of standard deviation, consider the MRI project's estimated returns listed in Table 5.1. Here are the steps:

1. Calculate the expected rate of return, $\hat{k}$:

$$\hat{k} = \sum_{i=1}^{n} P_i k_i$$
$$= 0.10(-10\%) + 0.20(0\%) + 0.40(10\%)$$
$$+ 0.20(20\%) + 0.10(30\%)$$
$$= 10.0\%.$$

2. Calculate the *variance* of the rate of return distribution:

$$\text{Variance} = \sum_{i=1}^{n} P_i(k_i - \hat{k})^2$$
$$= 0.10(-10\% - 10\%)^2 + 0.20(0\% - 10\%)^2$$
$$+ 0.40(10\% - 10\%)^2 + 0.20(20\% - 10\%)^2$$
$$+ 0.10(30\% - 10\%)^2$$
$$= 120.00.$$

3. Finally, take the square root of the variance to obtain the standard deviation:

$$\text{Standard deviation} = \sigma = \sqrt{\text{Variance}}$$
$$= \sqrt{120.00} = 10.95\% \approx 11.0\%.$$

Using the same procedure, the clinic investment listed in Table 5.1 was found to have a standard deviation of returns of about 18 percent. Since the clinic investment's standard deviation of returns is larger than that of the MRI investment, the clinic investment has more stand-alone risk than the MRI investment.

As a general rule, investments with higher expected rates of return have larger standard deviations than investments with smaller expected returns. This situation occurs in our MRI and clinic example. In situations where expected rates of return on investments differ substantially, standard deviation may not give a good picture of one investment's stand-alone risk relative to another. The *coefficient of variation (CV)*, which is defined as the standard deviation of returns divided by the expected return, measures the risk per unit of return, and hence standardizes the measurement of stand-alone risk. To illustrate, the MRI investment has a CV of 1.10, while the clinic's CV is 1.20:

$$\text{Coefficient of variation} = CV = \frac{\sigma}{\hat{k}}.$$
$$\text{MRI:} \quad CV_{MRI} = 11.0\%/10.0\% = 1.10.$$
$$\text{Clinic:} \quad CV_{Clinic} = 18.0\%/15.0\% = 1.20.$$

In this situation, the clinic investment has slightly more risk per unit of return, so it is riskier than the MRI as measured by both standard deviation and coefficient of variation. However, note that the clinic's stand-alone risk as measured by the coefficient of variation is not as great relative to the MRI as it is when measured by standard deviation. This difference in relative risk occurs because the clinic has a higher expected rate of return. Finally, note that coefficient of variation has no units—it is just a raw number.

Self-Test Questions:

What is stand-alone risk?

What are some measures of stand-alone risk? σ , CV

Is one measure better than another?

Risk in a Portfolio Context

The preceding section developed two risk measures—standard deviation and coefficient of variation—that apply to investments held in isolation. However, most investments are not held in isolation, but rather are held as part of a *portfolio* of investments. Individual investors hold portfolios of securities, while businesses hold portfolios of projects (different product or service lines). When investments are held as part of portfolios, the primary concern of investors is not the realized rate of return on an individual investment, but rather the realized rate of return on the entire portfolio. Similarly, the riskiness of each individual asset is not as important to the investor as is the aggregate riskiness of the portfolio. The whole nature of risk and how it is defined and measured changes when we consider that investments are not held by themselves (in isolation), but rather as parts of portfolios.

Portfolio returns

To help illustrate the concept of portfolio risk and return, consider the returns estimated for the five investment alternatives listed in Table 5.2.

The individual investment alternatives (Investments A, B, and C) could be projects under consideration by South West Clinics, Inc., or they could be stocks that you are evaluating for personal investment purposes. The remaining two alternatives in Table 5.2 are portfolios: Portfolio AB consists of 50 percent invested in Investment A and 50 percent in Investment B (say, $10,000 invested in A and $10,000 invested in B), while Portfolio AC is an equal-weighted portfolio of Investments A and C. As shown in the bottom of the table, Investments A and B have 10 percent expected rates of return, while the expected rate of return for Investment C is 15 percent. Investments A and B have identical stand-alone risk as measured by standard deviation and coefficient of variation, while Investment C has higher stand-alone risk.

Turning to Portfolios AB and AC, the expected rate of return on a portfolio, $\hat{k}_p$, is simply the weighted average of the expected returns on the assets that make up the portfolio, with the weights being the proportion of the total portfolio invested in each asset:

$$\hat{k}_p = \sum_{i=1}^{n} w_i(\hat{k}_i).$$

Here, w_i is the proportion of each investment in the overall portfolio and $\hat{k}_i$ is the expected rate of return on each investment. Thus, the expected rate of return on Portfolio AB is 10 percent:

$$\hat{k}_{AB} = 0.5(10\%) + 0.5(10\%) = 10\%.$$

Table 5.2   Estimated Returns for Three Stand-Alone Investments and Two Portfolios

Economic State	State's Probability of Occurrence	Rate of Return if State Occurs				
		A	B	C	AB	AC
Very poor	0.10	−10%	30%	−25%	10%	−17.5%
Poor	0.20	0	20	−5	10	−2.5
Average	0.40	10	10	15	10	12.5
Good	0.20	20	0	35	10	27.5
Very good	0.10	30	−10	55	10	42.5
	1.00					
Expected rate of return		10.0%	10.0%	15.0%	10.0%	12.5%
Standard deviation		11.0%	11.0%	21.9%	0.0%	16.4%
Coefficient of variation		1.10	1.10	1.46	0.0	1.31

while the expected rate of return on Portfolio AC is 12.5 percent:

$$\hat{k}_{AC} = 0.5(10\%) + 0.5(15\%) = 12.5\%.$$

Alternatively, the expected rate of return on a portfolio can be calculated by looking at the portfolio's return distribution. For example, the return distribution for Portfolio AC contained in Table 5.2 produces the same 12.5 percent expected rate of return as calculated above:

$$\begin{aligned} \hat{k}_{AC} &= 0.10(-17.5\%) + 0.20(-2.5\%) + 0.40(12.5\%) \\ &\quad + 0.20(27.5\%) + 0.10(42.5\%) \\ &= 12.5\%. \end{aligned}$$

Of course, after the fact, the actual, or realized, returns on Investments A and C will probably be different from their expected values, and hence the realized rate of return on Portfolio AC will likely be different from the 12.5 percent expected return.

Portfolio risk

When an individual or a business holds a portfolio of assets rather than a single asset, the relevant return is the return on the portfolio, as opposed to the return on any component asset. Similarly, the relevant risk is the overall riskiness of the portfolio, as measured by its standard deviation or coefficient of variation, as opposed to the riskiness of any component asset.

As just demonstrated, the expected rate of return on a portfolio of investments is simply the weighted average of the expected returns on the individual investments in the portfolio. However, unlike returns, the riskiness of a portfolio is generally *not* a weighted average of the riskiness of the individual components of the portfolio; the portfolio's riskiness may be smaller than the weighted average of the component's riskiness. Indeed, the riskiness of a portfolio may be less than the least risky component, or, under certain conditions, a portfolio of risky assets may even be riskless.

A simple example will help make this point clear. Suppose you are given the opportunity to flip a coin once; if it comes up heads, you win $10,000, but if it comes up tails, you lose $8,000. This is a reasonable bet—the expected dollar return is 0.5($10,000) + 0.5(−$8,000) = $1,000. However, it is a highly risky proposition, because you have a 50 percent chance of losing $8,000. Thus, because of risk aversion, most people would refuse to make the bet, especially if the $8,000 potential loss would result in financial disaster. Alternatively, suppose you are given the opportunity to flip the coin 100 times, and you would win $100 for each head but lose $80 for each tail. It is possible, although extremely unlikely, that you would flip all heads and win $10,000, and it is also possible, and also extremely unlikely, that you would flip all tails and lose $8,000. But the chances are very high that you would actually flip about 50 heads and about 50 tails, on net winning about $1,000. Even if you flipped a few more tails than heads, you would still make money on the gamble.

Although each individual flip is a very risky bet in the stand-alone sense, collectively you have a low-risk proposition, because you have diversified away most of the risk. In effect, you have created a portfolio of investments; each flip of the coin can be thought of as one investment, so you have a 100-investment portfolio. Furthermore, the return on each investment is independent of the returns on the other investments: you have a 50 percent chance of winning on each flip of the coin regardless of the results of the previous flips. By combining the flips into a single gamble, that is, into an investment portfolio, you can reduce the risk associated with each individual bet. In fact, if the gamble consisted of a very large number of flips, you could totally eliminate the risk inherent in the gamble, because the probability of a near-equal number of heads and tails would be extremely high, and the result would be a sure profit. Of course, the key to the portfolio benefits in this example is that the negative consequences of tossing a tail can be offset by the positive consequences of tossing a head.

To look more closely at portfolio risk, consider Portfolio AB in Table 5.2. Each individual investment (A and B) is quite risky when held in isolation, but a portfolio of the two investments has a rate of return of 10 percent in every possible state of the economy, and hence it offers a riskless 10 percent return. (This result is verified by the values of zero for Portfolio AB's standard deviation and coefficient of variation of returns.) The reason Investments A and B can be combined to form a riskless portfolio is that their returns move exactly counter to one another—in economic states when A's returns are relatively low, those of B are relatively high, and vice versa. The fact that gains on one investment in the portfolio exactly offset losses in the other results in a riskless portfolio.

The movement relationship of two variables (the tendency to move either together or in opposition) is called *correlation*, and the *correlation coefficient*, *r*, measures this relationship. Investments A and B can be combined to form a riskless portfolio because the returns on A and

B are perfectly negatively correlated, which is designated by $r = -1.0$. In every state where Investment A has a return higher than its expected return, Investment B has a return lower than its expected return, and vice versa. The opposite of perfect negative correlation is perfect positive correlation, with $r = +1.0$. Returns on two perfectly positively correlated investments move up and down together as the economic state changes. When the returns on two investments are perfectly positively correlated, combining the investments into a portfolio will not lower risk—the riskiness of the portfolio is merely the weighted average of the risks of the two components.

To illustrate the impact of perfect positive correlation, consider Portfolio AC in Table 5.2. Here, the standard deviation of the portfolio is simply the weighted average standard deviation of its components:

$$Standard\ deviation_{AC} = \sigma_{AC} = 0.5(11.0\%) + 0.5(21.9\%)$$
$$= 16.4\%.$$

There is no risk reduction in this situation: forming a portfolio does nothing to reduce risk when the returns on the two assets are perfectly positively correlated.

Portfolios AB and AC demonstrate that when the returns on two investments are perfectly negatively correlated ($r = -1.0$), all risk can be eliminated by forming a portfolio, but when the returns on two investments are perfectly positively correlated ($r = +1.0$), forming a portfolio is of no value in reducing risk. The obvious questions at this point are (1) what is the correlation among the returns on "real world" investments? and (2) what happens to portfolio risk when more than two assets are combined?

It is difficult to generalize about the correlations among investment alternatives, but the correlations between two randomly selected investments—whether they be real assets in a hospital's portfolio of projects or financial assets in an individual's investment portfolio—are almost never -1.0 or $+1.0$. In fact, it is almost impossible to find actual investment opportunities with returns that are negatively correlated with one another, or even to find investments with returns that are uncorrelated, or independent, and hence have $r = 0.0$. Since all investment returns are affected to a greater or lesser degree by general economic conditions, investment returns tend to be positively correlated with one another. However, since investment returns are not affected identically by general economic conditions, returns on most real world investments are not perfectly positively correlated.

The correlation between the returns of two randomly chosen investments will usually fall in the range of +0.4 to +0.8. Returns on investments that are similar in nature, such as two inpatient projects in a hospital or two stocks in the same industry, will typically have return correlations at the upper end of this range, while the returns on dissimilar real or financial assets will tend to have correlations at the low end of the range.

What happens when a portfolio is created with two investments that have positive, but not perfectly positive, returns correlation? Some risk can be eliminated by combining the two investments, but not all risk can be eliminated. While the portfolio may be less risky than the lower-risk component, some risk will still remain.[1]

Of course, businesses are not restricted to two projects, and individual investors are not restricted to holding two-asset portfolios; most companies have tens, or even hundreds or thousands, of individual projects (products or service lines), and most individual investors hold many different securities, or perhaps mutual funds, which themselves may be composed of hundreds of individual securities. Thus, what is most relevant to financial decision making is not what happens when two investments are combined into portfolios, but rather what happens when many investments are combined.

To illustrate the risk impact of creating portfolios of two, three, four, or many more investments, consider Figure 5.1. The figure illustrates the riskiness inherent in holding randomly selected portfolios of one asset, two assets, three assets, four assets, and so on. The plot is based on historical annual returns on common stock traded on the New York Stock Exchange (NYSE), but the conclusions reached are applicable to portfolios made up of any type of investment, including health care providers that offer many different types of services.

The riskiness inherent in holding an average one-asset portfolio is relatively high, as measured by the standard deviation of annual returns. The average two-asset portfolio has a lower standard deviation, so it is less risky to hold an average two-asset portfolio than to hold a single asset of average risk. The average three-asset portfolio has a still lower standard deviation of returns, so an average three-asset portfolio is even less risky than an average two-asset portfolio. As more and more assets are randomly added to create larger and larger portfolios, the riskiness of the portfolios decreases. However, (1) as more and more assets are added, the incremental risk reduction of adding even more assets decreases, and (2) regardless of how many assets are added, some risk always remains

Figure 5.1   Portfolio Size and Risk

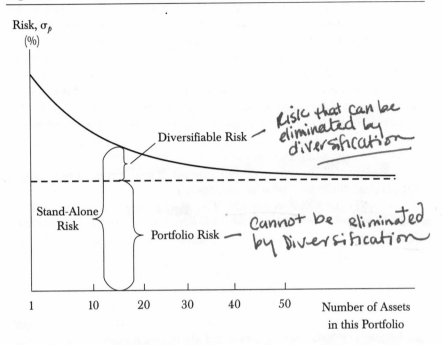

in the portfolio—even with a portfolio of thousands of assets, substantial risk remains.

The reason why all risk cannot be eliminated by creating a very large portfolio is because the returns on investment alternatives, although not perfectly so, are still positively correlated with one another. In other words, all investments, both real and financial, are affected to a lesser or greater degree by general economic conditions: if the economy booms, all investments tend to do well, while in a recession all investments tend to do poorly. Note that if there were zero correlation among investment returns, as in the multiple coin toss example, then a very large portfolio would be riskless (standard deviation of returns = 0%), or close to it. Since this is not the case, even very large portfolios are risky.

Diversifiable risk versus portfolio risk

Figure 5.1 shows that a large proportion of the stand-alone risk inherent in an investment can be eliminated if the asset is held as part of a large portfolio. For example, if a stock investor wanted to eliminate as much stand-alone risk inherent in owning NYSE stocks as possible, he or she would have to own about 2,000 stocks. Such a portfolio is called the *market portfolio,* because it consists of the entire stock market (or at least one entire segment of the stock market). Fortunately, it is not necessary for individual stock investors to own 2,000 stocks to gain the risk-reducing benefit inherent in holding portfolios. Most of the benefit can be obtained by holding about 50 randomly selected stocks. Such a large, randomly chosen portfolio is called a *well-diversified portfolio.* (A portfolio of, say, 50 health care stocks is not well diversified, because the stocks are in the same industry and hence are not randomly chosen.)

 That part of the stand-alone riskiness of an individual investment that can be eliminated by diversification (by holding a well-diversified portfolio) is called *diversifiable risk.* That part of the riskiness of an individual investment that cannot be eliminated by diversification is called *portfolio risk.* Thus, every investment, whether it be the stock of Beverly Enterprises held by an individual investor or an MRI system operated by a hospital, has some diversifiable risk that can be eliminated (by holding the asset as part of a well-diversified portfolio) and some portfolio risk that cannot be diversified away. Of course, some investments benefit more from portfolio risk-reducing effects than others but, in general, any investment will have some of its stand-alone risk eliminated by holding it as part of a well-diversified portfolio.

Diversifiable risk as seen by individuals investing in stocks is caused by events that are unique to a single firm, such as new product or service introductions, strikes, and lawsuits. Since these events are essentially random, their effects can be eliminated by diversification. When one stock in a portfolio does worse than expected because of a negative event unique to that firm, another stock in the portfolio will probably do better than expected due to a firm-unique positive event. On average, bad events will be offset by good events, so lower than expected returns will be offset by higher than expected returns, leaving the investor with an overall portfolio return closer to that expected than would be the case if only a single stock were held.

The same logic can be applied to a firm with a well-diversified portfolio of projects (products or services). Perhaps hospital returns generated from inpatient surgery are less than expected because of the trend toward outpatient procedures, but this might be offset by returns that are greater than expected on state-of-the-art diagnostic services. (Of course, if the hospital offered both inpatient and outpatient surgery, then it would be hedging itself against the trend toward more outpatient procedures because reduced demand for inpatient services would be offset by increased demand for outpatient services.)

The bottom line here is that the negative impact of random events that are unique to a particular firm, or to a particular product or service within a firm, can be offset by positive events in other firms, or in other products or services. Thus, the risk due to many random, unique events can be eliminated by portfolio diversification. Individual investors can diversify by holding many securities, and businesses can diversify by operating many projects. Unfortunately, not all risk can be diversified away. Portfolio risk, the risk that remains in diversified portfolios, stems from factors that systematically affect all stocks in a portfolio, such as wars, inflation, recessions, and high interest rates; or all goods or services produced by a business, such as with health care reform, which could lower reimbursement levels for all services offered by a hospital. Portfolio risk cannot be eliminated, so even well-diversified investors, whether they be individuals with large securities portfolios or diversified health companies with many different service lines, must deal with this type of risk.

Implications for investors

#6B

The ability of investors to eliminate some portion of the stand-alone riskiness inherent in individual investments has two significant implications for investors—especially individuals buying securities, but also businesses offering products and services.

1. It is not rational to hold a single investment. Much of the stand-alone riskiness inherent in individual investments can be eliminated by holding a well-diversified portfolio. Investors, who are risk averse, should seek to eliminate all diversifiable risk. Individual investors can easily diversify their personal investment portfolios either by buying many individual securities or by buying mutual funds that themselves hold diversified portfolios. Businesses cannot diversify their investments as easily as individuals, but businesses that offer a diverse line of products or services are less risky than businesses that rely on a single product or service.

2. Since the portfolio risk of an individual asset, and not its stand-alone risk, is the risk that "counts" to well-diversified investors, traditional stand-alone risk measures such as standard deviation and coefficient of variation of returns are not relevant to most individual and business

investors. Thus, it is necessary to rethink our definition and measurement of financial risk for individual assets.

Self-Test Questions:

What is a portfolio of assets? A well-diversified portfolio?

What happens to the risk of a single asset when it is held as part of a portfolio of assets?

Explain the differences between stand-alone risk, diversifiable risk, and portfolio risk.

What are the implications of portfolios for investors?

The Risk of Business Assets to
the Company: Corporate Risk

Firms typically offer a myriad of different products or services, and thus can be thought of as having a large number (hundreds or even thousands) of individual activities. For example, most HMOs offer health care services to a large number of diverse groups of enrollees in numerous service areas, and many hospitals and hospital systems offer a large number of inpatient, outpatient, and even home health services that cover a wide geographical area and treat a wide range of illnesses and injuries. Thus, health care managers operate a portfolio of individual products or services, called *projects*, so they manage a portfolio of projects. Furthermore, when investors buy the stock of a single company, they are really buying a portfolio of individual projects. So a well-diversified portfolio of 50 or more stocks is really a portfolio of tens of thousands of individual projects run by the companies whose stocks are held in the portfolio.

From this description, it is obvious that individual projects of a for-profit business actually reside in two different portfolios. First, a project is part of the firm's overall portfolio of projects. For example, the Women's Center at North Florida Regional Medical Center is one project of thousands that make up Columbia/HCA's portfolio of projects. Second, for stockholders, a project is one very small part of a well-diversified investment portfolio of securities. Investors who own Columbia/HCA stock own the Women's Center at North Florida Regional Medical Center along with thousands of other Columbia/HCA projects, plus tens of thousands of projects owned by other companies in their stock portfolios.

Thus, the portfolio riskiness of a business project depends on one's perspective. A health care manager sees project riskiness from the standpoint of the business's portfolio of projects, while a stock investor sees the riskiness inherent in holding the project as part of a well-diversified stock portfolio. Since the context is different for each portfolio, the riskiness of a given project is also different. In this section, the riskiness of business assets to the company is discussed. In the next section, the riskiness of business assets to stockholders is covered.

For now, put your manager's hat on. What is the riskiness of a project to the business? Since the project is part of the business's portfolio of assets, its stand-alone risk is not relevant because the project is not held in isolation. The relevant risk of any project to the business is its contribution to the business's overall risk, or the impact of the project on the variability of the firm's overall rate of return. Some of the stand-alone riskiness of the project will be diversified away by combining the project with the firm's other projects. The remaining risk, which focuses on the firm's portfolio of projects, is called *corporate risk*.

To illustrate corporate risk, assume that Project P represents the expansion into a new service area by AtlantiCare, a for-profit HMO with many existing projects. Table 5.3 contains the estimated rate of return distributions both for Project P and for AtlantiCare as a whole.[2] AtlantiCare's rate of return, like that of Project P, is uncertain and depends on future economic events. Overall, AtlantiCare's expected rate of return is 7.0 percent, with a standard deviation of 2.0 percent and a coefficient of variation of 0.3. Thus, looking at either the standard deviation or the coefficient of variation (stand-alone risk measures), Project P is riskier than the HMO in the aggregate; that is, Project P is riskier than AtlantiCare's *average project.*

However, the relevant risk of Project P is not its stand-alone risk, but rather its contribution to AtlantiCare's overall riskiness. Project P's corporate risk depends not only on its standard deviation of returns, but also on the correlation between the returns on Project P and the returns on the HMO's average project (AtlantiCare's rate of return distribution). If Project P's returns were negatively correlated with the returns on AtlantiCare's other projects (which they are not), then accepting it would reduce the riskiness of the HMO's aggregate returns; and the larger Project P's standard deviation, the greater the risk reduction. (An economic state resulting in a low return on AtlantiCare's average project would produce a high return on Project P, and vice versa, so the returns would offset one another and AtlantiCare's overall risk would be reduced.) In this situation, Project P would actually have negative risk relative to the HMO's average project, in spite of its high stand-alone risk. In actuality, however, Project P's returns are positively

Table 5.3   Estimated Return Distributions for Project P and
AtlantiCare

| | Probability of | Rate of Return | |
State of Economy	Occurrence	Project P	AtlantiCare
Very poor	0.05	2.5%	1.0%
Poor	0.20	5.0	6.0
Average	0.50	10.0	7.0
Good	0.20	15.0	8.0
Very good	0.05	17.5	13.0
Expected return		10.0%	7.0%
Standard deviation		4.0%	2.0%
Coefficient of variation		0.4	0.3
Correlation coefficient		0.80	

correlated with AtlantiCare's aggregate returns, and the project has twice the standard deviation, so accepting it would increase the risk of AtlantiCare's aggregate returns.

The quantitative measure of corporate risk is a project's *corporate beta,* or *corporate b,* which is the slope of the regression (scatter plot) line that results when the project's returns are plotted on the Y axis and the returns on the firm's average project are plotted on the X axis. Figure 5.2 contains this regression line, which is often called the *corporate characteristic line,* for Project P.

The slope (rise over run) of Project P's corporate characteristic line, which is Project P's corporate beta coefficient, is about 1.60, and it can be found algebraically as follows:

$$\text{Corporate } b_P = (\sigma_P/\sigma_F)r_{PF},$$

where

σ_P = standard deviation of Project P's returns,

σ_F = standard deviation of the firm's returns, and

r_{PF} = correlation coefficient between the returns on Project P and the firm's returns.

Thus,

$$\text{Corporate } b_P = (4.0\%/2.0\%)0.80 = 1.60.$$

A project's corporate beta measures the volatility of returns on the project relative to the firm as a whole (or relative to the firm's

Figure 5.2   Corporate Characteristic Line for Project P

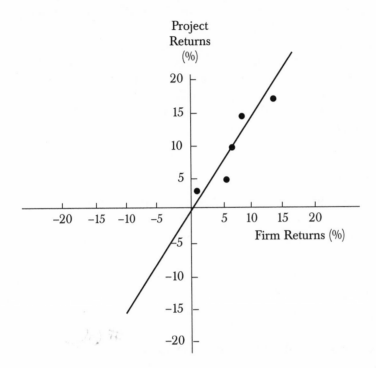

average project), which has a corporate beta of 1.0. (To estimate the corporate beta of the firm's average project, the firm's aggregate returns are plotted on both the X and Y axes, so the resulting slope of the corporate characteristic line is 1.0.)

If a project's corporate beta is 2.0, its returns are twice as volatile as the firm's returns; thus, adding such a project to the firm would increase the overall volatility of the firm's returns, and hence increase the riskiness of the business. A corporate beta of 1.0 indicates that the project's returns have the same volatility as the firm; and hence taking on the project would add identical risk to the firm's existing assets. A corporate beta of 0.5 indicates that the project's returns are less volatile than the firm's returns, so taking on the project would lower the overall risk of the firm. A negative corporate beta, which results when a project's returns are negatively correlated with the firm's returns, indicates that the returns on the project move counter-cyclical to the returns of the firm. The addition of such a project to the firm's portfolio of projects could reduce a firm's riskiness by a large amount, but such projects are very hard to find because most projects are in a single line of business, or in similar lines; their returns, therefore, are highly positively correlated.

With a corporate beta of 1.6, the returns on Project P are 1.6 times as volatile as the returns on AtlantiCare's average project. Economic events that would result in a return 10 percent less than expected on the HMO as a whole would produce a 16 percent less-than-expected return on Project P. Thus, adding project P to AtlantiCare's portfolio of projects would increase the risk of the HMO, and hence Project P would be judged to have more corporate risk than AtlantiCare's average project.

Self-Test Questions:

A business project in a for-profit firm is held as part of what two portfolios?

What is the riskiness of a project when held as part of a portfolio of projects?

What is a corporate beta? How is it calculated? Write out and explain the equation for corporate beta.

How are corporate betas interpreted?

The Risk of Business Assets to Stockholders: Market Risk

The last section discussed the riskiness of projects to a business. This section discusses the riskiness of business projects to stock investors. Why should a health care manager be concerned about how investors view risk? The answer is simple: stock investors are the suppliers of equity capital to investor-owned businesses, so they set the rates of return that such businesses must pay to raise equity capital. These rates, in turn, set the minimum profitability that investor-owned businesses must earn on the equity portion of their real asset investments. Even managers of not-for-profit firms should have an understanding of how stock investors view risk because market-set required rates of return also establish the opportunity costs inherent in making not-for-profit investments. (We will have much more to say about this in Chapter 8.)

The market risk of individual projects

Since stock investors hold well-diversified portfolios of stocks, the relevant riskiness of an individual project undertaken by a company in the portfolio is its contribution to the riskiness of a well-diversified stock portfolio. Thus, the riskiness of the Women's Center at North Florida Regional Medical Center to an individual investor who has a portfolio of 50 stocks, or to a trust officer managing a 150-stock portfolio, or to a 500-stock mutual fund owner is the contribution that the project makes to the riskiness of the overall stock portfolio. Some of the stand-alone riskiness of the project will be diversified away by combining the project with all the other projects in the stock portfolio. The remaining risk, which is portfolio risk, is called *market risk,* and it is defined as the contribution of a project to the riskiness of a well-diversified stock portfolio.

How should a project's market risk be measured? A project's *market beta,* or *market b,* measures the volatility of the project's returns relative to the returns on a well-diversified portfolio of stocks. Table 5.4 contains hypothetical estimates of the rate of return on a well-diversified portfolio of stocks, commonly called the *market portfolio,* or just *the market,* along with the returns on AtlantiCare's Project P. In practice, some stock index, say, the S&P 500 Index or the NYSE Index, is used as a proxy for the market portfolio. (The Standard & Poor's 500 is an index made up of 500 stocks across many industries, while the New York Stock Exchange Index is made up of the roughly 2,000 common stocks listed on the NYSE.)

The market beta of Project P is found by constructing the *market characteristic line* for the project, which is the regression (scatter plot) line that results from plotting the returns on Project P against the returns on the market. Project P's market characteristic line, which is shown in Figure 5.3, has a slope of 0.33, and hence Project P's market beta is 0.33.

Table 5.4   Estimated Return Distributions for Project P and the Market

State of the Economy	Probability of Occurrence	Rate of Return	
		Project P	The Market
Very poor	0.05	2.5%	−15.0%
Poor	0.20	5.0	5.0
Average	0.50	10.0	15.0
Good	0.20	15.0	25.0
Very good	0.05	17.5	45.0
Expected return		10.0%	15.0%
Standard deviation		4.0%	11.4%
Coefficient of variation		0.4	0.8
Correlation coefficient		0.94	

Figure 5.3   Market Charactersitc Line for Project P

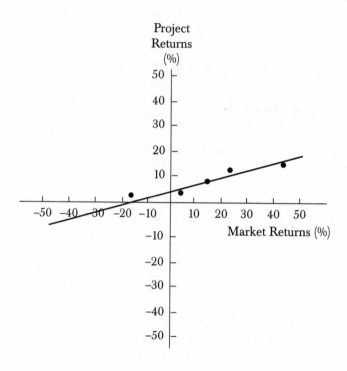

Note that Project P's market beta, *Market b_P*, can be calculated as follows:

$$Market\ b_P = (\sigma_P/\sigma_M)r_{PM},$$

where

> σ_P = standard deviation of Project P's returns,
>
> σ_M = standard deviation of the market's returns, and
>
> r_{PM} = correlation coefficient of returns between Project P and the market.

Thus, using the data from Table 5.4,

$$Market\ b_P = (4.0\%/11.4\%)0.94 = 0.33.$$

Project P's market beta measures its market risk, which is the risk relevant to AtlantiCare's well-diversified shareholders. Intuitively, a project's market beta measures the volatility of the project's returns relative to the returns on a well-diversified portfolio of stocks (the market portfolio), which has a beta of 1.0.

A project with a market beta of 2.0 has returns that are twice as volatile as the returns on the market, and adding it to a well-diversified portfolio will increase the portfolio's risk. A market beta of 1.0 indicates that the project's returns have the same volatility as the market; adding such a project would have no impact on the riskiness of the market portfolio. A market beta of 0.5 indicates that the project's returns are half as volatile as the returns on the market, and so adding such a project to a well-diversified portfolio would reduce its risk.

With a market beta of 0.33, Project P has only one-third the riskiness inherent in the market portfolio. If general economic conditions resulted in a return on the market portfolio that was 10 percent less than expected, the return on Project P would be only 3.3 percent less than expected. Thus, Project P has below-average market risk.

Since AtlantiCare's stockholders are assumed to hold well-diversified portfolios (with a beta of 1.0), the HMO's acceptance of Project P would reduce the riskiness of shareholder portfolios. (As you will see shortly, the beta of a portfolio is merely the weighted average of the betas of the individual components of the portfolio. Thus, adding a component with a lower beta than the portfolio average lowers the beta of the portfolio, and hence lowers the riskiness of the portfolio.)

Note that a negative market beta, which results when a project's returns are negatively correlated with the market's returns, indicates that the returns on the project move counter-cyclically to the returns on the market: when the market's return goes up, the project's return goes down, and vice versa. Negative beta projects are valuable to stockholders because of their risk reduction characteristics. However, negative market beta projects are rare since most projects' returns, as well as the market's returns, are positively correlated with the economy as a whole.

The market risk of firms

Even though an individual investor's stock portfolio can be thought of as a portfolio of many separate projects, the portfolio actually consists of the stocks of firms, so individual investors are most concerned with the risk and return characteristics of the companies themselves. Thus, individual investors are concerned with the company's, or stock's, market beta rather than the market betas of individual projects. A stock's market beta is the slope of the market characteristic line formed by regressing the firm's aggregate returns against the market's returns. For example, using the data in Tables 5.3 and 5.4, we find AtlantiCare's market beta to be 0.17. Since the average stock has a market beta of 1.0, AtlantiCare's market beta is very low, and adding the stock of AtlantiCare to a well-diversified portfolio would tend to lower the overall riskiness of the portfolio.

When individual investors assess the riskiness of individual stocks, the relevant measure is the stock's market beta, and the reference value is the market portfolio's overall beta of 1.0. When investor-owned firms conduct project market risk analyses, the question that is relevant to managers is how does the project's market risk compare to the market risk of the firm's average project? This question is answered by comparing the project's market beta to the firm's market beta. Our illustrative Project P, with a market beta of 0.33, has significantly more market risk than AtlantiCare's average project, which has a market beta of only 0.17.

Portfolio betas

Individual investors hold portfolios of stocks, each with its own market risk as measured by the stock's market beta coefficient, while businesses hold portfolios of projects, each with its own corporate and market betas. What impact does the beta of a portfolio component have on the overall portfolio's beta? The beta of any portfolio of investments is simply the weighted average of the individual investments' betas:

$$b_p = \sum_{i-1}^{n} w_i b_i.$$

Here, b_p is the beta of the portfolio, which measures the volatility of the entire portfolio, w_i is the fraction of the portfolio invested in one particular asset, and b_i is the beta coefficient of that asset.

To illustrate, Columbia/HCA Healthcare might have a market beta of 1.2, indicating that the returns on its stock are slightly more volatile that the returns on a well-diversified portfolio (with a beta of 1.0), and hence the stock is somewhat riskier than the average stock. But each project within Columbia/HCA Healthcare has its own market risk, as measured by each project's market beta. Some projects may have very high market betas, say, over 1.5, while other projects may have very low market betas, say, under 0.5. When all of the projects are combined, the overall market beta of the company is 1.2. For ease of discussion, assume that Columbia/HCA Healthcare has only the following three projects:

Project	Market Beta	Dollar Investment	Proportion
A	0.5	$ 15,000	15.0%
B	1.0	30,000	30.0
C	1.5	55,000	55.0
		$100,000	100.0%

The weighted average of the project market betas, which is the firm's market beta, is 1.2:

$$b_p = \sum_{i-1}^{n} w_i b_i.$$

$$= 0.15(0.5) + 0.30(1.0) + 0.55(1.5)$$

$$= 1.20.$$

Note that each project within Columbia/HCA Healthcare's fictitious portfolio of three projects also has a corporate beta that measures the volatility of the project's returns relative to that of the corporation as a whole. The weighted average of these project corporate betas must equal 1.00, which is the corporate beta of any business.

Self-Test Questions:

What is the relevant risk of a project to a stockholder?

What is a market beta, and how is it measured?

What is the difference between a project's market beta and the firm's market beta?

How is the beta of a portfolio related to the individual betas of the assets in the portfolio?

Relevance of the Three Risk Measures

Thus far, the chapter has discussed in some detail three measures of financial risk—stand-alone, corporate, and market—but it is still unclear which risk is the most relevant in financial decision making. It turns out that the risk that is relevant to any financial decision depends on the particular situation at hand. When the decision involves a single investment that will be held in isolation, stand-alone risk is the relevant risk. Here, the risk and return on the portfolio is the same as the risk and return on the single asset in the portfolio. In this situation, the riskiness faced by the investor, whether it be an individual considering a stock purchase or a business considering an MRI system investment, is defined in terms of returns less than expected, and the appropriate measure is the standard deviation or coefficient of variation of the return distribution.

In most investment decisions, however, the asset under consideration will not be held in isolation, but rather will be held as part of an investment portfolio. Individual investors normally hold portfolios of stocks, while businesses normally hold portfolios of real asset investments (projects). For individual investors holding stock portfolios, the most relevant risk is the asset's contribution to the overall riskiness of a well-diversified stock portfolio. This risk, which is called market risk, is measured by the asset's market beta.

For businesses, the most relevant risk depends on whether the business is for-profit or not-for-profit. For investor-owned businesses, the goal is shareholder wealth maximization, so risk must be measured in shareholder terms. Since stockholders tend to hold large portfolios of securities, and hence a very large portfolio of individual projects, the most relevant risk of a project under consideration by a for-profit firm is its contribution to a well-diversified stock portfolio (the market portfolio). Of course, this is the project's market risk.

Not-for-profit firms do not have stockholders, and their goals stem from a mission statement that generally involves service to society. In this situation, market risk is not relevant; the concern to managers is the impact of the project on the riskiness of the business, and this is measured by a project's corporate risk. Thus, the risk measure most relevant to projects in not-for-profit firms is a project's corporate beta.

Self-Test Question:

Explain the situations in which stand-alone, corporate, and market risk are the most relevant.

Interpretation of the Risk Measures

In closing this chapter, it is important to recognize that none of the risk measures discussed can be interpreted without some standard of reference. For example, if we are focusing on stand-alone risk, does

Project P's coefficient of variation of returns of 0.4 indicate high risk, low risk, or moderate risk? We don't know the answer without more information. However, knowing that AtlantiCare in the aggregate has a coefficient of variation of returns of 0.3 enables us to state that Project P has more stand-alone risk than the firm's average project.

Similarly, Project P's corporate beta of 1.6, when compared to AtlantiCare's overall corporate beta of 1.0 (by definition), indicates that the project has above-average corporate risk. Similarly, Project P's market beta of 0.33, when compared to AtlantiCare's market beta of 0.17, indicates that the project has above-average market risk. The point to remember is that in practice risk is always interpreted against some standard, for without a standard it is impossible to make judgments.

Which risk is most relevant to AtlantiCare? As discussed in the previous section, market risk is most relevant because AtlantiCare in an investor-owned business, and hence managers should be most concerned about the impact of new projects on stockholders' risk.

Self-Test Question:

How are risk measures interpreted?

Summary

This chapter has covered the very important concept of financial risk. Here is a summary of the key concepts:

- Risk definition and measurement is very important to financial decision making because people, in general, are *risk averse*, and hence require higher returns from investments having higher risk.

- *Financial risk* is associated with the prospect of returns less than the expected return. The higher the probability of a return being far less than expected, the greater the risk.

- The riskiness of investments held in isolation, called *stand-alone risk*, can be measured by the dispersion of the rate of return distribution about its expected value. The two most commonly used measures of stand-alone risk are the *standard deviation* and *coefficient of variation* of the return distribution.

- Most investments are not held in isolation, but rather as part of investment *portfolios*. Individual investors hold portfolios of securities and businesses hold portfolios of projects (products and services).

- When investments with returns that are less than perfectly positively correlated are combined, it may be possible to create a portfolio that is less risky than its components. The risk reduction occurs because the less than expected returns on some investments are offset by greater than expected returns on other investments. However, among real-world investments, it is impossible to eliminate all risk, because the returns on all assets are influenced to a greater or lesser degree by changes in overall economic conditions.

- That portion of the stand-alone risk of an investment that can be eliminated by holding the investment in a well-diversified portfolio is called *diversifiable risk*, while the risk that remains is called *portfolio risk*.

- There are two different types of portfolio risk. *Corporate risk* is the riskiness of business projects when they are considered as part of a business's portfolio of projects. *Market risk* is the riskiness of business projects (or of the stocks of entire businesses) when they are considered as part of an individual investor's well-diversified portfolio of securities.

- Corporate risk is measured by a project's *corporate beta*, which reflects the volatility of the project's returns relative to the returns of the aggregate business. The corporate risk of a project under consideration is a function of the project's standard deviation of returns, the standard deviation of returns on the business as a whole, and the correlation between the returns on the project and the returns on the business.

- Market risk is measured by a project's (or stock's) *market beta*, which reflects the volatility of a project's (or stock's) returns relative to the returns on a well-diversified portfolio of securities. The market risk of a project (or stock) under consideration is a function of the project's (or stock's) standard deviation of returns, the standard deviation of returns on a well-diversified portfolio of securities, and the correlation between the returns on the project (or stock) and the returns on the security portfolio.

- *Stand-alone risk* is most relevant to all investments held in isolation; *corporate risk* is most relevant to projects held by not-for-profit firms; and *market risk* is most relevant to projects held by investor-owned firms.

- The *overall beta coefficient of a portfolio* is the weighted average of the betas of the components of the portfolio, where the weights are the proportion of the overall investment in each component. Thus, the weighted average of corporate betas of all projects in a business must equal one, while the weighted average of all projects' market betas must equal the market beta of the firm's stock.

The risk concepts covered in this chapter will be used over and over throughout the book because defining and measuring risk is critical to making good financial decisions. Specifically, the risk concepts developed here will be used in Chapter 7, when setting required rates of return on stock investments, and in Chapter 11, when setting required rates of return on individual projects.

Notes

1. To be precise, a portfolio of two assets will have less risk than the lower-risk asset only when the correlation coefficient between the assets is less than the ratio of the asset's standard deviations, where the ratio is constructed with the lower standard deviation in the numerator. For example, for Portfolio AC in Table 5.2 to have less risk than either A or C, the correlation coefficient must be less than $\sigma_A/\sigma_C = 11.0\%/21.9\% = 0.50$.
2. The rates of return listed in Table 5.3 can be defined in several different ways. For our purposes here, it is not necessary to specify the exact nature of the rates of return. In later chapters, for instance, when we discuss capital budgeting analysis, we will provide specific rate of return definitions.

Selected Additional Reference

Brigham, E. F., and L. C. Gapenski. 1996. *Intermediate Financial Management,* Chapters 2 and 3. Fort Worth, TX: Dryden Press.

Case 5

University Physicians, Inc.

Financial Risk

University Physicians, Inc. (UP) is a not-for-profit corporation formed by physicians in the College of Medicine at Pacific Northwest University. UP, with over 400 physicians, provides the medical staff for University Hospital. In addition, UP staffs and administers a network of 25 ambulatory care clinics and centers at ten locations spread over most of northwest Oregon. In 1996, UP generated over $200 million in revenues from about 25,000 inpatient stays and 500,000 outpatient visits.

Over 70 percent of UP's revenues currently comes from inpatients, but this percentage has been declining, and by the year 2000 over half of UP's revenues are expected to stem from outpatient services. As improvements are made in technology and payers continue to pressure providers to cut costs, more and more inpatient services will revert to outpatient and home care. For example, in 1986, 80 percent of UP's ophthalmological surgeries took place in University Hospital, while in 1996, 80 percent were conducted in outpatient settings.

While UP has traditionally provided only specialty services, in 1990 it instituted a "personal physician services" program, whereby patients could receive both primary and specialty care from College of Medicine physicians. This was but the first step in UP's drive to develop an integrated delivery system offering a full range of patient services. Now that the system is in place, UP is contracting with managed care plans to provide virtually all medical services required by plan members. Furthermore, UP is examining the feasibility of contracting directly with employers, and hence bypassing managed care plans; but no decision has yet been made. Indeed, considerable opposition was expressed by various state insurance industry representatives when UP first announced the possibility of direct contracting. The insurance industry position is that direct contracting with employers to provide a complete health care benefit package is an insurance function, to be undertaken only by licensed insurance plans.

As part of its continuing education program, UP holds monthly "nonclinical grand rounds" for its physicians in which various staff members and outside specialists conduct seminars on nonclinical topics of interest. As part of this series, Brenda Cowan, UP's chief financial officer, has been invited to conduct two sessions on the financial risk inherent in integrated delivery systems. Her main concern is that physicians, although very sophisticated in clinical matters, have a very limited understanding of basic financial risk concepts, and will not appreciate the financial issues involved in integrated delivery systems without first gaining an understanding of basic risk concepts. Thus, she plans to devote the entire first session to basic risk concepts.

As preparation for the seminar, Cowan developed the return distributions for the five investments shown in Table 1. First, she hypothesized that there could be five possible economic states for the coming year, ranging from poor to excellent. Next, she estimated the one-year returns on each investment under each state. The five investments are T-bills; two real asset investment projects, A and B; an index fund designed to proxy the returns on the S&P 500 stocks; and an equity investment in University Physicians itself. T-bills are short-term (one-year or less maturity) U.S. Treasury instruments; Project A is a proposed sports medicine clinic; and Project B is a Medicaid-funded project for providing family health services to an underserved area in Portland. Note that Cowan developed the returns for Projects A and B and for UP as a whole by assessing the impact of each economic state on health care utilization and reimbursement patterns.

Table 1   Estimated One-Year Return Distributions on Five Investments

		Estimated Return on Investment				
State of the Economy	*Probability*	*One-Year T-Bill*	*Project A*	*Project B*	*S&P 500 Fund*	*University Physicians*
Poor	0.10	7.0%	−8.0%	18.0%	−15.0%	0.0%
Below average	0.20	7.0	2.0	23.0	0.0	5.0
Average	0.40	7.0	14.0	7.0	15.0	10.0
Above average	0.20	7.0	25.0	−3.0	30.0	15.0
Excellent	0.10	7.0	33.0	2.0	45.0	20.0

In addition to the returns on these alternative investments, Cowan developed the following questions to use as the structure for her presentation. See if you can answer her questions.

Questions

1. Why is the T-bill return independent of the state of the economy? Is the return on a one-year T-bill risk-free?

2. Calculate the expected rate of return on each of the five investment alternatives listed in Table 1. Based solely on expected returns, which of the potential investments appears best?

3. Now calculate the standard deviations and coefficients of variation of returns for the five alternatives.

   a. What type of risk do these statistics measure?

   b. Is the standard deviation or the coefficient of variation the better measure?

   c. How do the alternatives compare when risk is considered?

4. Suppose University Physicians forms a two-asset portfolio by investing in both Projects A and B.

   a. To begin, assume that the required investment is the same for both projects, say, $1,000,000 each.

      (1) What would be the portfolio's expected rate of return, standard deviation, and coefficient of variation?

      (2) How do these values compare with the corresponding values for the individual projects?

      (3) What characteristic of the two return distributions makes risk reduction possible?

   b. What do you think would happen to the portfolio's expected rate of return and standard deviation if the portfolio contained 75 percent of Project A? If it contained 75 percent of Project B?

5. Now consider a portfolio consisting of investments in Project A and the S&P 500 Fund.

   a. First, consider a portfolio containing equal investment in the two assets. Would this portfolio have the same risk reducing effect as the Project A/Project B portfolio considered in Question 4? Explain.

b. Construct a portfolio consisting of Project A and the S&P 500 Fund. What are the expected returns and standard deviations for a portfolio mix of 0 percent Project A, 10 percent Project A, 20 percent Project A, and so on, up to 100 percent Project A?

6. Suppose an individual investor starts with a portfolio consisting of one randomly selected stock.

a. What would happen to the portfolio's risk if more and more randomly selected stocks were added?

b. What are the implications for investors? Do portfolio effects have an impact on the way investors should think about the riskiness of individual securities? Would you expect this to affect companies' costs of capital?

c. Explain the differences between stand-alone risk, diversifiable (company-specific) risk, and market risk.

d. Assume that you choose to hold a single stock portfolio. Should you expect to be compensated for all of the risk that you bear?

7. Now change Table 1 by crossing out the state of the economy and probability columns, and replacing them with Year 1, Year 2, Year 3, Year 4, and Year 5. In other words, assume that the distributions represent historical returns earned on each asset in each of the last five years.

a. Plot four lines on a scatter diagram (regression lines) that show the returns on the S&P 500 Fund (the market) on the X axis and (1) T-bill returns, (2) Project A returns, (3) Project B returns, and (4) UP returns on the Y axis.

(1) What are these lines called?

(2) Estimate the slope coefficient of each line. What is the slope coefficient called, and what is its significance? (If you have a calculator with statistical functions or are using a spreadsheet, use linear regression to find the slope coefficients.)

(3) What is the significance of the distance between the plot points and the regression line, that is, the errors?

b. Plot two lines on a different scatter diagram that show the returns of UP (the firm) on the X axis, and (1) Project A returns and (2)

Project B returns on the Y axis.

(1) What are these lines called?

(2) Estimate the slope coefficient of each line. What is the slope coefficient called, and what is its significance? (If you have a calculator with statistical functions or are using a spreadsheet, use linear regression to find the slope coefficients.)

c. If you were an individual investor who could buy any of the assets in Table 1, which one(s) would you buy? Why? (Hint: To help answer this question, construct a Security Market Line graph and plot the returns on each asset on the graph. Also, note that University Physicians is actually a not-for-profit corporation, so it would be impossible to buy an equity interest in the firm. For this question, assume that UP is an investor-owned company.)

d. Now assume that you are the CEO of University Physicians and have to decide whether to invest in Project A, Project B, or both. Which project(s) would you choose if you could accept both? If you could only accept one of the two, which would you choose? Why? (Hint: To help answer this question, construct a "Corporate Market Line" graph, which plots corporate betas on the X axis, rather than market betas, and plot the returns for each project on the graph.)

8. a. What is the market risk of each project (A and B) *relative* to the aggregate market risk of University Physicians? (For this question, assume that UP is an investor-owned company.)

   b. What is the corporate risk of each project (A and B) relative to the aggregate corporate risk of University Physicians?

9. a. What is the efficient markets hypothesis (EMH)?

   b. What impact does this theory have on decisions concerning investments in securities?

   c. Is the EMH applicable to real asset investments such as the decision of University Physicians to invest in Project A or Project B?

   d. What impact does the EMH have on corporate financing decisions?

Part III

Capital Acquisition

6

Long-Term Debt Financing

In Part I, The Health Care Environment, we examined the nature of the health care industry, and in Part II, Basic Financial Management Concepts, we discussed discounted cash flow analysis and financial risk. Now, in Part III, we turn our attention to capital acquisition. The focus in this chapter is on debt financing. Then, in Chapter 7, we discuss the second primary source of capital: equity, or fund, financing.

Firms actually use a mix of short-term and long-term debt; the choice between the two types is called the *debt maturity decision*. In this chapter, we discuss long-term debt, because the primary focus of Parts IV, V, and VI of the text is long-term, or strategic, decision making. In Part VII, Working Capital Management, we discuss short-term debt, as well as those factors that influence the debt maturity decision.

An Overview of Business Financing

Any business must have assets if it is to operate, and in order to acquire assets, firms must raise *capital*. Capital comes in two basic forms, *debt* and *equity*. Historically, capital furnished by the owners (stockholders) of investor-owned businesses was called "equity" capital, while capital obtained by not-for-profit firms from grants, contributions, and retained earnings was called *fund* capital. Both types of capital serve the same purpose in financing businesses, so today the term "equity" is often used to represent non-liability capital regardless of ownership type.

Table 6.1 shows a simplified balance sheet for Criser Pharmaceutical Company, a medium-sized, investor-owned producer of prescription drugs, as of December 31, 1996.[1] Criser began life in 1966 as a partnership, and converted to a corporation in 1974. Its 1996 sales were $802 million, and the $560 million of assets shown in Table 6.1 were necessary to support these sales. Criser obtained the capital used to purchase its assets (1) by buying raw materials on credit from its suppliers (accounts payable); (2) by paying its employee's wages and government taxes periodically rather than daily (accruals); (3) by borrowing from banks (notes payable); (4) by borrowing from institutions, such as insurance companies and mutual funds, as well as from individuals (long-term bonds); (5) by selling common stock to investors; and finally (6) by earning more than the company paid out in dividends, and hence building up the retained earnings account.

All accounts listed on the right-hand side of the balance sheet above common stock are *liability*, or *creditor, accounts*. Although Criser's creditors have first claim against the firm's income and assets, creditors' claims are limited to fixed amounts. For example, most of the long-term debt bears interest at a rate of 9 percent per year, so the bondholders received interest of about 0.09($214) = $19.3 million in 1996. If Criser did extremely well and had profits of, say, $150 million, the bondholders would get only $19.3 million. However, if Criser lost money, the bondholders would probably still get their $19.3 million. If Criser's financial condition was so weak that it could not make the required payments to bondholders (or other creditors), the company would be in *default* and would face potential *bankruptcy*. If bankruptcy were to occur, Criser might be forced to sell off, or liquidate, some or all of its assets. The creditors would likely be paid, at least some amount, but the common stockholders would face the prospect of being completely wiped out.

Table 6.1   Criser Pharmaceutical Company: December 31, 1996
Balance Sheet (millions of dollars)

Assets		*Liabilities and Equity*	
Cash and marketable securities	$ 24	Accounts payable	$ 48
Accounts receivable	101	Accrued wages and taxes	5
Inventories	186	Notes payable	70
Total current assets	$311	Total current liabilities	$123
Gross fixed assets	$299	Long-term bonds	214
Accumulated depreciation	50	Common stock	50
Net fixed assets	$249	Retained earnings	173
Total assets	$560	Total liabilities and equity	$560

After all of the creditors have been paid, the remaining, or residual, income belongs to the common stockholders.[2] This income must be retained and reinvested by not-for-profit companies, but investor-owned firms may pay some or all of it out as dividends to the firms' shareholders. Most investor-owned firms, like Criser, retain some earnings to support growth and then pay the remainder out in dividends.

Criser's debt is held primarily by its suppliers, by banks, and by institutions such as mutual funds, insurance companies, and pension funds. The debt is rarely traded, because these investors tend to hold debt securities until they mature. Criser's common stock, on the other hand, is actively traded, and the stock price rises and falls depending (1) on how the company is doing at any point in time; (2) on what is happening to the economy as a whole; and (3) most important, on how investors expect the company to do in the future.

Self-Test Questions:

What are the two primary forms of capital used by businesses?

What is the difference between equity capital and fund capital? Is this difference meaningful?

The Cost of Money

Capital in a free economy is allocated through the price system. The interest rate is the price paid to borrow debt capital, whereas in the case of equity capital in for-profit firms, investors' returns come in the form of dividends and capital gains (or losses). The four most fundamental factors that affect the supply of and demand for investment capital, and hence the cost of money, are (1) investment opportunities; (2) time preferences for consumption; (3) risk; and (4) inflation.

To see how these factors operate, visualize the situation facing Lori Gibbs, an entrepreneur who is planning to found a new home health care agency. Lori does not have sufficient personal funds to start the firm, so she must go to the debt markets for additional capital. If Lori estimates that the business will be highly profitable, she will be able to pay creditors a higher interest rate than if the firm is barely profitable. Obviously, her ability to pay for borrowed capital depends on the firm's *investment opportunities.* The more productive Lori thinks the new firm will be, the higher her expected return on the investment, and hence the more she can offer to pay potential lenders for use of their savings.

How attractive Ms. Gibbs' offer will appear to lenders will depend in large part on their *time preferences for consumption.* For example, one potential lender, Jane Wright, might be saving for retirement, and she might be willing to loan funds at a relatively low rate because her preference is for future consumption. Another person, John Davis, might have a wife and several young children to clothe and feed, so he might be willing to lend funds out of current income, and hence forgo consumption, only if the interest rate is very high. Mr. Davis is said to have a high time preference for consumption and Ms. Wright a low time preference. Note also that if the entire population were living right at the subsistence level, time preferences for current consumption would necessarily be high, aggregate savings would be low, interest rates would be high, and capital formation would be difficult.

The *risk* inherent in the prospective home health care business, and thus in Ms. Gibbs' ability to repay the loan, would also affect the return investors would require: the higher the perceived risk, the higher the required rate of return. Investors would simply be unwilling to lend to high-risk businesses unless the interest rate was higher than on loans to low-risk businesses.

Finally, since the value of money in the future is affected by *inflation*, the higher the expected rate of inflation, the higher the interest rate demanded by savers. To simplify matters, our illustration implied that savers would lend directly to businesses needing capital, but in most cases the funds would actually pass through a *financial intermediary*, such as a bank or a mutual fund.

Self-Test Questions:

What is the price of debt and equity capital?

What four factors affect the cost of money?

Interest Rate Levels

Capital is allocated among potential borrowers by interest rates. Businesses with the most profitable investment opportunities are willing and able to pay the most for capital, so they tend to attract it away from less profitable businesses. Figure 6.1 shows how supply and demand interact to determine interest rates in two capital markets. Markets A and B represent two of the many capital markets in existence. The going interest rate, designated k, is initially 10 percent for the low-risk securities in Market A. Borrowers whose credit is strong enough to qualify for this market can obtain funds at a cost of 10 percent. Riskier borrowers must obtain higher-cost funds in Market B. Investors who are more willing to take risks invest in Market B, expecting to receive a 12 percent return, but also realizing that they might receive much less if the borrower fails.

If the demand for funds in a market declines, as it typically does during a business recession, the demand curves will shift to the left, as shown in Curve D_2 in Market A. The market-clearing, or equilibrium, interest rate in this example declines to 8 percent. Similarly, you should be able to visualize what would happen if the Federal Reserve tightened credit: the supply curve, S_1, would shift to the left, and this would raise interest rates and lower the level of borrowing in the economy.

Capital markets are interdependent. For example, if Markets A and B were in equilibrium before the demand shift to D_2 in Market A, then investors were willing to accept the higher risk in Market B in exchange for a *risk premium* of $12\% - 10\% = 2$ percentage points. After the shift to D_2, the risk premium would initially increase to $12\% - 8\% = 4$ percentage points. In all likelihood, this much larger premium would induce some of the lenders in Market A to move to Market B, which, in turn, would cause the supply curve in Market A to shift to the left (or up) and that in Market B to shift to the right. This transfer of capital between markets would raise the interest rate in Market A and lower it in Market B, thus bringing the risk premium back closer to its original level, 2 percentage points.

There are many capital markets in the United States. There are markets for short-term debt (*money markets*) and for long-term debt and equity (*capital markets*). These markets are further broken down into markets for home loans; farm loans; business loans for both taxable and tax-exempt firms; federal, state, and local government loans; and consumer loans. Within each category, there are regional markets as well as different types of submarkets. For example, within the business sector there are dozens of types of debt and also several sharply differentiated markets for common stocks. There is a price for each type of capital, and these prices change over time as shifts occur in supply and demand conditions.

Self-Test Questions:

How do interest rates serve to allocate debt capital among borrowers?

How does risk affect interest rates?

What happens to the market-clearing, or equilibrium, interest rate when the demand for loans increases? Decreases?

Figure 6.1   Interest Rates as a Function of Supply and Demand
for Funds

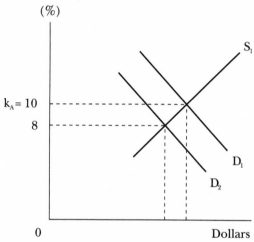

(a) Market A: Low-Risk Securities

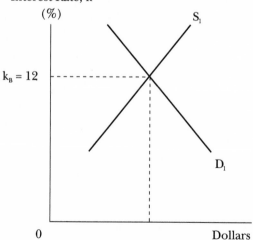

(b) Market B: High-Risk Securities

Source: E. F. Brigham and L. C. Gapenski. 1994. *Financial Management: Theory and Practice,* 7th
ed. Fort Worth, TX: The Dryden Press.

The Determinants of Market Interest Rates

Although prevailing interest rates result from supply and demand conditions in the debt markets, investors base their demand decisions on several factors. In general, the interest rate on a debt security, which is also its *required rate of return*, k, is composed of a real risk-free rate of interest, k^*, plus premiums that reflect inflation, the riskiness of the security, and the security's marketability (or liquidity). This relationship can be expressed as follows:

$$\text{Required rate of return} = k_d = k^* + IP + DRP + LP + MRP. \quad (6.1)$$

Here

k_d = required rate of interest on a given debt security.

k^* = real risk-free rate of interest, which is the rate that would exist on a riskless security if zero inflation were expected.

IP = inflation premium. IP is equal to the average expected inflation rate over the life of the security.

DRP = default risk premium. This premium reflects the possibility that the issuer will not pay interest or principal on a security at the stated time and in the stated amount.

LP = liquidity premium. This is a premium charged by lenders to reflect the fact that some securities cannot be converted to cash on short notice at a "fair market" price.

MRP = maturity risk premium. As we explain later, longer-term bonds are exposed to significant price declines if interest rates rise, so a maturity risk premium is charged by lenders to reflect this risk.

If we combine $k^* + IP$ and let this sum equal k_{RF}, then we have this expression for the required rate of return on a debt security:

$$k_d = k_{RF} + DRP + LP + MRP. \quad (6.2)$$

where k_{RF} = the nominal risk-free rate of interest. This is the interest rate on a security such as a U.S. Treasury bill, which is very liquid and free of most risks.[3] The components whose sum makes up the required rate on a given debt security are discussed in more detail in the following sections.

The real risk-free rate of interest (k*)

The *real risk-free rate of interest (k*)* is the interest rate that would exist on a riskless security if no inflation were expected, and it may be thought of as the rate of interest that would exist on short-term U.S. Treasury securities in an inflation-free world. The real risk-free rate is not static—it changes over time depending on economic conditions, especially on the rate of return borrowers expect to earn on productive assets and on people's time preferences for current versus future consumption. It is difficult to measure k^* precisely, but most estimates place it in the range of 2 to 4 percent.

The nominal risk-free rate of interest (k_{RF})

The *nominal risk-free rate (k_{RF})* is the real risk-free rate plus a premium for expected inflation: $k_{RF} = k^* + IP$. Conceptually, the nominal risk-free rate is the interest rate on a totally risk-free security—one that has no risk of default, no maturity risk, no liquidity risk, and no risk of loss if inflation increases. However, no such security exists in the United States. The closest thing to a truly risk-free security is a T-bill. Treasury bonds, which are longer-term government securities, are free of default and liquidity risks, but T-bonds are exposed to some risk due to changes in the level of interest rates. Nevertheless, we will generally use the T-bill rate to approximate the short-term risk-free rate, and the T-bond rate to approximate the long-term risk-free rate.

Inflation premium (IP)

Inflation has a major impact on interest rates because it erodes the purchasing power of the dollar and lowers the real rate of return on investments. Investors are well aware of the impact of inflation, so when they lend money, they build an *inflation premium (IP)* into the required rate of return that is equal to the expected inflation rate over the life of the security. For example, if the real risk-free rate of interest was $k^* = 3\%$, and if inflation was expected to be 4 percent (and hence IP = 4%) during the next year, then the rate of interest on one-year T-bills would be 7 percent.[4]

It is important to note that the rate of inflation built into interest rates is the *rate of inflation expected in the future*, not the rate experienced in the past. Thus, the latest reported figures might show an annual inflation rate of 3 percent, but that is for a past period. If people on the average expect a 6 percent inflation rate in the future, then 6 percent would be built into the current rate of interest. Note also that the inflation rate reflected in the interest rate on any security is the *average rate of inflation expected over the life of the security*. Thus, the inflation rate built into a one-year T-bill is the expected inflation rate for the next year, but the inflation rate built into a 30-year T-bond is the average rate of inflation expected over the next 30 years.

Default risk premium (DRP)

The risk that a borrower will *default* on a loan (fail to pay the full amount of interest or principal as scheduled) also affects the market interest rate on a security—the greater the default risk, the higher the interest rate lenders charge. Treasury securities have no default risk; thus, they carry the lowest interest rates on taxable securities in the United States. For corporate and municipal bonds, the higher the bond's rating, the lower its default risk, and, consequently, the lower its interest rate. Bond ratings will be discussed in detail later in the chapter. For now, merely note that bonds rated AAA are judged to have less default risk than bonds rated AA, AA bonds are less risky then A bonds, and so on.

Table 6.2 lists the interest rates on some representative long-term bonds with different ratings during March 1995. The difference between the interest rate on a T-bond and that on a corporate bond with similar maturity, liquidity, and other features is the *default risk premium (DRP)*. Therefore, if the bonds listed in table 6.2 were otherwise similar, the default risk premium would be DRP = 8.3% − 7.4 = 0.9 percentage points for AAA corporate bonds, 8.6% − 7.4% = 1.2 percentage points for AA corporate bonds, 8.8% − 7.4% = 1.4 percentage points for A corporate bonds, and so on. Bonds that are rated below BBB are called *junk bonds*, and such bonds tend to have large default risk premiums. The default risk premiums for tax-exempt health care bonds use AAA-rated bonds as the base, so they are not "pure" default risk premiums as in the case of corporate bonds, which can be compared to default-free Treasury securities.

Liquidity premium (LP)

A highly *liquid* asset is one that can be sold quickly at a predictable "fair market" price, and thus can be converted to a known amount of spendable cash on short notice. Active markets, which provide liquidity, exist for federal government bonds and for the stocks and bonds of larger corporations. Real estate, as well as securities issued by small companies, including health care businesses that issue municipal bonds, are *illiquid*—they can be sold to raise cash, but not quickly and not at a predictable price. If a security is illiquid, investors will add a *liquidity premium (LP)* when they establish the market rate on the security. It is very

Table 6.2   Representative Long-Term Interest Rates: March 1995

	Interest Rate	
Rating	*Taxable**	*Tax-Exempt†*
U.S. Treasury	7.4%	—
AAA	8.3	6.1%
AA	8.6	6.3
A	8.8	6.5
BBB	9.7	7.6
BB	10.6	8.8
B	11.6	10.2
CCC	13.4	11.8

* The non-Treasury taxable bonds are corporate issues.

† The tax-exempt bonds are municipal health care facility issues.

Sources: The *Wall Street Journal* and William R. Hough & Company.

difficult to measure liquidity premiums with precision, but a differential of at least two percentage points is thought to exist between the least liquid and the most liquid financial assets of similar default risk and maturity.

Maturity risk premium (MRP)

As we will demonstrate in the bond valuation section, the market prices of long-term bonds decline sharply when interest rates rise. Since interest rates can and do rise, all long-term bonds, even Treasury bonds, have an element of risk called *price risk.* For example, if you bought a 30-year Treasury bond in 1972 for $1,000 when the long-term interest rate was 7 percent, and held it until 1981, when T-bond rates were about 14.5 percent, the value of your bond would have declined to about $514. That would represent a loss of almost half your money, and it demonstrates that long-term bonds, even U.S. Treasury bonds, are not riskless.

As a general rule, the bonds of any organization, from the U.S. government to Columbia/HCA Healthcare, have more price risk the longer the maturity of the bond. Therefore, a *maturity risk premium (MRP),* which is higher the longer the years to maturity, must be included in the required interest rate. The effect of maturity risk premiums is to raise interest rates on long-term bonds relative to those on short-term bonds. This premium, like the others, is extremely difficult to measure, but it seems to vary over time, rising when interest rates are more volatile and uncertain and falling when they are more stable. In recent years, the maturity risk premium on 30-year T-bonds appears to have generally been in the range of one or two percentage points.

Self-Test Questions:

Write out an equation for the required interest rate on a debt security.

What is the difference between the real risk-free rate, k^*, and the nominal risk-free rate, k_{RF}?

Do the interest rates on Treasury securities include a default risk premium? A liquidity premium? Explain.

What is price risk? What type of debt securities would have the largest maturity risk premium?

The Term Structure of Interest Rates

At certain times, such as in 1995, short-term interest rates are lower than long-term rates, whereas at other times, such as in 1980, short-term rates are higher than long-term rates. The relationship between long- and short-term rates, which is called the *term structure of interest rates*, is important to health care managers, who must decide whether to borrow by issuing long- or short-term debt, and to investors, who must decide whether to buy long- or short-term bonds. Thus, it is important to understand (1) how the interest rates on long- and short-term bonds are related to one another, and (2) what causes shifts in their relative positions.

To examine the current term structure, look up the interest rates on bonds of various maturities by a single issuer in a source such as the *Wall Street Journal* or the *Federal Reserve Bulletin*. For example, the tabular section of Figure 6.2 presents interest rates for Treasury securities of different maturities on two dates. The set of data for a given date, when plotted on a graph, is called a *yield curve*. As can be seen in Figure 6.2, the yield curve changes both in position and in shape over time. Had we drawn the yield curve during January of 1982, it would have been essentially horizontal, for long-term and short-term bonds at that time had about the same rate of interest.

Figure 6.2 shows yield curves for U.S. Treasury securities, but we could have constructed them for similarly rated corporate bonds or for municipal (tax-exempt) bonds. In every case, the yield curves would be approximately the same shape, but would differ in vertical

Figure 6.2   U.S. Treasury Bond Interest Rates on Two Dates

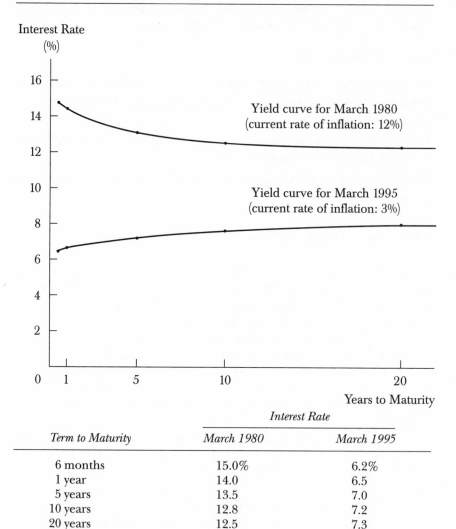

Term to Maturity	Interest Rate	
	March 1980	*March 1995*
6 months	15.0%	6.2%
1 year	14.0	6.5
5 years	13.5	7.0
10 years	12.8	7.2
20 years	12.5	7.3
30 years	12.4	7.4

position. For example, had we constructed the yield curve for Beverly Enterprises, it would fall above the Treasury curve because corporate interest rates include default risk premiums, while Treasury rates do not. Conversely, the curve for Baptist Medical Center, a not-for-profit hospital, would probably fall below the Treasury curve, because the tax-exemption benefit, which lowers the interest rate on tax-exempt securities, generally outweighs the default risk. In every case, however, the riskier the issuer, that is, the lower the bonds are rated, the higher the yield curve.

Historically, long-term rates have generally been above short-term rates, so usually the yield curve has been upward sloping. An upward-sloping curve would be expected if the inflation premium is relatively constant across all maturities because the maturity risk premium applied to long-term issues will push long-term rates above short-term rates. Since an upward-sloping yield curve is most prevalent, this shape is also called a *normal yield curve.* Conversely, a yield curve that slopes downward is called an *inverted,* or *abnormal, yield curve.* Thus, in Figure 6.2, the yield curve for March 1980 is inverted, but the one for March 1995 is normal.[5]

Self-Test Questions:

What is a yield curve, and what information is needed to create this curve?

What is the difference between a normal yield curve and an abnormal one?

Interest Rates and Business Decisions

The yield curve for March 1995, shown in Figure 6.2, shows how much the U.S. government had to pay at that time to borrow money for one year, five years, ten years, and so on. A taxable health care firm would have had to pay somewhat more, while a not-for-profit provider would probably have had to pay somewhat less, but assume for the moment that we are back in March 1995, and that the yield curve in Figure 6.2 applies to all companies. Now suppose that Baptist Medical Center has decided (1) to build a new outpatient clinic with a 20-year life which will cost $10 million and (2) to raise the $10 million by selling debt. If it borrowed in 1995 on a short-term basis—say, for one year—its interest cost for that year would be 6.5 percent, or $650,000, whereas if it used long-term (30-year) financing, its cost would be 7.4 percent, or $740,000. Therefore, at first glance, it would seem that Baptist should use short-term debt.

However, if the hospital uses short-term debt, it will have to renew the loan every year, and the rate charged on each renewal loan will reflect the then current short-term rate. Interest rates could return to their March 1980 levels, so by 1997 or 1998 the hospital could be paying 14 percent, or $1,400,000, per year. On the other hand, if Baptist used long-term financing in 1995, its interest costs would remain constant at $740,000 per year, so an increase in interest rates in the economy would not hurt it.

Does this suggest that firms should always avoid short-term debt? Not necessarily. If inflation remains low in the next few years, so will interest rates. If Baptist Medical Center had borrowed on a long-term basis for 7.4 percent in March 1995, it would be at a major disadvantage if its debt were locked in at 7.4 percent while its competitors that used short-term debt that cost 6.2 percent in March 1995 were able to continually renew that debt at a low rate. On the other hand, federal deficits might drive inflation and interest rates up to new record levels. In that case, all borrowers would wish that they had borrowed on a long-term basis in 1995.

Financing decisions would be easy if managers could develop accurate forecasts of future interest rates. Unfortunately, predicting future interest rates with consistent accuracy is somewhere between difficult and impossible—people who make a living by selling interest rate forecasts say it is difficult, but many others say it is impossible.

Even though it is difficult, if not impossible, to predict future interest rate *levels*, it is easy to predict that interest rates will *fluctuate*—they always have and they always will. This being the case, sound financial policy calls for using a mix of long- and short-term debt, as well as equity, in such a manner that the firm can survive in all but the most severe, and hence unlikely, interest rate environments. Furthermore, the optimal financial policy depends in an important way on maturities of the firm's assets—in general, to reduce risk, managers try to match the maturities of securities with the maturities of the assets being financed. We will return to this issue in Chapter 9 when we discuss capital structure decisions.

Self-Test Questions:

If short-term rates are lower than long-term rates, why might a business still choose to finance with long-term debt?

Explain the following statement: "A firm's financing policy depends in large part on the nature of its assets."

Common Debt Instruments

There are many types of long-term debt: amortized and nonamortized, publicly issued and privately placed, taxable and tax-exempt, secured and unsecured, marketable and nonmarketable, callable and noncallable, and so on. In this section, we briefly discuss the long-term debt instruments most commonly used by health care providers.

Term loans

A *term loan* is a contract under which a borrower agrees to make a series of interest and principal payments, on specified dates, to a lender. Investment bankers are generally not involved: term loans are negotiated directly between the borrowing firm and a financial institution—generally a bank, a mutual fund, an insurance company, or a pension fund. Thus, term loans are *private placements* as opposed to *public offerings*, which are typically used on bonds. Although the maturities of term loans vary from 2 to 30 years, most are for periods in the 3- to 15-year range. Term loans are usually amortized in equal installments over the life of the loan, so part of the principal of the loan is retired with each payment. For example, Sacramento Cardiology Group has a $100,000 five-year term loan with Bank of America to fund the purchase of new diagnostic equipment. The interest rate on the fixed-rate loan is 10 percent, which obligates the Group to five end-of-year payments of $26,379.75. Thus, loan payments total $131,898.75, of which $31,898.75 is interest and $100,000 is repayment of principal.

Term loans have three major advantages over public offerings—*speed, flexibility,* and *low issuance costs.* Because they are negotiated directly between the lender and the borrower, formal documentation is minimized. The key provisions of the loan can be worked out much more quickly, and with more flexibility, than can those for a public issue, and it is not necessary for a term loan to go through the Securities and Exchange Commission registration process. A further advantage of term loans over publicly held debt has to do with future flexibility: if a bond issue is held by many different bondholders, it is virtually impossible to alter the terms of the agreement, even though new economic conditions may make such changes desirable. With a term loan, the borrower can generally negotiate with the lender to work out modifications in the contract.

The interest rate on a term loan can be either fixed for the life of the loan or variable. If it is fixed, the rate used will be close to the rate on bonds of equivalent maturity for companies of comparable risk. If the rate is variable, it is usually set at a certain number of percentage points over an index rate such as the prime rate or the T-bill rate. Then, when the index rate goes up or down, so does the rate on the outstanding balance of the term loan.

Bonds

Like a term loan, a *bond* is a long-term contract under which a borrower agrees to make payments of interest and principal, on specific dates, to the holder of the bond. Although bonds are similar in some ways to term loans, a bond issue is generally registered with the Securities and Exchange Commission, advertised, offered to the public through investment bankers, and actually sold to many different investors. Indeed, thousands of individual and institutional investors may participate when a firm such as Columbia/HCA Healthcare sells a bond issue, while there is generally only one lender in the case of a term loan. Occasionally, a bond issue can be sold to one lender (or to just a few); in this case, the issue would be a private placement.

Although bonds are generally issued with maturities in the range of 20 to 30 years, shorter maturities, such as 7 to 10 years, are occasionally used, as are longer maturities. In fact, in 1995, Columbia/HCA Healthcare issued $200 million of noncallable 100-year bonds, following the issuance of 100-year bonds by Disney and Coca-Cola in 1993. These ultra-long-term bonds had not been used by any company since the 1920s.

Unlike term loans, a bond's interest rate is generally fixed, although in recent years, there has been an increase in the use of various types of floating rate bonds. Also unlike term loans, bonds typically pay only interest over the life of the bond, with the entire amount of principal being returned to lenders at maturity.

Mortgage bonds

With a *mortgage bond*, the issuer pledges certain real assets as security for the bond. To illustrate, Mid-Texas Healthcare System recently needed $50 million to purchase land and to build a new hospital. *First mortgage bonds* in the amount of $20 million, secured by a mortgage on the property, were issued. If the company defaults on the bonds, the bondholders could foreclose on the hospital and sell it to satisfy their claims.

Mid-Texas could, if it so chose, also issue *second mortgage bonds* secured by the same $50 million hospital. In the event of bankruptcy and liquidation, the holders of these second mortgage bonds would have a claim against the property only after the first mortgage bondholders had been paid off in full. Thus, second mortgages are sometimes called *junior mortgages*, or *junior liens*, because they are junior in priority to claims of senior mortgages, or first mortgage bonds.

Debentures

A *debenture* is an unsecured bond, and as such, it has no lien against specific property as security for the obligation. For example, Mid-Texas Healthcare System has $5 million of debentures outstanding. These bonds are not secured by real property, but are backed instead by the revenue-producing power of the corporation. Debenture holders are, therefore, general creditors whose claims are protected by property not otherwise pledged. In practice, the use of debentures depends on the nature of the firm's assets and its general credit strength. If a firm's credit position is exceptionally strong, it can issue debentures—it simply does not need specific security. Debentures are also issued by companies with only a small amount of assets suitable as collateral. Finally, companies that have used up their capacity to borrow in the lower-cost mortgage market may be forced to use higher-cost debentures.

Subordinated debentures

The term *subordinate* means "below" or "inferior." Thus, *subordinated debt* has a claim on assets in the event of bankruptcy only after senior debt has been paid off. Debentures may be subordinated either to designated notes payable—usually bank loans—or to all other debt. In the event of liquidation, holders of subordinated debentures cannot be paid until senior debt, as named in the debenture, has been paid. The subordinated debentures of a company that has used up its ability to employ mortgage bonds are normally quite risky, and these debentures carry interest rates that are much higher than the rate on top quality debt.

Municipal bonds

Municipal bonds are long-term debt obligations issued by states and their political subdivisions, such as counties, cities, port authorities, toll road or bridge authorities, and so on. Short-term municipal securities are used primarily to meet temporary cash needs, while municipal bonds are usually used to finance capital projects.

There are several types of municipal bonds. For example, *general obligation bonds* are secured by the full faith and credit of the issuing municipality, that is, they are backed by the full taxing authority of the issuer. Conversely, *special tax bonds* are secured by a specified tax such as a tax on utility services. *Revenue bonds* are bonds that are not backed by taxing power, but rather by the revenues derived from such projects as roads or bridges, airports, and water and sewage systems. Revenue bonds are of particular interest to not-for-profit health care providers, because they are legally entitled to issue such securities through government-sponsored health care financing authorities.

In the first half of 1995, not-for-profit health care firms sold 142 municipal bond issues totaling $4.9 billion. This was down significantly from the first half of 1994, when 246 issues were brought to market having a value of $8 billion. The slowdown in new health care issues was caused mainly by providers' concerns over coping with industry changes while carrying large amounts of debt. Recently, about 20 percent of the dollar volume of health care muni debt has had floating rates, while the remaining 80 percent has had fixed rates. Health care issuers tend to use more floating rate debt when interest rates are high, or when the yield curve has a steep upward slope, or both, since floating rates are tied to short-term interest levels. For example, in March 1995, A-rated hospitals had to pay 6.8 percent on long-term, fixed rate bonds, but only 5.7 percent on floating rate bonds. Of course, floating rate bonds are riskier to the issuer because interest rates could rise in the future, but virtually all such municipal debt has call provisions that permit issuers to replace the floating rate debt with fixed rate debt should conditions so dictate.

Most municipal bonds are sold in *serial* form; that is, a portion of the issue comes due periodically, anywhere from six months after issue to 30 years or more. Municipal bonds are typically issued in denominations of $5,000, or integral multiples of $5,000, and although most municipal bonds are tax exempt, some are taxable to investors.

In contrast to corporate issues, municipal issues are not required to be registered with the SEC. However, prior to bringing municipal debt to market, issuers are required to prepare an *official statement* that contains relevant financial information about the issuer and the nature of the bond issue. Prior to 1994, issuers were not required to provide periodic financial updates, so it was very difficult for investors to obtain credit information about municipal bonds after initial issue. However, in November 1994, the SEC introduced new rules that require issuers to (1) provide annual financial statements that update the information contained in the official statement and (2) release information on material events that could affect bonds' values as such events occur. This information will not be sent directly to investors, but rather will reside in data banks that can be easily accessed by investment bankers, mutual fund managers, and institutional investors. In effect, by making the information available to investment bankers who handle public trades, any individual who wants to buy or sell a municipal bond will also have access to current information affecting the bond's value.

Whereas the vast majority of federal government and corporate bonds are held by institutions, Table 6.3 shows that close to half of all hospital municipal bonds outstanding are held by individual investors. The primary attraction of most municipal bonds, as we discussed in Chapter 2, is their exemption from federal and state (in the state of issue)

Table 6.3   Holders of Hospital Municipal Bond Issues

Bondholder	Percent of All Holdings
Individuals	42%
Long-term (bond) mutual funds	14
Insurance companies	11
Commercial banks	8
Short-term (money market) mutual funds	8
Other (investment banks, partnerships, etc.)	17
	100%

Source: The *Wall Street Journal.* 1994. 9 February.

taxes. Looking back at Table 6.2, we see that the interest rate on an AAA-rated long-term corporate bond in March 1995 was 8.3 percent, while the rate on a similar risk health care muni was 6.1 percent. To an individual investor in the 40 percent federal-plus-state tax bracket, the muni bond's equivalent taxable yield is $6.1\%/(1 - 0.40) = 6.1\%/0.6 = 10.2\%$. It is easy to see why investors in high tax brackets are so enthusiastic about municipal bonds.

To illustrate the use of municipal bonds by a health care firm, consider the $56 million in municipal bonds issued in June 1995 by the Bay Area Health Facilities Authority. The Authority is a public body created under Florida's Health Facilities Authorities Law for the sole purpose of issuing health facilities municipal revenue bonds for qualifying health care providers. For this particular bond issue, the provider is Sabal Palm Medical Center, a not-for-profit hospital, and the primary purpose of the issue was to raise funds to build and equip a children's hospital facility. The bonds are secured solely by the revenues of Sabal Palm Medical Center, so the actual issuer, the Bay Area Health Facilities Authority, has no responsibility whatever regarding the interest or principal payments on the issue. The bonds are rated AAA, not on the basis of the financial strength of Sabal Palm Medical Center, but rather because the bonds are insured by the Municipal Bond Investors Assurance Corporation (MBIA). (Municipal bond insurance, which is called *credit enhancement*, will be discussed in more detail later in the chapter.) Table 6.4 shows the maturities and interest rates associated with the issue.

Note the following points:

1. The issue is a serial issue; that is, the $56,000,000 in bonds is composed of 13 series, or individual issues, with maturities ranging from about 2 years to 30 years.

Table 6.4   Sabal Palm Medical Center Municipal Bond Issue:
Maturities, Amounts, and Interest Rates

Maturity*	Amount	Interest Rate
1997	$ 705,000	5.20%
1998	740,000	5.30
1999	785,000	5.35
2000	825,000	5.40
2001	880,000	5.45
2002	925,000	5.50
2003	985,000	5.55
2004	1,050,000	5.60
2005	1,115,000	5.65
2006	1,190,000	5.70
2010	5,590,000	6.10
2015	9,435,000	6.20
2025	31,775,000	6.30
	$56,000,000	

* All serial issues mature on June 1 of the listed year.

2. Since the yield curve was normal, or upward sloping, at time of issue, the interest rates increase across series as the maturities increase.

3. The bonds that mature in 2010, 2015, and 2025 have sinking fund provisions (which we discuss shortly), whereby the hospital must place a specified dollar amount with a trustee each year to ensure that funds are available to retire the issues as they become due.

4. Although it is not shown in the table, the hospital's *debt service requirements*—that is, the total amount of principal and interest that it has to pay on the issue—are relatively constant over time. In effect, the debt payments are spread relatively evenly over time. The purpose of structuring the series in this way is to match the maturity of the asset with the maturities of the bonds. Think about it this way: the children's hospital has a life of about 30 years; during this time, it will be generating revenues more or less evenly, and its value will decline more or less evenly. Thus, the hospital has structured the debt series so that the debt service requirements can be met by the revenues associated with the

children's hospital. At the end of 30 years, the debt will be paid off, and Sabal Palm Medical Center will probably be planning for a replacement facility that would be funded, at least in part, by a new debt issue.

Current law limits the amount of tax-exempt bonds that can be issued by nonacute care providers to $150 million. Thus, while not-for-profit hospitals can issue an unlimited amount of municipal bonds, not-for-profit "nonhospital" facilities such as nursing homes, HMOs, and clinics are capped at $150 million. In addition, the cap applies to nonhospital facilities that are developed by acute care hospitals. The cap places an artificial limit on the ability of not-for-profit nonhospital corporations to obtain favorable financing, and hence to consolidate and form integrated delivery systems, so lobbyists for the managed care and nursing home industries, as well as others, have been arguing for a change in the law to eliminate the restriction.

Private placement of bonds

Most bonds, including Treasury, corporate, and municipal bonds, are sold through investment bankers to the public at large. For example, the largest hospital municipal bond issue in 1994 was a $675 million municipal mortgage revenue issue sold by the New York State Medical Care Facilities Financing Agency for New York Hospital. The issue was marketed to the public at large, including institutional investors, by Goldman Sachs & Co., the top underwriter of tax-exempt health care issues. However, smaller bond issues, typically $10 million or less, can be sold directly to a single buyer (or small group of buyers). Issues placed directly with lenders, called *private placements*, have the same advantages as term loans, which we discussed in an earlier section.

Although the interest rate on private placements is generally higher than the interest rate set on public issues, the up-front costs of placing the issue are less with private placements. Moreover, since there is direct negotiation between the borrower and lender, the opportunity is greater to structure bond terms that are more favorable to the borrower than the terms routinely contained in public debt issues.

To illustrate a private placement, in 1995, Pacific Shores Hospital sold $5 million of ten-year municipal bonds to a regional bank at an interest rate of 6.4 percent. When the up-front costs were added in, the *all-in cost* of the issue was 6.5 percent. The interest rate on a public issue would have been only 6.0 percent, but the addition of selling fees, bond insurance, and other up-front costs would raise the all-in cost of a public issue to 6.75 percent. Thus, the bank received an interest rate that was 50 basis points (0.5 percentage points) above the rate it would have earned if it had bought the bonds in a public sale, and the hospital saved 25 basis points on the issue when all costs are considered. The reason why private placements can be structured so that both borrower and lender "win" is that the savings in issuance costs can be allocated to the benefit of both parties.

Self-Test Questions:

Describe the primary features of the following long-term debt securities:

1. Term loan

2. Bond

3. First mortgage bond; junior mortgage

4. Debenture; subordinated debenture

5. Municipal bond

What are the key differences between a private placement and a public issue?

Debt Contract Provisions

A firm's managers are most concerned about (1) the effective cost of debt, including issuance costs, and (2) any provisions which might restrict the firm's future actions. In this section, we discuss features that could affect either the cost of the firm's debt or its future flexibility.

Bond indentures

An *indenture,* a legal document that may be several hundred pages in length, spells out the rights of both bondholders and the issuing corporation. The indenture includes a set of *restrictive covenants* that cover such points as the conditions under which the issuer can pay off the bonds prior to maturity, the financial condition that the company must maintain to issue additional debt, and restrictions against the payment of dividends unless earnings meet certain specifications. Overall, these covenants relate to the *agency problem* that arises between bondholders and managers that we discussed in Chapter 2.

The *trustee* is an official or institution (usually a bank) who represents the bondholders and makes sure that the terms of the indenture are being carried out. The trustee is responsible for trying to keep the covenants from being violated and for taking appropriate action if a violation does occur. What constitutes "appropriate action" varies with the circumstances. It might be that to insist on immediate compliance would result in bankruptcy and possibly large losses on the bonds. In such a case, the trustee might decide that the bondholders would be better served by giving the company a chance to work out its problems, and thus avoid forcing it into bankruptcy.

Call provisions

A *call provision* gives the issuer the right to call a bond for redemption, that is, the right to pay off the bondholders in entirety and retire the issue. If it is used, the call provision generally states that the company must pay an amount greater than the initial amount borrowed. The additional sum required is defined as the *call premium*. Note that many callable bonds offer a period of call protection. For example, some bonds are not callable until five or ten years after the original issue date. This type of call provision is known as a *deferred call*.

To illustrate call provisions, consider Sabal Palm Medical Center's bond issue contained in Table 6.4. All bonds that mature in 2006 and later are subject to call after December 31, 2005. If the call is made in 2006 and 2007, the call premium is 2 percent, or $20 for each $1,000 in face value. The premium drops to 1.5 percent for calls in 2008 and 2009, 1 percent for calls in 2010 and 2011, 0.5 percent for calls in 2012 and 2013, and zero for any calls beyond 2013.

The call privilege is valuable to the issuer, but potentially detrimental to bondholders, especially if the bond is issued in a period when interest rates are cyclically high. In general, bonds are called when interest rates have fallen, because the issuer usually replaces the old, high-interest issue with a new lower-interest issue. Thus, investors are forced to reinvest the principal returned in new securities at lower rates. The added risk to investors causes the interest rate on a new issue of callable bonds to exceed that on a new issue of noncallable bonds.

Put provisions

Whereas call provisions protect issuers against falling interest rates, *put provisions* protect investors against rising interest rates. If interest rates rise in the economy, or on a particular issue due to deteriorating credit quality, the value of fixed rate debt declines. However, the inclusion of a put provision allows bondholders, at their option, to return the bonds to the issuer and receive the par, or principal amount, in return. Thus, if interest rates rise, bondholders can exercise the put and reinvest the proceeds in new, higher-yielding bonds. Note, however, that put provisions, when used, often are not effective until some time after issue. Also, some put provisions can be exercised only on a specified date or a few specified dates.

While call provisions increase the riskiness of a debt issue as seen by investors, put provisions decrease investors' risk. Thus, bond issues with put provisions have interest rates that are slightly lower than the rates set on comparable issues without put provisions.

Sinking funds

A *sinking fund* is a provision that provides for the systematic retirement of a bond issue. Typically, sinking fund provisions require the issuer to retire a portion of its bonds each year. On some occasions, the issuer may be required to deposit money with a trustee, who invests the funds and then uses the accumulated sum to retire the entire bond issue when it matures. Sometimes the stipulated sinking fund payment is tied to the sale or earnings of the current year, but usually it is a mandatory fixed amount. If it is mandatory, a failure to meet the sinking fund requirement causes the bond issue to be thrown into default, which could force the issuer into bankruptcy.

Although a sinking fund is designed to protect the bondholders by assuring that the issue is retired in an orderly fashion, it must be recognized that, like a call provision, a sinking fund may at times work to the detriment of bondholders. On balance, however, securities that provide for a sinking fund and continuing redemption are regarded as being safer than bonds without sinking funds, so adding a sinking fund provision to a bond issue will lower the interest rate on the bond.

Self-Test Questions:

What is a bond indenture? A restrictive covenant?

What is a call (put) provision? What impact does a call (put) provision have on an issue's required rate of return (interest rate)?

What is a sinking fund? How are bonds retired for sinking fund purposes?

What impact does a sinking fund have on an issue's required rate of return? How do sinking fund provisions differ from call provisions?

Bond Ratings

Since the early 1900s, bonds have been assigned quality ratings that reflect their probability of going into default. The two major rating agencies are Moody's Investors Service (Moody's) and Standard & Poor's Corporation (S&P), which rate both corporate and municipal bonds. These agencies' rating designations are shown in Table 6.5. In the discussion to follow, reference to the S&P code is intended to imply the Moody's code as well. Thus, for example, triple B bonds means both BBB and Baa bonds; double B bonds, both BB and Ba bonds; and so on.

Bonds with a BBB and higher rating are called *investment grade*, and they are the lowest-rated bonds that many banks and other institutional investors are permitted by law to hold. Double B and lower bonds are speculations; they are *junk bonds* with a fairly high probability of going into default, and many financial institutions are prohibited from buying them.

Bond rating criteria

Although the rating assignments are subjective, they are based on both qualitative characteristics, such as "quality of management" and quantitative factors, such as a firm's financial strength. Analysts at the rating

Table 6.5   Bond Ratings

Credit Risk	Moody's	Standard & Poor's
Prime	Aaa	AAA
Excellent	Aa	AA
Upper medium	A	A
Lower medium	Baa	BBB
Speculative	Ba	BB
Very speculative	B	B
	Caa	CCC
		CC
Default	Ca	D
	C	

Note: Both Moody's and S&P use "modifiers" for bond rates below triple A. S&P uses a plus and minus system; thus A+ designates the strongest A-rated bonds and A— the weakest. Moody's uses a 1, 2, or 3 designation, with 1 denoting the strongest and 3 the weakest; thus, within the double-A category, Aa1 is the best, Aa2 is average, and Aa3 is the weakest. Triple-A bonds have no modifiers in either system.

agencies have consistently stated that no precise formula is used to set a firm's rating—many factors are taken into account, but not in a mathematically precise manner. Statistical studies have borne out this contention. Researchers who have tried to predict bond ratings on the basis of quantitative data have had only limited success, indicating that the agencies do indeed use a good deal of subjective judgment to establish a firm's rating.

Table 6.6 presents a financial glimpse of stand-alone hospitals recently rated by Standard & Poor's. Note that these hospitals are not part of chains, nor did they use credit enhancement, as discussed in the next major section. Standard & Poor's indicated that during this time of structural change in the health care industry, other business fundamentals besides financial indicators must be considered when assigning a credit rating, including location, market position, operating efficiency, and attractiveness to managed care plans.

Importance of bond ratings

Bond ratings are important both to firms and to investors. First, a bond's rating is an indicator of its default risk, so the rating has a direct, measurable influence on the default risk premium set by investors, and hence on the bond's interest rate and the firm's cost of debt capital. Second, most corporate (taxable) bonds are purchased by institutional investors, not by individuals, and many of these institutions are restricted to investment-grade securities. Also, most individual investors who buy

Table 6.6   Standard & Poor's 1993 New Hospital Ratings

| | | *Average* | | | |
| | | | | | |
Rating	*Number of Hospitals*	*Bed Size*	*Occupancy Rate*	*Profit Margin*	*Debt Ratio*
AA	6	621	81%	9.3%	26%
AA−	3	554	65	5.3	25
A+	15	494	77	5.7	40
A	19	290	62	5.5	36
A−	32	247	64	5.0	38
BBB+	20	224	58	4.6	41
BBB	19	269	68	2.4	59
BBB−	9	192	68	5.5	38

Source: Standard & Poor's Corporation *CreditWeek Municipal.*

municipal bonds are unwilling to take high risks in their bond purchases. Thus, if a firm's bonds fall below BBB, it will have a harder time trying to sell new bonds, because the number of potential purchasers is reduced.

As a result of their higher risk and more restricted market, lower-grade bonds have much higher interest rates than do high-grade bonds. This point was highlighted in Table 6.2, which shows that investors require higher rates of return on both corporate and municipal bonds with lower ratings.

Changes in ratings

A change in a firm's bond rating will have a significant effect on its ability to borrow long-term capital, and on the cost of that capital. Rating agencies review outstanding bonds on a periodic basis, occasionally upgrading or downgrading a bond as a result of the issuer's changed circumstances. Also, an announcement that a company plans to sell a new debt issue, or to merge with another company and pay for the acquisition by exchanging bonds for the stock of the acquired company, will trigger an agency review and possibly will lead to a rating change. If a firm's situation has deteriorated somewhat, but its bonds have not been reviewed and downgraded, then it may choose to use a term loan or short-term debt rather than to finance through a public bond issue. This will perhaps postpone a rating agency review until the situation has improved.

To illustrate a ratings change, on February 22, 1994, Moody's raised its rating on Hospital Corporation of America's $750 million of senior unsecured bonds from Ba to Baa, and thus pushed HCA's debt into the investment grade category. In the announcement, Moody's stated that the upgrade reflects "the significant improvement in bondholder debt protection resulting from the merger with Columbia Healthcare Corporation."

Self-Test Questions:

What are the two major rating agencies?

What are some criteria the rating agencies use when assigning ratings?

What impact does bond rating have on the cost of debt to the issuing firm?

Credit Enhancement

Credit enhancement, or *bond insurance,* which is available only for municipal bonds, is a relatively recent development for upgrading a bond's rating to AAA. Credit enhancement is offered by several credit insurers, the three largest being the Municipal Bond Investors Assurance (MBIA) Corporation, AMBAC Indemnity Corporation, and Financial Guaranty Insurance Corporation, a subsidiary of General Electric Capital Corporation. Currently, almost 60 percent of all new health care municipal issues carry bond insurance.

Here is how credit enhancement works. Regardless of the inherent credit rating of the issuer, the bond insurance company guarantees that bondholders will receive the promised interest and principal payments. Thus, bond insurance protects investors against default by the issuer. Because the insurer gives its guarantee that payments will be made, the bond carries the credit rating of the insurance company, not the issuer. For example, in our discussion on the bonds issued by Sabal Palm Medical Center, we noted that the bonds were rated AAA because of MBIA insurance. The hospital itself has an A rating, and hence bonds issued without credit enhancement would be rated A. The guarantee by MBIA resulted in the AAA rating.

Credit enhancement gives the issuer access to the lowest possible interest rate, but not without a cost. Bond insurers typically charge an up-front fee of about 0.2 to 0.5 percent of the total debt service over the life of the bond. Of course, the lower the hospital's inherent credit rating, the higher the cost of bond insurance. About 70 percent of newly issued insured municipal bonds have an underlying credit rating of AA or A. The remainder are still of investment grade, rated BBB.

Thus far, issuers have defaulted on very few insured bonds. For example, in its 20-year existence, MBIA has had to cover only two defaults: a $30 million hospital issue and a $12 million housing issue. However, many insurance analysts question the ability of the bond insurers to cover default payments should a severe recession occur. Furthermore, the market as a whole has some reservations about bond insurance because interest rates on AAA insured issues tend to be slightly higher than rates on bonds that carry an uninsured AAA rating.

Self-Test Questions:

What does the term "credit enhancement" mean?

Why would health care issuers seek bond insurance?

Debt Valuation

Now that you know the basic facts about long-term debt, the next step is to understand how investors value debt securities. Your reaction at this point might be: "Why should I have to worry about security valuation when what I really want to learn is health care financial decision making?" Security valuation concepts are important to health care financial decision making for many reasons. Here are just a few:

1. The life blood of any business is capital. In fact, one of the most common reasons for small business failures is insufficient capital. Therefore, it is vital that health care managers understand how investors make investment allocation decisions.

2. For investor-owned firms, stock price maximization is an important goal, if not the most important, so health care managers of for-profit firms must know how investors value the firm's securities to understand how managerial actions affect stock price.

3. For health care managers to make financially sound investment decisions regarding real assets (plant and equipment), it is necessary to estimate the business's cost of capital, and security valuation is a necessary skill in this process. We will discuss the cost of capital in Chapter 8.

4. One decision that all health care managers must face is the appropriate mix of debt and equity financing. An understanding of stock and bond valuation is critical to this decision, so the concepts presented in this chapter will be used again in Chapter 9.

5. Real assets are valued in the same general way as securities. Thus, security valuation provides health care managers with an excellent foundation to learn real asset valuation, the heart of capital investment decision making within firms. The concepts presented here are crucial to a good understanding of Chapters 10 and 11.

The general valuation model

In most situations, individuals and institutions buy assets for one reason: to receive the cash flows that the asset is expected to produce. Since the values of most assets stem from streams of expected cash flows, all such assets are valued by the same four-step process:

1. *Estimate the expected cash flow stream.* Estimating the cash flow stream involves estimating both the expected cash flow in each period and the riskiness of the cash flows. For some types of

assets, such as Treasury securities, the estimation process is quite easy—the interest and principal repayment stream is known with some certainty. For other types of assets, such as the stock of a biotechnology start-up company that is not yet paying dividends, the estimation process can be very difficult.

2. *Set the required rate of return.* The required rate of return on the cash flow stream is established on the basis of the stream's riskiness and the returns available on alternative investments of similar risk. Again, in some situations it will be fairly easy to assess the riskiness of the estimated cash flow stream; in other situations it may be quite difficult. Once the riskiness is assessed, the opportunity cost principle is applied. By investing in one asset, the funds are no longer available to invest in alternative assets of similar risk. This opportunity loss sets the required rate of return on the asset being valued.

3. *Discount the expected cash flows.* Each cash flow is now discounted at the asset's required rate of return.

4. *Sum the present values.* The final step is to sum the present values of the individual cash flows to find the value of the asset.

The following time line formalizes the valuation process:

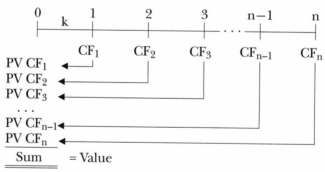

Here, CF_t is the expected cash flow in each Period t, k is the required rate of return (opportunity cost rate) on the asset, and n is the number of periods for which cash flows are expected. The periods can be months, quarters, semiannual periods, or years, depending on the frequency of the cash flows expected from the asset.

Note that the general valuation model can be applied to both *financial assets* (or *securities*), such as stocks and bonds, and *real* (or *physical*) *assets,* such as buildings, equipment, and even whole businesses. Each of the asset types requires a somewhat different application of the general valuation model, but the basic approach remains the same. We will first apply the general valuation model to a specific type of security, bonds. Later, we will apply the model to other types of securities and to real assets.

Some basic definitions

To begin, we need to discuss some basic bond terminology:

1. *Par value.* The par value, or just *par*, is the stated face value of the bond; it is often set at $1,000 or $5,000. The par value generally represents the amount of money the firm borrows and promises to repay at some future date.

2. *Maturity date.* Bonds generally have a specified maturity date on which the par value will be repaid. For example, Biomatic Corporation, a biotechnology firm, issued $50 million worth of $1,000 par value bonds on January 1, 1996. The bonds will mature on December 31, 2010, so they had a 15-year maturity at the time they were issued. Most bonds have original maturities of from 10 to 40 years, but the effective maturity of a bond declines each year after it was issued. Thus, at the beginning of 1997, Biomatic's bonds will have a 14-year maturity, and so on.

3. *Coupon rate.* A bond requires the issuer to pay a specific amount of interest each year (or, more typically, each six months). The rate of interest is called the *coupon interest rate*, or just *coupon rate*. The rate may be variable, in which case it is tied to some index, such as two percentage points above the prime rate. More commonly, the rate will be fixed over the maturity of the bond. For example, Biomatic's bonds have a 10 percent coupon rate, so each $1,000 bond pays 0.10($1,000) = $100 in interest each year. The dollar amount of annual interest, in this case $100, is called the *coupon payment*. The term *coupon* goes back to the time when bonds were *bearer bonds*. Bearer bonds had small coupons attached, one for each interest payment. To collect the interest, bondholders would send the coupon to the issuer, or take it to a bank, where it would be exchanged for the dollar payment. Today, all bonds are *registered bonds*, and interest payments are automatically sent to the registered owner.

4. *New issues versus outstanding bonds.* As we shall see, a bond's value is determined by its coupon payments—the higher the coupon payments,

other things held constant, the higher its value. At the time a bond is issued, its coupon rate is generally set at a level that will cause the bond to sell at its par value. In other words, the coupon rate is set at the going interest rate. A bond that has just been issued is called a *new issue.* Once the bond has been on the market for a while, about a month, it is classified as an *outstanding bond,* or a *seasoned issue.* New issues sell close to par, but since a bond's coupon payments are generally constant, when economic conditions change, and hence interest rates change, a seasoned bond will sell for more or less than its par value.

5. *Debt service payments.* Firms that issue bonds are concerned with their total debt service payments, which includes both interest expense and repayment of principal. For Biomatic, the debt service payment is 0.10($50 million) = $5 million per year until maturity. In 2010, the firm's debt service payment will be $5 million in interest plus $50 million in principal repayment, for a total of $55 million. In Biomatic's case, only interest is paid until maturity, so the entire principal amount must be repaid at that time. Many issues, such as Sabal Palm Medical Center's muni bonds discussed earlier, are structured so that the debt service requirements are constant over time. In this situation, the issuer pays back a portion of the principal during each year.

The basic bond valuation model

Bonds call for the payment of a specific amount of interest for a specific number of years, and for the repayment of par on the bond's maturity date. Thus, a bond represents an annuity plus a lump sum, and its value is found as the present value of this cash flow stream:

$$
\text{Value} = V = \frac{I}{(1+k_d)^1} + \frac{I}{(1+k_d)^2} + \cdots + \frac{I}{(1+k_d)^n}
$$
$$
+ \frac{M}{(1+k_d)^n}
$$
$$
= \sum_{t=1}^{n} I\left(\frac{1}{1+k_d}\right)^t + M\left(\frac{1}{1+k_d}\right)^n. \tag{6.3}
$$

Here

I = Dollars of interest paid each year = Coupon rate × Par value.

M = par, or maturity value.

k_d = required rate of return on the bond. As discussed earlier in the chapter, $k_d = k^* + IP + DRP + LP + MRP$.

n = number of years until maturity. n declines each year after the bond is issued.

Here are the cash flows from Biomatic's bonds on a time line:

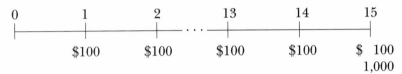

If the bonds had just been issued, and the coupon rate was set at the current interest rate for bonds of this risk, then $k_d = 10\%$. Since the value of the bond is merely the present value of the bond's cash flows, discounted to Time 0 at a 10 percent discount rate, the value of the bond at issue was $1,000:

Present value of a 15-period, $100 payment annuity at 10 percent	= $ 760.61
Present value of a $1,000 lump sum discounted 15 periods	= 239.39
Value of bond, V,	= $1,000.00

The value of the bond can be found using most financial calculators as follows:

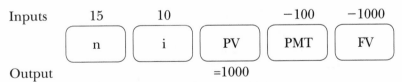

Input n = 15, i = 10, PMT = −100, and FV = −1,000, and then press the PV key to get the answer, 1,000. (We treated the cash flows as outflows so that the value would be displayed as a positive number.) Also, note that in bond valuation, all five of the time-value-of-money keys on a calculator are used, since bonds involve both an annuity payment and a lump sum.

If k_d remained constant at 10 percent over time, what would be the value of the bond one year after it was issued? Now, the term to maturity

is only 14 years—that is, n = 14. We see that the bond's value remains at
$1,000:

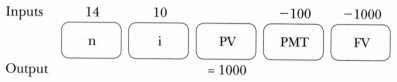

Inputs   14   10   −100   −1000

| n | i | PV | PMT | FV |

Output   = 1000

Now suppose that interest rates in the economy fell after the
Biomatic bonds were issued, and, as a result, k_d decreased from 10
percent to 5 percent. The coupon rate and par value are fixed by
contract, so they remain unaffected by changes in interest rates, but
now the discount rate is 5 percent rather than 10 percent. At the end of
the first year, with 14 years remaining, the value of the bond would be
$1,494.93:

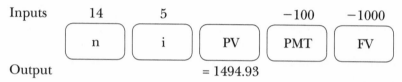

Inputs   14   5   −100   −1000

| n | i | PV | PMT | FV |

Output   = 1494.93

The arithmetic of the bond value increase should be clear, but what
is the logic behind it? The fact that k_d has fallen to 5 percent means that
if you had $1,000 to invest, you could buy new bonds like Biomatic's
(every day some 10 to 20 companies sell new bonds), except that these
new bonds would only pay $50 in interest each year. Naturally, you would
favor $100 to $50, so you would be willing to pay more than $1,000 for
Biomatic's bonds. All investors would recognize this and, as a result, the
Biomatic bonds would be bid up in price to $1,494.93, at which point
they would provide the same rate of return as new bonds of similar risk—
5 percent.

Assuming that interest rates stay constant at 5 percent over the next
14 years, what would happen to the value of a Biomatic bond? It would
fall gradually from $1,494.93 at present to $1,000 at maturity, when the
company will redeem each bond for $1,000. We can illustrate the point
by calculating the value of the bond one year later, when it has 13 years
remaining to maturity:

Inputs   13   5   −100   −1000

| n | i | PV | PMT | FV |

Output   = 1469.68

The value of the bond with 13 years to maturity is $1,469.68.

Notice that if you purchased the bond at a price of $1,494.93, and then sold it one year later with interest rates still at 5 percent, you would have a capital loss of $25.25. Your rate of return on the bond over the year consists of an *interest*, or *current*, *yield* plus a *capital gains yield*:

Current yield	=	$100/$1,494.93	=	0.0669 = 6.69%
Capital gains yield	=	−$25.25/$1,494.93	=	−0.0169 = −1.69%
Total rate of return, or yield	=	$74.75/$1,494.93	=	0.0500 = 5.00%

Had interest rates risen from 10 to 15 percent during the first year after issue rather than fallen, the value of Biomatic's bonds would have declined to $713.78 at the end of the first year. If interest rates held constant at 15 percent, the bond would have a value of $720.84 at the end of the second year, so the total yield to investors would be:

Current yield	=	$100/$713.78	=	0.1401 = 14.01%
Capital gains yield	=	$7.06/$713.78	=	0.0099 = 0.99%
Total rate of return, or yield	=	$107.06/$713.78	=	0.1500 = 15.00%

Figure 6.3 graphs the values of the Biomatic bond over time, assuming that interest rates (1) remain constant at 10 percent, (2) fall to 5 percent and then remain at that level, and (3) rise to 15 percent and remain constant at that level. Of course, interest rates do not remain level, so a bond's price fluctuates as (1) interest rates in the economy fluctuate and (2) the bond's term to maturity decreases. Figure 6.3 illustrates the following important points:

1. Whenever the going rate of interest, k_d, is equal to the coupon rate, a bond will sell at its par value.
2. When interest rates fall after a bond is issued, the bond's value rises above its par value, and the bond is said to sell at a *premium*.
3. When interest rates rise after a bond is issued, the bond's value falls below its par value, and the bond is said to sell at a *discount*.
4. Bond prices and interest rates are inversely related. Increasing rates lead to falling prices, and decreasing rates lead to increasing prices.
5. The price of a bond will always approach its par value as its maturity date approaches, provided the firm does not default on the bond.

Figure 6.3   Time Path of the Value of a 15-Year, 10% Coupon,
$1,000 Par Value Bond When Interest Rates are 5%,
10%, and 15%

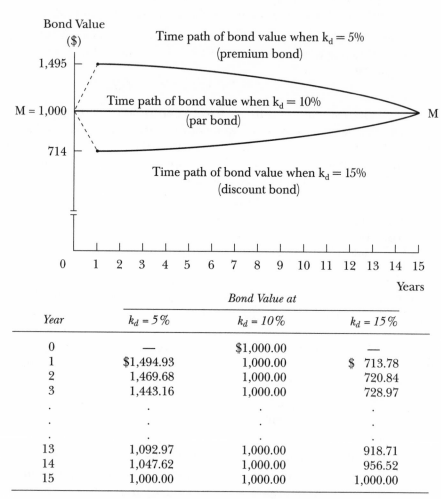

Year	$k_d = 5\%$	$k_d = 10\%$	$k_d = 15\%$
0	—	$1,000.00	—
1	$1,494.93	1,000.00	$ 713.78
2	1,469.68	1,000.00	720.84
3	1,443.16	1,000.00	728.97
.	.	.	.
.	.	.	.
.	.	.	.
13	1,092.97	1,000.00	918.71
14	1,047.62	1,000.00	956.52
15	1,000.00	1,000.00	1,000.00

Source: E. F. Brigham and L.C. Gapenski. 1994. *Financial Management: Theory and Practice,* 7th
ed. Fort Worth, TX: The Dryden Press.

Yield to maturity on a bond

Up to this point, we have assumed that k_d is known, and we have solved
for the value of the bond. In reality, investors' required rates of return

on securities are not observable, but security prices can be easily determined, as least on those securities that are actively traded, by looking in the local newspaper or the *Wall Street Journal.* Suppose the Biomatic bond had 14 years remaining to maturity, and the bond was selling at a price of $1,494.93. What rate of interest, or *yield to maturity (YTM)*, would you earn if you bought the bond at this price and held it to maturity? To find the answer, 5 percent, use your financial calculator as follows:

Inputs	14		1,494.93	−100	−1000
	n	i	PV	PMT	FV
Output		= 5.00			

The yield to maturity is identical to the total rate of return discussed in the previous section. In other words, the YTM is the expected rate of return on the bond if it is held to maturity and there is no chance that the firm will default on the bond payments. The YTM for a bond that sells at par consists entirely of an interest yield, but if the bond sells at a discount or premium, the YTM consists of the current yield plus a positive or negative capital gains yield.

Bond values with semiannual compounding

Virtually all bonds issued in the United States actually pay interest semiannually, or every six months. To apply the valuation concepts to semiannual bonds, we must modify the bond valuation procedures as follows:

1. Divide the annual interest payment, I, by 2 to determine the dollar amount paid each six months.
2. Multiply the number of years to maturity, n, by 2 to determine the number of semiannual interest periods.
3. Divide the annual required rate of return, k_d, by 2 to determine the semiannual required rate of return.

These changes result in the following equation for valuing a bond that pays semiannual interest:

$$\text{Value} = V = \sum_{t=1}^{2n} \frac{I}{2}\left(\frac{1}{1+k_d/2}\right)^t + M\left(\frac{1}{1+k_d/2}\right)^{2n}. \qquad (6.3a)$$

To illustrate the use of the semiannual bond valuation model, assume that the Biomatic bonds pay $50 every six months rather than $100 at the end of each year. Thus, each interest payment is only half as large, but there are twice as many of them. When the going rate of interest is 5 percent, the value of Biomatic's bonds with 14 years left to maturity is $1,499.12.

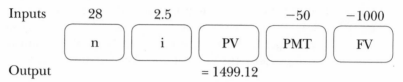

Similarly, if the bond were actually selling for $1,400 with 14 years to maturity, its YTM would be 5.80 percent.

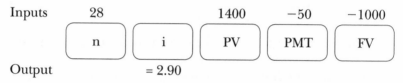

Note that the value for i, 2.90 percent, is the periodic (semiannual) YTM, so it is necessary to multiply it by 2 to get the annual YTM, which everyone uses in practice. Astute students will note that the effective annual YTM on the bond is somewhat greater than the 5.80 percent nominal YTM. However, it is convention in the bond markets to quote all rates on a nominal basis, so the procedures outlined in this section are correct when bonds, almost all of which have semiannual coupons, are being compared. However, when the returns on securities that have different periodic payments are being compared, all returns should be expressed as effective annual rates.

Interest rate risk

Interest rates change over time, which gives rise to two types of risk that fall under the general classification of *interest rate risk*. First, an increase in interest rates leads to a decline in the values of outstanding bonds. Since interest rates can rise, bondholders face the risk of losses on their holdings. This risk is called *price risk*. Second, many bondholders buy bonds to build funds for some future use. These bondholders reinvest the interest and principal cash flows as they are received. If interest rates fall, the bondholders will earn a lower rate on reinvested cash flows, which will have a negative impact on the future value of their holdings. This risk is called *reinvestment rate risk*.

To illustrate price risk, suppose you bought some of Biomatic's 10 percent bonds when they were issued at a price of $1,000. As illustrated earlier, if interest rates rise, the value of your bonds will fall. An investor's exposure to price risk depends on the maturity of the bonds. Figure 6.4, which shows the values of 1-year and 14-year bonds at several different market interest rates, illustrates price risk. Notice how much more sensitive the price of the 14-year bond is to changes in interest rates. For bonds with similar coupons, the longer the maturity of the bond, the greater its price changes in response to a given change in interest rates. Thus, even if the default risk on two bonds is the same, the one with the longer maturity is exposed to more price risk.

Although a 1-year bond exposes the buyer to less price risk than a 14-year bond, the 1-year bond carries with it more reinvestment rate risk. That is, if your holding period is more than one year, investment in a 1-year bond means that you would have to reinvest the principal and interest at the end of the first year. If interest rates fall, the return that you can get at that time is less than the return earned during the first year. Reinvestment rate risk is the second dimension of interest rate risk.

It is clear that bond investors face both price risk and reinvestment rate risk as a result of interest rate fluctuations over time. Which risk is most meaningful to a particular investor depends on the circumstances, but in general, interest rate risk, including both price and reinvestment rate risk, is reduced by matching the maturity of the bond with the anticipated investment horizon. For example, suppose Hilldale Community Hospital received a $5,000,000 contribution that it will use in five years to build a new neonatal care center. By investing the contribution in five-year bonds, the hospital would minimize its interest rate risk because it would be matching its investment horizon. Price risk would be minimized because the bond will mature in five years, and hence investors will receive par value regardless of prevailing interest rates. Reinvestment rate risk is also minimized because only the interest on the bond would have to be reinvested, a less risky situation than if both principal and interest had to be reinvested.

Hedging interest rate risk

Most financial and real asset transactions occur in the *spot*, or *cash*, *market*, in which the asset is delivered immediately (or within a few days). *Futures*, or *futures contracts*, on the other hand, call for the purchase or sale of a financial or real asset at some future date, but the price is fixed today. Futures markets are used for both speculation and hedging. *Speculation* involves betting on future price (or interest rate) movements, while *hedging* is done by both individuals and companies to protect

Figure 6.4   Value of Long- and Short-Term 10% Annual Coupon
Rate Bonds at Different Market Interest Rates

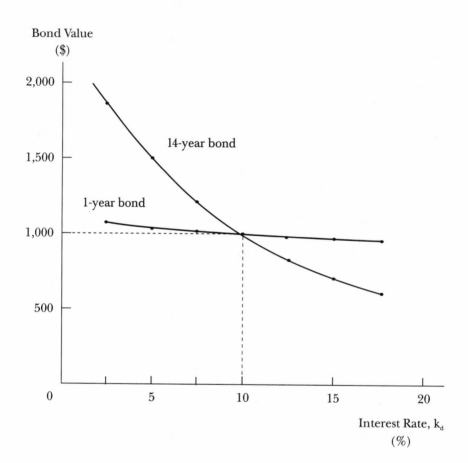

| Current Market | Bond Value | |
Interest Rate, k_d	*1-Year Bond*	*14-Year Bond*
2.5%	$1,073.17	$1,876.82
5.0	1,047.62	1,494.93
7.5	1,023.26	1,212.23
10.0	1,000.00	1,000.00
12.5	977.78	838.45
15.0	956.52	713.78
17.5	936.17	616.25

against price (or interest rate) changes that could adversely affect the profitability of some underlying transaction.

For example, suppose Midwest Medical Supply (MMS) Corporation plans to issue new bonds but will be unable to undertake the transaction for several months. In this situation, the cost of the issue will be adversely affected if interest rates rise during the waiting period. To protect against this adverse event, MMS can take a position in the futures market that will increase in value if interest rates do indeed rise. Then, the higher cost of the new issue will be offset by the profit earned on the firm's futures position.[6]

Self-Test Questions:

What is the general valuation model?

How are bonds valued?

What is meant by a bond's yield to maturity?

Differentiate between price risk and reinvestment rate risk.

How can interest rate risk be hedged?

Summary

This chapter provided an overview of business financing, described the nature of financial markets, and discussed how interest rates are determined. The chapter also described the characteristics of the major types of long-term debt securities, along with how such securities are valued. The key concepts covered are listed here:

• Any business must have assets if it is to operate, and in order to acquire assets, the firm must raise *capital.* Capital comes in two basic forms, *debt* and *equity (fund)* capital.

• There are many different types of *financial markets.* Each market serves a different set of customers or deals with a different type of security.

• Capital is allocated through the price system—a price is charged to "rent" money. Lenders charge *interest* on funds they lend, while equity investors receive dividends and capital gains in return for letting the firm use their money.

• Four fundamental factors affect the cost of money: (1) *investment opportunities;* (2) *time preferences for consumption;* (3) *risk;* and (4) *inflation.*

- The *nominal interest rate* on a debt security, k_d, is composed of the real risk-free rate, k^*, plus premiums that reflect inflation (IP), default risk (DRP), liquidity (LP), and maturity risk (MRP):

$$k_d = k^* + IP + DRP + LP + MRP.$$

- The relationship between the yields on securities and the securities' maturities is known as the *term structure of interest rates,* and the *yield curve* is a graph of this relationship.

- *Term loans* and *bonds* are long-term debt contracts under which a borrower agrees to make a series of interest and principal payments on specific dates to the lender. A term loan is generally sold to one (or a few) lenders, while a bond is typically offered to the public and sold to many different investors.

- There are many different types of bonds, including *mortgage bonds, debentures, and municipal bonds.* The return required on each type of bond is determined by prevailing interest rates, the bond's riskiness, and tax consequences.

- *Revenue bonds* are municipal bonds in which the revenues derived from such projects as roads or bridges, airports, water and sewage systems, and not-for-profit health care facilities are pledged as security for the bonds.

- A bond's *indenture* is a legal document that spells out the rights of the bondholders and of the issuing corporation. A *trustee* is assigned to make sure that the terms of the indenture are carried out.

- A *call provision* gives the issuing corporation the right to redeem the bonds prior to maturity under specified terms, usually at a price greater than the maturity value (the difference is a *call premium*). A firm will typically call a bond issue and refund it if interest rates fall substantially.

- A *put provision* gives the bondholder the right to return the bonds to the issuer prior to maturity and receive the maturity value. Bondholders will typically exercise a put provision when interest rates rise.

- A *sinking fund* is a provision that requires the corporation to retire a portion of the bond issue each year. The purpose of the sinking fund is to provide for the orderly retirement of the issue. No call premium is paid to the holders of bonds called for sinking fund purposes.

- Bonds are assigned *ratings* that reflect the probability of their going into default. The higher a bond's rating, the lower its interest rate.

- *Credit enhancement*, or *bond insurance*, upgrades a municipal bond rating to AAA. Regardless of the inherent credit rating of the issuer, the bond insurance company guarantees that bondholders will receive the promised interest and principal payments.

- Bonds call for the payment of a specific amount of *interest* for a specific number of years, and for the *repayment of par* on the bond's maturity date. Like most assets, a bond's value is simply the present value of the expected cash flow stream.

- The annual rate of return on the bond consists of an *interest*, or *current*, *yield* plus a *capital gains yield*. If the bond is selling at a *discount*, the capital gains yield is positive; if the bond is selling at a *premium*, the capital gains yield is negative.

- A bond's *yield to maturity (YTM)* is the rate of return earned on a bond if it is held to maturity (and no default occurs). The YTM for a bond that sells at par consists entirely of an interest yield, but if the bond sells at a discount or premium, the YTM consists of the current yield plus a positive or negative capital gains yield.

- Bondholders face *price risk* because bond values change when interest rates change. An investor's exposure to price risk depends on the maturity of the bonds.

- Bondholders face *reinvestment rate risk* when the investment horizon exceeds the maturity of the bond issue.

- The *futures market* can be used to *hedge*, or protect, the firm against price (or interest rate) changes that would have an adverse impact on the profitability of some underlying transaction.

Notes

1. For an illustration of a not-for-profit firm's balance sheet, see Table 12.2 in Chapter 12.
2. Some investor-owned companies also issue *preferred stock*, which has some characteristics of debt and some characteristics of common equity, although it typically does not carry ownership rights. Preferred stock will be discussed in Chapter 7.

3. *Treasury bills (T-bills)* are debt instruments issued by the federal government that have maturities of one year or less. *Treasury notes (T-notes)* have original maturities of two to ten years, and *Treasury bonds (T-bonds)* have original maturities over ten years. Note that when T-notes or T-bonds that were issued years ago have but six months to maturity, they are still called notes or bonds. The designation is based on the maturity of the security when issued, and not the maturity today.

4. To be precise, the rate should be $k_{RF} = (1 + k^*)(1 + IP) - 1.0 = (1.03)(1.04) - 1.0 = 1.0712 - 1.0 = 0.0712 = 7.12\%$. However, the difference between the precise calculation and the approximation given by $k_{RF} = k^* + IP$ is generally small, so the approximation method is often used in practice.

5. For a discussion of the forces that influence the shape of the yield curve, see E. F. Brigham and L. C. Gapenski, *Financial Management: Theory and Practice* (Fort Worth, TX: Dryden Press, 1997), chap. 3.

6. For a more complete discussion of interest rate risk and how such risk can be minimized, see E. F. Brigham and L. C. Gapenski, *Intermediate Financial Management* (Fort Worth, TX: Dryden Press, 1996), chap. 25.

Selected Additional References

Aderholdt, J. M. and C. R. Pardue. 1989. "A Guide to Taxable Debt Financing Alternatives." *Healthcare Financial Management* (July): 58–66.

Carlile, L. L., and B. M. Serchuk. 1995. "The Coming Changes in Tax-Exempt Health Care Finance." *Journal of Health Care Finance* (Fall): 1–42.

Cleverley, W. O., and P. C. Nutt. 1984. "The Decision Process Used for Bond Rating—and Its Implications." *Health Services Research* (December): 615–37.

Culler, S. D. 1993. "Assessing Hospital Credit Risk: A Banker's View." *Topics in Health Care Financing* (Summer): 35–43.

———. 1993. "A Creditor's Perspective on the Hospital Industry." *Topics in Health Care Financing* (Summer): 12–20.

Elrod, J. L., Jr. 1986. "Can Municipal Bond Futures Contracts Minimize Financial Risk?" *Healthcare Financial Management* (April): 40–44.

Harris, J. P., and J. B. Price. 1988. "Finding Money under Your Nose Using New Capital Techniques," *Healthcare Financial Management* (July): 24–30.

Kaufman, K., and M. L. Hall. 1990. *The Capital Management of Health Care Organizations.* Ann Arbor, MI: Health Administration Press, chap. 5.

LeBuhn, J. 1994. "Primary Market Derivatives: Satisfying Investor Appetites." *Journal of Health Care Finance* (Winter): 11–21.

Mullner, R., D. Matthews, J. D. Kubal, and S. Andes. 1983. "Debt Financing: An Alternative for Hospital Construction Funding." *Healthcare Financial Management* (April): 18–24.

Nemes, J. 1991. "Dealing with the Authorities." *Modern Healthcare* (14 October): 22–29.

Odegard, B. M. 1988. "Tax-Exempt Financing under the Tax Reform Act of 1986." *Topics in Healthcare Financing* (Summer).

Prince, T. R., and R. Ramanan. 1994. "Bond Ratings, Debt Insurance, and Hospital Operating Performance." *Topics in Health Care Financing* (Fall): 36–50.

Sims, W. B.. 1984. "Financing Strategies for Long-Term Care Facilities." *Healthcare Financial Management* (March): 42–54.

Smith, S. D. 1994. "The Use of Interest Rate Swaps in Hospital Capital Finance." *Journal of Health Care Finance* (Winter): 35–44.

Sterns, J. B. 1994. "Emerging Trends in Health Care Finance." *Journal of Health Care Finance* (Winter): 1–10.

West, D. A. 1983. "Debt Financing in the 1980s: Is the Risk for Non-Profit Hospitals Too Great?" *Healthcare Financial Management* (April): 56–62.

Woodward, M. A. 1993. "Interest Rate Swaps: Financial Tool of the '90s." *Healthcare Financial Management* (November): 56–64.

Appendix 6A: Refunding Decisions

A great deal of long-term debt was sold in the early 1980s at interest rates going up to 18 percent on AA-rated corporate bonds and 14 percent on AA-rated municipal bonds. Since the period of call protection on much of that debt ended after five or ten years, and since interest rates generally fell during the remainder of the 1980s and early 1990s, many issuers elected to lower their interest expense by conducting bond *refundings*. In a refunding, the old bond issue is called and replaced with a new issue having a lower interest rate. There are costs involved in refunding, but there is also one major benefit: the issuer reduces the dollar amount of interest payments that it must make in the future. A refunding analysis is a classical application of discounted cash flow cost/benefit analysis— the issuer should refund the bond if the present value of the refunding savings exceeds the present value of the costs of refunding.

The easiest way to examine the refunding decision is through an example. Midwest Medical Supply (MMS) Corporation has outstanding a $60 million bond issue which has a 15 percent annual coupon and 20 years remaining to maturity. This 30-year issue, which was sold ten years ago, had flotation costs of $3 million, which the firm has been amortizing on a straight line basis over the 30-year original life of the issue. (Flotation costs, which will be discussed in Chapter 7, are the printing, accounting, legal, and investment banker expenses associated with new securities issues.) The bond has a call provision with ten-year call deferral, so the bond can now be called, but a 10 percent call premium is required. The firm's investment bankers have assured the company that it can sell a new $60-$70 million issue of 20-year annual coupon bonds at an interest rate of 12 percent. Flotation costs on a new issue would amount to $4 million. MMS's marginal federal-plus-state tax rate is 40 percent. Should the company refund the $60 million of 15 percent bonds?

The following steps outline the decision process; the steps are summarized in worksheet form in Table 6A.1.

1. *Determine the investment outlay required to refund the issue.*
   a. *Call premium.*

$$\text{Before tax: } 0.10(\$60,000,000) = \$6,000,000.$$
$$\text{After tax: } \$6,000,000(1-T) = \$6,000,000(0.60)$$
$$= \$3,600,000.$$

Although MMS must spend $6 million on the call premium, this is a tax-deductible expense in the year the call is made. Since the company is in the 40 percent marginal tax bracket, it saves $0.40(\$6,000,000) = \$2,400,000$ in taxes, for an after-tax cost of only $3,600,000. This amount is shown as a cost, or outflow, on Line 1 of Table 6A.1.

   b. *Flotation costs on the new issue.*

   Flotation costs on the new issue are $4,000,000, as shown on Line 2 of the worksheet. For tax purposes, flotation costs must be

Table 6A.1   Bond Refunding Worksheet

	Amount before Tax	Amount after Tax	Present Value at 7.2%
Investment Outlay at t = 0			
1. Call premium on old issue	($6,000,000)	($3,600,000)	($ 3,600,000)
2. Flotation costs on new issue	(4,000,000)	(4,000,000)	(4,000,000)
3. Tax savings on old issue flotation costs	2,000,000	800,000	800,000
4. Net investment outlay			($ 6,800,000)
Annual Flotation Cost Tax Effects at t = 1–20			
5. Benefit from new issue flotation costs	$ 200,000	$ 80,000	$ 834,505
6. Lost benefit on old issue flotation costs	(100,000)	(40,000)	(417,252)
7. Present value of amortization tax effects			$ 417,253
Savings Due to Refunding at t = 1–20			
8. Interest payment on old issue	$9,000,000	$5,400,000	
9. Interest payment on new issue	7,200,000	4,320,000	
10. Net interest savings		$1,080,000	$11,265,817
NPV of Refunding Decision			
11. NPV of refunding decison			$ 4,883,070

amortized (or spread) over the 20-year life of the new bond, and then used to reduce taxable income in each year. Therefore, the annual taxable income deduction is $4,000,000/20 = $200,000. Since MMS is in the 40 percent tax bracket, it has a tax savings of 0.40($200,000) = $80,000 a year for 20 years. In a refunding analysis, all cash flows must be discounted at the after-tax cost of new debt, which is 12%(1 − T) = 12%(0.6) = 7.2%. The present value of the new issue flotation cost tax savings, when discounted at 7.2 percent, is $834,505, which is shown as a savings, or inflow, on Line 5. Note that when choosing a discount rate to apply to a series of cash flows, the primary consideration is the riskiness of the cash flow stream. In a bond refunding, the cash flows are relatively safe—they are fixed by contract—so a relatively low discount rate should be chosen. What market rate reflects relatively low risk? The answer is the rate of return required on MMS's bonds, so it is chosen as the basis for the discount rate used in the refunding analysis.

c. *Flotation costs on the old issue.*

The flotation costs on the old issue were amortized and deducted from taxable income, just as we have done (item b.) on the new issue flotation costs. However, if the refunding takes place, MMS can immediately expense for tax purposes that portion of the old issue flotation costs that have not yet been expensed. Since ten years have passed since the old 30-year bond was originally issued, only one-third of the $3 million flotation costs have been expensed, leaving two-thirds, or $2 million, unexpensed. This immediate deduction from taxable income would create a 0.40($2,000,000) = $800,000 tax savings, or inflow, which is shown on Line 3. However, if the refunding takes place, MMS loses the opportunity to continue to expense the old flotation costs over time, so the $2,000,000/20 = $100,000 reduction in annual taxable income is lost. Thus, MMS loses the annual tax savings of 0.40($100,000) = $40,000 for the next 20 years. The present value of this lost savings, which is an opportunity cost of refunding, is $417,252, which is shown on Line 6. Note that because of the refunding, the remaining old flotation costs provide an immediate tax savings, rather than annual savings, over the next 20 years. Thus, the $800,000 − $417,252 = $382,748 net savings simply reflects the difference between the present value of tax benefits to be received in the future without the refunding versus the immediate benefit if the refunding takes place.

d. *Total after-tax investment outlay.*
The total investment outlay required at Time 0 to refund the bond issue is $6,800,000, which is shown on Line 4.

2. *Determine the net effect of flotation cost amortization.*
The net effect of the amortization of flotation costs on the old and new debt issues is $417,253 on a present value basis. This amount is shown on Line 7.

3. *Determine the annual interest savings.*

a. *Interest expense on old issue.*
The annual after-tax interest on the old issue is $5,400,000, which is shown on Line 8:

$$0.15(\$60,000,000)(0.60) = \$5,400,000.$$

b. *Interest expense on new issue.*
The annual after-tax interest on the new issue is $4,320,000, which is shown on Line 9:

$$0.12(\$60,000,000)(0.60) = \$4,320,000.$$

c. *Annual interest savings.*
The annual interest savings is $1,080,000, which is shown on Line 10:

$$\$5,400,000 - \$4,320,000 = \$1,080,000.$$

d. *PV of annual savings.*
The present value of $1,080,000 per year for 20 years, when discounted at 7.2 percent, is $11,265,817. This amount is also shown on Line 10.

3. *Determine the net present value (NPV) of the refunding.*

Net investment outlay	($ 6,800,000)
Amortization tax effects	417,253
Interest savings	11,265,817
NPV of refunding	$ 4,883,070

Because the net present value of the refunding is positive, the present value of the inflows exceeds the present value of the outflows. Thus, it would be profitable for MMS to refund the old bond issue.

Several other points should be noted. First, since the refunding is advantageous to the firm, it must be disadvantageous to bondholders; they must give up their 15 percent bonds and reinvest the proceeds in securities that have a lower interest rate. This points out the danger of a call provision to bondholders, and it also explains why bonds without a call provision command higher prices (and hence lower rates) than callable bonds. Second, although it is not emphasized in the example, we assumed that the firm raises the investment required to undertake the refunding operation (the $6,800,000 shown on Line 4) as debt. This should be feasible, because the refunding operation will reduce the firm's interest charges. Typically, firms raise the investment outlay by increasing the amount of the new issue. In our example, MMS might sell $67,000,000 of new bonds. Third, we set up the example so that the new issue had the same maturity as the remaining life of the old issue. Often, the old bonds have only a relatively short term to maturity (say, 5 to 10 years), while the new bonds have a longer maturity (say, 25 to 30 years). In this situation, a replacement chain analysis is required.[1] Fourth, not-for-profit firms conduct refunding analyses in exactly the same way as that presented in Table 6A.1. The only difference is that the tax rate is zero, and hence there are no direct tax effects to consider in the analysis.

Finally, refunding decisions are well suited for analysis with a spreadsheet program. The spreadsheet is easy to set up, and once it is, it is easy to vary the assumptions about the interest rate on the new issue and to see how such changes affect the refunding decision. To illustrate a spreadsheet format, we set up the analysis on a time line in Table 6A.2. All of the cash flows are after-tax amounts. The logic behind the flows is the same as presented earlier, and the net present value of the Line 8 net cash flows, when discounted at 7.2 percent, is $4,883,070, the same value we developed in Table 6A.1.

One closing point must be addressed: although our analysis shows that the refunding would be profitable now, it might be even more profitable if the issuer waits and refunds later. If interest rates continue to fall, then it might pay for MMS to delay the refunding. The mechanics of calculating the NPV of refunding is relatively simple, but the decision on when to refund is not simple at all because it requires a forecast of future interest rates. Thus, the refund now versus refund later decision is more a matter of judgment than of quantitative analysis.

Table 6A.2   Bond Refunding Time Line

	0	1	20
1. Call premium on old issue	($3,600,000)		
2. Flotation costs on new issue	(4,000,000)		
3. Tax savings on old issue flotation costs	800,000		
4. Benefit from new issue flotation costs		$ 80,000	$ 80,000
5. Lost benefit on old issue flotation costs		(40,000)	(40,000)
6. After tax payment on old issue		5,400,000	5,400,000
7. After tax payment on new issue		4,320,000	4,320,000
8. Net cash flow	($6,800,000)	$1,120,000	$1,120,000

Net present value (NPV) of the net cash flows when discounted at 7.2% = $4,883,070.

To illustrate the timing decision, assume that MMS's managers forecast that long-term interest rates have a 50 percent probability of remaining at their present level of 12 percent over the next year. However, there is a 25 percent probability that rates could fall to 10 percent, and a 25 percent probability that rates could rise to 14 percent. The refunding analysis could then be repeated, as previously, but assuming that it would take place one year from now, when the old bonds have only 19 years to maturity. (We assume also that the new issue would have a 19-year maturity.) We performed the analysis and found this NPV distribution one year from now:

Probability	*Interest Rate*	*NPV of Refunding One Year from Now*
25%	10%	$13,737,916
50	12	4,607,124
25	14	(3,067,344)

Note that if rates rose to 14 percent next year, and the NPV of refunding turned out to be negative, MMS would not refund the issue, so the realized NPV at a 14 percent interest rate would be $0. Thus, the expected NPV of refunding next year is $5,738,041, versus $4,883,070 if refunding takes place now:

$$0.25(\$13,737,916) + 0.50(\$4,607,124) + 0.25(\$0) = \$5,738,041.$$

Even though the expected NPV of refunding in one year is higher, MMS's managers would probably decide to refund today. First, when $5,738,041 is discounted back one year to today at some rate, say, a 10 percent rate, the NPV of refunding in one year drops to $5,216,401. More important, the NPV of refunding in one year is only an expected NPV, because it depends on future interest rates, while the NPV of refunding today is known with some certainty. MMS's managers would opt to delay funding only if the expected NPV today from refunding later is sufficiently above the refund now NPV to compensate for the risks involved.

Clearly, the decision to refund now versus refund later is complicated by the fact that there would be numerous opportunities to refund in the future rather than just a single opportunity one year from now. Furthermore, the decision must be based on a large set of interest rate forecasts, a daunting task in itself. Fortunately, managers making bond refunding decisions are advised by sophisticated investment bankers, who can now use the values of derivative securities to estimate the value of a bond's embedded call option. If the call option is worth more than the NPV of refunding today, the issue should not be immediately refunded. Rather, the issuer should either delay the refunding to take advantage of the information obtained from the derivative market or actually create a derivative transaction to lock in the value of the call option.

Note

1. A replacement chain analysis is required because (1) if the debt is not refunded, the firm will have to incur flotation costs again in 5 to 10 years, but (2) if the debt is refunded, those flotation costs are pushed out 25 or 30 years into the future. The difference in timing of future flotation costs must be accounted for in the analysis by a replacement chain. When the two issues have the same maturity, there is no difference in the timing of future flotation costs, and hence this aspect of the analysis can be ignored.

Case 6A

Big Bend Health Systems (A): Bond Valuation

Big Bend Health Systems, Inc., is an investor-owned hospital chain that owns and operates nine hospitals in Texas and New Mexico. George Waterman, a recent graduate of a prominent health services adminis-tration program, has just been hired by El Paso General, Big Bend's largest hospital. Like all new management personnel, Waterman must undergo three months of intensive indoctrination at the system level before joining the hospital.

Waterman began his indoctrination in January 1997. His first as-signment at the parent was to review Big Bend's latest annual report. This was a stroke of luck for Waterman, because his father owned several bonds issued by Big Bend, and Waterman was especially interested in whether or not his father had made a good investment. To glean more information about the firm's bonds, Waterman examined Note E to Big Bend's Consolidated Financial Statements, which lists the firm's long-term debt obligations, including its first mortgage bonds, installment contracts, and term loans. Table 1 contains information on three of the first mortgage bonds listed in Big Bend's annual report.

Table 1 Big Bend Health Systems: Partial Long-Term Debt Listing

Face Amount	Coupon Rate	Maturity Year	Years to Maturity
$ 48,000,000	4½	2001	5
$ 32,000,000	8¼	2011	15
$100,000,000	12⅝	2021	25

Unfortunately, Big Bend's chief financial officer (CFO), Maria Martinez, found out about Waterman's interest in the firm's debt financing. "As long as you are so interested in our firm's financial structure," she said, "here are some questions that I've developed as part of a debt financing presentation to our executive committee. See if you can answer them."

Waterman took this as a challenge, as he was convinced that he knew as much about debt financing as most finance MBAs. Apparently he was right, because he answered the questions with no difficulty. See how you do!

Questions

1. To begin, assume it is now January 1, 1997, and that each bond in Table 1 matures on December 31 of the year listed. Furthermore, assume that each bond has a $1,000 par value, each had a 30-year maturity when it was issued, and all three bonds currently have a 10 percent required nominal rate of return.

    a. Why do the bonds' coupon rates vary so widely?

    b. What would be the value of each bond if it had annual coupon payments?

    c. Big Bend's bonds, like virtually all bonds, actually pay interest semiannually. What is each bond's value under these conditions? Are the bonds currently selling at a discount or at a premium?

    d. What is the effective annual rate of return implied by the values obtained in Part (c)?

    e. Would you expect a semiannual payment bond to sell at a higher or lower price than an otherwise equivalent annual payment bond? Look at the values calculated in Parts (b) and (c) for the five-year bond; are the prices shown consistent with your expectations? Explain.

2. Now, regardless of your answers to Question 1, assume that the 5-year bond is selling for $800.00, the 15-year bond is selling for $865.49, and the 25-year bond is selling for $1,220.00. *(Use these prices, and assume semiannual coupons, for all of the remaining questions in this case.)*

    a. What is the nominal (as opposed to effective annual) yield to maturity (YTM) on each bond?

    b. What is the effective annual YTM on each issue?

    c. In comparing bond yields with the yields on other securities, should the nominal or effective YTM be used? In comparing yields among bonds, should the nominal or effective YTM be used? Explain.

    d. Explain in words the meaning of the term "yield to maturity."

3. Suppose Big Bend has a second bond with 25 years left to maturity (in addition to the one listed in Table 1), which has a coupon rate of 7⅜ percent and a market price of $747.48.

    a. What is (1) the nominal and (2) the effective annual YTM on this bond?

    b. What is the current yield on each of the 25-year bonds?

    c. What is each bond's expected price on January 1, 1998, and its capital gains yield for 1997, assuming no change in interest rates? (Hint: Remember that the nominal required rate of return on each bond is 10.18 percent.)

    d. What would happen to the price of each bond over time? (Again, assume constant future interest rates.)

    e. What is the expected total (percentage) return on each bond during 1997?

    f. If you were a tax-paying investor, which of the 25-year bonds would you prefer? Why? What impact would this preference have on the prices, and hence YTMs, of the two bonds?

4. Consider the riskiness of the bonds.

    a. Explain the difference between price risk and reinvestment rate risk.

    b. Which of the bonds listed in Table 1 has the most price risk? Why?

    c. Assume that you bought 5-year, 15-year, and 25-year bonds, all with a 10 percent coupon rate and semiannual coupons, at their $1,000 par values. Which bond's value would be affected most if interest rates rose to 13 percent? Which would be affected least?

    d. Assume that your investment horizon (or expected holding period) is 25 years. Which of the bonds listed in Table 1 has the greatest reinvestment rate risk? Why? Is there a type of bond you could buy to eliminate reinvestment rate risk?

e. Assume that you plan to keep your money invested, and to reinvest all interest receipts, for five years. Furthermore, assume you bought the five-year bond for $800, and interest rates suddenly fell to 5 percent and remained at that level for five years.

   (1) Set up a time line that can be used to calculate the actual realized rate of return on the bond. (Hint: Each interest receipt must be compounded to the terminal date and summed, along with the maturity value. Then, the rate of return that equates this terminal value to the initial price of the bond is the bond's realized return.) How does your answer compare with the bond's YTM?

   (2) What would have happened if interest rates had risen to 15 percent rather than fallen to 5 percent? How would the results have differed if you had bought the 25-year bond rather than the five-year bond?

f. Today, many bond market participants are speculators as opposed to long-term investors. If you thought interest rates were going to fall from current levels, what bond maturity would you buy to maximize short-term capital gains?

5. Now assume that the 15-year bond is callable after five years at $1,050.

   a. What is its yield to call (YTC)? (Hint: Set up the cash flows on a time line. If the bond is called, investors will receive interest payments for five years, and then receive $1,050 [$1,000 in principal and call premium of $50] at the end of five years. The YTM on this cash flow stream is the bond's YTC.)

   b. Do you think it is likely that the bond will be called?

6. Now consider another bond issued by Big Bend that has not yet been discussed. This bond has a par value of $1,000 and pays interest once a year at a 10 percent rate. The bond has a mandatory sinking fund provision that requires the firm to redeem one-fifth of the outstanding issue in each year beginning in Year 3 and continuing until the entire issue is retired in Year 7. If the required rate of return on this bond is 8.0 percent, what is the current (Year 0) value of the bond?

7. Discuss the basic differences between the bonds issued by investor-owned corporations and those issued by not-for-profit firms through municipal financing authorities.

8. Explain how investors set required rates of return on debt securities. (Hint: Think in terms of the real risk-free rate plus any risk borne by investors.)

9. What is the term structure of interest rates? What is a yield curve? Why is the yield curve important to both investors and managers?

10. Briefly describe the bond rating system. Be sure to include the names of the major rating agencies, the actual ratings used, the criteria for assigning ratings, and the importance of ratings to both investors and managers.

Case 6B

American Surgical, Inc.: Refunding Decisions

Robert Williams, financial vice president of American Surgical, Inc., a major manufacturer of surgical and dental instruments, has just begun reviewing the minutes of the company's final 1996 board of directors meeting. The major topic discussed at the meeting was whether American Surgical should refund any of its currently outstanding bond issues. Of particular interest is a $50 million, 30-year, 11.5 percent, first-mortgage bond issued approximately five years ago. Several of the board members had taken markedly different positions on the question, and at the conclusion of the meeting, John Danforth, chairman of the board, asked Williams to prepare a report analyzing the alternative points of view.

The bonds in question had been issued in January of 1992, when interest rates were relatively high. It was necessary to issue the bonds at that time, despite the high interest rates, because American Surgical needed immediately to complete the modernization and expansion of its manufacturing facilities if it was to meet rapidly growing demand for its products. At that time, Williams and the board strongly believed interest rates were at a peak and would decline in the future, but they were unsure when rates would fall or by how much. Now, almost five years later, with lower rates, American Surgical can sell A-rated bonds that yield significantly less than 11.5 percent.

Since Williams had anticipated a decline in interest rates when the company sold the $50 million issue, he had insisted that the bonds be made callable after five years. (If the bonds had not been callable, American Surgical would have had to pay an interest rate of only 10.8 percent, 70 basis points less than the actual 11.5 percent. If the bonds had been immediately callable, rather than having a deferred call, the coupon rate would have had to be pegged at 11.7 percent.) The bonds can be called on January 1, 1997 (Year 5), but an initial call premium of one year's interest payment, or $115 per bond, would have to be paid. This premium declines by $11.5\%/25 = 0.46$ percentage points, or $4.60, each year. Thus, if the bonds were called on January 1, 2002, the call premium would be $(11.5/25)(20) = 9.2\%$, or $92, where 20 represents the number of years remaining to maturity. The flotation costs on this issue amounted to 1.5 percent of the face amount, or $750,000. The firm's federal-plus-state tax rate is 40 percent.

Williams estimates that American Surgical can sell a new issue of 25-year first mortgage bonds at an interest rate of 10.0 percent. The call of the old and sale of the new bonds could take place five to seven weeks after the decision to refund has been made; this time is required to give legal notice to bondholders and to arrange the $50 million or more needed to pay them off. The flotation cost on the refunding issue would be 1 percent of the new issue's face amount, and funds from the new issue would be available from the underwriters the day they were needed to pay off the old bonds.

Williams had proposed at the last directors' meeting that the company call the 11.5 percent bonds at first opportunity and refund them with a new 10.0 percent issue. Although the refunding cost would be substantial, he believed that the interest savings of 150 basis points per year for 25 years on a $50 million issue would be well worth the cost. Williams did not anticipate adverse reactions from any of the board members; however, three of them voiced strong doubts about the refunding proposal. The first was Pamela Rosenberg, a long-term member of American Surgical's board and chairman of Rosenberg, Mathias & Company, an investment banking house catering primarily to institutional clients such as insurance companies and pension funds. Rosenberg argued that calling the bonds for refunding would not be well received by the major institutions that hold the firm's outstanding bonds. According to Rosenberg, the institutional investors who hold the bonds purchased them on the expectation of receiving the 11.5 percent interest rate for at least ten years, and these investors would be very disturbed by a call after only five years. Since most of the leading institutions hold some of American Surgical's bonds, and since the firm typically sells new bonds to finance its growth every four or five years, it would be most unfortunate if institutional investors developed a feeling of ill will toward the company.

A second director, Vincent Marchiano, who was a relatively new member of the board and president of a local bank, also opposed the call but for an entirely different reason. Marchiano believed that the decline in interest rates was not yet over. He said a study by his bank suggested that the long-term interest rate on highly rated mortgage bonds might fall to as low as 8 percent next year. Under questioning from the other board members, however, Marchiano admitted that the interest rate decline could in fact be over and that interest rates might begin to move back up again. When pressed, Marchiano produced the following probability distribution that the bank's economists had developed for interest rates on A-rated first mortgage bonds one year from now, on January 1, 1998:

Probability	Interest Rate on A-Rated First Mortgage Bonds
0.1	8.0%
0.2	9.0
0.4	10.0
0.2	11.0
0.1	12.0

The third director, Kim Mitchell, stated that she was not against the refunding, but wondered whether it was wise to sell the new bonds and call the old bonds at essentially the same time. Mitchell was worried that something might go wrong, keeping American Surgical from obtaining the cash generated by the sale of the new bonds in time to pay for the repurchase of the old bonds. Therefore, she suggested that American Surgical issue the new bonds two to three weeks before the refunding of the old bonds to ensure that sufficient cash would be on hand when the old bonds were repurchased. Mitchell also pointed out that the funds generated by the sale of the new bonds could be invested in T-bills yielding 5 percent during this overlap period. Finally, she noted that interest rates had been quite volatile lately, and that if rates rose before the new issue could be sold, but after the firm had committed to the refunding, the refunding would be a disaster. Therefore, she wondered if American Surgical could "lock in a profit," and thus protect itself against rising interest rates, by assuming a position in the futures market.

As Williams's assistant, you have been asked to draft responses to the following questions.

Questions

1. What discount rate should be used to perform the refunding analysis? Why?

2. Calculate the net present value of the refunding if American Surgical goes ahead with the new bond issue on January 1, 1997. (For ease of calculation, assume that both the old and the new bonds have annual coupons.)

3. Give a critique of each of the positions taken by the various board members. As a part of your answer, calculate the expected NPV of refunding next year based on Marchiano's probability distribution of interest rates. Remember, however, that if American Surgical refunds next year, the old bonds will have 24 years left to maturity. Assume for purposes of this question that American Surgical could issue the new bonds with a 24-year maturity. Also, remember that American Surgical would not act next year if the refunding had a negative NPV at that time.

4. When should American Surgical refund the bonds?

5. How would the nature of the probability distribution of expected future interest rates affect the decision to refund now or to wait? (Hint: To answer this question, consider (1) the expected value of the distribution, (2) the standard deviation of the distribution, and (3) any skewness that might occur in the distribution.)

6. Suppose the major bond rating agencies downgraded American Surgical's credit rating from A to triple-B before American Surgical could initiate the refunding, resulting in the following changes:

   (1). The coupon rate on the new bond is 10.5 percent.

   (2). The flotation cost on the new issue is 1.5 percent of the issue's face value, or $750,000.

   How would these factors affect the refunding decision?

7. If the yield curve had been downward sloping, and if Williams felt that "the market knows more than I do" about the future course of interest rates, how might this affect his decision to recommend immediate refunding versus deferred refunding? (Hint: The yield curve depicts the relationship between yield to maturity and term to maturity at a single point in time. According to the expectations theory of term structure, the shape of the curve reflects investors' expectations of future interest rates.)

8. Another bond that American Surgical is considering refunding is a $25 million, 30-year issue sold about 25 years ago in January 1972. At the time this bond was issued, American Surgical was in poor financial condition and was considered to be a relatively poor credit risk. To raise the $25 million, American Surgical was forced to issue subordinated debentures with a B rating and a coupon rate of 11.3 percent, which was quite high at the time. The flotation cost on this issue was 2 percent of the face amount, or $500,000. This issue is callable, with five-year call protection, and the call premium is determined in the same manner as on the bond discussed in the case. Robert Williams estimates that American Surgical could refund this $25 million issue with a 25-year, 10.5 percent coupon subordinated debenture that would require a flotation cost of $250,000. Assume that this $25 million of capital will be needed into the indefinite future, so whether the bond is refunded now or in five years, it will subsequently be refunded every 25 years with a 25-year, 10.5 percent bond, with each successive replacement bond remaining outstanding to its maturity. Is the refunding analysis you used in Question 2 appropriate for this bond? Explain how the analysis could be modified to make it better, and if you are using the spreadsheet model, complete the numerical analysis.

9. Describe how American Surgical could use the futures market to protect against a possible interest rate increase between the time the decision is made to refund the old issue and the time the refunding actually takes place. If you are using the spreadsheet model, plot the relationship between the refunding NPV and the interest rate on the new issue. Determine the breakeven interest rate; that is, the new issue interest rate that results in a refunding NPV of $0.

10. Do you think that a lower tax rate, say 20 percent, would make the refunding more or less attractive? If you are using the spreadsheet model, graph the relationship between refunding NPV and tax rate.

11. Now assume that the refunding is being evaluated by a not-for-profit hospital. Redo the Question 2 analysis, using the same data, but assume (1) that the relevant interest rates are 75 percent of the rates given to account for the fact that the debt would be tax exempt, and (2) that the call premium is calculated in the standard way, that is, one year's interest if the call is made at the end of Year 5. (Hint: There are no tax implications for a not-for-profit hospital.)

7

Equity (Fund) Financing

In Chapter 6, we discussed long-term debt financing, including how interest rates are set in the economy, the features of various long-term debt securities, and how debt securities, particularly bonds, are valued. The second primary source of long-term capital to health care firms is equity financing, which consists of preferred and common stock for investor-owned firms and fund capital for not-for-profit firms. In this chapter, we discuss the same general issues as in Chapter 6, but the focus is on equity financing. In addition, we will provide some supplemental information on how securities are sold, or the investment banking process.

Preferred Stock

Preferred stock, which can be issued only by investor-owned firms, is a hybrid—it is similar to bonds in some respects, and to common stock in other ways. Accountants classify preferred stock as equity, so it is shown on the balance sheet as an equity account. However, from a financial management perspective, preferred stock is probably closer in nature to debt than to equity. Preferred stock imposes a fixed charge on the company, and hence it increases the firm's financial leverage. However, unlike interest on debt, if a preferred dividend is missed, preferred stockholders do not have the legal right to force a firm into bankruptcy.

Basic features

Preferred stock usually has a stated *par*, or *face*, *value*, often $100. The dividend on preferred stock, which is almost always paid quarterly, is stated either as some percentage of par or as so many dollars per share. For example, in 1995, OnLine Health Resources, a company that develops "expert" software programs to help physicians make diagnoses, sold 50,000 shares of $100 par value preferred stock, raising a total $5 million of new capital. This issue had a stated dividend of 10 percent, so the annual dollar dividend was $10, or $2.50 each quarter. Preferred dividends are set when the stock is issued, so OnLine's preferred dividend will remain at $10 per year regardless of interest rate changes over time. Thus, if the required rate of return on OnLine's preferred increases to 12 percent, the value of the stock will fall, just as with bonds.

Although preferred stock contains a promise to pay the stated dividend, issuers do not have the contractual obligation to make the payment. Thus, like common stock, preferred stock dividends are declared each quarter by the firm's board of directors, and if the firm's financial condition deteriorates, the board can elect to *omit*, or *pass*, the dividend. However, most preferred issues are *cumulative*, meaning that the cumulative total of all unpaid preferred dividends must be paid before dividends can be paid on the firm's common stock. Unpaid preferred dividends are called *arrearages*, so all arrearages must be paid before common dividends can be paid.

Preferred stock typically carries no voting privileges, so preferred stockholders have no ownership rights. However, most preferred issues stipulate that preferred stockholders can elect a minority of directors— say, 3 out of 12—if the preferred dividends are passed. Even though nonpayment of preferred dividends will not bankrupt a company, companies issue preferred stock with every intention of paying the dividends. Passing a dividend usually precludes the payment of common dividends and places preferred stockholders on the board. Furthermore, companies with preferred dividends in arrears have a difficult time selling new debt, and find it almost impossible to sell new common or preferred stock.

Investors regard preferred stock as being riskier than debt for two reasons: (1) preferred dividends will be omitted before interest payments because default on interest payments has more serious consequences; and (2) in the event of bankruptcy and liquidation, preferred stockholders' claims are junior (subordinate) to debtholders' claims. Accordingly, investors require a higher rate of return on a firm's preferred stock than on its bonds. However, preferred stock has tax advantages to corporate buyers because 70 percent of the preferred dividends received by a corporation are exempt from corporate taxes. Thus, a corporate buyer of OnLine's preferred stock in the 40 percent tax bracket would pay 40 percent taxes on 30 percent of the preferred dividend, for an effective tax rate of only $(0.40)(0.30) = 0.12 = 12$ percent. If the corporate buyer purchased OnLine's debt, it would have to pay taxes on the interest earned at the full 40 percent rate. Corporate demand for tax-advantaged preferred stock tends to lower returns on preferred stocks to the point where before-tax returns are actually lower on preferred stocks than on lower-risk bonds. For this reason, almost all ordinary preferred stock is sold to corporate, rather than individual, investors.

Almost half of all preferred stock sold in recent years is *convertible*, meaning that the preferred stock can be converted, or exchanged, into a set number of shares of common stock. The number of common shares obtained by conversion is fixed when the preferred is issued so that immediate conversion makes no financial sense. Over time, however, if the price on the firm's common stock rises, a point is reached when the holders of the preferred stock will be better off if they convert the preferred into common.

Some older preferred stocks are similar to perpetual bonds in that they have no maturity date. However, most preferred stock issued in recent years has had either sinking fund or call provisions that limit the life of the issue. For example, many preferred shares have a sinking fund that calls for the retirement of 2 percent of the issue each year, meaning that the average maturity of the issue is 25 years, and that the issue will be totally refunded in 50 years.

Preferred stock valuation

Most preferred stocks entitle their owners to regular, fixed dividend payments. If the stock is perpetual preferred, meaning that the payments are expected to last forever, then the stock can be valued using a simple perpetuity formula:

$$V_p = \frac{D_p}{k_p}. \tag{7.1}$$

Here, V_p is the value of the preferred stock, D_p is the preferred dividend, and k_p is the required rate of return on the stock. For example, OnLine's preferred dividend is $10 per year. If interest rates have risen since the stock was issued, and the required rate of return is now 12 percent, the value of the stock is $83.33:

$$V_p = \frac{\$10}{0.12} = \$83.33.$$

The required rate of return on the issue would be determined in the same manner as for debt, as we discussed in Chapter 6. Note that the value could also be determined using quarterly data, with a quarterly dividend of $10/4 = $2.50 and a quarterly required rate of return of 12%/4 = 3%:

$$V_p = \frac{\$2.50}{0.03} = \$83.33.$$

In general, the current price, P_p, of the preferred stock is known, and investors want to find the rate of return on the issue. This can be done easily by rearranging Equation 7.1:

$$k_p = \frac{D_p}{P_p}. \qquad (7.1a)$$

For example, the rate of return on OnLine's preferred stock, if it is currently selling for $85, is 11.8 percent:

$$k_p = \frac{\$10}{\$85} = 11.8\%.$$

Using the quarterly dividend of $2.50 and a price of $85 gives a quarterly rate of return of 2.94 percent, which converts to a nominal annual rate of 11.8 percent and an effective annual rate of 12.3 percent, which considers the effect of quarterly compounding.

If the preferred stock being valued is not perpetual, but rather has limited life due to sinking fund or call provisions, it would be valued using the debt valuation techniques described in Chapter 6.

Self-Test Questions:

Should preferred stock be considered as equity or debt financing? Explain.

Who are the major purchasers of nonconvertible preferred stock? Why?

How is perpetual preferred stock valued? How is finite-life preferred stock valued?

Legal Rights and Privileges of Common Stockholders

Common stockholders are the owners of for-profit corporations, and as such they have certain rights and privileges. The most important of these rights are discussed in this section.

Claim on residual earnings

The reason why most people buy common stocks is to gain the right to a proportionate share of the residual earnings of the firm. A firm's net income, which is the residual earnings after all expenses have been paid, belongs to the firm's common stockholders. Some portion of net income will typically be paid out in *dividends* each quarter, so stockholders receive quarterly cash payments. In addition, the portion of net income that is retained within the firm will be invested in new assets, which presumably will increase the firm's earnings, and hence dividends, over time.

An increasing dividend stream means that the firm's stock will be more valuable in the future than it is today, because dividends will be higher, say, in five years, than they are today. Thus, common stockholders typically expect to be able, at some time in the future, to sell the stock they purchased at a higher price than they paid for it, and hence to realize a *capital gain*. To illustrate the payment of dividends, consider Table 7.1, which lists the annual per share dividend payment and earnings, as well as the average annual stock price, for Big Sky Healthcare from 1985 through 1995. Over the ten growth periods, Big Sky's dividend grew by 275 percent, or at an average annual growth rate of 14.1 percent. At the same time, the firm's stock price grew by 247 percent, which is an average annual growth rate of 13.2 percent.

Note that Big Sky's dividend growth was not a constant 14.1 percent each year. Many firms hold the dividend constant for several years to

Table 7.1   Big Sky Healthcare: Dividends, Earnings, and Stock Prices, 1985–1995

Year	Annual Per Share Dividend	Annual Per Share Earnings	Annual Average Stock Price
1985	$0.20	$0.48	$ 7.70
1986	0.23	0.55	10.95
1987	0.23	0.52	11.00
1988	0.23	0.58	10.40
1989	0.48	0.85	15.30
1990	0.52	1.10	18.70
1991	0.58	1.25	20.60
1992	0.58	0.45	19.50
1993	0.65	1.35	23.20
1994	0.70	1.50	24.40
1995	0.75	1.55	26.70

allow earnings to climb to a point where they can support a higher dividend payment. For example, Big Sky kept its dividend at $0.23 a share from 1986 through 1988, while earnings per share were flat at about $0.55.

In general, managers are very reluctant to reduce dividends, because investors interpret lower dividends as a signal that management forecasts poor times ahead. Thus, when Big Sky saw its earnings per share tumble from $1.25 in 1991 to $0.45 in 1992, it maintained its $0.58 per share dividend. Big Sky was able to pay a cash dividend that exceeded earnings in 1992 because the firm's cash flow, which is roughly equal to Net income + Depreciation, easily supported the dividend. When earnings picked up again in 1993, Big Sky increased its dividend to $0.65.

Over the entire period, Big Sky has proved to be a good investment for stockholders. For example, assume that you bought the stock for $7.70 in 1985, received a $0.20 dividend payment, and then sold the stock one year later for $10.95. For simplicity, assume that the dividend payment, rather than occurring quarterly, was paid at the end of the one-year holding period. Thus, you paid $7.70, and one year later you received $10.95 + $0.20 = $11.15. The total return earned was Total profit/Amount of investment = ($11.15 − $7.70)/$7.70 = 0.448 = 44.8%. (Or, using a financial calculator, enter PV = 7.70 [or −7.70], FV = 11.15, n = 1, and press i to get 44.8 percent.) Note, however, that investors who bought Big Sky's stock in 1987 or 1991 and then sold it one year later would have had a capital loss rather than a capital gain on the sale. Of course, they would have received quarterly dividends over the one-year holding period. We will have much more to say about stock valuation later in the chapter.

Control of the firm

Common stockholders have the right to elect the firm's directors, who in turn elect the officers who will manage the business. In small firms, the major stockholder typically assumes the positions of president and chairman of the board of directors. In large, publicly owned firms, managers typically have some stock, but their personal holdings are insufficient to allow them to exercise voting control. Thus, the managements of most publicly owned firms can be removed by the stockholders if they decide that a management team is not effective.

Various state and federal laws stipulate how stockholder control is to be exercised. First, corporations must hold an election of directors periodically, usually once a year, with the vote taken at the annual meeting. Frequently, one-third of the directors are elected each year for a three-year term. Each share of stock has one vote; thus, the owner of 1,000 shares has 1,000 votes. Stockholders can appear at the annual meeting and vote in person, but typically they transfer their right to vote to a second party by means of a *proxy*. Management always solicits stockholders' proxies and usually gets them. However, if the common stockholders are dissatisfied with current management, an outside group may solicit the proxies in an effort to overthrow management and take control of the business. This is known as a *proxy fight*.

The preemptive right

Common stockholders often have the right, called the *preemptive right*, to purchase any new shares sold by the firm. In some states, the preemptive right is mandatory; in others, it can be specified in the corporate charter.

The purpose of the preemptive right is twofold. First, it protects the present stockholders' power of control. If it were not for this safeguard, the management of a corporation under criticism from stockholders could secure its position by issuing a large number of additional shares and purchasing these shares itself. Management would thereby gain control of the corporation and frustrate the current stockholders.

The second, and more important, reason for the preemptive right is that it protects stockholders against a dilution of value. For example, suppose HealthOne HMO has 1,000 shares of common stock outstanding, each with a price of $100, making the total market value of the firm $100,000. If an additional 1,000 shares were sold at $50 a share, or for $50,000, this would raise the total market value of HealthOne's stock to $150,000. When the total market value is divided by the new total shares outstanding, a value of $75 a share is obtained. HealthOne's old stockholders thus lose $25 per share, and the new stockholders have an instant profit of $25 per share. Thus, selling common stock at a price below the market value would dilute its price and would transfer wealth from the present stockholders to those who purchase the new shares. The preemptive right prevents such occurrences.

Self-Test Questions:

In what forms do common stock investors receive returns?

How do common stockholders exercise their right of control?

What is the preemptive right, and what is its purpose?

Types of Common Stock

Although most firms issue only one type of common stock, in some instances *classified stock* is used to meet the special needs of the company. Generally, when special classifications of stock are used, one type is designated *Class A*, another *Class B*, and so on. Small, new companies seeking to obtain funds from outside sources frequently use different types of common stock. For example, when Genetic Research, Inc. went public in 1995, its Class A stock was sold to the public and paid a dividend but carried no voting rights for five years. Its Class B stock was retained by the organizers of the company and carried full voting rights for five years, but dividends could not be paid on the Class B stock until the company had established its earning power by building up retained earnings to a designated level. The firm's use of classified stock allowed the public to take a position in a conservatively financed growth company without sacrificing income, while the founders retained absolute control during the crucial early stages of the firm's development. At the same time, outside investors were protected against excessive withdrawals of funds by the original owners. As is often the case in such situations, the Class B stock was also called *founders' shares*.

Note that "Class A," "Class B," and so on, have no standard meanings. Most firms have no classified shares, but a firm that does could designate its Class B shares as founders' shares and its Class A shares as those sold to the public, while another could reverse these designations. Other firms could use the A and B designations for entirely different purposes.

Self-Test Question:

Name several types of common stock, and explain their uses.

Procedures for Selling New Common Stock

If stock is to be sold to raise new capital, the new shares may be sold in one of five ways: (1) on a pro rata basis to existing stockholders through a rights offering; (2) through investment bankers to the general public in a public offering; (3) to a single buyer (or a very small number of buyers) in a private placement; (4) to employees through employee stock purchase plans; or (5) through a dividend reinvestment plan.

Rights offerings

As discussed earlier, common stockholders often have the *preemptive right* to purchase any additional shares sold by the firm. If the preemptive right is contained in a particular firm's charter, the company must offer any newly issued common stock to existing stockholders. If the charter does not prescribe a preemptive right, the firm can choose to sell to its existing stockholders or to the public at large. If it sells to the existing stockholders, the stock sale is called a *rights offering*. Each stockholder is issued an option to buy a certain number of new shares at a price below the existing market price, and the terms of the option are listed on a certificate called a *stock purchase right*, or simply a *right*. If a stockholder does not wish to purchase any additional shares in the company, then he or she can sell the rights to some other person who does want to buy the stock.[1]

Public offerings

If the preemptive right exists in a company's charter, it must sell new stock through a rights offering. If the preemptive right does not exist, the company may choose to offer the new shares to the general public through a *public offering*. We discuss procedures for public offerings in detail in a later section.

Private placements

In a *private placement*, securities are sold to one or a few investors, generally institutional investors. Private placements are most common with bonds, but they also occur with stocks. The primary advantages of private placements are lower issuance costs and greater speed, since the shares do not have to go through the SEC registration process.

The primary disadvantage of a private placement is that the securities generally will not have gone through the SEC registration process, so they must be sold initially to a large, "sophisticated" investor, usually an insurance company, mutual fund, or pension fund. Furthermore, in the event that the original purchaser wants to sell the securities, they must be sold to other large, "sophisticated" investors. However, the SEC currently allows any institution with a portfolio of $100 million or more to buy and sell private placement securities. Since there are thousands of institutions with assets that exceed this limit, private placements are becoming more and more popular with issuers.

Employee purchase plans and ESOPs

Many companies have plans that allow employees to purchase stock on favorable terms. First, under executive incentive *stock option plans*, key managers are given options to purchase stock. These managers generally have a direct, material influence on the company's fortunes, so if they perform well, the stock price will go up and the options will become valuable. Second, there are plans for lower-level employees. For example, Texas HealthPlans, Inc., a regional investor-owned HMO, permits employees who are not participants in its stock option plan to allocate up to 10 percent of their salaries to its *stock purchase plan*, and the funds are then used to buy newly issued shares at 85 percent of the market price on the purchase date. Often the company's contribution (in this case, the 15 percent discount) is not vested in an employee until five years after the purchase date. Thus, the employee cannot realize the benefit of the company's contribution without working an additional five years. This type of plan is designed both to improve employee performance and to reduce turnover.

A third type of plan is related to the second one, but here the stock bought for employees is purchased out of a share of the company's profits. Under an *Employee Stock Ownership Plan (ESOP)*, companies can claim a tax credit equal to a percentage of wages, provided that the funds are used to buy newly issued stock for the benefit of employees. The amount of the credit varies from year to year, depending on the whims of Congress: currently it is $\frac{1}{2}$ of 1 percent of total wages. Firms have been jumping on the ESOP bandwagon in record numbers in recent years—over 10,000 companies now have ESOPs covering over 12 million employees.

Dividend reinvestment plans

During the 1970s, many large companies instituted *dividend reinvestment plans (DRIPs)*, whereby stockholders can automatically reinvest their dividends in the stock of the paying corporation. There are two types of DRIPs: (1) plans that involve only "old" stock that is already outstanding, and (2) plans that involve newly issued stock. In either case, the stockholder must pay income taxes on the amount of the dividends, even though stock, rather than cash, is received.

Under both types of DRIP, stockholders must choose between continuing to receive cash dividends or using the cash dividends to buy more stock in the corporation. Under the "old" stock type of plan, a bank, acting as a trustee, takes the total funds available for reinvestment from each quarterly dividend, purchases the corporation's stock on the open market, and allocates the shares purchased to the participating stockholders on a pro rata basis. The brokerage costs of buying the shares are low because of volume purchases, so these plans benefit small stockholders who do not need cash for current consumption.

The "new" stock type of DRIP provides for dividends to be invested in newly issued stock; hence, these plans raise new capital for the firm. No fees are charged to participating stockholders, and some companies offer the new stock at a discount of 3 to 5 percent below the prevailing market price. The companies absorb these costs as a trade-off against the issuance costs that would be incurred if the stock were sold through investment bankers rather than through the DRIP.

Self-Test Questions:

What is a rights offering?

What is a private placement? What are its primary advantages over a public offering?

Briefly describe employee stock purchase plans and ESOPs.

What is a dividend reinvestment plan?

The Market for Common Stock

Some companies are so small that their common stock is not actively traded—it is owned by only a few people, usually the companies' managers. Such companies are said to be *privately held*, or *closely held*, and the stock is said to be *closely held stock*.

The stocks of smaller, publicly owned firms are not listed on any exchange; they trade in the *over-the-counter (OTC)* market. The companies and their stocks are said to be *unlisted*. However, most larger, publicly owned companies apply for listing on an exchange. These companies and their stocks are said to be *listed*. As a general rule, companies are first listed on a regional exchange, such as the Pacific or Midwest, then they move up to the American (AMEX), and finally, if they grow large enough, to the "Big Board," the New York Stock Exchange (NYSE). For example, American Healthcare Management, a King of Prussia, Pennsylvania-based company that owns or manages 16 hospitals in nine states, listed on the NYSE in 1993. The firm, which had previously traded on the AMEX, believed that listing on the NYSE would increase the trading of its shares and make the company more visible to the investment community, and that this presumably would have a positive impact on the price of its stock. Thousands of stocks are traded in the OTC market, but in terms of market value of both outstanding and daily transactions, the NYSE dominates, with about 60 percent of the business.

Institutional investors such as pension funds, insurance companies, and mutual funds own about 40 percent of all common stocks. However, the institutions buy and sell relatively actively, so they account for about 80 percent of all transactions. Thus, the institutions have a heavy influence on the prices of individual stocks—in a real sense, institutional investors determine the price levels of individual stocks.

Stock market transactions can be classified into three distinct categories:

1. *Initial public offerings by privately held firms: the new issue market.* A small company is typically owned by its management and a handful of private investors. At some point, if the company is to grow further, its stock must be sold to the general public—this action is defined as *going public.* The market for stock that is in the process of going public is often called the *new issue market,* and the issue is called an *initial public offering (IPO).* To illustrate, 41 health care providers went public in 1995, raising about 3.5 billion dollars. In the largest offering, American Oncology Resources, a Houston-based company that manages 12 oncology practices with 90 physicians in nine states, raised $100 million.

2. *Additional shares sold by established publicly owned companies: the primary market.* In 1994, Evergreen Healthcare, which operates 79 nursing homes in ten states, sold 3.1 million shares of new common stock, thereby raising $31.2 million of new equity financing. Since the shares sold were newly created, Evergreen's issue was defined as a *primary market* offering, but since the firm was already publicly held, the offering was not an IPO. Firms prefer to obtain equity by retaining earnings because of the issuance costs and market pressure associated with the sale of new common stock. Still, if a company requires more equity funds than can be generated from retained earnings, a stock sale may be required.

3. *Outstanding shares of established, publicly owned companies: the secondary market.* If the owner of 100 shares of Columbia/ HCA Healthcare sells his or her stock, the trade is said to have occurred in the *secondary market.* Thus, the market for

outstanding shares, or *used shares*, is defined as the secondary market. Over 12 million shares of Columbia/HCA were bought and sold on the NYSE in 1995, but the company did not receive a dime from these transactions.

Self-Test Questions:

What is an initial public offering (IPO)?

What are the differences between Columbia/HCA Healthcare selling shares in the primary market versus its shares being sold in the secondary market?

Regulation and the Investment Banking Process

In this section, we describe the regulation of securities markets, the way securities are issued, and the role that investment bankers play in the issuance process.

Regulation of securities markets

Sales of new securities, and also sales in the secondary markets, are regulated by the *Securities and Exchange Commission (SEC)* and, to a lesser extent, by each of the 50 states. Here are the primary elements of SEC regulation:

1. The SEC has jurisdiction over all interstate offerings of new securities to the public in amounts of $1.5 million or more.

2. Newly issued securities must be registered with the SEC at least 20 days before they are publicly offered. The *registration statement* provides financial, legal, and technical information about the company to the SEC, and the *prospectus* summarizes this information for investors. SEC lawyers and accountants analyze both the registration statement and the prospectus; if the information is inadequate or misleading, the SEC will delay or stop the public offering.

3. After the registration has become effective, new securities may be offered, but any sales solicitation must be accompanied by the prospectus. Preliminary, or *"red herring," prospectuses* may be distributed to potential buyers during the 20-day waiting period, but no sales may be finalized during this time. The "red herring" prospectus contains all of the key information that will appear in

the final prospectus except the price, which is generally set after the market closes the day before the new securities are actually offered to the public.

4. If the registration statement or prospectus contains misrepresentations or omissions of material facts, any purchaser who suffers a loss may sue for damages. Severe penalties may be imposed on the issuer or its officers, directors, accountants, engineers, appraisers, underwriters, and all others who participated in the preparation of the registration statement or prospectus.

5. The SEC also regulates all national stock exchanges. Companies whose securities are listed on an exchange must file annual reports similar to the registration statement with both the SEC and the exchange.

6. The SEC has control over corporate *insiders*. Officers, directors, and major stockholders must file monthly reports of changes in their holdings of the stock of the corporation.

7. The SEC has the power to prohibit manipulation by such devices as pools (large amounts of money used to buy or sell stocks to artificially affect prices) or wash sales (sales between members of the same group to record artificial transaction prices).

8. The SEC has control over the form of the proxy and the way the company uses it to solicit votes.

States also have some control over the issuance of new securities within their boundaries. This control is usually exercised by a "corporation commissioner" or someone with a similar title. State laws relating to security sales are called *blue sky laws*, because they were put into effect to keep unscrupulous promoters from selling securities that offered the "blue sky" but that actually had few or no assets to back them up.

The securities industry itself realizes the importance of stable markets, sound brokerage firms, and the absence of price manipulation. Therefore, the various exchanges, as well as other industry trade groups, work closely with the SEC to police transactions and to maintain the integrity and credibility of the system. These industry groups also cooperate with regulatory authorities to set net worth and other standards for securities firms, to develop insurance programs to protect the customers of brokerage houses, and the like.

In general, government regulation of securities trading, as well as industry self-regulation, is designed to ensure that investors receive information that is as accurate as possible, that no one artificially manipulates the market price of a given security, and that corporate insiders do not take advantage of their position to profit in their companies' securities at the expense of others. Neither the SEC, the state regulators, nor the industry itself can prevent investors from making foolish decisions or from having bad luck, but they can and do help investors obtain the best data possible for making sound investment decisions.

The investment banking process

The investment banking process takes place in two stages.

Stage I decisions

At Stage I, the firm itself makes some initial, preliminary decisions, including the following:

1. *Dollars to be raised.* How much new capital is needed?

2. *Type of securities used.* Should common stock, bonds, some other security, or a combination of securities be used? Further, if common stock is to be issued, should it be done as a rights offering, by a direct sale to the general public, or by a private placement? If a public offering, Decisions 3 and 4 must be made.

3. *Competitive bid versus negotiated deal.* Should the company simply offer a block of its securities for sale to the highest bidding investment banker, or should it negotiate a deal with an investment banker? These two procedures are called *competitive bids* and *negotiated deals,* respectively. Only about 100 of the largest firms listed on the NYSE, whose securities are already well known to the investment banking community, are in a position to use the competitive bidding process. The investment banks must do a large amount of investigative work in order to bid on an issue unless they are already quite familiar with the firm, and such costs would be too high to make it worthwhile unless the banker were sure of getting the deal. Therefore, except for the largest firms, offerings of stocks or bonds are generally on a negotiated basis.

4. *Selection of an investment banker.* If the issue is to be negotiated, the firm must select an investment banker. This can be an important decision for a firm that is going public. On the other hand, an older firm that has already "been to market" will have an established relationship with an investment banker. However, it is easy to change bankers if the firm is dissatisfied.

Stage II decisions

Stage II decisions, which are made jointly by the firm and its selected investment banker, include the following:

1. *Reevaluating the initial decisions.* The firm and its banker will reevaluate the initial decisions regarding the size of the issue and the type of securities to use.

2. *Setting the contractual basis of the issue.* The firm and its investment banker must decide whether the banker will work on a *best-efforts* basis or will *underwrite* the issue. In a best-efforts sale, the banker does not guarantee that the securities will be sold or that the company will get the cash it needs, only that it will put forth its best efforts to sell the issue. On an underwritten issue, the company does get a guarantee because the banker agrees to buy the entire issue and then resell the stock to its customers. Bankers bear significant risk in underwritten offerings, for if the price of the security falls between the time the security is purchased from the issuer and the time of resale to the public, the investment banker must bear the loss.

3. *Negotiating banker's compensation and estimating other expenses.* The investment banker's compensation must be negotiated. Also, the firm must estimate the other issuance expenses it will incur in connection with the issue—lawyers' fees, accountants' costs, printing and engraving, and so on. In an underwritten issue, the banker will buy the issue from the company at a discount below the price at which the securities are to be offered to the public, with this "spread" being set to cover the banker's costs and to provide a profit. In a best-efforts sale, fees to the investment banker are normally set as some percentage of the dollar volume sold.

   Table 7.2 gives an indication of the issuance costs associated with public issues of bonds and common stock. As the table shows, costs as a percentage of the proceeds are higher for stocks than for bonds, and costs are higher for small than for large issues. The relationship between size of issue and issuance cost is due primarily to the existence of fixed costs—certain costs must be incurred regardless of the size of the issue, so the percentage cost is quite high for small issues.

4. *Setting the offering price.* If the company is already publicly owned, the offering price will be based on the existing market price

Table 7.2   Issuance Costs as a Percentage of Gross Proceeds

Size of Issue (Millions of Dollars)	Bonds			Common Stock		
	Underwriting Commission	*Other Expenses*	*Total Costs*	*Underwriting Commission*	*Other Expenses*	*Total Costs*
Under 1.0	10.0%	4.0%	14.0%	13.0%	9.0%	22.0%
1.0–1.9	8.0	3.0	11.0	11.0	5.9	16.9
2.0–4.9	4.0	2.2	6.2	8.6	3.8	12.4
5.0–9.9	2.4	0.8	3.2	6.3	1.9	8.2
10.0–19.9	1.2	0.7	1.9	5.1	0.9	6.0
20.0–49.9	1.0	0.4	1.4	4.1	0.5	4.6
50.0 and over	0.9	0.2	1.1	3.3	0.2	3.5

Notes:

a. Issuance costs tend to rise somewhat when interest rates are cyclically high, indicating that money is in relatively tight supply; when this happens investment bankers have a relatively hard time placing issues with investors. Thus, the figures shown in this table represent averages, as the costs actually vary somewhat over time.

b. The issuance costs listed for common stocks are for new stock offerings by publicly owned firms. Issuance costs on initial public offerings are significantly higher, ranging from 31.7 percent for small issues to 16.3 percent on issues over $10 million.

Sources: U.S. Securities and Exchange Commission. 1974. *Cost of Flotation of Registered Equity Issues.* Washington, DC: Government Printing Office (December); R. Hansen. 1986. "Evaluating the Costs of a New Equity Issue." *Midland Corporate Finance Journal* (Spring); and J. R. Ritter. 1987. "The Costs of Going Public." *Journal of Financial Economics* (December).

of its stock or the yield on its bonds. The investment banker will have an easier job if the issue is priced relatively low, but the issuer of the securities naturally wants as high a price as possible. Some conflict of interest on price therefore arises between the investment banker and the issuer. If the issuer is financially sophisticated and makes comparisons with similar security issues, the investment banker will be forced to price close to the market.

Selling procedures

Once the company and its investment banker have decided how much money to raise, the types of securities to issue, and the basis for pricing the issue, they will prepare and file a registration statement and a prospectus. It generally takes about 20 days for the issue to be approved by the SEC. The final price of the stock (or the interest rate on a bond issue) is set at the close of business the day the issue clears the SEC, and the securities are offered to the public the following day.

Investors are required to pay for securities within ten days, and the investment banker must pay the issuing firm within four days of the official commencement of the offering. Typically, the banker sells the securities within a day or two after the offering begins; but on occasion, the banker miscalculates, sets the offering price too high, and thus is unable to move the issue. At other times, the market declines during the offering period, forcing the banker to reduce the price of the stock or bonds. In either instance, on an underwritten offering the firm receives the dollar amount that was agreed on, so the banker must absorb any losses incurred.

Because they are exposed to large potential losses, investment bankers typically do not handle the purchase and distribution of issues single-handedly unless the issue is a very small one. If the sum of money involved is large, investment bankers form *underwriting syndicates* in an effort to minimize the risk each banker carries. The banking house that sets up the deal is called the *lead,* or *managing, underwriter.*

In addition to the underwriting syndicate, on larger offerings still more investment bankers are included in a *selling group,* which handles the distribution of securities to individual investors. The selling group includes all members of the underwriting syndicate, plus additional dealers who take relatively small percentages of the total issue from the members of the underwriting syndicate. Thus, the underwriters act as *wholesalers,* while members of the selling group act as *retailers.* The number of houses in a selling group depends partly upon the size of the issue, but also on the number and types of buyers. For example, the selling group that handled a recent $92 million municipal bond issue for Adventist Health System/Sunbelt consisted of three members, while the one that sold $1 billion in junk (B-rated) bonds for National Medical Enterprises consisted of eight members.[2]

Self-Test Questions:

What are the key features of securities markets regulation?

What types of decisions must be made by the issuer and its investment banker?

What is the difference between an underwritten and a best-efforts issue?

Are there any conflicts that might arise between the issuer and the investment banker when setting the offering price on a stock issue?

Equity in Not-for-Profit Firms

Investor-owned firms have two sources of equity financing: retained earnings and new stock sales. Not-for-profit firms can, and do, retain earnings, but they do not have access to the equity markets; that is, they cannot sell stock to raise equity capital. Not-for-profit firms can, however, raise equity capital through *government grants* and *charitable contributions*. Federal, state, and local governments are concerned about the provision of health care services to the general population. Therefore, these entities often make grants to not-for-profit providers to help offset the costs of services rendered to patients who cannot pay for those services. Sometimes these grants are nonspecific, but often they are to provide specific services, such as neonatal intensive care to needy infants.

As for charitable contributions, individuals, as well as companies, are motivated to contribute to health care organizations for a variety of reasons, including concern for the well-being of others, the recognition that often accompanies large contributions, and tax deductibility. Since only contributions to not-for-profit firms are tax-deductible, this source of funding is, for all practical purposes, not available to investor-owned health care organizations. Although charitable contributions are not a substitute for profit retentions, charitable contributions can be a significant source of fund capital. For example, in 1994, the Association for Health Care Philanthropy reported total gifts to not-for-profit hospitals of $3.8 billion, of which $2.1 billion represented cash contributions.

Most not-for-profit hospitals received their initial, start-up equity capital from religious, educational, or governmental entities, and today some hospitals continue to receive funding from these sources. However, since the 1970s, these sources have provided a much smaller proportion of hospital funding, forcing not-for-profit hospitals to rely more on retained earnings and charitable contributions. Furthermore, federal programs, such as the Hill-Burton Act, which provided large amounts of funds for hospital expansion following World War II, have been discontinued, and state and local governments, which are also facing significant financial pressures, are finding it more and more difficult to fund grants to health care providers.

Finally, as we discussed in Chapter 2, there is a growing trend among legislative bodies and tax authorities to force not-for-profit hospitals to "earn" their favorable tax treatment by providing a certain amount of charity care to indigent patients. Even more severe, some cities have pressured not-for-profit hospitals to make "voluntary" payments to the city to make up for the lost property tax revenue. All of these trends tend to reduce the ability of not-for-profit health care organizations to raise equity capital by grants and contributions; hence, the result is increased reliance on making money "the old fashioned way," by earning it.

On the surface, it appears that investor-owned firms have a significant advantage in raising equity capital. In theory, new common stock can be issued at any time and in any amount. Conversely, charitable contributions are much less certain. The planning, solicitation, and collection periods can take years, and pledges are not always collected, so funds that were counted on may not materialize. Also, the proceeds of new stock sales may be used for any purpose, but charitable contributions may be *restricted*, in which case they can be used only for a designated purpose. Note, however, that managers of investor-owned firms do not have complete freedom to raise capital in the equity markets. If market conditions are poor and the stock is selling at a low price, then a new stock issue can be harmful to the firm's current stockholders. Additionally, as we will discuss in Chapter 9, a new stock issue can be viewed by investors as a signal by management that the firm's stock is overvalued, so new stock issues tend to have a negative impact on the firm's stock price.

Self-Test Question:

What are the sources of equity (fund capital) to not-for-profit firms?

Required Rates of Return on Stock Investments

In Chapter 6, in our discussion of financial risk, we saw that a company's (stock's) market beta is the appropriate measure of its portfolio risk. Now we must specify the relationship between risk and return: for a given beta, what rate of return will investors require on a stock in order to compensate them for assuming the risk? The answer to that question is given by the *Capital Asset Pricing Model (CAPM)*, which defines the equilibrium relationship between market risk and return.[3]

To begin, let us define the following terms:

$\hat{k}_i$ = expected rate of return on the ith stock.

k_i = required rate of return on the ith stock. Note that if $\hat{k}_i$ is less than k_i, you would not purchase this stock, or you would sell it if you owned it. If $\hat{k}_i$ were greater than k_i, you would want to buy the stock, and you would be indifferent if $\hat{k}_i = k_i$.

k_{RF} = risk-free rate of return, in this context generally measured by the return on long-term U.S. Treasury bonds.

b_i = beta coefficient of the ith stock. The beta of an average stock is $b_A = 1.0$.

k_M = required rate of return on a portfolio consisting of all stocks, which is the market portfolio. k_M is also the required rate of return on an average ($b_A = 1.0$) stock.

RP_M = market risk premium = $(k_M - k_{RF})$. This is the additional return over the risk-free rate required to compensate an investor for assuming average ($b_A = 1.0$) risk.

RP_i = risk premium on the ith stock = $(k_M - k_{RF})b_i$. The stock's risk premium is less than, equal to, or greater than the premium on an average stock, depending on whether its beta is less than, equal to, or greater than 1.0. If $b_i = b_A = 1.0$, then $RP_i = RP_M$.

The *market risk premium (RP$_M$)* depends on the degree of aversion that investors in the aggregate have to risk. If at one point in time, T-bonds yielded $k_{RF} = 8\%$ and an average share of stock had a required rate of return of $k_M = 12\%$, the market risk premium would be 4 percentage points:

$$RP_M = k_M - k_{RF} = 12\% - 8\% = 4 \text{ percentage points.}$$

It follows that if one stock were twice as risky as another, its risk premium would be twice as high and, conversely, if its risk were only half as much, its risk premium would be half as large. Further, we can measure a stock's relative riskiness by its beta coefficient. Therefore, if we know the market risk premium, RP_M, and the stock's risk as measured by its beta coefficient, b_i, we can find its risk premium as the product $(RP_M) b_i$. For example, if $b_i = 0.5$ and $RP_M = 4\%$, then RP_i is 2 percent:

$$\text{Risk Premium for Stock } i = RP_i = (RP_M) b_i$$
$$= (4\%)(0.5) = 2.0\%.$$

To summarize, given estimates of k_{RF}, k_M, and b_i, we can find the required rate of return on Stock i:

$$k_i = k_{RF} + (k_M - k_{RF}) b_i \qquad (7.2)$$
$$= k_{RF} + (RP_M) b_i$$
$$= 8\% + (12\% - 8\%)(0.5)$$
$$= 8\% + 4\%(0.5) = 10\%.$$

If some other stock were riskier than Stock i and had $b_j = 2.0$, then its required rate of return would be 16 percent:

$$k_j = 8\% + (4\%)2.0 = 16\%.$$

An average stock, with $b = 1.0$, would have a required return of 12 percent, the same as the market return:

$$k_A = 8\% + (4\%)1.0 = 12\% = k_M.$$

Equation 7.2 is called the *Security Market Line (SML)* equation, and it is often expressed in graph form, as in Figure 7.1, which shows the SML when $k_{RF} = 8\%$ and $k_M = 12\%$. Note the following points:

1. Required rates of return are shown on the vertical axis, while risk as measured by beta is shown on the horizontal axis.

2. Riskless securities have $b_i = 0$; therefore, k_{RF} appears as the vertical axis intercept in Figure 7.1.

3. The slope of the SML reflects the degree of risk aversion in the economy. The greater the average investor's aversion to risk (1) the steeper the slope of the SML, (2) the greater the risk premium for any stock, and (3) the higher the required rate of return on stocks.

4. The values we worked out for stocks with $b_i = 0.5$, $b_i = 1.0$, and $b_i = 2.0$ agree with the values shown on the graph for k_{Low}, k_A, and k_{High}.

Both the Security Market Line and a company's position on it change over time due to changes in interest rates, investors' risk aversion, and individual companies' beta. Thus, the SML, as well as a company's risk, must be evaluated on the basis of current information.

A word of caution

A word of caution about betas and the Capital Asset Pricing Model (CAPM) is in order. To begin, the CAPM is based on a very restrictive set of assumptions that does not conform well to real world conditions. Second, although these concepts are logical, the entire theory is based on *ex ante*, or expected, conditions, yet we have available only *ex post*, or historical, data. Thus, the betas we calculate show how volatile a stock has been in the *past*, but conditions may change, and its *future volatility*—the item of real concern to investors—might be quite different from its past volatility. Although the CAPM represents a very important contribution to risk and return theory, it does have some potentially serious problems when applied in practice. We will come back to this point in Chapter 8.

Figure 7.1   The Security Market Line

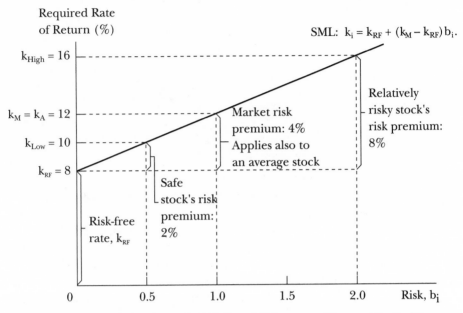

Source: E. F. Brigham and L. C. Gapenski. 1994. *Financial Management: Theory and Practice*, 7th ed. Fort Worth, TX: The Dryden Press.

Self-Test Questions:

What is the Capital Asset Pricing Model (CAPM)?

What is the appropriate measure of risk in the CAPM?

Write out the equation for and graph the Security Market Line (SML).

Describe the SML in words.

Common Stock Valuation

Common stocks provide expected future cash flows, and a stock's value is found in the same way as the values of most other assets—namely, as the present value of the expected future cash flow stream. The expected cash flows consist of two elements: (1) the dividends expected in each year, and (2) the price investors expect to receive when they sell the stock. The expected final stock price includes the return of the original investment plus an expected capital gain.

We begin by defining the following terms:

D_t = dividend the stockholder *expects* to receive at the end of Year t. D_0 is the most recent dividend, which has already been paid; D_1 is the first dividend expected, and it is assumed to be paid at the end of one year; D_2 is the dividend expected at the end of two years; and so forth. D_1 represents the first cash flow a new purchaser of the stock will receive. Note that D_0, the dividend that has just been paid, is known with certainty. However, all future dividends are expected values, so the estimate of D_t may differ among investors.[4]

P_0 = actual *market price* of the stock today.

$\hat{P}_t$ = expected price of the stock at the end of each Year t (pronounced "P hat t"). $\hat{P}_0$ is the *intrinsic value* of the stock today as seen by a particular investor based on his or her estimate of the stock's expected dividend stream and riskiness; $\hat{P}_1$ is the price expected at the end of one year; and so on. Thus, whereas P_0 is fixed and is identical for all investors, $\hat{P}_0$ will differ among investors depending on each investor's assessment of the stock's riskiness and dividend stream. The caret, or "hat," is used to indicate that $\hat{P}_t$ is an expected value. $\hat{P}_0$, the investor's estimate of the intrinsic value today, could be above or below P_0, the current stock price, but an investor would buy the stock only if his or her estimate of $\hat{P}_0$ were equal to or greater than P_0.

g = *expected growth rate* in dividends. Different investors may use different g's to evaluate a firm's stock.

k_s = *required rate of return* on the stock, considering both its riskiness and the returns available on other investments. In the last section, we discussed how the CAPM can be used to estimate k_s.

$\hat{k}_s$ = *expected rate of return* which an investor who buys the stock expects to receive. $\hat{k}_s$ (pronounced "k hat s") could be above or below k_s, but one would buy the stock only if $\hat{k}_s$ were equal to or greater than k_s.

$\bar{k}_s$ = *actual*, or *realized, rate of return*. You may expect to obtain a return of $\hat{k}_s$ = 15 percent if you buy Columbia/HCA

Healthcare stock today, but if the market goes down, you may end up next year with a realized return that is much lower than that expected, and perhaps even negative.

D_1/P_0 = expected *dividend yield* on a stock during the coming year. If the stock is expected to pay a dividend of $1 during the next 12 months, and if its current price is $10, then the expected dividend yield is $1/$10 = 0.10 = 10%.

$\dfrac{\hat{P}_1 - P_0}{P_0}$ = expected *capital gains yield* on the stock during the coming year. If the stock sells for $10 today, and if it is expected to rise to $10.50 at the end of the year, then the expected capital gain is $\hat{P}_1 - P_0$ = $10.50 − $10.00 = $0.50, and the expected capital gains yield is $0.50/$10 = 0.050 = 5.0%.

Expected dividends as the basis for stock values

In our discussion of long-term debt in Chapter 6, we found the value of a bond as the present value of interest payments over the life of the bond plus the present value of the bond's maturity (or par) value. Stock prices are likewise determined as the present value of a stream of cash flows, and the basic stock valuation equation is similar to the bond valuation equation. What are the cash flows that stocks provide to their holders? First, think of yourself as an investor who buys a stock with the intention of holding it (in your family) forever. In this case, all that you (and your heirs) will receive is a stream of dividends, and the value of the stock today is calculated as the present value of an infinite stream of dividends:

$$\hat{P}_0 = PV \text{ of expected future dividends}$$

$$= \frac{D_1}{(1 + k_s)^1} + \frac{D_2}{(1 + k_s)^2} + \frac{D_3}{(1 + k_s)^3} + \ldots + \frac{D_\infty}{(1 + k_s)^\infty}. \quad (7.3)$$

What about the more typical case, in which one expects to hold the stock for a finite period and then sell it—what will be the value of $\hat{P}_0$ in this case? The value of the stock is again determined by Equation 7.3. To see this, recognize that for any individual investor, expected cash flows consist of expected dividends plus the expected sale price of the stock. However, the sale price the current investor receives will depend on the dividends some future investor expects. Therefore, for all present and future investors in total, expected cash flows must be based on expected future dividends. To put it another way, unless a firm is liquidated or sold to another concern, the cash flows it provides to its stockholders consist only of a stream of dividends; therefore, the value of a share of its stock must be established as the present value of that expected dividend stream.

Equation 7.3 is a generalized stock valuation model in the sense that the time pattern of D_t can be anything: D_t can be rising, falling, or constant, or it can even fluctuate randomly, and Equation 7.3 will still hold. Often, however, the projected stream of dividends follows a systematic pattern, in which case we can develop a simplified (that is, easier to evaluate) version of the general stock valuation model expressed in Equation 7.3. In the following sections we consider two special cases: constant growth and nonconstant growth followed by constant growth.

Constant growth

A *constant growth stock* is one whose dividend is expected to grow at a constant rate forever. Thus, if a constant growth stock's last dividend, which has already been paid, was D_0, its dividend in any future Year t may be forecast as $D_t = D_0(1 + g)^t$, where g is the constant expected rate of growth. For example, if Memphis Home Health, Inc. just paid a dividend of $1.82 (that is, $D_0 = \$1.82$) and if investors expect a constant growth rate of 10 percent, the estimated dividend one year hence will be $D_1 = \$1.82(1.10) = \$2.00$; D_2 will be $2.00(1.10) = \$2.20$; and the estimated dividend five years hence will be $D_t = D_0(1 + g)^t = \$1.82(1.10)^5 = \$2.93$.

Although the dividends of few, if any, firms actually grow at a constant rate, many companies' dividend growth rates are close enough to constant to make the assumption useful in real world valuation. Of course, the value of a constant growth stock, like that of any stock, can always be found by estimating the future dividends as set forth above, calculating the present value of, say, the first 50 dividends and then summing these present values. However, if g is constant, Equation 7.3 may be simplified as follows:[5]

$$\hat{P}_0 = \frac{D_0(1 + g)}{k_s - g} = \frac{D_1}{k_s - g}. \tag{7.4}$$

If $D_0 = \$1.82$, $g = 10\%$, and $k_s = 16\%$, the value of the stock would be $33.33:

$$\hat{P}_0 = \frac{\$1.82(1.10)}{0.16 - 0.10} = \frac{\$2.00}{0.06} = \$33.33.$$

Equation 7.4 is called the *constant growth model*. A necessary condition for the derivation of Equation 7.4 is that k_s is greater than g. If the equation is used when k_s is not greater than g, the results will be meaningless. Note, though, that constant growth stocks have dividends that are expected to grow at a constant growth rate forever. Some stocks may have g greater than k_s for short periods, but we would not expect g to exceed k_s forever (for the life of the company).

Growth in dividends occurs primarily as a result of growth in earnings per share (EPS). Earnings growth, in turn, results from a number of factors, including inflation and the amount of earnings the company retains and reinvests. If output volume is stable, and if both sales prices and input costs increase at the inflation rate, then EPS also will grow at the inflation rate. EPS will also grow as a result of the reinvestment of earnings. If the firm's earnings are not all paid out as dividends (that is, if some fraction of earnings is retained), the dollars of investment behind each share will rise over time, which should lead to growth in earnings and dividends.

Expected rate of return on a constant growth stock

We can solve Equation 7.4 for k_s, again using the hat to denote that we are dealing with an expected rate of return.[6]

$$\begin{array}{ccc} \text{Expected} & \text{Expected} & \text{Expected growth} \\ \text{rate of} \; = & \text{dividend} \; + & \text{rate, or capital} \\ \text{return} & \text{yield} & \text{gains yield} \end{array}$$

$$\hat{k}_s \quad = \quad \frac{D_1}{P_0} \quad + \quad g. \qquad (7.4a)$$

Thus, if you buy a stock for a price $P_0 = \$33.33$, and if you expect the stock to pay a dividend $D_1 = \$2.00$ one year from now and to grow at a constant rate $g = 10\%$ in the future, your expected rate of return is 16.0 percent:

$$\hat{k}_s = \frac{\$2.00}{\$33.33} + 10.0\% = 6.0\% + 10.0\% = 16.0\%.$$

In this form, we see that $\hat{k}_s$ is the *expected total return* and that it consists of an *expected dividend yield, $D_1/P_0 = 6.0\%$*, plus an *expected growth rate* or *capital gains yield, $g = 10\%$*.

Suppose this analysis had been conducted on January 1, 1996, so $P_0 = \$33.33$ is the January 1, 1996, stock price and $D_1 = \$2.00$ is the dividend expected at the end of 1996. What is the value of $\hat{P}_1$, the stock price at the end of 1996 (or the beginning of 1997)? We would again apply Equation 7.4, but this time we would use the 1997 dividend, $D_2 = D_1(1 + g) = \$2.00(1.10) = \$2.20$:

$$\hat{P}_1 = \frac{D_2}{k_s - g} = \frac{\$2.20}{0.06} = \$36.67.$$

Now notice that $\hat{P}_1 = \$36.67$ is 10 percent greater than $P_0 = \$33.33$: $\$33.33(1.10) \approx \$36.67$. Thus, we would expect to make a capital gain of $\$36.67 - \$33.33 = \$3.34$ during 1996, and hence a capital gains yield of 10 percent:

$$\text{Capital gains yield} = \frac{\text{Capital gain}}{\text{Beginning price}} = \frac{\$3.34}{\$33.33}$$
$$= 0.100 = 10.0\%.$$

We could extend the analysis on out, and in each future year the expected capital gains yield would always equal g, the expected dividend growth rate.

The expected dividend yield in 1997 (Year 2) could be found as follows:

$$\text{Dividend yield} = \frac{D_2}{\hat{P}_1} = \frac{\$2.20}{\$36.67} = 0.060 = 6.0\%.$$

The dividend yield for 1998 (Year 3) could also be calculated, and again it would be 6 percent. Thus, *for a constant growth stock,* the following conditions must hold:

1. The dividend is expected to grow forever at a constant rate, g.
2. The stock price is expected to grow at this same rate.
3. The expected dividend yield is a constant.
4. The expected capital gains yield is also a constant, and it is equal to g.
5. The expected total rate of return, $\hat{k}_s$, is equal to the expected dividend yield plus the expected growth rate: $\hat{k}_s = D_{n+1}/P_n + g$.

The term *expected* should be clarified—it means expected in a statistical sense. Thus, if we say the growth rate is expected to remain constant at 10 percent, we mean that the growth in each year can be represented by a probability distribution with an expected value of 10 percent, not that we literally expect the growth rate to be exactly equal to 10 percent in each future year. In this sense, the constant growth assumption is reasonable for many large, mature companies.

Nonconstant growth followed by constant growth

Some firms exhibit constant dividend growth, or at least growth close enough to apply the constant growth model. However, many firms do not. For example, firms that are in their infancies, such as biotechnology firms today, may be growing much faster than the average firm. However, at some point in time, as the industry matures, the growth of these firms will slow down to the growth of an average firm. Also, some firms, such as Beverly Enterprises, are currently paying no dividends, so their current dividend growth is zero. But, at some time in the future, investors expect Beverly to start paying dividends.[7] If a firm is not expected to exhibit more-or-less constant growth in dividends in the future, then the constant growth model cannot be used.

To find the value of a nonconstant growth stock, assuming that the growth rate will eventually stabilize, we proceed in four steps:

1. Estimate the stock's dividend stream, stopping with the first dividend in the constant growth phase.

2. Find the PV of the dividends during the period of nonconstant growth.

3. Find the price of the stock at the end of the nonconstant growth period, at which point it has become a constant growth stock, and discount this price back to the present.

4. Add the dividend and price components to find the value of the stock, $\hat{P}_0$.

To illustrate the process for valuing nonconstant growth stocks, suppose the following facts exist:

k_s = stockholders' required rate of return = 16%.

N = years of nonconstant growth = 3.

g_n = rate of growth in dividends during the nonconstant growth period = 30%. (Note that the growth rate during the nonconstant growth period could vary from year to year.)

g_c = rate of constant growth after the nonconstant period = 10%.

D_0 = last dividend paid = $1.82.

The valuation process is diagrammed in Figure 7.2, and it is explained in the steps now set forth:

1. Find the expected dividends during the nonconstant growth phase (Years 1, 2, and 3 in this case) plus the first dividend of the steady-state

constant growth phase (Year 4) by multiplying each dividend by one plus the growth rate expected in the coming year:

$$D_0 = \$1.82.$$
$$D_1 = D_0(1.30) = \$1.82 \ (1.30) = \$2.366.$$
$$D_2 = D_1(1.30) = \$2.366(1.30) = \$3.076.$$
$$D_3 = D_2(1.30) = \$3.076(1.30) = \$3.999.$$
$$D_4 = D_3(1.10) = \$3.999(1.10) = \$4.399.$$

2. Find the present values of the dividends that occur during the non-constant growth phase, remembering that D_0 just occurred, so it does not contribute to the stock's value:

$$PV \ D_1 = \$2.366/(1.16)^1 = \$2.040.$$
$$PV \ D_2 = \$3.076/(1.16)^2 = \$2.286.$$
$$PV \ D_3 = \$3.999/(1.16)^3 = \$2.562.$$

3. The stock price expected at the end of Year 3 (the beginning of Year 4) can be found using the constant growth model, because dividends are expected to grow at a constant rate of 10 percent in Year 4 and beyond. Note that this price captures the value of all the dividends beyond Year 3. Calculate the stock price at the end of Year 3, and then discount this value to Year 0:

$$\hat{P}_3 = \frac{D_4}{k_s - g} = \frac{\$4.399}{0.16 - 0.10} = \$73.317.$$
$$PV\hat{P}_3 = \$73.32/(1.16)^3 = \$46.971.$$

4. Add the present values to find the value of the stock today:

$$\hat{P}_0 = \$2.040 + \$2.286 + \$2.562 + \$46.971$$
$$= \$53.859 \approx \$53.86.$$

When all these steps are combined, we find the value of the stock to be $53.86.

Self-Test Questions:

What are the two elements of a stock's expected rate of return?

Write out and explain the valuation model for a constant growth stock.

Explain how to find the value of a nonconstant growth stock.

Figure 7.2   Valuing a Nonconstant Growth Stock

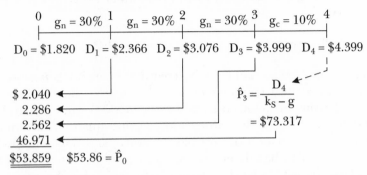

Source: E. F. Brigham and L. C. Gapenski. 1994. *Financial Management: Theory and Practice,* 7th ed. Fort Worth, TX: The Dryden Press.

Market Equilibrium, Market Efficiency, and the Risk/Return Trade-Off

The concepts of market equilibrium, market efficiency, and the risk/return trade-off are extremely important both to investors and to health care managers.

Market equilibrium

Investors will want to buy a stock if its expected rate of return exceeds its required rate of return, that is, when its value exceeds its current price. Conversely, investors will want to sell a stock when its required rate of return exceeds its expected rate of return, that is, when its current price exceeds its value. When more investors want to buy a stock than to sell it, its price is bid up, and when more investors want to sell a stock than to buy it, its price falls. In equilibrium, these two conditions must hold:

1. The expected rate of return on the stock must equal the required rate of return, or $\hat{k}_s = k_s$.

2. The market price of a stock must equal its value, or $P_0 = \hat{P}_0$.

If these conditions do not hold, then trading will occur until they do. Of course, stock prices are not constant. A stock's price can swing wildly as new information becomes available to the market that changes investors' expectations concerning the stock's dividend stream and risk. But evidence suggests that stock prices, especially those of large companies that are actively traded, adjust rapidly to disequilibrium situations. The key to the continual movement of security prices toward equilibrium is market efficiency.

Market efficiency

A market, say, the market for U.S. Treasury securities, is *informationally efficient* if (1) all information relevant to the values of the securities can be obtained easily and at low cost, and (2) the market contains many buyers and sellers who act on this information. In this situation, current prices contain all information of possible relevance, and hence future price movements will be based solely on new information as it becomes known.

The *Efficient Markets Hypothesis (EMH),* which has three forms, formalizes the theory of informational efficiency:

1. The *weak form* of the EMH holds that all information contained in past price movements is fully reflected in current market prices. Therefore, information about recent trends in a security's price, or a bond's yield, is of no value in choosing which security will "outperform" the market.

2. The *semistrong form* of the EMH holds that current market prices reflect all *publicly available* information. Therefore, it makes no sense to spend hours and hours analyzing economic data and financial reports because whatever information you might find, good or bad, has already been absorbed by the market and imbedded in current prices.

3. The *strong form* of the EMH holds that current market prices reflect *all relevant* information, whether publicly available or privately held. If this form holds, then even investors with "inside information," such as corporate officers, would find it impossible to earn abnormal returns, that is, returns in excess of that justified by the riskiness of the investment.

The EMH is a hypothesis, not a proven law, so it is not necessarily true. However, hundreds of empirical tests have been conducted to try to prove (or disprove) the EMH, and the results are relatively consistent. Most tests support the weak and semistrong forms of the EMH for well-developed markets, such as the U.S. markets for large firms' stocks and bond issues and for Treasury securities. Supporters of these forms of the EMH note that there are some 100,000 or so full-time, highly trained, professional analysts and traders operating in these markets. Furthermore, many of these analysts and traders work for companies such as

Citibank, Fidelity Investments, Merrill Lynch, Prudential Insurance, and the like, which have billions of dollars available to take advantage of undervalued securities. Finally, as a result of disclosure requirements and electronic information networks, new information about these heavily followed securities is almost instantaneously available. Therefore, security prices in these markets adjust almost immediately as new developments occur, and it is very difficult, if not impossible, to "beat the market."[8]

However, many theorists, and even more Wall Street analysts, believe that pockets of inefficiency do exist. In some cases, entire markets may be inefficient. For example, the markets for the securities issued by small companies may be inefficient because there are neither enough analysts ferreting out information on these companies, nor sufficient numbers of investors trading these securities. Also, many people even believe that individual securities traded in efficient markets are occasionally priced inefficiently, or that investor emotions can drive prices too high during raging bull markets or too low during rampant bear markets. In spite of such anomalies, most people believe that the prices of securities traded in the major U.S. markets pretty much reflect all publicly available information.

Virtually no one, however, believes that strong form efficiency holds. Studies of legal purchases and sales by people with inside information, such as corporate officers, indicate that insiders can make abnormal profits by trading on that information. It is even more apparent that insiders can make abnormal profits if they trade illegally on specific information that has not been disclosed to the public, such as a takeover bid, a research and development breakthrough, and the like.

The EMH has implications both for investors and for corporate managers. Since security prices do appear in general to reflect all public information, most actively followed and traded securites are in equilibrium and fairly valued. This does not mean that new information could not cause a security's price to soar or to plummet, but it does mean that stocks and bonds, in general, are neither undervalued nor overvalued. Therefore, investors with no inside information can only expect to earn a return on an investment that compensates them for the risks involved.

What bearing does the EMH have on financial management decisions? Since security prices generally reflect all available information, and hence are fairly valued, it makes little sense for managers to try to "time" the issuance of securities to catch market highs or lows. Since the EMH also applies to bond markets, bond prices—and hence interest rates—reflect all current public information. Thus, it is impossible to forecast future interest rates consistently: interest rates change in response to new information, and this information could either lower or raise rates.

In closing, note that managers may have information about their own firms that is unknown to the general public. This condition is called *asymmetric information,* and it can have a profound effect on managerial decisions. For example, suppose a drug manufacturer has made a breakthrough in AIDS research, but it does not want to announce the development until it completes the final series of in-house tests. The firm might want to delay any new securities offerings because securities can probably be sold under more favorable terms once the announcement is made. This scenario does not mean that markets are inefficient, but rather that markets are not strong-form efficient. Managers can and should act on inside information for the benefit of the firm, but inside information cannot legally be used for the managers' own benefit.

The risk/return trade-off

Most financial decisions involve alternative courses of action, generally having different risk and return characteristics. In all such situations, one might be tempted to accept the alternative with the higher expected return, but this would be incorrect. In efficient markets, those alternatives that offer higher returns also entail higher risk. The correct question to ask when making financial decisions, then, is not which alternative has the higher return, but which alternative has the higher return after adjusting for risk. In other words, which alternative has the higher return over and above the return commensurate with the riskiness of each alternative.

To illustrate, suppose Beverly Enterprises' stock has an expected rate of return of 14 percent, while its bonds yield 9 percent. Does this mean that investors should flock to buy Beverly's stock and ignore the firm's bonds? Of course not—the higher expected rate of return on the stock merely reflects the fact that the stock is riskier than the bonds. Those investors who are not willing to assume much risk will buy Beverly's bonds, while those who are less risk-averse will buy the stock. From the perspective of Beverly's managers and other stakeholders, financing with stock is less risky than using debt, so the firm is willing to pay the higher cost of equity to limit the firm's risk exposure.

The moral of this story is simple. Three key questions are involved in every financial decision: (1) What is the expected return? (2) What is the risk? (3) Is the return commensurate with the risk? For decisions that involve the major capital (stock and bond) markets, which are efficient, expected returns will usually be just sufficient to compensate for the risks. However, product markets (that is, markets for real assets such as MRI systems) are usually not efficient, and hence large returns (or large losses) can be experienced. However, when excess returns are found in product markets, competition will usually bring these returns down to efficient market returns in the long run, with the final result being returns that are just commensurate with the risks involved.

Self-Test Questions:

What two conditions must hold for a stock to be in equilibrium?

What are the three forms of the Efficient Markets Hypothesis (EMH), and what are their differences?

What are the implications of the EMH for managerial decisions?

Explain the meaning of the term "risk/return trade-off."

Summary

This chapter contained a wealth of material on equity financing, including required rates of return and valuation. In addition, the chapter discussed financial markets and regulation. A knowledge of the issues discussed here is essential to an understanding of health care financial management. The key concepts covered are listed here:

- *Preferred stock* is a hybrid security: it has some features like debt and other features like equity.

- The most important *common stockholder* rights are (1) a claim on the firm's residual earnings; (2) voting control; and (3) the preemptive right.

- A *proxy* is a document that gives one person the power to act for another person, typically the power to vote shares of common stock. A *proxy fight* occurs when an outside group solicits stockholders' proxies in order to vote a new management team into office.

- Common stockholders often have the right to purchase any additional shares sold by the firm. This right, called the *preemptive right,* protects the control of the present stockholders and prevents dilution of the value of their stock.

- Although most firms use only one type of common stock, in some instances several *classes of stock* are issued.

- A *closely held corporation* is one that is owned by a few individuals who are typically associated with the firm's management.

- A *publicly owned corporation* is one that is owned by a relatively large number of individuals who are not actively involved in its management.

- New common stock may be sold in five ways: (1) on a pro rata basis to existing stockholders through a *rights offering;* (2) through investment bankers to the general public in a *public offering*; (3) to a single buyer, or a small number of buyers, in a *private placement;* (4) to employees through an *employee purchase plan;* and (5) to shareholders through a *dividend reinvestment plan.*

- Securities markets are regulated by the *Securities and Exchange Commission (SEC).*

- An *investment banker* assists in the issuing of securities by helping the firm determine the size of the issue and the type of securities to be used, by establishing the selling price, by selling the issue, and, in some cases, by maintaining an after-market for the stock.

- Not-for-profit firms do not have access to the equity markets. However, *charitable contributions*, which are tax-deductible to the donor, and *governmental grants*, constitute unique equity sources for not-for-profit firms.

- The *Capital Asset Pricing Model (CAPM)* is an equilibrium model that describes the relationship between market risk and required rates of return.

- The *Security Market Line (SML)* describes the risk/return relationship for individual assets. The required rate of return for any Stock i is equal to the risk-free rate plus the market risk premium times the stock's beta coefficient: $k_i = k_{RF} + (k_M - k_{RF})b_i$.

- The *value* of a share of stock is found by *discounting* the stream of *expected dividends* by the stock's required rate of return.

- The value of a stock whose dividends are expected to grow at a constant rate for many years is found by applying the *constant growth model*:

$$\hat{P}_0 = \frac{D_0(1 + g)}{k_g - g} = \frac{D_1}{k_g - g}.$$

- The *expected rate of return* on a stock consists of an *expected dividend yield* plus an *expected capital gains yield*. For a constant growth stock, both the expected dividend yield and the expected capital gains yield are constant, and the expected rate of return can be found by this equation:

Expected rate of return		Expected dividend yield		Expected growth rate, or capital gains yield
$\hat{k}_s$	$=$	$\dfrac{D_1}{P_0}$	$+$	$g.$

- The valuation of *nonconstant growth stocks* is somewhat more complicated than the valuation of constant growth stocks.

- The *Efficient Markets Hypothesis (EMH)* holds that (1) stocks are always in equilibrium and fairly valued, (2) it is impossible for an investor to consistently "beat the market," and (3) managers should not try to forecast future interest rates or "time" security issues.

- In some situations, a company's managers may know more about their firm's future prospects than do investors. This situation is called *asymmetric information.* If this condition holds, then managers may use the private information for the benefit of the firm, but not for their own personal benefit.

- In efficient markets, alternatives that offer higher returns must also have higher risk; this is the *risk/return trade-off.* The implication is that investments must be evaluated on the basis of both risk and return.

Notes

1. For more details on the mechanics of a rights offer, see E. F. Brigham and L. C. Gapenski, *Intermediate Financial Management* (Fort Worth, TX: Dryden Press, 1996), chap. 12.
2. Large security issues are announced in the *Wall Street Journal* and other publications by advertisements, called *tombstones,* placed by the underwriters. Check several recent issues of the *Journal* to see if there are any health care issues advertised.
3. The CAPM is a relatively complex subject, and we present only the basic conclusions in this text. For more detailed discussions, see E. F. Brigham and L. C. Gapenski, *Intermediate Financial Management* (Fort Worth, TX: Dryden Press, 1996), chap. 3.
4. Stocks generally pay dividends quarterly, so theoretically we should evaluate them on a quarterly basis. However, in stock valuation, most analysts work

on an annual basis because the data generally are not precise enough to warrant the refinement of a quarterly model. For additional information on the quarterly model, see C. M. Linke and J. K. Zumwalt, "Estimation Biases on Discounted Cash Flow Analysis of Equity Capital Cost in Rate Regulation." *Financial Management* (Autumn 1984): 15–21.

5. Equation 6.4 is derived in Appendix 4A of E. F. Brigham and L. C. Gapenski, *Intermediate Financial Management* (Fort Worth, TX: Dryden Press, 1996).

6. The k_s value of Equation 7.4 is a *required* rate of return, but when we transform to obtain Equation 7.4a, we are finding an *expected* rate of return. Obviously, the transformation requires that $k_s = \hat{k}_s$. This equality holds if the stock market is in equilibrium, a condition that will be discussed later in the chapter.

7. What is the value of the stock of a firm that is never expected to pay dividends? Since the value of a stock is the present value of the expected dividend stream, the answer is zero.

8. If markets were not efficient, the better managers of stock and bond mutual funds would be able to outperform the broad averages. In fact, few managers, if any, can consistently better the broad averages, and on average mutual fund managers underperform the market.

Selected Additional References

Dunn, K. C., G. B. Shields, and J. B. Stern. 1991. "The Dynamics of Leveraged Buy-Outs, Conversions, and Corporate Reorganizations of Not-For-Profit Health Care Institutions." *Topics in Health Care Financing* (Spring): 5–20.

Flaherty, M. P. 1991. "Planned Giving Programs as a Source of Financing: Creating a 'Win-Win' Situation for a Health Care Organization and Its Donors." *Topics in Health Care Financing* (Spring): 70–81.

Shields, G. B., and G. C. McKann. 1991. "Raising Health Care Capital Through the Public Equity Markets." *Topics in Health Care Financing* (Fall): 21–36.

Sykes, C. S., Jr. 1991. "The Role of Equity Financing in Today's Health Care Environment." *Topics in Health Care Financing* (Fall): 1–4.

Wallace, C. 1985. "Not-For-Profits Competing for Capital by Selling Stock in Alternative Ventures." *Modern Healthcare* (16 August): 32–38.

Case 7

Big Bend Health Systems (B): Stock Valuation

Big Bend Health Systems, Inc., is an investor-owned hospital chain that owns and operates nine hospitals in Texas and New Mexico. George Waterman, a recent graduate of a prominent health services administration program, has just been hired by El Paso General, Big Bend's largest hospital. Like all new management personnel, Waterman must undergo three months of intensive indoctrination at the system level before joining the hospital.

In Case 6A (Big Bend Health Systems [A]), Waterman conducted an analysis of the firm's bonds and presented his findings to the firm's executive committee. Big Bend's chief financial officer (CFO), Maria Martinez, was very impressed with the quality of Waterman's presentation. Furthermore, the other members of the committee stated that they learned a great deal about debt financing from Waterman's presentation, and that they would like to see a similar presentation on equity financing. Since Waterman would be leaving corporate headquarters to start his hospital assignment in less than four weeks, Martinez immediately assigned Waterman the task of analyzing the firm's equity situation and preparing another presentation for the executive committee. Waterman began by reexamining the firm's Annual Report to get some basic data. Then he searched the *Wall Street Journal, Value Line,* and other potential sources of financial data to obtain some market data as well as analysts' forecasts for the firm. Table 1 contains the information that Waterman developed.

As before, Martinez did not want Waterman to go off on a tangent, so she provided him with a list of questions to answer. Also as before,

Table 1   Big Bend Health Systems: Selected Stock Data

Year	Earnings Per Share	Dividends Per Share
Historical Data		
1991	$1.14	$0.21
1992	1.32	0.32
1993	1.54	0.35
1994	1.56	0.36
1995	1.80	0.39
1996	2.00	0.48

Assumed Current (January 1, 1997) Data
Current stock price: $8.00
Estimated dividend growth rates:
  Next 5 years: 12.0%
  Long-term steady state: 6.0%
Market data:
  Yield on long-term Treasury bonds: 8.0%
  Merrill Lynch estimate of market returns (k_M): 13.0%
Value Line beta coefficient: 1.2

Waterman welcomed the challenge of working on a task that was traditionally assigned to finance MBAs rather than graduates in health and
hospital administration. Put yourself in Waterman's shoes and see how
you would fare if assigned this task.

Questions

1. What were Big Bend's earnings and dividend growth rates over the entire 1991–1996 period? What were the average annual compounded
   growth rates?

2. a. What was the firm's payout ratio in 1996? (Hint: The payout ratio is
       the percentage of earnings paid out to stockholders as dividends.)

   b. What was the firm's average payout over the past six years?

   c. If the payout ratio of an average investor-owned hospital company
       was about 50 percent, is Big Bend's payout about average, below
       average, or above average? What is the primary factor that influ-
       ences whether a firm has a high, low, or average payout ratio?

3. a. What is the Capital Asset Pricing Model (CAPM)?

b. Sketch the Security Market Line (SML) using the data presented in Table 1.

c. What would happen to the SML if investors' risk aversion increased and the required rate of return on the market rose to 16 percent?

d. What would happen to the SML if inflation expectations increased by 1 percentage point? (Hint: Investors would add 1 percentage point to their required rates of return on all assets.)

e. Return to the base case data in Part (b). According to the SML, what is the required rate of return on Big Bend's stock? Plot that point on your SML graph.

4. *Value Line* estimated the firm's long-term dividend growth rate to be 6.0 percent. Further, the 1996 dividend (D_0) was $0.48, and the end of year (December 31, 1996, or January 1, 1997) stock price (P_0) was $8. Assume for now that the 6.0 percent long-run growth rate also applies to the next five years, so the firm is expecting a constant dividend growth rate.

a. What is the expected rate of return on Big Bend's stock on January 1, 1997?

b. What is the expected dividend yield and expected capital gains yield?

c. What is the relationship between dividend yield and capital gains yield over time under constant growth assumptions?

d. What conditions must hold to use the constant growth model? Do many "real world" stocks satisfy the constant growth assumptions?

e. Plot the expected rate of return found in Part (a) on the SML graph from Question 3. Based on the data developed so far, would you buy the firm's stock?

5. Now consider the fact that *Value Line* actually predicted that Big Bend's dividends would grow at a 12 percent rate for the next five years, and then the growth rate would fall to a steady-state 6 percent into the foreseeable future.

a. Under these conditions, what is the value of Big Bend's stock at the beginning of 1997?

b. Assume that the value you calculated was the actual stock price on January 1, 1997. What is the expected stock price at the end of

1997 assuming that the stock is in equilibrium?

c. What are the expected dividend yield, capital gains yield, and total return for 1997?

d. Repeat the Part (c) analysis for 1998. What happens to the expected dividend and capital gains yields from 1997 to 1998? What are the expected dividend and capital gains yields for 2002?

6. Suppose Big Bend's dividend was expected to remain constant at $0.48 for the next five years, and then to grow at a constant 6 percent rate. (In other words, the growth rate for the first five years would be zero.)

a. Under these conditions, what is the value of Big Bend's stock at the beginning of 1997?

b. Assume that the value you calculated was the actual stock price on January 1, 1997. What is the expected stock price at the end of 1997 assuming that the stock is in equilibrium?

c. What are the expected dividend yield, capital gains yield, and total return for 1997?

d. Repeat the Part (c) analysis for 1998. What happens to the expected dividend and capital gains yields from 1997 to 1998? What are the expected dividend and capital gains yields for 2002?

7. Big Bend's stock price was actually $8.00 at the beginning of 1997. Using the growth rates given in Table 1 (and also used in Question 5), what is the stock's expected rate of return?

Part IV

Cost of Capital and Capital Structure

8

Cost of Capital

The cost of capital is an extremely important concept in health care financial management. All firms, whether investor-owned or not-for-profit, have to raise funds to buy the assets required to meet their strategic objectives. Hospitals, nursing homes, clinics, group practices, and so on, all need assets to provide services. The funds to acquire the assets come in many shapes and forms, including contributions, profit retention, equity sales to stockholders, and debt capital supplied by creditors such as banks, bondholders, lessors, and suppliers. Most of the capital raised by organizations has a cost, either explicit, such as the interest payments on debt, or implicit, such as the opportunity cost associated with equity (fund) capital. Since many business decisions require the cost of capital as an input, it is necessary for managers to both understand the cost of capital concept and know how to estimate the costs of capital for their own firms.

An Overview of the Cost of Capital Estimation Process

The goal of the cost of capital estimation process is to estimate the firm's *overall, or weighted average, cost of capital (WACC)*, which is then used as the hurdle rate to evaluate capital investment opportunities. For example, assume that Bayside Memorial Hospital has a cost of capital of 10 percent. If a new investment, say, an MRI, is expected to return at least 10 percent, then it is financially attractive to the hospital. If the MRI is expected to return less than 10 percent, accepting it will have an adverse effect on the hospital's financial soundness.

Capital, as the term is used in the weighted average cost of capital, refers to the right-hand side of the balance sheet because the liabilities and equity listed here represent the sources of funds used to acquire the assets shown on the left-hand side. Once the specific sources of capital to be included in the WACC have been identified, the next step is to estimate the cost of each of the sources, or the *component costs* of capital. Finally, the component costs are combined to estimate the firm's WACC.

The exact form of the WACC estimate depends on the purpose of the estimate. The WACC is used primarily in making capital investment decisions—a firm's investment in new plant and equipment will be financed by some mix of debt and equity (fund) capital, and the investment must provide a return to the capital suppliers—so the discussion in this chapter will focus on estimating the WACC for that purpose.

Capital components

The first task in estimating a firm's WACC is to decide which sources of capital on the right-hand side of the balance sheet should be included in the estimate. To begin, consider a firm's short-term, non-interest bearing liabilities: accounts payable and accruals. These items arise from normal operations: if volume increases, then typically more supplies will be purchased and accounts payable will increase. Similarly, volume increases lead to increased labor expenses and higher accrued wages. Higher volume usually also leads to higher profits, and hence higher accrued taxes for investor-owned firms.

Because funds from accounts payable and accruals automatically rise and fall with volume changes, these accounts are called *spontaneous liabilities.* As you will see in Chapter 10 when we discuss project evaluation, any funds generated by spontaneous liabilities are used to offset the cost of the project. Furthermore, spontaneous liabilities typically do not have an explicit cost. For these reasons, spontaneous liabilities are usually not included in a firm's WACC estimate.

The next capital component to consider is short-term notes payable, often bank loans. This account is not generated spontaneously; rather, it results from managerial decisions to use short-term interest-bearing debt financing. If a firm uses notes payable financing only as temporary financing to support seasonal or cyclical fluctuations in volume, then it should not be included in the WACC estimate. However, if a firm uses short-term debt as part of its permanent financing mix, then such debt should be included in the firm's WACC estimate. As we will discuss in Chapter 14, the use of short-term debt to finance permanent assets is highly risky, and it is not common under normal conditions. Therefore, in this chapter, we will assume that interest-bearing short-term debt is used only to support seasonal or cyclical increases in current assets, so we shall exclude it from the WACC estimate.

The remainder of the capital components—long-term debt, preferred stock (if used), common stock (or fund capital for not-for-profit organizations)—are the primary sources of permanent capital for most firms, so they are the components that are routinely included in a firm's WACC estimate.

Taxes

In developing the costs for the different capital components, the issue of taxes arises for investor-owned companies. Should the component costs be estimated on a before- or after-tax basis? In Chapter 9, you will see that the use of debt financing creates a tax benefit, because interest expense is tax-deductible, while the use of equity financing has no impact on taxes. The tax benefit associated with debt financing can be incorporated either in the cash flows of the project being analyzed or in the WACC estimate. Because it is generally easier to incorporate the tax benefit of debt financing in the WACC estimate, we will use this approach throughout the book. Thus, the tax benefits associated with debt financing will be recognized in the component cost of debt estimate, resulting in an after-tax cost of debt. For not-for-profit firms, the benefits arising from the issuance of tax-exempt debt will be incorporated directly by estimating a relatively low component cost of debt.

Capital pass-through payments

Capital pass-through payments are separate payments made by some third party payers to compensate health care providers—mainly hospitals—for capital costs. Whereas only investor-owned firms gain the benefit of tax deductibility of interest, all providers, regardless of ownership, may benefit from capital pass-through payments. When used by payers, capital pass-through payments are typically made for depreciation expense, interest expense, and lease and rental payments.

Whereas capital pass-through payments were important sources of capital to many providers in the past, its importance is diminishing over time as more and more payers adopt reimbursement methods that do not include capital pass-through payments. Thus, we will not emphasize capital pass-through in the examples in this book. However, we will use footnotes to highlight those situations where capital pass-through, if being received by the provider, does affect the analysis.

Historical versus marginal costs

Two very different sets of costs can be measured: *historical*, or *embedded*, *costs*, which reflect the cost of funds raised in the past, and *new*, or *marginal*, *costs*, which measure the cost of funds raised in the future. Historical costs are important in many ways. For example, payers that reimburse on a cost basis are concerned with embedded costs. However, our primary purpose in developing a firm's WACC is to use it in making capital investment decisions, which involve future asset acquisitions and future capital financing. Thus, for our purposes, the relevant costs are the marginal costs of new funds to be raised in the future (normally during some planning period, say, a year), and not the cost of funds raised in the past.

Self-Test Questions:

What is the basic concept of the weighted average cost of capital (WACC)?

What financing sources are typically included in a firm's WACC?

Should the component costs be estimated on a before-tax or an after-tax basis?

Should the component costs reflect historical or marginal costs?

Cost of Debt

It is unlikely that a firm's managers will know at the start of a planning period the exact types and amounts of debt that will be issued in the future; the type of debt actually used will depend on the specific assets to be financed and on market conditions as they develop over time. Even so, a firm's managers do know what types of debt are typically used by the firm. For example, Bayside Memorial Hospital typically uses bank debt to raise short-term funds to finance seasonal or cyclical working capital needs, and it uses 30-year tax-exempt bonds to raise long-term debt capital. Since Bayside does not use short-term debt to finance permanent assets, its managers include only long-term debt in their WACC estimate, and they assume that this debt will consist solely of 30-year tax-exempt bonds.

Suppose Bayside's managers are developing the hospital's WACC estimate for the coming year. How should they estimate the hospital's component *cost of debt*? Most managers would begin by discussing current and prospective interest rates with their firms' investment bankers, the institutions that help companies bring security issues to market. Assume that the municipal bond analyst at Suncoast Securities, Inc., Bayside's investment banker, states that new 30-year tax-exempt health care issues currently require semiannual interest payments of $35 ($70 annually) for each $1,000 par value bond issued. Thus, municipal bond investors currently require a $70/$1,000 = 7.0% return on their investment.

The true cost of the issue to Bayside would be higher than 7.0 percent, however, because the hospital must incur expenses to sell the bonds. Such expenses, which are called *issuance*, or *flotation costs*, consist of accounting costs, legal fees, printing costs, and the fees paid to governmental entities and investment bankers. The impact of flotation costs on the cost of debt can be easily estimated by solving for k_d in the following bond valuation equation:

$$\text{Net proceeds} = \sum_{t=1}^{2n} \frac{\text{Semiannual interest payment}}{(1 + k_d/2)^t}$$
$$+ \frac{\text{Par value}}{(1 + k_d/2)^{2n}}. \tag{8.1}$$

where k_d = annual flotation-adjusted cost of debt and n = life of bond.[1] To illustrate, if Bayside's flotation costs were estimated to be 1.0 percent of the gross amount of the issue, then the flotation cost on each $1,000 par value bond would be 0.01($1,000) = $10, and the net proceeds would be $1,000 − $10 = $990. Thus, the hospital's flotation-adjusted annual cost of debt would be 7.08 percent:

$$\$990 = \sum_{t=1}^{60} \frac{\$35}{(1 + k_d/2)^t} + \frac{\$1,000}{(1 + k_d/2)^{60}}$$
$$k_d/2 = 3.54\%$$
$$k_d = 7.08\%.$$

As we discussed in Chapter 6, bond valuation can be done quite easily using a financial calculator. On most types of financial calculators, simply enter PV = 990 (or −990), PMT = 35, FV = 1,000, and n = 60. Then, press the i key, and 3.54 is displayed. Since this is the semiannual rate, multiply by 2 to obtain the annual rate.

A question arises here about whether the nominal yield to maturity or the effective annual rate should be used in the cost of debt estimate. In general, the difference will be inconsequential, so most firms opt for the easier approach, which is simply to use the nominal rate. (The effective annual rate in this example is $1.0354^2 − 1.0 = 7.21\%$ versus a 7.08 percent nominal rate.) More importantly, most capital budgeting analyses use end-of-year cash flows to proxy cash flows that occur throughout the year, in effect creating nominal cash flows. For consistency, we prefer to use a nominal cost of capital—the cash flows will be understated, but so will the cost of capital.

Note that flotation costs on bond issues are typically small, so their impact on the cost of debt estimate is often inconsequential, especially when one considers the uncertainty inherent in the entire cost of capital estimation process. In this example, the flotation-adjusted cost of debt is only eight basis points higher than the unadjusted cost of debt.[2] Therefore, it is common practice to ignore flotation costs when estimating the component cost of debt. Bayside follows this practice, so they would estimate the component cost of debt as 7.0 percent:

$$\text{Tax-exempt component cost of debt} = k_d = 7.0\%.$$

If Bayside's currently outstanding debt were actively traded, then the current yield to maturity on this debt could be used to estimate the cost of new debt. For example, Bayside has a tax-exempt debt issue outstanding that has a 20-year life, a 6 percent coupon, and currently sells in the secondary market for $905. The yield to maturity on this issue is 6.9 percent:

$$\$905 = \sum_{t=1}^{40} \frac{\$30}{(1 + k_d/2)^t} + \frac{\$1,000}{(1 + k_d/2)^{40}}$$

$$k_d/2 = 3.44\%$$

$$k_d = 6.88\% \approx 6.9\%.$$

Using the yield to maturity on an outstanding issue to estimate the cost of new debt provides a good estimate for k_d when the remaining life of the old issue approximates the anticipated maturity of the new issue. If this is not the case, then yield curve differentials might cause the estimate to be biased. For example, if the yield curve is upward sloping, the yield to maturity on a 15-year issue would understate the actual cost of a new 30-year issue.

A taxable health care organization would use the techniques just described to estimate its before-tax cost of debt. However, the tax benefits of interest payments must then be incorporated into the estimate. To illustrate, consider Ann Arbor Health Systems, Inc., an investor-owned company that operates 16 acute care hospitals in Michigan, Indiana, and Ohio. The company's investment bankers indicate that a new 30-year taxable bond issue would require a yield of 11.7 percent. Since the firm's federal-plus-state tax rate is 40 percent, its component cost of debt estimate is also 7.0 percent:

$$\text{Taxable component cost of debt} = k_d(1 - T)$$
$$= 11.7\%(1 - 0.40)$$
$$= 11.7\%(0.60) = 7.0\%.$$

Note that the component cost of debt to an investor-owned firm is an after-tax cost, because the effective cost to the firm is reduced by the $(1 - T)$ term. By reducing Ann Arbor's component cost of debt from 11.7 percent to 7.0 percent, we have incorporated the benefit associated with interest payment tax deductibility into the cost of debt.[3]

In general, the effective cost of debt is roughly comparable between investor-owned and not-for-profit firms of similar risk. Investor-owned firms have the benefit of tax deductibility of interest payments, while not-for-profit firms have the benefit of being able to issue tax-exempt debt.

Self-Test Questions:

What are some methods used to estimate a firm's cost of debt?

What is the impact of flotation costs on the cost of debt? Are these costs generally material?

For investor-owned firms, how is the before-tax cost of debt converted to an after-tax cost?

Should the nominal or effect annual rate be used as the cost of debt estimate? Explain.

Cost of Equity (Fund) Capital

Equity capital is raised by investor-owned firms by selling new common stock and by retaining earnings for use by the firm rather than paying them out as dividends to shareholders. Not-for-profit firms raise equity capital through contributions and grants, and by generating an excess of revenues over expenses, none of which can be paid out as dividends. In the following sections, we describe how to estimate the costs of the various forms of equity capital, both to investor-owned and not-for-profit firms.[4]

Self-Test Question:

What are the sources of equity capital for health care firms?

Cost of Retained Earnings to Investor-Owned Firms

The two sources of equity capital to investor-owned firms—retentions and new common stock sales—have slightly different costs. The difference arises because flotation costs must be incurred on new common stock sales, while the retention of earnings does not require such costs.

The cost of debt is based on the return that investors require on debt securities, and the *cost of retained earnings* to investor-owned firms can be defined similarly: it is the rate of return that investors require on the firm's common stock. At first glance, it might appear that retained earnings are a costless source of capital to investor-owned firms. After all, dividend payments must be paid on new shares of stock that are issued, but no such payments are required on funds that are obtained by retaining earnings. The reason why a cost of capital must be assigned to retained earnings involves the *opportunity cost principle*. An investor-owned firm's net income literally belongs to its common stockholders. Employees are compensated by wages, suppliers are compensated by cash payments for supplies, bondholders are compensated by interest payments, governments are compensated by tax payments, and so on. The residual earnings of a firm, its net income, belongs to the stockholders and serves to "pay the rent" on the stockholder-supplied capital.

Management can either pay out earnings in the form of dividends or retain earnings for reinvestment in the business. If part of the earnings are retained, an opportunity cost is incurred: stockholders could have received these earnings as dividends and then invested this money in stock, bonds, real estate, commodity futures, and so on. Thus, the firm should earn on its retained earnings at least as much as its stockholders themselves could earn on alternative investments of similar risk. If the firm cannot earn as much as the stockholders can in similar risk investments, then the firm's net income should be paid out as dividends rather than retained for reinvestment within the firm. What rate of return can stockholders expect to earn on other investments of equivalent risk? The answer is k_s, the required rate of return on equity. Investors can earn this return either by buying more shares of the firm in question or by buying stock of similar firms.

Whereas debt is a contractual obligation with an easily estimated cost, it is not nearly as easy to estimate k_s, the cost of retained earnings. Two primary methods are used to estimate k_s: the Capital Asset Pricing Model (CAPM) and the discounted cash flow (DCF) model. These methods should not be regarded as mutually exclusive, for neither approach dominates the estimation process. In practice, both approaches should be used to estimate k_s, and then the final value should be chosen on the basis of the analyst's confidence in the data at hand.

Capital Asset Pricing Model (CAPM) Approach

The *Capital Asset Pricing Model (CAPM)*, which we introduced in Chapter 7, is a widely accepted finance model that specifies the equilibrium risk/return relationship on common stocks. Basically, the model assumes that investors consider only one risk factor when setting required rates of returns—the volatility of returns on the stock compared with the volatility of returns on a well-diversified portfolio called the *market portfolio*, or just the *market*. The measure of risk in the CAPM is the stock's *beta*, or *beta coefficient*, which measures the relative volatility of the stock's returns. The market, which is a large collection of stocks such as the S&P 500 Index, has a beta of 1.0. A stock with a beta of 2.0 has twice the volatility of returns as the market, while a stock with a beta of 0.5 has only half the volatility of returns as the market. Since return volatility is a measure of risk, a low beta stock, defined as having a beta less than 1.0, is less risky than the market, while a high beta stock, defined as having a beta more than 1.0, is more risky than the market.

Within the CAPM, the actual equation that relates risk to return is called the *Security Market Line (SML)*:

$$k_s = \text{Risk-free rate} + \text{Risk premium}$$
$$= k_{RF} + (k_M - k_{RF})b.$$

Here,

k_{RF} = risk-free rate, the required rate of return on riskless securities.

k_M = required rate of return on the market.

b = beta coefficient of the stock in question.

$(k_M - k_{RF})$ = market risk premium, the premium above the risk-free rate that investors require to buy a stock with average risk.

$(k_M - k_{RF})b$ = stock risk premium, the premium above the risk-free that investors require to buy the stock in question.

Given estimates of (1) the risk-free rate, k_{RF}; (2) the beta of the firm's stock, b; and (3) the required rate of return on the market, k_M, we can estimate the required rate of return on the firm's stock. This estimate, in turn, can be used as the estimate for the firm's cost of retained earnings.

Estimating the risk-free rate

The starting point for the CAPM cost of equity estimate is k_{RF}, the risk-free rate. Unfortunately, there is no security in the United States that is truly riskless. Treasury securities are essentially free of default risk, but long-term T-bonds will suffer capital losses if interest rates rise, and a portfolio invested in short-term T-bills will provide a volatile earnings stream because the rate paid on T-bills varies over time.

Since we cannot in practice find a truly riskless rate on which to base the CAPM, what rate should we use? Our preference—and this preference is shared by most analysts—is to use the rate on long-term Treasury bonds. There are many reasons for favoring the T-bond rate, including the fact that T-bill rates are very volatile because they are directly affected by actions taken by the Federal Reserve Board. Perhaps the most persuasive argument is that common stocks are generally viewed as long-term securities, and although a particular stockholder may not have a long investment horizon, the majority of stockholders do invest on a long-term basis. Therefore, it is reasonable to think that stock returns embody long-term inflation expectations similar to those embodied in bonds, rather than the short-term inflation expectations embodied in bills. On this account, the cost of equity should be more highly correlated with T-bond rates than with T-bill rates. T-bond rates can be found in local newspapers, in the *Wall Street Journal*, and in the *Federal Reserve Bulletin*. Generally, we use the yield on 20-year T-bonds as the proxy for the risk-free rate.

Estimating the required rate of return on the market

The required rate of return on the market, and its derivative, the market risk premium, $RP_M = k_M - k_{RF}$, can be estimated on the basis of (1) ex post, or historical, returns, or (2) ex ante, or forward-looking, returns.

1. *Ex post risk premiums.* The most complete, accurate, and up-to-date ex post risk premium study is available annually from Ibbotson Associates, which examines market data over long periods of time to find the average annual rates of return on stocks, T-bills, T-bonds, and a set of high-grade corporate bonds.[5] For example, Table 8.1 summarizes some results from Ibbotson Associates' 1995 study, which covers the period 1926–1994.

Table 8.1   Selected Historical Returns Data, 1926–1994

	Annual Average	Standard Deviation
Total Return Data		
Common stocks (large company)	12.2%	20.3%
Long-term corporate bonds	5.7	8.4
Long-term Treasury bonds	5.2	8.8
Treasury bills	3.7	3.3
Inflation rate	3.2	4.6
Risk Premium Data		
Common stocks over T-bills	8.4%	NA*
Common stocks over T-bonds	7.0	NA
T-bonds over T-bills	1.0	NA

*Not available.

Source: Ibbotson Associates. *1995 Yearbook.*

Note that common stocks provided the highest average return over the 69-year period, while Treasury bills gave the lowest. T-bills barely covered inflation over the period, but common stocks provided a substantial real return. However, the superior returns on stock investments had its cost—stocks were by far the riskiest of the investments listed as judged by standard deviation (which measures dispersion about the mean), and they would also rank as riskiest within a market risk framework. To further illustrate the risk differentials, the range on annual returns on stocks was from −43.3 to 54.0 percent, while the range on T-bills was only 0.0 to 14.7 percent. The study provides strong empirical support for the basic premise that we discussed in earlier chapters—namely, that in efficient markets, higher returns can be obtained only by bearing greater risk.

The study also reported the risk premiums, or differences, among the various securities. For example, Ibbotson Associates found the average risk premium of stocks over T-bonds to be 7.0 percentage points. However, although not reported, these premiums have large standard deviations, so one must use them with caution. Also, it should be noted that the choice of the beginning and ending periods can have a major impact on the calculated risk premiums. Ibbotson Associates used the longest period available to them, but had their data begun some years earlier or later, or had it ended earlier, their results would have been significantly affected. Indeed, in many years their data would indicate *negative* risk premiums, which would lead to the conclusion that Treasury securities have a higher required return than common stocks—a conclusion that is contrary to both financial theory and common sense. All of this suggests that historical risk premiums should be approached with caution. As one businessman muttered after listening to a professor give a lecture on the CAPM: "Beware of academics bearing gifts!"

2. *Ex ante risk premiums.* The ex post approach to risk premiums used by Ibbotson Associates assumes that investors expect future results, on average, to equal past results. However, as we noted, the historical risk premium varies greatly depending on the period selected and, in any event, investors today probably expect results in the future to be different from those achieved during the Great Depression of the 1930s, during the World War II years of the 1940s, and during the peaceful boom years of the 1950s, all of which are included (and given equal weight with more recent results) in the Ibbotson Associates data. The questionable assumption that future expectations are equal to past realizations, together with the sometimes nonsensical results obtained in historical risk premium studies, has led to the search for ex ante risk premiums.

The most common approach to ex ante premiums uses the Discounted Cash Flow (DCF) model to estimate the expected market rate of return, $\hat{k}_M = k_M$; then calculates RP_M as $k_M - k_{RF}$; and finally uses this estimate of RP_M in the CAPM. This procedure recognizes that, if markets are in equilibrium, the expected rate of return on the market portfolio is also its required rate of return. Thus, if we can estimate $\hat{k}_M$, we also have an estimate of k_M.

Many financial services companies publish forecasts based on DCF methodology for the expected rate of return on the market, $\hat{k}_M$. For example, Merrill Lynch puts out such a forecast in its bimonthly publication *Quantitative Analysis*. One can subtract the current T-bond rate from such a market forecast to obtain an estimate of the current market risk premium, RP_M.

Estimating beta

The last parameter needed for a CAPM cost of retained earnings estimate is the beta coefficient. Recall from Chapter 5 that a stock's beta is a measure of its volatility relative to that of an average stock, and that betas are generally estimated from the stock's characteristic line, that is, estimated by running a linear regression between past returns on the stock in question and past returns on some market index. We will define betas developed in this manner as *historical betas*.

Unfortunately, historical betas show how risky a stock was *in the past*, whereas investors are interested in *future* risk. It may be that a given company appeared to be quite safe in the past, but that things have changed and its future risk is judged to be higher than its past risk, or vice versa. The hospital industry presents a good example. Prior to 1983, when the industry operated on a cost-plus basis, investor-owned hospitals were among the bluest of the blue chips. However, when prospective payment began, the industry became much riskier. HMOs, on the other hand, were doing poorly a few years ago, but now many of them appear to be quite healthy. Therefore, one would think that the HMOs' risk has declined while the hospital industry's has increased.

Now consider the use of beta as a measure of a company's risk. If we use a historical beta in a CAPM framework to measure the firm's cost of retained earnings, we are implicitly assuming that its future risk is the same as its past risk. This would be a troublesome assumption for a hospital in 1983. But what about most companies in most years? As a general rule, is future risk sufficiently similar to past risk to warrant the use of historical betas in a CAPM framework? For individual firms, historical betas are often not very stable, so past risk is often *not* a good predictor of future risk.

Since historical betas may not be good predictors of future risk, researchers have sought ways to improve them. This has led to the development of two other types of betas: (1) adjusted betas and (2) fundamental betas. *Adjusted betas* recognize the fact that true betas tend to move toward 1.0 over time.[6] Therefore, one can begin with a firm's pure historical statistical beta, make an adjustment for the expected future movement toward 1.0, and produce an adjusted beta that on average will be a better predictor of the future beta than would the unadjusted historical beta.

Finally, *fundamental betas* extend the adjustment process to include such fundamental risk variables as the use of debt financing, sales volatility, and the like.[7] These betas are constantly adjusted to reflect changes in a firm's operations and capital structure, whereas with historical betas (including adjusted ones) such changes might not be fully reflected until several years after the company's "true" beta has changed.

Adjusted betas are obviously heavily dependent on unadjusted historical betas, and so are fundamental betas as they are actually calculated. Therefore, the plain old historical beta, calculated as the slope of the characteristic line, is important even if one goes on to develop a more exotic version. With this in mind, it should be noted that several different sets of data can be used to calculate historical betas, and the different data sets produce different results. Here are some points to note:

- Betas can be based on historical periods of different lengths. For example, data for the past one, two, three, and so on, years may be used. Most people who calculate betas today use five years of data, but this choice is arbitrary, and different lengths of time usually alter significantly the calculated beta for a given company.[8]

- Returns may be calculated on holding periods of different lengths—a day, a week, a month, a quarter, a year, and so on. For example, if it has been decided to analyze data on NYSE stocks over a five-year period, then we might obtain $52(5) = 260$ weekly returns, or $1(5) = 5$ annual returns. The set of returns on each stock, however large it turns out to be, would then be regressed on the corresponding market returns to obtain the stock's beta. In statistical analysis, it is generally better to have more rather then fewer observations, because using more observations generally leads to greater statistical confidence. This suggests the use of weekly returns and, say, five years of data, for a sample size of 260, or even daily returns for a still larger sample size. However, the shorter the holding period, the more likely the data are to exhibit random "noise," and the greater the number of years of data, the more likely it is that the company's market risk will have changed. Thus, the choice of both the number of years of data and the length of the holding period involves a trade-off between a desire to have many observations versus a desire to have recent and consequently more relevant data.

- The value used to represent "the market" is also an important consideration, and one that can have a significant effect on the calculated beta. Most beta calculators today use the New York Stock Exchange Composite Index (based on about 2,000 stocks, weighted by the value of each company), but others use the S&P 500 Index or some other group, including one (the Wilshire Index) with over 5,000 stocks. In theory, the broader the index, the better the beta: indeed, the index should really include returns on all risky assets, including stocks, bonds, leases, private businesses, real estate, and even "human capital." As a practical matter, however, we cannot get accurate returns data on most types of assets, so measurement problems largely restrict us to stock indexes.

The bottom line of all of this is that one can calculate betas in many different ways and, depending on the methods used, different betas, and hence different costs of retained earnings, will result. Where does this leave managers regarding the proper beta? They must "pay their money and take their choice." Some managers will calculate their own betas, using whichever procedure seems most appropriate under the circumstances. Others will use betas calculated by organizations such as Merrill Lynch or Value Line, perhaps using one service or perhaps averaging the betas of several services. The choice is a matter of judgment and data availability, for there is no "right" beta. With luck, the betas derived from different sources will, for a given company, be close together. If they are not, then our confidence in the CAPM cost of retained earnings estimate will be diminished.

Table 8.2 contains the betas of some representative investor-owned health care firms as provided by Value Line. Value Line uses the New York Stock Exchange Composite Index as its proxy for the market, 260 weekly observations, and it adjusts the betas for their tendency to move toward 1.0 over time. On the basis of this very limited selection, it appears that health care firms carry above-average market risk for stockholders. Drug producers carry the lowest risk, with betas of 1.05, while HMOs and high-technology firms carry very high risk, with betas over 1.50.

Illustration of the CAPM approach

To illustrate the CAPM approach, consider Ann Arbor Health Systems, which has a beta coefficient, b, of 1.10. Furthermore, assume that the

Table 8.2 Beta Coefficients for Selected Heath Care Companies

Company	Primary Line of Business	Beta
Alza	Drug delivery systems	1.60
Baxter International	Medical supplies	1.15
Beverly Enterprises	Nursing homes	1.35
Bristol-Myers Squibb	Diversified drugs	1.05
Chiron	Biotechnology	1.60
Community Psychiatric Centers	Psychiatric hospitals	1.35
Lincoln National	Diversified insurance	1.05
Manor Care	Nursing homes	1.15
National Medical Enterprises	Acute care hospitals	1.30
Omnicare	Clinical supplies	1.15
PacifiCare Systems	HMO	1.55
Upjohn	Diversified drugs	1.05
U.S. Healthcare	HMO	1.55
U.S. Surgical	Medical equipment	1.40

Source: Value Line Investment Survey. 1995.

current yield on T-bonds, k_{RF}, is 8.5 percent, and that the best estimate for the current market risk premium, RP_M, is 5.0 percentage points. (In other words, the current required rate of return on the market, k_M, is 13.5 percent.) We now have estimated all of the required input parameters, and we can complete the SML equation as follows:

$$k_s = k_{RF} + (k_M - k_{RF})b$$
$$= 8.5\% + (13.5\% - 8.5\%)1.10$$
$$= 8.5\% + (5.0\%)1.10 = 14.0\%.$$

Thus, according to the CAPM, Ann Arbor's required rate of return on retained earnings is 14.0 percent.

In words, what does the 14.0 percent estimate for k_s imply? In essence, equity investors believe that Ann Arbor's stock, with a beta of 1.10, is slightly more risky than the average stock, with a beta of 1.00. With a risk-free rate of 8.5 percent, and a market risk premium of 5.0 percentage points, an average company, with $b = 1.0$, has a required rate of return on retained earnings of

$$k_s = k_{RF} + (k_M - k_{RF})b$$
$$= 8.5\% + (5.0\%)1.00 = 13.5\%.$$

Thus, according to the CAPM, equity investors require 50 basis points more return for investing in Ann Arbor Health Systems, with $b = 1.10$, rather than an average stock, with $b = 1.0$.

It should be obvious to you that there is a great deal of uncertainty in the CAPM estimate of k_s. Some of this uncertainty stems from the fact that there is no assurance that the CAPM is correct, that is, that the CAPM accurately describes the risk/return choices of stock investors. Additionally, there is a great deal of uncertainty in the input parameter estimates, especially the required rate of return on the market and the beta coefficient. Because of these uncertainties, it is highly unlikely that Ann Arbor's true, but unobservable, k_s is 14.0 percent. Thus, instead of picking single values for each parameter, it may be better to develop high and low estimates, and then to combine all of the high estimates and all of the low estimates to develop a range, rather than a point estimate, for k_s.

Discounted cash flow (DCF) approach

The second procedure for estimating the cost of retained earnings is the *discounted cash flow (DCF) method.* We know that the intrinsic value of a stock, $\hat{P}_0$, is the present value of its expected dividend stream:

$$\hat{P}_0 = \frac{D_1}{(1 + k_s)^1} + \frac{D_2}{(1 + k_s)^2} + \frac{D_3}{(1 + k_s)^3} + \ldots + \frac{D_\infty}{(1 + k_s)^\infty}. \quad (8.2)$$

If the dividend is expected to grow each year at a constant rate, g, then Equation 8.2 reduces to the *constant growth model*:

$$\hat{P}_0 = \frac{D_1}{k_s - g}. \quad (8.3)$$

Stock prices are generally in equilibrium, which means that the stock price, P_0, is the same as its intrinsic value, $\hat{P}_0$, so we can rewrite Equation 8.3 as

$$P_0 = \frac{D_1}{k_s - g}. \quad (8.3a)$$

Finally, Equation 8.3a can be solved for k_s, giving this equation:

$$\hat{k}_s = k_s = \frac{D_1}{P_0} + g. \quad (8.3b)$$

This is the form of the DCF model that often is used to estimate the cost of retained earnings.[9]

Estimating the current stock price

As in the CAPM approach, there are three input parameters in the DCF model. Current stock price is readily available for firms that are actively traded. Ann Arbor Health Systems' stock is traded in the over-the-counter (OTC) market, so its stock price generally can be found in the *Wall Street Journal.* At the time of the analysis, Ann Arbor's stock price was $40.

Estimating the next dividend payment

Next year's dividend payment is also relatively easy to estimate. If you are one of Ann Arbor's managers, you can look in the firm's five-year financial plan for the dividend estimate. If you are an outsider, dividend data on larger publicly traded firms are available from brokerage houses and investment advisory firms. Also, current (D_0) dividend information is published in the *Wall Street Journal,* and it can be used as a basis for estimating next year's dividend (D_1). Ann Arbor Health Systems is followed by several analysts at major brokerage houses, and their consensus estimate for next year's dividend payment is $2.50, so for purposes of this analysis, $D_1 = \$2.50$.

Estimating the growth rate

The growth rate, g, is the most difficult of the DCF model parameters to estimate. Here we discuss several methods for estimating g.

1. *Historical growth rates.* If growth rates in earnings and dividends have been relatively stable in the past, and if investors expect these trends to continue, then the past realized growth rate may be used as an estimate of the expected future growth rate. To illustrate, consider Table 8.3, which gives earnings per share (EPS) and dividends per share (DPS) data from 1986 to 1995 for Ann Arbor Health Systems. Note these points:

   a. We show 10 years (nine growth periods) of data in Table 8.3, but we could have used 15 years or 5 years, or some other historical time period. There is no rule about the appropriate number of years to analyze when calculating historical growth rates. However, the period chosen should reflect, to the extent possible, the conditions expected in the future.

   b. The easiest historical growth rate to calculate is the compound rate between two dates, called the *point-to-point rate.* For example, EPS grew at an annual rate of 6.8 percent from 1986 to 1995, and DPS grew at a 7.2 percent rate during this same period. (To obtain g_{EPS} using a financial calculator, enter 2.95 [or −2.95] as PV, 5.35 as FV, 9 as n [because with ten data points we have nine growth periods], and then press i to obtain the growth rate, 6.8 percent.) Note that the point-to-point growth rate could change radically if we used two other points. For example, if we calculate

Table 8.3   Ann Arbor Health Systems: Historical EPS and DPS Data

Year	EPS	DPS
1986	$2.95	$1.24
1987	3.07	1.32
1988	3.22	1.32
1989	3.40	1.52
1990	4.65	1.72
1991	5.12	1.92
1992	5.25	2.00
1993	5.20	2.20
1994	5.12	2.20
1995	5.35	2.32

the five-year EPS growth rate from 1990 to 1995, we would obtain only 2.8 percent. This radical change occurs because the point-to-point rate is extremely sensitive to the beginning and ending years chosen.

c. To alleviate the problem of beginning and ending year sensitivity, some analysts use the *average-to-average method,* which reduces the sensitivity of the growth rate to beginning and ending year values. The 1986–1988 average EPS is ($2.95 + $3.07 + $3.22)/3 = $3.08, the average 1993–1995 EPS is ($5.20 + $5.12 + $5.35)/3 = $5.22, and the number of years of growth between the two averages is 1987–1994 = 7. The average-to-average DPS growth rate is 8.2 percent, and the average-to-average EPS growth rate is 7.8 percent. Note that we are calculating compound annual growth rates, which are much easier to interpret than a single growth rate over the entire period.

d. A third way, and in our view the best way, to estimate historical growth rates is by *log-linear least squares regression.*[10] The regression method gives consideration to all data points in the series; thus, it is the least likely to be biased by a randomly high or low beginning or ending year. The only practical way to estimate a least squares growth rate is with a computer or a financial calculator. Using a spreadsheet's data regression capability, we find the growth rate in earnings to be 7.9 percent, while the growth rate in dividends is 7.7 percent.

e. If earnings and dividends are growing at approximately the same rate, there is no problem, but if these two growth rates are unequal, we do have a problem. First the DCF model calls for the expected *dividend* growth rate. However, if EPS and DPS are growing at different rates, something is going to have to change: these two series cannot grow at two different rates indefinitely. There is no rule for handling differences in historical g_{EPS} and g_{DPS}, and when they differ, this simply demonstrates in yet another way the problems with using historical growth as a proxy for expected future growth. Like many aspects of financial management, judgment is required when estimating growth rates.

Table 8.4 summarizes the historical growth rates we have just discussed. It is obvious that one can take a given set of historical data and, depending on the years and the calculation method used, obtain a large number of quite different growth rates. Now recall our purpose in making these calculations: we are seeking the future dividend growth rate that investors expect. If past growth rates have been stable, then investors might base future expectations on past trends. This is a reasonable proposition; but, unfortunately, one rarely finds much historical stability. Therefore, the use of historical growth rates in a DCF analysis must be applied with judgment and also used (if at all) in conjunction with other growth estimation methods as discussed next.

2. *Retention growth.* The *retention growth method* is another method for estimating the growth rate in dividends:

$$g = \text{Retention ratio(Expected ROE).} \tag{8.4}$$

Equation 8.4 produces a constant growth rate, and when we use it we are, by implication, making four important assumptions: (1) we expect the payout ratio, and thus the retention ratio, to remain constant; (2) we expect the return on equity on new investment to equal the firm's current ROE, which implies that we expect the return on equity to remain constant; (3) the firm is not expected to issue new common stock or, if it does, we expect this new stock to be sold at a price equal to its book value; and (4) future projects are expected to have the same degree of risk as the firm's existing assets.

Suppose that Ann Arbor Health Systems has had an average return on equity of about 14 percent over the past ten years. The ROE has been relatively steady, but even so it has ranged from a low of 8.9 percent to a high of 17.6 percent during this period. In addition, the firm's dividend payout ratio has averaged 0.45 over the past ten years, so its retention ratio has averaged $1.0 - 0.45 = 0.55$. Using Equation 8.4, the retention growth method gives a g estimate of 7.7 percent:

$$g = 0.55(14\%) = 7.7\%.$$

This figure, together with the historical EPS and DPS growth rates examined earlier, might lead us to conclude that Ann Arbor Health

Table 8.4   Ann Arbor Health Systems: Historical Growth Rates, 1986–1995

Method	EPS	DPS	Average
Point-to-point	6.8%	7.2%	7.0%
Average-to-average	7.8	8.2	8.0
Log-linear regression	7.9	7.7	7.8

System's expected dividend growth rate is in the range of 7.0 to 8.0 percent.

3. *Analysts' forecasts.* A third growth rate estimation technique calls for using security analysts' forecasts. Analysts forecast and then publish growth rate estimates for most of the larger publicly owned companies. For example, *Value Line* provides such forecasts on about 1,700 companies, and all of the larger brokerage houses provide similar forecasts. Further, several companies compile analysts' forecasts on a regular basis and provide summary information such as the median and range of forecasts on widely followed companies. These growth rate summaries, such as the one compiled by Lynch, Jones & Ryan in its *Institutional Brokers Estimate System (IBES)*, can be ordered for a fee and obtained either in hard-copy format or as on-line computer data.

However, analysts' forecasts often assume nonconstant growth. For example, assume that analysts were forecasting that Ann Arbor Health Systems would have a 12.0 percent annual growth rate in earnings and dividends over the next five years, and a steady-state growth rate of 6.5 percent following the high-growth period. A simple way to handle this situation is to use the nonconstant growth forecast to develop a proxy constant growth rate. Computer simulations indicate that dividends beyond Year 50 contribute very little to the value of any stock—the present value of dividends beyond Year 50 is virtually zero, so for practical purposes, we can ignore anything beyond that point. If we consider only a 50-year horizon, we can develop a weighted average growth rate and use it as a constant growth rate for cost of capital purposes. For Ann Arbor Health Systems, we assumed a growth rate of 12.0 percent for five years followed by a growth rate of 6.5 percent for 45 years, which produced an arithmetic average annual growth rate of $0.10(12.0\%) + 0.90(6.5\%) = 7.2\%$.

Illustration of the DCF approach

To illustrate the DCF approach, consider the data developed for Ann Arbor Health Systems. The company's current stock price, P_0, is $40, and its next expected annual dividend, D_1, is $2.50. Thus, the firm's DCF estimate of k_s, according to Equation 8.3b, is

$$k_s = \frac{D_1}{P_0} + g. \tag{8.3b}$$
$$= \frac{\$2.50}{\$40} + g = 6.25\% + g.$$

With a g estimate range of 7–8 percent, we will use the midpoint, 7.5 percent, as our estimate. Thus, our DCF estimate for Ann Arbor Health System's cost of retained earnings is 6.25% + 7.5% = 13.75% ≈ 13.8%.

Comparison of the CAPM and DCF methods

We have discussed two methods for estimating the required rate of return on retained earnings, CAPM and DCF.[11] Our CAPM estimate was 14.0 percent and our DCF estimate was 13.8 percent. In our view, there is sufficient consistency in the results to warrant the use of 13.9 percent as our estimate of the cost of retained earnings for Ann Arbor Health Systems. If the two methods produced widely different estimates, then Ann Arbor's managers would have to use their judgment regarding the relative merits of each estimate, and then choose the estimate that seemed most reasonable under the circumstances. In general, this choice would be made on the basis of the managers' confidence in the input parameters of each approach.

Self-Test Questions:

What is the best proxy for the risk-free rate in the CAPM? Why?

What are the three types of beta that can be used in the CAPM?

What are three common methods for estimating the future dividend growth rate?

How would you choose between widely different estimates of k_s?

Cost of Fund Capital to Not-for-Profit Firms

Not-for-profit firms raise equity, or fund, capital in two basic ways: (1) by receiving contributions and grants, and (2) by earning an excess of revenues over expenses (retained earnings). In recent years considerable controversy has arisen over the "cost" of this capital to not-for-profit firms. In this section we first discuss some views regarding the cost of fund capital, and then we illustrate how the cost might be estimated.

What is the cost of fund capital?

Our primary purpose in this chapter is to develop a weighted average cost of capital that can be used in capital budgeting decisions. Thus, the estimated "costs" represent the cost of using capital to purchase fixed assets, rather than for alternative uses. What is the cost of using fund capital for real asset investment? There are at least four positions that can be taken on this question.[12]

1. It has been argued that fund capital has zero cost. The rationale here is that (1) contributors do not expect a monetary return on their contributions, and that (2) the firm's stakeholders, especially the patients who pay more for services than warranted by the firm's tangible costs, do not require an explicit return on the capital retained by the firm.

2. The second position is that fund capital has some cost, but that the cost is not very high. When a not-for-profit firm receives contributions or retains earnings, it can always invest these funds in marketable securities (highly liquid, safe securities) rather than purchase real assets. Thus, fund capital has an opportunity cost that should be acknowledged, and this cost is roughly equal to the return available on a portfolio of short-term, low-risk securities such as T-bills.

3. The third position rests not so much on the inherent cost of fund capital, but more on the correct premise that a not-for-profit firm must earn a return on its fund capital if it is to expand its services over time.[13] For example, assume that a hospital in a growing city must increase its total assets by 5 percent per year to keep pace with increased patient demand. To purchase the required assets without increasing the percentage of debt used to finance the assets, it must grow its fund capital at a 5 percent rate. In this way it can finance asset growth by growing both debt and equity at the same 5 percent rate, and hence can hold the relative amount of debt constant. If the hospital earned zero return on its fund capital, its equity base would remain constant over time, and the only way it could add new assets would be to take on additional debt without matching equity, and hence drive up its debt ratio. Of course, at some point lenders would be unwilling to provide additional debt financing, so no new assets could be added.

   If inflation exists, a not-for-profit firm must earn a return on its fund capital just to replace its existing asset base as assets wear out or become obsolete. The return is required because new assets will cost more than the old ones being replaced, so depreciation cash flow in itself will not be sufficient to replace assets as needed. The bottom line here is that not-for-profit firms must earn a return on fund capital, and the greater the growth rate in total assets, including that caused by inflation, the greater the return that must be earned.

4. Finally, others have argued that fund capital to not-for-profit firms has about the same cost as the cost of retained earnings to similar investor-owned firms. The rationale here also rests on the opportunity cost concept as discussed earlier in point 2, but the opportunity cost is now defined as the return available from investing fund capital in alternative investments of *similar risk*.

   Which of the four positions is correct? Think about it this way. Suppose Bayside Memorial Hospital, a not-for-profit corporation, receives $500,000 in contributions in 1996 and also retains $4,500,000 in earnings, so it has $5 million of new fund capital available for investment. The $5 million could be used to purchase assets related to its core business, such as an outpatient clinic or diagnostic equipment; or it could be temporarily invested in securities with the intent of purchasing health care assets some time in the future; or the $5 million could be used to retire debt; or it could be used to pay management bonuses; or it could be placed in a non-interest-bearing account at the bank; and on and on. By using this capital to invest in real assets, Bayside is deprived of the opportunity to use this capital for other purposes, so an opportunity cost must be assigned.

   What opportunity cost should be assigned? The answer is that the hospital's investment in real assets should return at least as much as the return available on securities investments of similar risk. What return is available on securities with similar risk to hospital assets? The answer is the return that is expected from investing in the stock of an investor-owned hospital company, such as Ann Arbor Health Systems. After all, instead of using fund capital to purchase real health care assets, Bayside could always use the funds to buy the stock of a hospital company such as Ann Arbor Health Systems and delay the real asset purchase until some time in the future. Note that we do not mean to imply here that not-for-profit firms should never invest in a project that will "lose" money. Not-for-profit firms do invest in negative profit projects that benefit its stakeholders, but managers must be aware of the financial opportunity costs inherent in such investments. We will have more to say about this issue in Chapter 10.

   In general, the opportunity cost principle applies to all fund capital: it has a cost to the firm that equals the cost of retained earnings to similar investor-owned firms. However, if contributions are made for a specific purpose, such as a children's wing to a hospital, then those funds do indeed have zero cost. Since their use is restricted to a particular project, the firm does not have the opportunity to invest those funds in other alternatives.

Measuring the cost of fund capital

We have defined the cost of fund capital to not-for-profit firms as the return available on the stocks of similar investor-owned companies. Thus, if Bayside Memorial Hospital and Ann Arbor Systems were equivalent in all respects, then we could use the 13.9 percent estimate for Ann Arbor's cost of retained earnings as our estimate for Bayside's cost of fund capital. However, it is impossible to find identical investor-owned and not-for-profit firms—even when they are in the same line of business and about the same size, they will often use different amounts of debt financing, and one is taxable and the other is not. Because of these dissimilarities, it is necessary to adjust the cost estimate before it can be used by not-for-profit organizations.

The adjustment is accomplished by using *Hamada's equation*, which was developed by Robert Hamada in 1969. Hamada combined the Capital Asset Pricing Model (CAPM) with Modigliani and Miller's capital structure model (which we will discuss in the next chapter) to obtain the following equation:[14]

$$b_{Firm} = b_{Assets}[1 + (1 - T)(D/S)]. \tag{8.5}$$

Here b_{Firm} is the market-determined beta of the firm, b_{Assets} is the inherent market beta of the assets assuming that the firm uses no debt financing, T is the tax rate, D is the market value of the firm's debt, and S is the market value of the firm's equity. In essence, b_{Assets} measures the inherent market risk of the assets, and b_{Firm} measures the market risk of the assets when operated by a firm with a given capital structure and tax rate.

To illustrate the use of Hamada's equation, remember that the market beta of Ann Arbor Health Systems is 1.10 and its tax rate is 40 percent. Also, Ann Arbor's target capital structure consists of 60 percent debt and 40 percent equity. Assuming that the firm is at (or close to) its target capital structure, then these weights represent the firm's current market value structure. To begin the adjustment, use Equation 8.5 to obtain the market beta for Ann Arbor's hospital assets:

$$b_{Firm} = b_{Assets}[1 + (1 - T)(D/S)]$$
$$1.10 = b_{Assets}[1 + (1 - 0.40)(0.60/0.40)]$$
$$1.10 = b_{Assets}(1.90)$$
$$b_{Assets} = 1.10/1.90 = 0.58.$$

Now, if 0.58 is the inherent market beta of Ann Arbor's hospital assets, what is the implied market beta of those assets *as employed by*

Bayside Memorial Hospital, which uses 50 percent debt financing and is tax-exempt? To find the answer, we must again use Hamada's equation, but this time we know the asset beta and are solving for the firm's beta:

$$b_{Firm} = b_{Assets}[1 + (1 - T)(D/S)]$$
$$= 0.58[1 + (1 - 0)(0.50/0.50)]$$
$$= 0.58(2.0) = 1.16.$$

Finally, remembering that the risk-free rate is 8.5 percent and the required rate of return on the market is 13.5 percent, we use the Security Market Line (SML) to estimate Bayside's cost of fund capital:

$$k_s = k_{RF} + (k_M - k_{RF})b$$
$$= 8.5\% + (13.5\% - 8.5\%)1.16$$
$$= 8.5\% + (5.0\%)1.16 = 14.3\%.$$

Because of tax and leverage (debt financing) differences, Bayside's cost of fund capital, 14.3 percent, is slightly greater than Ann Arbor's cost of retained earnings, 13.9 percent.

Before we close this section, a word of caution is in order. There are a lot of issues that cast doubt on the accuracy of the adjustment process just described. Here are only a few. (1) Beta measures the risk to an investor-owned firm's stockholders, which is not the same as the risk to a not-for-profit firm's stakeholders, so using market betas to measure the risk inherent in fund capital can be considered only a very rough approximation. (2) There is no market value of a not-for-profit firm's fund capital, so the *D/E* ratio is not really defined for not-for-profit firms. (3) The derivation of Hamada's equation requires many unrealistic assumptions. Thus, we should view the adjustment process with some skepticism, which means that the cost of fund capital estimate is only a rough approximation. Nevertheless, the estimate is the best we have, and a cost of capital developed in this way is better than ignoring the fact that an opportunity cost is inherent in the use of fund capital.

Self-Test Questions:

Why is there a cost associated with fund capital?

What is the cost of fund capital?

Explain why Hamada's equation should be used in the process of estimating the cost of fund capital.

Cost of Newly Issued Common Stock
(Investor-Owned Firms)

The cost of retained earnings (or fund capital) as estimated in the last four sections is appropriate when retained earnings (or contributions) are being used to finance new projects. However, if an investor-owned firm is expanding so rapidly that its retained earnings have been exhausted, then it can raise equity by selling newly issued common stock, which has a higher cost than retained earnings. Specifically, the sale of new common stock, as with the sale of debt, involves flotation costs. These costs lower the net usable dollars produced by new stock issues, and this in turn increases the cost of the funds. We ignored flotation costs in our estimate of the cost of debt because flotation costs were small, but we cannot ignore them when new stock is issued.

When the firm sells new common stock, it nets $P_0(1 - F)$, where F is the percentage flotation cost expressed in decimal form. For example, if Ann Arbor Health Systems, whose stock sells for $40 a share, must incur flotation costs of $F = 20\%$, then it will net only $40(1 - 0.20) = $32 on each new share sold. Note that F consists of issuance expenses such as printing costs, accounting and legal fees, and investment banker commissions, as well as price effects resulting from market pressure and information asymmetries. (We will discuss information asymmetry effects in Chapter 9.)

To begin, the constant growth DCF model, modified to include flotation costs, is used to calculate the DCF $\hat{k}_e$, the cost of equity raised by selling new common stock:

$$P_0(1 - F) = \frac{D_1}{k_e - g}. \tag{8.6}$$

Solving Equation 8.6 for $\hat{k}_e$ produces this equation:

$$\hat{k}_e = k_e = \frac{D_1}{P_0(1 - F)} + g. \tag{8.6a}$$

This procedure recognizes that the purchaser of a share of newly issued stock will expect the same dividend stream as the holder of an old share, but the company will, because of flotation expenses, receive less money from the sale of the new share, $P_0(1 - F)$, than the value of the old share, P_0. Therefore, the money raised from the sale of new stock will have to "work harder" to produce the earnings needed to provide the dividend stream. As a result, $k_e > k_s$.

Using Equation 8.6a, and a growth estimate of 7.5 percent, we obtain Ann Arbor Health System's DCF cost of new common equity:

$$k_e = \frac{D_1}{P_0(1 - F)} + g$$

$$= \frac{\$2.50}{\$40(1 - 0.20)} + 7.5\% = 7.8\% + 7.5\% = 15.3\%.$$

The DCF value for k_e is 15.3 percent versus the DCF k_s = 13.8% for retained earnings that we estimated earlier using the same 7.5 percent growth rate, so the flotation cost adjustment factor is +1.5 percentage points:

$$\text{Flotation cost adjustment factor} = DCF\ k_e - DCF\ k_s$$

$$= 15.3\% - 13.8\%$$

$$= 1.5\ \text{percentage points.}$$

This means that, according to the DCF method, new outside equity costs about 1.5 percentage points more than retained earnings.

Notice that only one method (DCF) is commonly used to estimate the flotation cost adjustment factor, whereas two methods are used to estimate k_s. However, we will not use the DCF estimate for k_e as our final estimate. Rather, we will add the flotation cost adjustment factor to our final k_s estimate to obtain our final estimate for k_e. For Ann Arbor, our final estimate of the cost of retained earnings was 13.9 percent, so our final estimate for k_e is 15.4 percent:

$$\text{Final } k_e = \text{ Final } k_s + \text{ Flotation cost adjustment factor}$$

$$= 13.9\% + 1.5\% = 15.4\%.$$

Self-Test Questions:

Explain why the cost of new common stock is higher than the cost of retained earnings.

How is the flotation cost adjustment factor estimated?

The Weighted Average Cost of Capital

Thus far, we have discussed how to estimate the costs of debt, retained earnings and fund capital, and new common stock. Now we must combine these elements to form a weighted average cost of capital (WACC). Each firm has in mind a target capital structure, defined as the particular mix of debt and common equity that causes its WACC to be minimized. Furthermore, when a firm raises new capital, it generally tries to finance in a way that will keep the actual capital structure reasonably close to its target over time. Here is the general formula for the weighted average cost of capital (WACC) for all firms:[15]

$$\text{WACC} = w_d k_d (1 - T) + w_s (k_s \text{ or } k_e \text{ or } k_f). \qquad (8.7)$$

Here w_d and w_s are the target weights for debt and common equity, respectively. The cost of the debt component of the WACC will be an average if the firm uses several types of debt for its permanent financing, or Equation 8.7 could be expanded to include multiple debt terms. Investor-owned firms would use their marginal tax rate for T, while T would be zero for not-for-profit firms. The common equity cost used in the WACC will be either the cost of retained earnings, k_s, the cost of new common stock, k_e, or, for not-for-profit firms, the cost of fund capital, k_f.

One point should be made immediately: *The WACC is the weighted average cost of each new dollar of capital raised at the margin*—it is not the average cost of all the dollars the firm has raised in the past, nor is it the average cost of all the dollars the firm will raise during the current year. We are primarily interested in obtaining a cost of capital for use in capital budgeting, and for such purposes a *marginal cost* is required. That means, conceptually, that we must estimate the cost of each dollar the firm raises during the year. Each of those dollars will consist of some debt and some common equity, and the equity will be either retained earnings, new common stock, or fund capital.

To illustrate, Ann Arbor Health Systems has a target capital structure calling for 60 percent debt and 40 percent common equity. As we estimated earlier, the company's before-tax cost of debt, k_d, is 11.7 percent ignoring flotation costs; its tax rate, T, is 40 percent; its cost of common equity from retained earnings, k_s, is 13.9 percent; and its cost of equity from new common stock sales, k_e, is 15.4 percent.

Now suppose the firm needs to raise \$100. Conceptually, to keep its capital structure on target, it must obtain \$60 as debt and \$40 as common equity. In any one year, the firm may raise all its required capital by issuing debt or by retaining earnings. But over the long run, Ann Arbor plans to use 60 percent debt financing and 40 percent equity financing, and these weights must be used in the WACC estimate regardless of the actual financing plans for the near term. The weighted average cost of the \$100, assuming the equity portion is from retained earnings, is calculated using Equation 8.7 as follows:

$$\begin{aligned}
\text{WACC (retained earnings)} &= w_d k_d (1 - T) + w_s(k_s) \\
&= 0.60(11.7\%)(1 - 0.40) \\
&\quad + 0.40(13.9\%) \\
&\approx 9.8\%.
\end{aligned}$$

Every dollar of new capital that Ann Arbor obtains consists of 60 cents of debt with an after-tax cost of 7.0 percent and 40 cents of common equity with a cost of 13.9 percent. The average cost of each new dollar is 9.8 percent.

The weights could be based on the accounting values shown on the firm's balance sheet (book values), or on the market values of the different securities shown on the balance sheet, or on management's estimation of the firm's optimal capital structure, which becomes the firm's target market value weights. The correct weights are the firm's target weights, and the methodology for estimating a firm's target weights is discussed in Chapter 9.

The marginal cost of capital (MCC) schedule

Could Ann Arbor Health Systems raise an unlimited amount of new capital at the 9.8 percent cost? The answer is *no*. As companies raise larger and larger sums during a given time period, the costs of both the debt and the equity components begin to rise, and as this occurs, the weighted average cost of new dollars also rises. Thus, just as corporations cannot hire unlimited numbers of workers at a constant wage, neither can they raise unlimited amounts of capital at a constant cost. At some point, the cost of each new dollar will increase above 9.8 percent. This occurs when Ann Arbor expands so rapidly that its retained earnings for the year are not sufficient to meet its needs for new equity, forcing it to sell new common stock. Since we previously estimated the cost of new equity, k_e, to be 15.4 percent, Ann Arbor's WACC using new common stock as the equity component is

$$\begin{aligned}
\text{WACC (new stock)} &= w_d k_d (1 - T) + w_s(k_e) \\
&= 0.60(11.7\%)(1 - 0.40) + 0.40(15.4\%) \\
&\approx 10.4\%.
\end{aligned}$$

Thus, we see that the WACC is 9.8 percent so long as retained earnings are used as the common equity component, but it jumps to 10.4 percent as soon as the firm exhausts its retained earnings and is forced to sell new common stock.

How much new capital can Ann Arbor Health Systems raise before it exhausts its retained earnings and is forced to sell new common stock? Assume that the company expects to have total earnings of $9 million for the year, and that it has a policy of paying out about 45 percent of its earnings as dividends. Thus, its *retention ratio*, which is the proportion of net income retained within the firm, is 1 − Payout ratio = 1 − 0.45 = 0.55. Therefore, the addition to retained earnings will be 0.55($9,000,000) = $4,950,000 during the year. How much *total financing*, debt plus this $4.95 million of retained earnings, can be done before the retained earnings are exhausted and the firm is forced to sell new common stock? In effect, we are seeking some amount of capital, X, which is defined as a *break point* and which represents the total financing that can be done before Ann Arbor is forced to sell new common stock. We know that 40 percent of X will be the new retained earnings, while 60 percent will be debt financing. We also know that retained earnings will amount to $4.95 million. Therefore,

$$0.4X = \text{Retained earnings} = \$4,950,000.$$

Solving for X, which is the *retained earnings break point*, we obtain

$$\text{Break point} = X = \frac{\text{Retained earnings}}{\text{Equity proportion}} = \frac{\$4,950,000}{0.40}$$
$$= \$12,375,000.$$

Thus, the company can raise a total of $12,375,000 of new capital, consisting of $4,950,000 of retained earnings and $12,375,000 − $4,950,000 = $7,425,000 of new debt supported by these new retained earnings, without altering its capital structure:

New debt supported by retained earnings	$ 7,425,000	60%
Retained earnings	4,950,000	40
Total expansion supported by retained earnings	$12,375,000	100%

The top panel (a) of Figure 8.1 graphs Ann Arbor's *marginal cost of capital (MCC) schedule*, ignoring depreciation cash flow. Each dollar has a weighted average cost of 9.8 percent until the company has raised a total of $12,375,000. However, if the firm raises $12,375,001 or more, each additional (or marginal) dollar will contain 40 cents of equity *obtained by selling new common equity at a cost of 15.4 percent*, so the firm's WACC rises from 9.8 to 10.4 percent.

Figure 8.1   Ann Arbor Health Systems: Marginal Cost of Capital
(MCC) Schedules

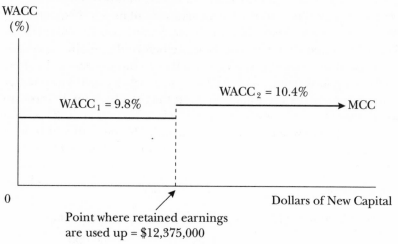

(a) MCC Schedule
   Not Considering Depreciation

WACC
(%)

WACC$_1$ = 9.8%

WACC$_2$ = 10.4%   → MCC

0   Point where retained earnings
     are used up = $12,375,000

     Dollars of New Capital

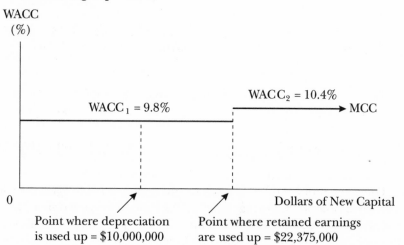

(b) MCC Schedule
   Considering Depreciation

WACC
(%)

WACC$_1$ = 9.8%

WACC$_2$ = 10.4%   → MCC

0   Dollars of New Capital

Point where depreciation   Point where retained earnings
is used up = $10,000,000   are used up = $22,375,000

Cost of depreciation-generated funds

Although we have ignored it thus far, the very first increment of internal funds used to finance any year's investments in new assets is funds generated by depreciation. Of course, depreciation is an allowance for the annual reduction in value of a firm's fixed assets. Thus, for an ongoing firm, depreciation-generated funds would be used first to replace worn-out and obsolete assets, and then any remaining funds would be available to purchase new assets or to return to investors.

For capital budgeting purposes, should depreciation-generated funds be considered "free" capital, should they be ignored completely, or should a charge be assessed against them? The answer is that a charge should indeed be assessed against depreciation-generated funds, and the cost used should be the weighted average cost of capital before outside equity is used. The reasoning here is that the firm, if it so desired, could distribute the depreciation-generated funds to its stockholders and creditors, the parties who financed the assets in the first place, so these funds definitely have an opportunity cost. Remember that depreciation is a return *of* capital, rather than a return *on* capital, so depreciation cash flow "belongs" to the original capital suppliers, which includes both stockholders and debtholders.

For example, suppose Ann Arbor Health Systems has $10 million of depreciation-generated funds available. Suppose further that the firm has no projects available to it, not even projects to replace worn-out equipment, that return 9.8 percent or more. From the stockholders' perspective, the firm should not raise new capital, and it should not even retain any earnings for internal investment, because stockholders would be better off receiving the earnings as dividends and investing the funds themselves at $k_s = 13.9\%$, or having the company repurchase its stock. Going on, Ann Arbor should not even invest its depreciation-generated $10 million. If it did, it would receive a return less than 9.8 percent, and hence could not pay its investors their required rates of return. If it distributed the $10 million to investors, with $4 million going to stockholders and $6 million to bondholders, these investors could invest the funds received in alternative investments of similar risk and earn their required rates of return. The conclusion from all of this is that depreciation-generated capital has an opportunity cost that is equal to the weighted average cost of capital before external equity is used.

Since depreciation-generated funds have the same cost as the firm's WACC when retained earnings are used for the equity component, it is not necessary to consider them when estimating the WACC. However, depreciation does influence the point at which a firm's marginal cost of capital schedule increases due to flotation costs on new stock sales. As shown in the bottom panel (b) of Figure 8.1, depreciation-generated funds push the point where the WACC increases out to the right by the amount of depreciation, in this case $10 million. Thus, the effect of depreciation is to move Ann Arbor's retained earnings break point from $12.375 million to $22.375 million.

The MCC schedule beyond the retained earnings break point

There is a jump, or break, in Ann Arbor's MCC schedule at $22,375,000 of new capital. Could there be other breaks in the schedule? Yes, the cost of capital could also rise due to increases in the cost of debt as the firm issues more and more debt or as a result of increases in flotation costs as the firm issues more and more common stock. As a result, firms face increasing MCC schedules such as the one shown in Figure 8.2. Here we have identified a specific retained earnings break point, but because of estimation difficulties, we have not attempted to identify precisely any additional break points. However, (1) we have shown the MCC schedule to be upward sloping, reflecting a positive relationship between capital raised and capital costs, and (2) we have indicated our inability to measure these costs precisely by using a band of costs rather than a single line. Note that this band exists even at the first dollar of capital raised: our component costs are only estimates that become more uncertain as the firm requires more and more capital, and thus the band widens as the amount of new capital needed increases.

We have shown that an investor-owned firm actually has two (or maybe more) steps on its marginal cost of capital schedule. Which of the values on the schedule should be used for capital budgeting purposes? In general, a firm's managers will estimate the firm's MCC schedule as we have just discussed. Then, its managers will estimate the firm's need for capital, that is, the dollars of capital that will likely be invested during the planning period. The firm's cost of capital is then defined as the marginal cost of capital at that point on the MCC schedule. Thus, if Ann Arbor Health Systems estimates that it will raise and invest $15 million of capital, its cost of capital will be 9.8 percent, but if the firm estimates its investment requirements to be $30 million, its cost of capital is 10.4 percent.

The marginal cost of capital (MCC) schedule for not-for-profit firms

The MCC schedule for not-for-profit firms is developed using Equation 8.7 in the same way as for investor-owned firms, but with a few minor

Figure 8.2   Ann Arbor Health Systems: MCC Schedule beyond
the Retained Earnings Break Point

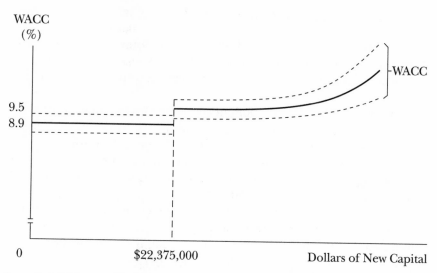

Source: E. F. Brigham and L. C. Gapenski. 1991. *Financial Management: Theory and Practice*, 6th
ed. Hinsdale, IL: The Dryden Press.

differences. To illustrate, the WACC for Bayside Memorial Hospital,
assuming a 50 percent debt/50 percent equity optimal capital structure,
and using the values for the other variables that we developed earlier, is
about 10.6 percent:

$$
\begin{aligned}
\text{WACC} &= w_d k_d (1 - T) + w_s (k_s \text{ or } k_e \text{ or } k_f) \\
&= 0.50(7.0\%)(1.0) + 0.50(14.3\%) \\
&\approx 10.6\%.
\end{aligned}
$$

Since not-for-profit firms do not incur flotation costs, there is no retained
earnings break point, and hence the MCC schedule is a flat line with
only one cost rate. Thus, for Bayside's depreciation cash flow, and for all
reasonable amounts of new capital, the MCC is 10.6 percent.

Self-Test Questions:

What is the general formula for a firm's WACC?

What weights should be used in the WACC formula? Why?

What is the MCC schedule?

What are the differences in WACCs and MCC schedules between investor-owned and not-for-profit firms?

An Economic Interpretation of the WACC

In this chapter, we have focused on the methodologies for estimating a firm's cost of capital. In closing, it is worthwhile to step back from the mathematics of the process and examine the interpretation of the cost of capital.

First, note that the component cost estimates that make up a firm's cost of capital (the costs of debt and equity) are based on the returns that investors require to supply capital to the firm. Investors' required rates of return, in turn, are based on the opportunity costs borne by investing in the debt and equity of the firm in question, rather than in alternative investments of similar risk.

The opportunity costs to investors, when combined into the firm's cost of capital, establish the opportunity cost to the firm. If the firm cannot earn this rate of return on new capital investments, the capital should be returned to investors for reinvestment elsewhere.

The required rates of return set by investors are based on perceptions regarding the riskiness of their investments (the riskiness of their expected cash flow streams), which, in turn, are based on the inherent riskiness of the business and the amount of debt financing used by the firm. (More debt usage leads to more risk to both debtholders and equityholders, and hence to higher-component required rates of return.) Thus, the firm's inherent business risk and capital structure are embedded in the cost of capital estimate.

The primary purpose of estimating a firm's cost of capital is to help make capital budgeting decisions. That is, the cost of capital will be used as the capital budgeting *hurdle rate*, or minimum return necessary for a project to be attractive financially. The firm can always earn its cost of capital by investing in selected stocks and bonds that in the aggregate have the same risk as the firm's assets, so it should not invest in real assets unless it can earn at least as much. But remember: the cost of capital has embedded in it the aggregate risk and capital structure of the firm or, put another way, the risk and capital structure of the firm's average project. Thus, the firm's cost of capital can be applied without modification only to those projects under consideration that have average risk and average debt capacity, where average is defined as that applicable to the firm's currently held assets in the aggregate. If a new project under consideration has risk or debt capacity that differs significantly from that of the firm's average asset, then the firm's cost of capital must be adjusted to account for this differential when the project is being evaluated.

To illustrate the concept, Bayside's cost of capital, 10.6 percent, is probably appropriate for use in evaluating a new outpatient clinic that has risk and debt capacity similar to the hospital's average project, which involves the provision of health care services. However, it would not be appropriate to apply Bayside's 10.6 percent cost of capital, without adjustment, to a new project that involves establishing a for-profit food management subsidiary, because this project does not have the same risk or debt capacity as the hospital's average asset. We will discuss how to make adjustments to a firm's cost of capital, when appropriate, in Chapter 11.

Self-Test Question:

Explain the economic interpretation and use of the WACC.

Summary

This chapter showed how the firm's cost of capital is estimated. The key concepts covered are listed next.

- The cost of capital to be used in capital budgeting decisions is the *weighted average* of the various types of capital the firm uses, typically debt and common equity.

- The *component cost of debt* is the *after-tax* cost of new debt. For taxable firms, it is found by multiplying the before-tax cost of new debt by $(1 - T)$, where T is the firm's marginal tax rate, so the component cost of debt is $k_d(1 - T)$. For not-for-profit firms, the debt is often tax-exempt, but no other tax effects apply, so the component cost of debt is merely the tax-exempt k_d.

- The *cost of common equity* to investor-owned firms is the cost of retained earnings as long as the firm has retained earnings, but the cost of equity becomes the cost of new common stock once the firm has exhausted its retained earnings.

- For not-for-profit firms, the *cost of fund capital* can be approximated by the cost of retained earnings of similar investor-owned firms.

- The *cost of retained earnings* is the rate of return investors require on the firm's common stock, and it is usually estimated by two methods:

(1) the Capital Asset Pricing Model (CAPM) approach and (2) the discounted cash flow (DCF) approach.

- To use the *CAPM approach*, we (1) estimate the firm's beta, (2) multiply this beta by the market risk premium to determine the firm's risk premium, and (3) add the firm's risk premium to the risk-free rate to obtain the firm's cost of retained earnings:

$$k_s = k_{RF} + (k_M - k_{RF})b.$$

- The best proxy for the *risk-free rate* is the yield on long-term T-bonds.

- There are three types of betas that can be used in the CAPM: (1) *historical*, (2) *adjusted*, and (3) *fundamental*.

- The market risk premium can be estimated either *historically (ex post)* or *prospectively (ex ante)*.

- To use the *DCF approach*, we solve for k_s in the stock valuation equation. Under constant growth, this is done by adding the firm's expected growth rate to its expected dividend yield:

$$k_s = \hat{k}_s = D_1/P_0 + g.$$

- The growth rate can be estimated from historical data by using the *retention growth model*, g = Retention ratio(Expected ROE), or from securities analysts' forecasts.

- *Hamada's equation* can be used to convert the beta of an investor-owned firm to a proxy beta for a not-for-profit firm:

$$b_{Firm} = b_{Assets}[1 + (1 - T)(D/S)].$$

- The *cost of new common equity*, k_e, is higher than the cost of retained earnings because the firm must incur *flotation expenses* to sell new stock.

- Each firm has a *target capital structure*, and the target weights are used to estimate the firm's weighted average cost of capital (WACC):

$$\text{WACC} = w_d k_d (1 - T) + w_s(k_s \text{ or } k_e \text{ or } k_f).$$

- The *marginal cost of capital (MCC)* is defined as the cost of the last dollar of new capital the firm raises. The MCC increases as the firm raises more and more capital during a given period.

- The *MCC schedule* is a graph of the MCC plotted against dollars of new capital needed.

- When making *capital investment decisions*, the firm will use as a *hurdle rate* the value on the MCC schedule that corresponds to the total amount of capital expected to be invested.

The concepts developed in this chapter will be used extensively throughout the book, especially in capital structure decisions (Chapter 9) and in capital budgeting decisions (Chapters 10 and 11).

Notes

1. The impact of flotation costs on the cost of debt to an investor-owned firm is more difficult to calculate because the dollar amount of flotation costs can be amortized and expensed for tax purposes over the life of the issue. The ability to expense flotation costs for tax purposes reduces such costs for taxable firms.
2. A *basis point* is 1/100th of a percentage point. Basis points are often used by investment bankers to measure differences in yields. For example, the difference between yields of 8.0 percent and 7.4 percent is 60 basis points.
3. If a hospital receives capital pass-through payments, its cost of debt is reduced. To illustrate, assume that 25 percent of Ann Arbor's patient revenue comes from third party payers that make capital pass-through payments, but, on average, they reimburse the hospital for only 80 percent of the interest expense attributed to their patients. In this situation, the effective capital pass-through rate would be $0.80(25\%) = 20\%$. To incorporate the interest expense pass-through benefit into the component cost of debt, the cost is reduced by the effective pass-through rate. Thus, Ann Arbor's after-tax, after-pass-through component cost of debt would be

$$
\begin{aligned}
\text{Component cost of debt} &= k_d(1 - T)(1 - P) \\
&= 11.7\%(1 - 0.40)(1 - 0.20) \\
&= 11.7\%(0.48) = 5.62\% \approx 5.6\%.
\end{aligned}
$$

where P = Effective pass-through rate.
4. Preferred stock is used by only a few firms in the health care industry, so we will not include preferred stock in our WACC examples. If preferred stock is used as a source of permanent financing, then it should be included in the WACC estimate, and its cost would be estimated using procedures like those discussed for the cost of debt.
5. See *Stocks, Bonds, Bills and Inflation: 1995 Yearbook* (Chicago: Ibbotson Associates, 1995). Also, note that Ibbotson Associates now recommends using the T-bond rate as the proxy for the risk-free rate when using the CAPM. Before 1988, Ibbotson Associates recommended that the T-bill rate be used.
6. See M. E. Blume, "Betas and Their Regression Tendencies," *Journal of Finance* (June 1973), 785–796.

7. See B. Rosenberg and J. Guy, "Beta and Investment Fundamentals," *Financial Analysts Journal* (May-June 1976), 60–72. Rosenberg, a professor at the University of California at Berkeley, later set up a company that calculates fundamental betas by a proprietary procedure and then sells them to institutional investors.

8. A commercial provider of betas once admitted that his firm, and others, did not know what the right period was to use, but that they decided to use five years in order to reduce the apparent differences between various services' betas—large differences reduced everyone's credibility!

9. There are many possible forms of the DCF model, including the quarterly growth model, which considers quarterly dividends rather than assuming annual dividends, and the nonconstant growth model, which permits different dividend growth rates in future periods. Even so, many analysts still use the constant growth model, because more complex models do not necessarily give better answers when the input parameters are very uncertain.

10. Log-linear regression is a standard time-series linear regression in which the data points are plotted as natural logarithms. The advantage of a log-linear regression is that the slope of the regression line is the average annual growth rate assuming continuous compounding. In a standard time-series linear regression of EPS or DPS, the slope of the regression line is the average annual dollar change. For a more complete discussion of log-linear regression, see R. C. Radcliffe, *Investment: Concepts, Analysis, and Strategy* (Glenview, IL: Scott, Foresman, 1996).

11. A third method—the bond yield plus risk premium method—can also be used. See E. F. Brigham and L. C. Gapenski, *Intermediate Financial Management* (Fort Worth, TX: Dryden Press, 1996), chap. 6.

12. For one of the classic works on this topic, see D. A. Conrad, "Returns on Equity to Not-For-Profit Hospitals: Theory and Implementation," *Health Services Research* (April 1984), 41–63. Also, see the follow-up articles by Pauly; Conrad; and Silvers and Kauer in the April 1986 issue of *Health Services Research.*

13. For an excellent discussion of this issue, see W. O. Cleverley, "Return on Equity in the Hospital Industry: Requirement or Windfall?" *Inquiry* (Summer 1982), 150–59.

14. For more information on Hamada's equation, see R. S. Hamada, "Portfolio Analysis, Market Equilibrium, and Corporation Finance," *Journal of Finance* (March 1969), 13–31; or E. F. Brigham and L. C. Gapenski, *Intermediate Financial Management* (Fort Worth, TX: Dryden Press, 1996), chap. 11.

15. If the firm receives capital pass-through payments, the generalized WACC formula is

$$\text{WACC} = w_d k_d (1 - T)(1 - P) + w_s(k_s \text{ or } k_e \text{ or } k_f), \tag{8.7a}$$

where P is the effective pass-through rate. Also, if the firm uses preferred stock as part of its permanent financing mix, then a $w_p k_p$ term must be added to the WACC formula, where w_p is the target weight of preferred stock and k_p is the cost preferred stock.

Selected Additional References

Boles, K. E. 1986. "Implications of the Method of Capital Cost Payment on the Weighted Average Cost of Capital." *Health Services Research* (June): 191–211.

Sloan, F. A., J. Valvona, and M. Hassan. 1988. "Cost of Capital to the Hospital Sector." *Journal of Health Economics* (March): 25–45.

Smith, D. G. and J. R. C. Wheeler. 1989. "Accounting Based Risk Measures for Not-for-Profit Hospitals." *Health Services Management Research* (November): 221–26.

Wheeler, J. R. C., and D. G. Smith, "The Discount Rate for Capital Expenditure Analysis in Health Care." *Health Care Management Review* (Spring): 43–51.

Case 8

PLM Healthcare, Inc.: Cost of Capital

PLM Healthcare, Inc. was founded in 1983 in Los Angeles as a taxable partnership by Shana Peterson, M.D., Roger Lane, R.N., and Christy Markowitz, L.P.T. Its purpose was to provide an "at home" alternative to hospitals and ambulatory care facilities for basic health care services provided by physicians, registered nurses, licensed practical nurses, and physical therapists.

The partnership enjoyed enormous success from the very first day, and even its founders were surprised at how easy it was to establish and run the business. The founding coincided with the search by third party payers for alternative, and potentially less costly, delivery settings. Also, the AIDS epidemic provided a patient clientele that was totally unexpected. On the basis of their success in the metropolitan Los Angeles area, the partnership expanded services into San Francisco and San Diego, then moved into other metropolitan areas in California, and finally began operations in 11 cities in Arizona, Oregon, and Washington. They also expanded their services at each location to include occupational and speech therapy.

The founders had sufficient personal resources to start the enterprise, and they had enough confidence in the business to commit most of their own funds to the new venture. However, after only two years, the capital requirements brought on by rapid growth exhausted their personal funds, and they were forced to borrow heavily. Soon, although they still needed external capital to finance growth, the partnership's ability to borrow at reasonable rates was exhausted. Thus, in 1988 they incorporated the business, and in 1990 they sold common stock to the public through an initial public offering (IPO). The founders still retain a large, but minority, ownership position in the firm, and currently the stock trades in the over-the-counter market, although there has been some talk of listing on the Pacific Stock Exchange.

PLM Healthcare is widely recognized as one of the regional leaders in an emerging growth industry, and it won an award in 1994 for being one of the 100 best-managed medium-sized companies in the United States. The company has two operating divisions: (1) the Healthcare Services Division and (2) the Information Systems Division. The Healthcare Services Division operates PLM's home health care services at the company's 22 locations. Since sales and earnings in this division are relatively predictable, the business risk of this division is about average. The Information Systems Division sells to other home health care companies the computer software system that PLM designed to control its own operations. This system combines inventory control, visit scheduling, clinical record keeping, billing and collections, and payroll into an integrated package. Although the system is excellent, this division competes head-to-head with some major software firms, as well as with information services and management consulting firms. Because of this competition, and the rapid technological changes inherent in the information services industry, PLM's management considers the Information Services Division to have more business risk than the Healthcare Services Division.

Although the firm's growth has been exceptional, it has been more random than planned. The founders would simply decide on a location for a new office, run an advertisement in a local newspaper for health care professionals and clerical employees, send in an experienced manager from one of the established offices, and begin to make money almost immediately. Formal decision structures were almost nonexistent, but the company's head start and its bright, energetic founders easily overcame any deficiencies in its managerial decision-making processes. Recently, however, competition has become stiffer. Other investor-owned home health care firms have sprung up like weeds, especially in major cities, and several hospitals in the firm's area of operations, including not-for-profits, have begun to offer home health care services.

Because of this increasing competition, PLM's board of directors has concluded that the firm must apply state-of-the-art techniques in its corporate managerial processes, as well as in its operations. As a first step, the board has directed the financial vice president to develop an estimate for the firm's cost of capital. The financial VP, in turn, has directed PLM's treasurer, Mark Rubin, to have a cost of capital estimate on his desk in two weeks. Rubin has an accounting background, and his primary task since taking over as treasurer has been cash and short-term liability management. Thus, he is somewhat apprehensive about this new assignment, especially since one of the board members is a well-regarded UCLA finance professor.

Rubin began by reviewing PLM Healthcare's 1996 financial statements, which are presented in Table 1 in simplified form. Next, he assembled the following data:

1. PLM's long-term debt consists of 12 percent coupon, BBB-rated, semiannual payment bonds with 15 years remaining to maturity. The bonds recently traded at a price of $1,153.72 per $1,000 par value bond. The bonds are callable in five years at par value plus a call premium of one year's interest, for a total of $1,120.

2. The founders have an aversion to short-term debt, so PLM uses such debt only to fund cyclical working capital needs. The company typically issues 30-year bonds to meet its long-term debt needs.

3. PLM's federal-plus-state tax rate is 40 percent.

Table 1   PLM Healthcare: 1996 Financial Statements (millions of dollars)

Balance Sheet

Cash and marketable securities	$ 2.5	Accounts payable	$ 1.1
Accounts receivable	5.9	Accruals	1.0
Inventory	1.3	Notes payable	0.2
Current assets	$ 9.7	Curent liabilities	$ 2.3
Net fixed assets	32.9	Long-term debt	20.0
		Common stock	20.3
Total assets	$42.6	Total claims	$42.6

Income Statement

Net revenues	$80.6
Cash expenses	71.8
Depreciation	2.8
Taxable income	$ 6.0
Taxes	2.4
Net income	$ 3.6
Dividends	1.8
Additions to retained earnings	$ 1.8

4. The firm's last dividend (D_0) was $0.18, and some analysts predict the firm's dividend growth rate to be in the range of 7 to 11 percent into the foreseeable future. However, other analysts predict a growth rate of 25 percent over the next five years, followed by a long-term (steady state) growth rate of 6 percent. PLM's common stock now sells at a price of $5 per share. The company has 10.0 million common shares outstanding.

5. Over the last few years, PLM has averaged a 20 percent return on equity (ROE) and has paid out about 50 percent of its net income as dividends.

6. The current yield curve on U.S. Treasury securities is as follows:

Term to Maturity	Yield
3 months	5.5%
6 months	6.0
9 months	6.3
1 year	6.5
5 years	7.0
10 years	7.4
15 years	7.7
20 years	7.9
25 years	8.0
30 years	8.1

7. A prominent investment banking firm has recently estimated the expected rate of return on the S&P 500 portfolio to be 13.0 percent.

8. The firm's historical beta, as measured by several analysts who follow the stock, falls in the range of 1.1 to 1.3.

9. The required rate of return on an average (A-rated) company's long-term debt is 9.5 percent.

10. PLM is forecasting retained earnings of $2,000,000 and depreciation of $3,000,000 for the coming year.

11. The firm's investment bankers believe that a new common stock issue would involve total flotation costs—including underwriting costs, market pressure from increased supply, and market pressure from negative signaling effects—of 30 percent.

12. The firm's market value target capital structure calls for 35 percent long-term debt and 65 percent common stock.

13. None of PLM's third party payers makes capital pass-through payments to the firm.

14. Mark Rubin is aware of a third method (in addition to the capital asset pricing and discounted cash flow models) for estimating a firm's cost of retained earnings: the bond yield plus risk premium method. Here, a risk premium is added to the firm's own before-tax cost of debt estimate to obtain an estimate of the cost of retained earnings. Note that the risk premium used here is not the market risk premium, which is applied to the risk-free rate. Rather, the risk premium reflects the difference between the cost of debt to an average firm and its cost of retained earnings.

15. About 60 percent of PLM's operating assets are used by the Healthcare Services Division and 40 percent by the Information Systems Division. Management's best estimate of the beta of its Healthcare Services Division is 1.0.

Assume that Mark Rubin has hired you as a consultant to develop PLM's overall marginal cost of capital (MCC) schedule. You will have to meet with the financial VP and, possibly, with the president and the full board of directors (including the founders and the UCLA finance professor) to present your findings and answer any questions they might have. Note that the divisional presidents are concerned that a single cost of capital will be applied across the company, regardless of any divisional risk and debt capacity differences. Rubin has asked you to be sure to address their concerns. Specifically, he wants you to develop divisional costs of capital in addition to PLM's MCC schedule.

The managers at PLM Healthcare are very concerned about the threat posed by home health care businesses started by not-for-profit hospitals, because they have both cost (in the sense that they do not need to pay dividends) and tax advantages. In particular, Pine Hills Community Hospital, a not-for-profit hospital in Sacramento, appears to be ready to start a competing business. To help assess the threat, Rubin has asked you to use the information that you are developing for PLM, along with some Pine Hills data, to estimate the MCC schedule for Pine Hills' home health care business. Pine Hills' target capital structure is thought to be 50 percent tax-exempt long-term debt, which currently has a cost of 7.2 percent, and 50 percent fund capital.

Finally, one of PLM's directors has expressed concern over the difference between the firm's target capital structure and the current structure as reported on the balance sheet. Rubin wondered if this should be a matter of concern.

9

Capital Structure Decisions

$\mathbf{I}$n Chapter 8, when we discussed a firm's weighted average cost of capital, we noted that the weights used represent the firm's optimal, or target, mix of debt and equity financing. However, one of the most perplexing issues facing health care managers is the *capital structure* decision. How much debt financing, as opposed to equity (or fund) financing, should a firm use? Do hospitals have different optimal capital structures than home health agencies or ambulatory surgery centers and, if so, what are the factors that lead to these differences?

We will begin our discussion of the capital structure decision by examining the impact of debt (or preferred stock) financing on a firm's risk and return. Next, we will discuss the important concepts of business and financial risk. Then, we will present the most important capital structure theories, which attempt to define the relationship between the use of debt financing and the value of the firm. Finally, we will discuss how managers make capital structure decisions in practice.

Impact of Debt Financing on Risk and Return

One of the most important concepts in capital structure decisions is the impact of debt (or preferred stock) financing on a business's accounting return and financial risk. The best way to present this concept is by using an illustration. Assume that you are about to start a new company. Let's call it Super Health, Inc. The business requires $200,000 in assets to get into operation, and there are only two financing alternatives available to you: (1) all equity (all common stock) and (2) 50 percent equity and 50 percent debt.

Table 9.1 contains the business's projected financial statements under the two financing alternatives. To begin, consider the balance sheets shown in the top portion of the table. The business will require $100,000 in current assets and $100,000 in fixed assets to begin operations. Since the asset requirement depends on the nature and size of the business rather than on how the business will be financed, the asset side of the balance sheet is unaffected by the financing scheme. However, the capital, or claims, side of the balance sheet is influenced by the type of financing. Under the all-equity alternative, you will put up the entire $200,000 needed to purchase the assets. If 50 percent debt financing is used, you will contribute only $100,000 of your own funds, and the remaining $100,000 will be obtained from creditors, say, a bank loan with a 10 percent interest rate.

Now consider the impact of the two financing alternatives on the business's projected income statement. Revenues are projected to be

Table 9.1   Super Health, Inc.: Projected Financial Statements under Two Financing Alternatives

	Stock	*Stock/Debt*
Balance Sheet		
Current assets	$100,000	$100,000
Fixed assets	100,000	100,000
Total assets	$200,000	$200,000
Bank loan (10% cost)	$ 0	$100,000
Common stock	200,000	100,000
Total claims	$200,000	$200,000
Income Statement		
Revenues	$150,000	$150,000
Operating costs	100,000	100,000
Operating income	$ 50,000	$ 50,000
Interest expense	0	10,000
Taxable income	$ 50,000	$ 40,000
Taxes (40%)	20,000	16,000
Net income	$ 30,000	$ 24,000
ROE	15%	24%
Total dollar return to investors	$ 30,000	$ 34,000

$150,000 and operating costs are forecasted at $100,000, so the firm's operating income is expected to be $50,000. Since the method of financing does not affect revenues and operating costs, the operating income projection is the same under both financing alternatives. However, interest expense must be paid if debt financing is used, so the stock/debt alternative results in a 0.10($100,000) = $10,000 annual interest charge, while no interest expense occurs if the firm is financed entirely by stock. The result is taxable income of $50,000 under the all-equity alternative, and lower taxable income of $40,000 under the stock/debt alternative. Since the business anticipates being taxed at a 40 percent federal-plus-state rate, the expected tax liability is 0.40($50,000) = $20,000 under the all-equity alternative and 0.40($40,000) = $16,000 for the stock/debt alternative. Finally, when taxes are deducted from the income stream, the business projects $30,000 in net income if it is all-equity financed and $24,000 in net income if 50 percent debt financing is used.

At first glance, the use of debt financing appears to be the inferior alternative. After all, if you use 50 percent debt financing, the business's projected net income will fall by $30,000 − $24,000 = $6,000. But the conclusion that debt financing is bad requires closer examination. What is most important to you, the owner of Super Health, is not the business's net income, but rather the return that you expect to earn on your equity investment. Perhaps the most meaningful measure of return to a firm's owners (stockholders) is the rate of return on equity, or just return on equity (ROE), which is defined as Net income/Common stock. This measure tells stock investors (owners) the percentage return on their investment. Under all-equity financing, your projected ROE is $30,000/$200,000 = 0.15 = 15%, but with 50 percent debt financing, projected ROE increases to $24,000/$100,000 = 24%. The key here is that although net income decreases with debt financing, so does the amount of capital you need to put up, and the capital requirement decreases proportionally more than does net income.

The result of all this is that the use of debt financing increases your expected rate of return on invested capital. Why does this positive result happen? There is no magic here. The key is in the tax code—interest expense is tax-deductible for investor-owned firms. To understand the impact of the tax deductibility of interest, take another look at the Table 9.1 income statements. The total dollar return to all investors, including both you and the bank, is $30,000 in net income if all-equity financed, but $24,000 in net income plus $10,000 of interest = $34,000 when 50 percent debt financing is used. Where did the "extra" $4,000 come from? The answer is "from the tax man." Taxes are $20,000 if the business is all-equity financed, but only $16,000 when debt financing is used, and $4,000 less in taxes means $4,000 more for investors. Because debt financing reduces taxes, more of a firm's operating income is available for distribution to investors (including both stockholders and creditors).

It now appears that the financing decision on your business is clear. Given only the two alternatives, you should use the 50 percent debt alternative, because it provides you (the stockholder) with the higher return. Unfortunately, like the proverbial no free lunch, there is a catch. The use of debt financing not only increases the return to equity holders; it also increases their risk. To demonstrate the risk-increasing characteristics of debt financing, consider Table 9.2. Here we recognize that Super Health, like all businesses, is risky. You really do not know precisely what the first year's revenues and operating costs will be. Assume, for illustrative purposes, that Revenues − Operating costs = Operating income could be as low as $0 or as high as $100,000 in the business's first year of operation. Furthermore, assume that there is a 25 percent chance of the worst and the best cases occurring, and a 50 percent chance that the Table 9.1 forecast, with an operating income of $50,000, will be realized.

The assumptions regarding uncertainty in the future profitability of the business lead to three different ROEs for each financing alternative. The expected ROEs (the sum of the probability-outcome products) are

Table 9.2 Super Health, Inc.: Partial Income Statements in an Uncertain World

	Stock			*Stock/Debt*		
Probability	.25	.50	.25	.25	.50	.25
Operating income	$0	$50,000	$100,000	$ 0	$50,000	$100,000
Interest expense	0	0	0	10,000	10,000	10,000
Taxable income	$0	$50,000	$100,000	($10,000)	$40,000	$ 90,000
Taxes (40%)	0	20,000	40,000	(4,000)	16,000	36,000
Net income	$0	$30,000	$ 60,000	($ 6,000)	$24,000	$ 54,000
ROE	0%	15%	30%	−6%	24%	54%
Expected ROE		15%			24%	
Standard deviation of ROE		10.6%			21.2%	

the same as when we ignored uncertainty; that is, 15 percent if the firm is all-equity financed and 24 percent when 50 percent debt financing is used. However, the uncertainty in operating income produces uncertainty, and hence risk, in stockholder returns. If we measure risk to the stockholders by the standard deviation of ROE, we see that the return is more risky when you use 50 percent debt financing. To be precise, your risk is twice as much in the 50 percent debt financing alternative: 21.2 percent standard deviation of ROE versus 10.6 percent standard deviation in the zero debt alternative.

The increase in risk is apparent without even calculating the standard deviations. If you use only stock financing, the worst you can do is an ROE of zero. However, with 50 percent debt financing, you could realize an ROE of −6 percent. (Here the assumption is made that the business's $10,000 loss could be used to offset your personal income, so you can realize a $4,000 tax savings.) In fact, with no operating income to pay the $10,000 interest to the bank in the worst case scenario, you as the owner would either have to put up additional personal funds to pay the interest due or declare the business bankrupt. Clearly, the use of 50 percent debt financing has increased the riskiness of your equity investment in the firm.

This simple example illustrates two key points about the use of debt financing:

1. The use of debt financing increases the percentage return (ROE) to the firm's stockholders. Note, however, that for the use of debt financing to increase stockholder returns, the inherent return on the business must be greater than the interest rate on the debt. The basic return on the business in the Super Health illustration is 25 percent ($50 in operating income divided by $200 in assets), and debt financing costs only 10 percent, so the use of debt financing increases ROE.

2. At the same time that return is increased, the use of debt financing also increases the risk to stockholders. In the example, we saw that 50 percent debt financing doubled the risk to stockholders (as measured by standard deviation of ROE).

The ultimate decision on which financing alternative should be chosen is not clear cut. One alternative (no debt) has a lower expected ROE, but also lower risk. The second alternative (50 percent debt) offers a higher expected ROE, but only at the price of higher risk. To complicate matters even more, there is actually an almost unlimited number of debt level choices available to you, not just the 50/50 mix used in the illustration.

Later sections will try to resolve your dilemma involving whether or not to use debt financing, and, if so, how much, but first we need to introduce some other concepts.

Self-Test Questions:

What is the impact of debt (or preferred stock) financing on a business's risk and return?

Why does the use of debt (or preferred stock) financing leverage up (increase) the return to stockholders?

Business and Financial Risk

In Chapter 5, we discussed several different dimensions of risk, including stand-alone risk and portfolio (corporate and market) risk. Now we introduce two new dimensions: (1) business risk, or the riskiness to common stockholders if the firm uses no debt financing; and (2) financial risk, the additional risk placed on common stockholders as a result of the firm's decision to use debt (or preferred stock) financing. Here, the term "financial risk" has a very specific connotation, as opposed to Chapter 5, where we used the term generically to mean the risk arising from business transactions as opposed to other types of risk such as risk to life and limb. Note that the concepts of business and financial risk apply just as much to not-for-profit businesses as they do to for-profit businesses, but that in not-for-profits the risk concepts apply to the firm's non-creditor stakeholders, rather than to common stockholders.

Business risk

Business risk is the inherent riskiness of a business as seen by its common stockholders, and it is measured by the uncertainty inherent in a firm's ROE, assuming that the firm uses no debt financing. To illustrate the concept of business risk, consider Santa Fe Healthcare, Inc., a *debt-free* investor-owned hospital chain that operates in the Southwestern United States. Figure 9.1 provides some insights into the company's business risk. The top graph gives both security analysts and Santa Fe's management an idea of the historical variability of ROE, and consequently how the firm's ROE might vary in the future. This graph also shows that Santa Fe's ROE is growing slowly, so the relevant variability of ROE is the dispersion about the trend line rather than the overall standard deviation of historical ROE.

Figure 9.1   Sante Fe Healthcare: Trend in ROE, 1985–1995, and
Subjective ROE Distribution, 1995

(a) Trend in Return on Equity (ROE)

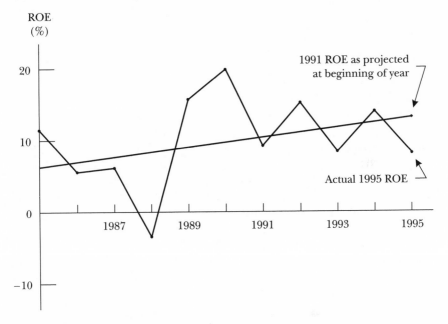

(b) Subjective Probability Distribution of (ROE)

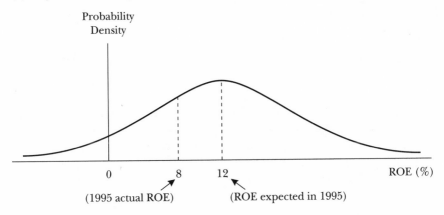

The lower graph shows the beginning-of-year subjectively estimated probability distribution of Santa Fe's ROE for 1995, based on the trend line in the top section of Figure 9.1. As both graphs indicate, Santa Fe's actual ROE in 1995 was only 8 percent, well below the expected value of 12 percent.

Santa Fe's past fluctuations in ROE were caused by many factors—changes in the economy, actions by competing hospitals, changes in payer mix, payment policies of third party payers, changing labor costs, and so on. Similar events will undoubtedly occur in the future, and when they do, Santa Fe's realized ROE will almost always be higher or lower than the projected level. Furthermore, there is always the possibility that some event might occur that permanently depresses the company's earning power. For example, the government could move to a single payer system with dramatically reduced hospital reimbursement rates.

Since Santa Fe uses no debt financing, the uncertainty regarding its future ROE is defined as the company's basic business risk. The key point here is that we are trying to measure the riskiness of the business before it is influenced by the use of debt financing. Business risk varies not only from industry to industry, but also among firms in a given industry. Furthermore, business risk can change over time. For example, acute care hospitals were regarded for years as having little business risk, but events in the 1980s and 1990s (primarily the move of governmental payers to prospective payment and the vulnerability of hospitals to large managed care plan discounts) altered the hospitals' profitability situation, producing sharp declines in their ROEs and greatly increasing the industry's business risk.

Business risk depends on a number of factors, including the following:

1. *Demand variability.* The more stable the demand for a firm's products or services, other things held constant, the lower its business risk.

2. *Sales price variability.* Firms whose products or services are sold in markets with highly volatile prices are exposed to more business risk than firms whose sales prices are more stable.

3. *Input cost variability.* Firms whose input costs (labor, materials, and capital) are highly uncertain are exposed to a high degree of business risk.

4. *Ability to adjust output prices for changes in input costs.* Some firms are better able than others to raise their own output prices when input costs rise. The greater the ability to adjust output prices

to reflect cost conditions, the lower the degree of business risk, other things held constant.

5. *The extent to which costs are fixed: operating leverage.* If a high percentage of a firm's costs are fixed, and hence do not decline when demand falls off, then the firm is exposed to a relatively high degree of business risk. This factor is called operating leverage, and it is discussed in more detail in following paragraphs.

Each of these factors is determined partly by the firm's industry characteristics, but each of them is also controllable to some extent by management. For example, most firms can, through their marketing policies, take actions to stabilize both unit sales and sales prices. However, this stabilization may require firms to spend a great deal on advertising, price concessions, or both, to get commitments from their customers to purchase fixed quantities at fixed prices in the future.

As noted above, business risk depends in part on the extent to which a firm builds fixed costs into its operations: if fixed costs are high, even a small decline in sales can lead to a large decline in ROE, so, other things held constant, the higher a firm's fixed costs, the greater its business risk. Higher fixed costs are generally associated with more highly technical, capital-intensive firms and industries. Thus, hospitals have higher fixed costs, relative to total costs, than do home health care agencies. Also, businesses, such as many health care providers that employ highly skilled workers who must be retained and paid even during periods of low demand, have a relatively high proportion of fixed costs.

If a high percentage of a firm's total costs are fixed, then the firm is said to have a high degree of *operating leverage.* In physics, leverage implies the use of a lever to raise a heavy object with a small force. In politics, if people have leverage, their smallest word or action can accomplish a lot. In business terminology, a high degree of operating leverage, other factors held constant, implies that a relatively small change in sales results in a large change in ROE, even when no debt financing is used.

To what extent can firms control their operating leverage? To a large extent, operating leverage is determined by industry characteristics. Companies such as drug manufacturers, hospitals, and ambulatory care clinics simply must have heavy investments in fixed assets and labor, which results in high fixed costs and operating leverage. On the other hand, companies such as home health agencies generally have significantly lower fixed costs and hence lower operating leverage. Still, although industry factors do exert a major influence, all firms do have some control over their operating leverage. For example, a hospital can expand its diagnostic imaging capability by either buying a new imaging device or by leasing it on a per procedure basis.[1] If the device were purchased, the hospital would incur fixed costs, but the device's per procedure operating costs would be relatively low. If leased, the hospital would have lower fixed costs, but the variable (per procedure) costs for the device would be higher. Thus, by its financing decisions (and also by its capital investment decisions), a firm can influence its operating leverage, and hence its basic business risk.

The concept of operating leverage was, in fact, originally developed for use in capital investment decisions. Competing projects that involve alternative methods for producing a given product or service often have different degrees of operating leverage and thus different breakeven points and different degrees of risk. Santa Fe and many other companies regularly undertake a type of breakeven analysis (the sensitivity analyses discussed in Chapter 11) for each proposed project as a part of their regular capital budgeting process. Still, once a firm's operating leverage has been established, this factor exerts a major influence on the capital structure decision.

Financial risk

Financial risk is the additional risk placed on the common stockholders as a result of the decision to use debt (or preferred stock) financing. Conceptually, a firm has a certain amount of risk inherent in its operations. This is its business risk, which is defined as the uncertainty inherent in projections of future ROE, assuming that the firm is all-equity financed. However, the use of debt financing, or *financial leverage*, concentrates (increases) the risk seen by common stockholders. Since the return to debtholders is fixed by contract and is independent of fluctuations in the firm's revenues and costs, creditors do not bear any of the firm's business risk. To illustrate, think back about the situation presented earlier in the Super Health illustration. The business could be financed either by $200,000 of equity or $100,000 of equity and $100,000 of debt. Using debt financing concentrates the riskiness of the business (which is fixed) on a smaller equity base, and hence increases the risk to the equityholders.

Business and financial risk can be easily measured. Refer again to Table 9.2. The standard deviation of ROE to Super Health if it used no debt financing, $\sigma_{ROE(U)}$, where U stands for unleveraged (no debt), is a measure of the business risk seen by stockholders. The standard deviation of ROE at any positive debt level, $\sigma_{ROE(L)}$, where L stands for leveraged (some debt), is a measure of the stand-alone risk borne by stockholders. Because the use of debt financing increases the risk to stockholders, $\sigma_{ROE(L)}$ is always greater than $\sigma_{ROE(U)}$, and the financial risk seen by stockholders is $\sigma_{ROE(L)} - \sigma_{ROE(U)}$. Applying these measures to Super Health, we see that the business risk to stockholders is $\sigma_{ROE(U)}$ = 10.6%, the stand-alone risk borne by stockholders under 50 percent debt financing is $\sigma_{ROE(L)}$ = 21.2%, and the financial risk to stockholders is $\sigma_{ROE(L)} - \sigma_{ROE(U)}$ = 21.2% − 10.6% = 10.6%.

Operating leverage and financial leverage normally work in the same way; they both increase expected ROE, but they also increase the risk borne by stockholders. Operating leverage affects the business risk seen by stockholders, while financial leverage affects the financial risk borne by stockholders.

Self-Test Questions:

What is business risk? How can it be measured?

What are some determinants of business risk?

What is operating leverage?

What is financial risk? How can it be measured?

What are the similarities between operating leverage and financial leverage?

Capital Structure Theory

The preceding discussion points out the fact that the use of debt financing increases the expected return to stockholders, but it also increases their risk. In a not-for-profit setting, the use of debt financing increases the return on the firm's fund capital, but it also increases the risk to the firm's noncreditor stakeholders. The obvious question at this point is whether the benefit of debt financing (increased expected return) exceeds the cost of debt financing (increased risk). Capital structure theory attempts to define the relationship between the amount of debt financing and the value of a firm (stock price), and thus its goal is to determine whether the use of financial leverage is beneficial to stockholders. Although capital structure theory does not provide a complete answer to the optimal capital structure question, it does provide many insights into the value of debt financing versus equity (or fund) financing. Thus, an understanding of capital structure theory will aid managers in making capital structure decisions.

The Modigliani-Miller Models

Until 1958, capital structure theories were little more than loose assertions about investor behavior rather than carefully constructed models which could be tested by formal statistical studies. In what has been called the most influential set of financial papers ever published, *Franco Modigliani and Merton Miller (M-M)* addressed the capital structure issue in a rigorous, scientific fashion, and set off a chain of research that continues to this day.[2]

Assumptions

To begin, Modigliani and Miller made the following assumptions, some of which were later relaxed.

1. Firms' business risk can be measured by the standard deviation of earnings before interest and taxes (σ_{EBIT}). Firms with the same degree of business risk are said to be in a *homogeneous risk class*.

2. All present and prospective investors have identical estimates of each firm's future EBIT; that is, investors have *homogeneous expectations* about expected future corporate earnings and the riskiness of those earnings.

3. Stocks and bonds are traded in *perfect capital markets*. This assumption implies, among other things, that there are no brokerage costs and that investors (both individual and institutions) can borrow at the same rate as corporations.

4. The debt of firms and individuals is *riskless*, so the interest rate on debt is the risk-free rate. Furthermore, this situation holds regardless of how much debt a firm (or an individual) uses.

5. All cash flows are *perpetuities*; that is, the firm is a zero-growth firm with an "expectationally constant" EBIT, and its bonds are perpetuities. "Expectationally constant" means that investors expect EBIT to be constant, but the realized, or after the fact, level could be different from the expected level.

M-M without taxes

Modigliani and Miller first performed their analysis under the assumption that there are no corporate or personal income taxes. On the basis of the preceding assumptions, and in the absence of taxes, they proposed and then algebraically proved two propositions:[3]

Proposition I

The value of any firm, V, is established by capitalizing, or discounting, its expected net operating income (EBIT when $T = 0$) at a constant rate that is appropriate for the firm's risk class:

$$V_L = V_U = \frac{\text{EBIT}}{\text{WACC}} = \frac{\text{EBIT}}{k_{sU}}. \tag{9.1}$$

Here the subscripts L and U designate levered (a firm that uses debt financing) and unlevered (a firm that uses no debt financing) firms in a given risk class, and the constant rate, $k_{sU} = \text{WACC}$, is the required rate of return for an unlevered, or all-equity firm.

Since V as established by Proposition I is a constant regardless of the level of debt financing, *then under the M-M model with no taxes, the value of a firm is independent of its leverage.* This also implies (1) that the weighted average cost of capital to any firm is completely independent of its capital structure and (2) that the WACC for all firms in a risk class is equal to the cost of equity to an unlevered firm in that same risk class regardless of the amount of debt financing used.

Proposition II

The cost of equity to a levered firm, k_{sL}, is equal to (1) the cost of equity to an unlevered firm in the same risk class, k_{sU}, plus (2) a risk premium that depends on both the differential between the costs of equity and debt to an unlevered firm and the amount of leverage used:

$$k_{sL} = k_{sU} + \text{Risk Premium} = k_{sU} + (k_{sU} - k_d)(D/S). \tag{9.2}$$

Here D = market value of the firm's debt, S = market value of the firm's equity, and k_d = constant cost of debt. *Proposition II states that as the firm's use of debt increases, its cost of equity also rises, and in a mathematically precise manner.*

Taken together, the two M-M propositions imply that the inclusion of debt in a firm's capital structure will not increase its value, because the benefits of the less costly (as compared to equity) debt financing will be exactly offset by an increase in the riskiness, and hence in the cost, of the firm's equity. *Thus, M-M theory implies that in a world without taxes, both the value of a firm and its overall cost of capital are unaffected by its capital structure.*

M-M used an *arbitrage proof* to support their propositions.[4] They showed that, under their assumptions, if two companies differed only (1) in the way they are financed and (2) in their total market values, then investors would sell shares of the higher-valued firm, buy those of the lower-valued firm, and continue this process until the companies had exactly the same market value. Thus, the actions of investors would ensure that the two firms had identical market values, and hence stock prices. Once the values are proved to be equal, the two M-M propositions are the logical result.[5]

Note that each of the assumptions listed at the beginning of this section is necessary for the arbitrage proof to work. For example, if the companies are not identical in business risk, then the arbitrage process cannot be invoked. We will discuss further implications of the assumptions later in the chapter.

M-M with corporate taxes

Modigliani and Miller's original work, published in 1958, assumed zero taxes. In 1963, M-M published a second article that included corporate tax effects. With corporate income taxes, the authors concluded that leverage will increase a firm's value, because interest on debt is a tax-deductible expense, and hence, as shown earlier in the Super Health example, more of a levered firm's operating income flows through to investors.

When corporations are subject to income taxes, the Modigliani and Miller propositions are as follows.

Proposition I

The value of a levered firm is equal to (1) the value of an unlevered firm in the same risk class plus (2) the gain from leverage, which is the present value of the tax savings and which equals the corporate tax rate, T, times the amount of debt the firm uses, D:[6]

$$V_L = V_U + TD. \qquad (9.1a)$$

The important point here is that when corporate taxes are introduced, the value of the levered firm exceeds that of the unlevered firm by the amount TD. Note also that the differential increases as the use of debt increases, so a firm's value is maximized at virtually 100 percent debt financing.

To find the value for V_U in Equation 9.1a, recognize that M-M assumed that all firms are in a zero-growth situation; that is, EBIT is expected to remain constant, and all earnings are paid out as dividends. Under this assumption, the total market value of a firm's common stock, S, is a perpetuity whose value is found as follows:

$$S = \frac{\text{Dividends}}{k_s} = \frac{\text{Net income}}{k_s} = \frac{(\text{EBIT} - k_d D)(1 - T)}{k_s}. \quad (9.3)$$

With zero debt, $D = \$0$ and the total value of the firm is its equity value, so

$$S = V_U = \frac{\text{EBIT}(1 - T)}{k_{sU}}. \quad (9.3a)$$

Proposition II

The cost of equity to a levered firm is equal to (1) the cost of equity to an unlevered firm in the same risk class plus (2) a risk premium that depends on the differential between the costs of equity and debt to an unlevered firm, the amount of financial leverage used, *and the corporate tax rate*:

$$k_{sL} = k_{sU} + (k_{sU} - k_d)(1 - T)(D/S). \quad (9.2a)$$

Notice that Equation 9.2a is identical to the corresponding without-tax equation, 9.2, except for the term $(1 - T)$ in 9.2a. Since $(1 - T)$ is less than 1.0, the imposition of corporate taxes causes the cost of equity to rise at a slower rate than it did in the absence of taxes. It is this characteristic, along with the fact that the effective cost of debt is reduced, that produces the Proposition I result, namely the increase in firm value as leverage increases.[7]

Illustration of the M-M models

To illustrate the Modigliani and Miller models, assume that the following data and conditions hold for New England Clinical Laboratories, Inc., an old, established firm that operates in several no-growth areas in rural Maine, New Hampshire, and Vermont:

- New England currently has no debt; it is an all-equity company.
- Expected EBIT = $2,400,000. EBIT is not expected to increase over time, so New England is in a no-growth situation.
- New England pays out all of its income as dividends, because no retained earnings are required to finance growth. (Worn-out assets are replaced using depreciation cash flow.)

- If New England begins to use debt, it can borrow at a rate $k_d = 8\%$. This borrowing rate is constant, and it is independent of the amount of debt used. Any money raised by selling debt would be used to retire common stock, so New England's assets and EBIT would remain constant.

- The risk of New England's assets, and thus its EBIT, is such that its shareholders require a rate of return, k_{sU}, of 12 percent if no debt is used.

With zero taxes

To begin, assume that there are no taxes so $T = 0\%$. At any level of debt, Proposition I (Equation 9.1) can be used to find New England's value, $20 million:

$$V_L = V_U = \frac{\text{EBIT}}{k_{sU}} = \frac{\$2.4\text{million}}{0.12} = \$20.0\text{million}.$$

Now, the total market value of the firm is the sum of the market values of the firm's debt and equity:

$$V = S + D.$$

So, if New England uses $10 million of debt, its stock value must be $10 million:

$$S = V - D = \$20 \text{ million} - \$10 \text{ million} = \$10 \text{ million}.$$

We can also find New England's cost of equity, k_{sL}, and its WACC at a debt level of $10 million. First we use Proposition II (Equation 9.2) to find k_{sL}, New England's levered cost of equity:

$$
\begin{aligned}
k_{sL} &= k_{sU} + (k_{sU} - k_d)(D/S) \\
&= 12\% + (12\% - 8\%)(\$10 \text{ million}/\$10 \text{ million}) \\
&= 12\% + 4.0\% = 16.0\%.
\end{aligned}
$$

Now we can find the company's weighted average cost of capital:

$$
\begin{aligned}
\text{WACC} &= (D/V)(k_d)(1 - T) + (S/V)k_s \\
&= (\$10/\$20)(8\%)(1.0) + (\$10/\$20)(16.0\%) = 12.0\%.
\end{aligned}
$$

New England's value and cost of capital based on the M-M model with zero taxes at various debt levels are shown in Figure 9.2. Here we see that in an M-M world without taxes, financial leverage does not matter:

the value of the firm and its overall cost of capital are independent of the amount of debt financing.

With corporate taxes

To illustrate the M-M model with corporate taxes, assume that all of the previous assumptions hold except these two:

1. Expected EBIT = $4,000,000.
2. New England has a 40 percent federal-plus-state tax rate, so $T = 40\%$.

Figure 9.2   Effects of Financial Leverage: MM Model without Corporate Taxes (millions of dollars)

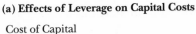

(a) Effects of Leverage on Capital Costs

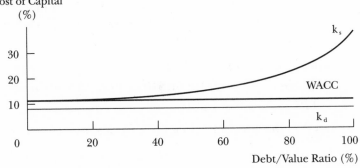

(b) Effect of Leverage on Firm Value

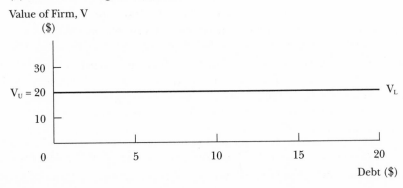

Note that, other things held constant, the introduction of corporate taxes would lower New England's value by $(1 - T)$, so we increased its EBIT from \$2.4 million to \$4 million to make the comparison between the two models easier.

When New England has zero debt but pays taxes, Equation 9.3a can be used to find its value, \$20 million:

$$V_U = \frac{\text{EBIT}(1 - T)}{k_{sU}} = \frac{\$4 \text{ million}(0.6)}{0.12} = \$20.0 \text{ million.}$$

With \$10 million of debt in a world with taxes, we see by Proposition I (Equation 9.1a) that New England's total market value rises to \$24 million.

$$V_L = V_U + TD = \$20 \text{ million} + 0.4(\$10 \text{ million}) = \$24 \text{ million.}$$

Therefore, the value of New England's stock must be \$14 million:

$$S = V - D = \$24 \text{ million} - \$10 \text{ million} + \$14 \text{ million.}$$

We can also find New England's cost of equity, k_{sL}, and its WACC at a debt level of \$10 million. First, we use Proposition II (Equation 9.2a) to find k_{sL}, the levered cost of equity:

$$
\begin{aligned}
k_{sL} &= k_{sU} + (k_{sU} - k_d)(1 - T)(D/S) \\
&= 12\% + (12\% - 8\%)(0.6)(\$10 \text{ million}/\$14 \text{ million}) \\
&= 12\% + 1.71\% = 13.71\%.
\end{aligned}
$$

Now we can find the company's weighted average cost of capital:

$$
\begin{aligned}
\text{WACC} &= (D/V)(k_d)(1 - T) + (S/V)k_s \\
&= (\$10/\$24)(8\%)(0.6) + (\$14/\$24)(13.71\%) = 10.0\%.
\end{aligned}
$$

New England's value and cost of capital at various debt levels with corporate taxes are shown in Figure 9.3. Here we see that in a Modigliani-Miller world with corporate taxes, financial leverage does matter: the value of the firm is maximized and its overall cost of capital is minimized if it uses virtually 100 percent debt financing. Further, we see that the increase in value is due solely to the tax deductibility of interest payments, which causes both the cost of debt and the increase in the cost of equity with leverage to be reduced by $(1 - T)$.

Self-Test Questions:

What is the single most important conclusion of the M-M zero-tax model?

What is the single most important conclusion of the M-M model with corporate taxes?

Figure 9.3   Effects of Financial Leverage: MM Model with
Corporate Taxes (millions of dollars)

(a) Effects of Leverage on Capital Costs

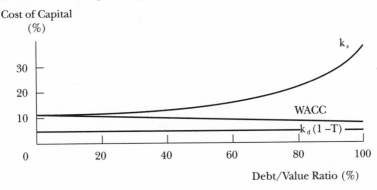

(b) Effect of Leverage on Firm Value

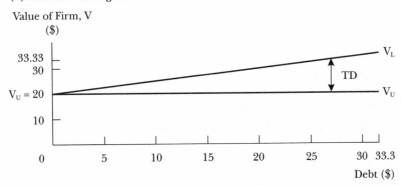

What is the underlying cause of the "gain from leverage" in the M-M
model with corporate taxes?

The Miller Model

Although Modigliani and Miller included *corporate* taxes in the second
version of their model, they did not extend the model to analyze the
effects of *personal* taxes. However, in 1976, Merton Miller did introduce
a model designed to show how leverage affects firms' values when both
personal and corporate taxes are taken into account.[8] To explain Miller's
model, let us begin by defining T_c as the corporate tax rate, T_s as the

personal tax rate on income from stocks, and T_d as the personal tax rate on income from debt. Note that stock returns come partly as dividends and partly as capital gains, so T_s is a weighted average of the effective tax rates on dividends and capital gains, while essentially all debt income comes from interest, which is taxed at investors' top rates.

With personal taxes included, *and under the remaining assumptions used in the earlier M-M models,* the value of an unlevered firm is found by modifying Equation 9.3a as follows:

$$V_U = \frac{\text{EBIT}(1 - T_c)(1 - T_s)}{k_{sU}}. \tag{9.4}$$

The $(1 - T_s)$ term adjusts for personal taxes. Therefore, the numerator shows how much of the firm's cash flow is left after the unlevered firm itself pays corporate income taxes and its investors subsequently pay personal taxes on their dividend income. In effect, the numerator of Equation 9.4 is the perpetual after-all-taxes dividend stream to investors. Since the introduction of personal taxes lowers the usable income to investors, personal taxes reduce the value of the unlevered firm, other things held constant.

The Miller model, which can be derived using an arbitrage proof similar to the one used in the earlier M-M models, is as follows:

$$\text{Miller Model: } V_L = V_U + \left[1 - \frac{(1 - T_c)(1 - T_s)}{(1 - T_d)} \right] D. \tag{9.5}$$

The Miller Model, which defines the value of a levered firm in a world with both corporate and personal taxes, has several important implications:

1. The term in brackets,

$$\left[1 - \frac{(1 - T_c)(1 - T_s)}{(1 - T_d)} \right]$$

   when multiplied by D, represents the gain from leverage. The bracketed term replaces the factor $T = T_c$ in the earlier M-M model with corporate taxes, $V_L = V_U + TD$.

2. If we ignore all taxes, that is, if $T_c = T_s = T_d = 0$, then the bracketed term reduces to zero, so in that case Equation 9.5 is the same as the original M-M model without taxes.

3. If we ignore personal taxes, that is, if $T_s = T_d = 0$, then the bracketed term reduces to $[1 - (1 - T_c)] = T_c$, so Equation 9.5 reduces to the M-M model with corporate taxes.

4. If the effective personal tax rates on stock and bond incomes were equal, that is if $T_s = T_d$, then $(1 - T_s)$ and $(1 - T_d)$ would cancel, and the bracketed term would again reduce to T_c.

5. If $(1 - T_c)(1 - T_s) = (1 - T_d)$, then the bracketed term would go to zero, and the value of using leverage would also be zero. This implies that the tax advantage of debt to the firm would be exactly offset by the personal tax advantage of equity. Under this condition, capital structure would have no effect on a firm's value or its cost of capital, so we would be back to Modigliani and Miller's original zero-tax theory.

6. Because the actual capital gains tax rate in the highest bracket is less than the tax rate on ordinary income (28 percent versus 36 percent in 1995), and because taxes on capital gains are deferred, the effective tax rate on stock income is normally less than the effective tax rate on bond income. This being the case, what would the Miller model predict as the gain from leverage? To answer this question, assume that the tax rate on corporate income is $T_c = 34\%$, the effective rate on bond income is $T_d = 36\%$, and the effective rate on stock income is $T_s = 25\%$ (28 percent plus some gain from deferral of capital gains taxes). Using these values in the Miller model, we find that a levered firm's value increases over that of an unlevered firm by 23 percent of the market value of corporate debt:

$$\text{Gain from leverage} = \left[1 - \frac{(1 - T_c)(1 - T_s)}{(1 - T_d)} \right] D$$
$$= \left[1 - \frac{(1 - 0.34)(1 - 0.25)}{(1 - 0.36)} \right] D$$
$$= [1 - 0.77]D = 0.23D.$$

Note that with these data the M-M model with corporate taxes would indicate a gain from leverage of $T_c D = 0.34D$, or 34 percent of the amount of corporate debt. Thus, with these assumed tax rates, adding personal taxes to the model lowers the benefit derived from corporate debt financing. In general, whenever the effective tax rate on stock income is less than the effective rate on bond income, the Miller model produces a lower gain from leverage than is produced by the M-M with corporate taxes model.

In his paper, Miller argued that firms in the aggregate would issue a mix of debt and equity securities such that the before-tax yields on corporate securities and the personal tax rates of the investors who bought these securities would adjust until an equilibrium was reached. At the equilibrium, $(1 - T_d)$ would equal $(1 - T_c)(1 - T_s)$, so, as we noted earlier in Point 5, the tax advantage of debt to the firm would be exactly offset by personal taxation, and capital structure would have no effect on a firm's value or its cost of capital. Thus, according to Miller, the conclusions derived from the original Modigliani-Miller zero-tax model are correct!

Others have extended and tested Miller's analysis. Generally, these extensions disagree with Miller's conclusion that there is no advantage to the use of corporate debt. In the United States, the effective tax rate on stock income is probably less than the effective tax rate on bond income, so it appears that $(1 - T_c)(1 - T_s)$ is less than $(1 - T_d)$, and there is an advantage to the corporate use of debt financing. However, Miller's work does show that personal taxes offset some of the benefits of corporate debt, so the tax advantages of corporate debt are less than were implied by the earlier M-M model that considered only corporate taxes.

Self-Test Questions:

How does the Miller model differ from the M-M model with corporate taxes?

What are the implications of the Miller model under various tax assumptions?

What is the primary implication of the Miller model given the current tax situation in the United States?

Criticisms of the M-M and Miller Models

The conclusions of each of the three models just discussed follow logically from their initial assumptions: if the assumptions are correct, then the resulting conclusions must be reached. However, both academics and managers have voiced concern over the validity of the Modigliani and Miller and Miller models, and virtually no firms follow the recommendations of any of the models. The M-M zero-tax model leads to the conclusion that capital structure does not matter, but we observe some regularities in structure within industries. Furthermore, when used with "reasonable" tax rates, both the M-M model with corporate taxes and the Miller model lead to the conclusion that firms should use 100 percent debt financing. That situation is not observed in practice except by firms whose equity has been eroded by operating losses. People who disagree with the M-M and Miller models and their suggestions for financial policy generally attack the models on the grounds that their assumptions do not reflect real world conditions. Some of the main objections include the following:

1. Modigliani and Miller and, later, Miller assume that personal and corporate leverage are perfect substitutes. However, an individual investing in a levered firm has less loss exposure, which means a more *limited liability*, than if he or she used "homemade" leverage. This increased personal risk exposure would tend to restrain investors from engaging in arbitrage, and that could cause the models to be incorrect.

2. Brokerage costs were assumed away in the M-M and Miller models. However, brokerage and other transaction costs do exist, and they too impede the arbitrage process.

3. M-M initially assumed that corporations and investors can borrow at the risk-free rate. Although risky debt has been introduced into the analysis by others with no significant change in results, to reach the M-M and Miller conclusions it is still necessary to assume that both corporations and investors can borrow at the same rate. Although major institutional investors probably can borrow at the corporate rate, many institutions are not allowed to borrow to buy securities. Furthermore, most individual investors must borrow at higher rates than those paid by large corporations.

4. The M-M and Miller models assume that there are no costs associated with financial distress. Further, they ignore agency costs. These topics are discussed in the next section.

Self-Test Questions:

Should we accept one of the models presented thus far as being correct? Why or why not?

Which of the assumptions used in the models is most likely, in your view, to cause the models to be invalid?

Financial Distress and Agency Costs

Some of the assumptions inherent in the M-M and Miller models can be relaxed, and when this is done, their basic conclusions remain unchanged.[9] However, as we discuss next, when financial distress and agency costs are added, the M-M and Miller results are altered significantly.

Financial distress costs

A number of firms experience financial distress each year, and some of them are forced into bankruptcy. Financial distress includes but is not restricted to bankruptcy, and when it occurs, several things can happen:

- Arguments between claimants often delay the liquidation of assets. Bankruptcy cases can take many years to settle, and during this time equipment loses value, buildings are vandalized, inventories become obsolete, and so on.

- Lawyer's fees, court costs, and administrative expenses can absorb a large part of the firm's value. Together, the costs of physical deterioration plus legal fees and administrative expenses are called the *direct costs of bankruptcy.*

- Managers and other employees generally lose their jobs when a firm fails. Knowing this, the management of a firm that is in financial distress often takes actions that keep it alive in the short run, but that dilute its long-run value. For example, a hospital in financial distress may fail to modernize, or may sell off valuable nonessential assets at bargain prices to raise cash or cut costs so much that the quality of its services is impaired and the firm's long-run market position is eroded.

- Both customers and suppliers of organizations that are experiencing financial difficulties are aware of the problems that can arise, and they often stop dealing with firms that are experiencing financial distress. These actions further damage troubled firms. Nonoptimal managerial actions associated with financial distress, as well as the costs imposed by customers, suppliers, and capital providers, are called the *indirect costs of financial distress.* Of course, these costs may be incurred by a firm in financial distress even if it does not go into bankruptcy; bankruptcy is just one point on the continuum of financial distress.

All things considered, the direct and indirect costs associated with financial distress are high, but financial distress typically occurs only if a firm uses debt financing—debt-free firms do not usually experience financial distress. *Therefore, the greater the use of debt financing, and the larger the fixed interest charges, the greater the probability that a decline in earnings will lead to financial distress, and hence the higher the probability that the costs of financial distress will be incurred.*

An increase in the probability of financial distress raises a firm's cost of equity capital, k_s, and hence lowers the current value of the firm's stock. Furthermore, the probability of financial distress increases with leverage, causing the expected present value cost of financial distress to rise as more and more debt financing is used. The effects of financial distress are also felt by a firm's bondholders. Firms experiencing financial distress have a higher probability of defaulting on debt payments, so the expectation of financial distress influences bond investors' required rates of return: the higher the probability of financial distress, the higher the required return on debt. Thus, as a firm uses more and more debt financing, and hence increases the probability of financial distress, its cost of debt, k_d, also increases.

Agency costs

We introduced the concept of agency costs in Chapters 2 and 6. One type of agency cost is associated with the use of debt, and it involves the relationship between a firm's stockholders and its bondholders. In the absence of any restrictions, a firm's management might be tempted to take actions that would benefit stockholders at the expense of bondholders. For example, if a firm were to use only a small amount of debt financing, then this debt would have relatively little risk, and hence a high rating and a low interest rate. Yet, having sold the low-risk debt, the firm could then issue more debt secured by the same assets as the original debt. This would raise the risks faced by *all bondholders*, cause k_d to rise, and consequently cause the original bondholders to suffer capital losses.

Similarly, suppose that after issuing a substantial amount of debt, the firm decided to restructure its assets, selling off assets with low business risk and acquiring assets that were more risky but that also had higher expected rates of return. If things worked out well, the stockholders would benefit. If things went sour, most of the loss in a highly leveraged firm would fall on the creditors. In other words, the stockholders would be playing a game of "heads, I win; tails, you lose" with the creditors.

Because of the possibility that stockholders might try to take advantage of creditors in these and other ways, creditors are protected by restrictive covenants in loan agreements. These covenants hamper the corporation's legitimate operations to some extent. Furthermore, the company must be monitored to ensure that the covenants are being obeyed, and the costs of monitoring are passed on to the stockholders in the form of higher debt costs. The costs of lost efficiency plus monitoring are what we mean here by *agency costs*, and these costs increase the cost of debt to the firm and reduce the value of the equity, and thus reduce the advantage of debt financing. As with financial distress costs, the greater the amount of debt financing, the greater the amount of agency costs.

Firm value and the cost of capital with financial distress and agency costs

If the M-M model with corporate taxes were correct, a firm's value would rise continuously as it moved from zero debt toward 100 percent debt: the equation $V_L = V_U + TD$ shows that TD, hence V_L, is maximized if D is at a maximum. Recall that the rising component of value, TD, results directly from the tax shelter provided by interest on the debt. However, the following factors, which were ignored in the M-M model, could cause V_L to decline as the level of debt rises: (1) the present value of costs associated with potential future financial distress and (2) the present value of agency costs. Therefore, the M-M model's relationship between a firm's value and its use of leverage should look like this when financial distress and agency costs are added:

$$V_L = V_U + TD - \begin{matrix} PV \text{ of expected} \\ \text{financial} \\ \text{distress costs} \end{matrix} - \begin{matrix} PV \text{ of} \\ \text{agency} \\ \text{costs.} \end{matrix} \qquad (9.6)$$

The relationship expressed in Equation 9.6 is graphed in Figure 9.4. The tax shelter effect totally dominates until the amount of debt reaches Point A. After Point A, financial distress and agency costs become increasingly important, offsetting some of the tax advantages. At Point B, the marginal tax shelter benefits of additional debt are exactly offset by the marginal disadvantages of debt, and beyond Point B, the marginal disadvantages outweigh the marginal *benefits*.

Equation 9.5, the Miller model, can also be modified to reflect financial distress and agency costs. The equation would be identical to Equation 9.6, except that the gain-from-leverage term, TD, would reflect the addition of personal taxes. In either the M-M or Miller models, the gain from leverage can at least be roughly estimated, but the value reduction resulting from potential financial distress and agency costs is almost entirely subjective. We know that these costs must increase as leverage rises, but we simply do not know the specific functional relationships.

Figure 9.4   Net Effect of Financial Leverage on the Value of
the Firm

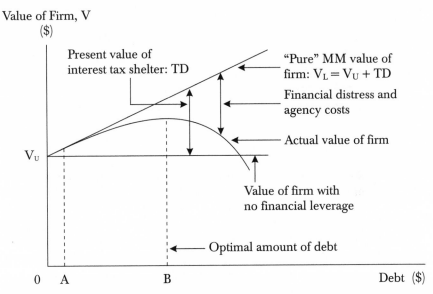

Source: E. F. Brigham and L. C. Gapenski. 1994. *Financial Management: Theory and Practice,* 7th
ed. Fort Worth, TX: The Dryden Press.

Self-Test Questions:

Describe some types of financial distress and agency costs.

How are financial distress and agency costs related to the use of financial
leverage?

How are the basic M-M models with corporate taxes, and the Miller
model, affected by the addition of financial distress and agency costs?

Trade-off Models

Both the M-M with corporate taxes and Miller models as modified to
reflect financial distress and agency costs are described as *trade-off models.*
That is, the optimal capital structure is found, at least conceptually, by
balancing the tax shield benefits of leverage against the financial distress
and agency costs of leverage, so the costs and benefits are "traded off"
against one another.

Implications of the trade-off models

The trade-off models are not capable of specifying precise optimal capital structures, but they do enable us to make three statements about debt usage:

1. Higher-risk firms, as measured by the variability of returns on the firm's assets, ought to borrow less than lower-risk firms, other things equal. The greater this variability, the greater the probability of financial distress at any level of debt, and hence the greater the expected costs of distress. Thus, firms with lower business risk can borrow more before the expected costs of distress offset the tax advantages of borrowing.

2. Firms that employ tangible assets such as real estate and standardized equipment should borrow more than firms whose value is derived either from intangible assets such as patents and goodwill or from growth opportunities. The costs of financial distress depend not only on the probability of incurring distress, but also on what happens if distress occurs. Specialized assets, intangible assets, and growth opportunities are more likely to lose value if financial distress occurs than are standardized, tangible assets.

3. Firms that are currently paying taxes at the highest rate, and that are likely to continue to do so in the future, should carry more debt that firms with current and/or prospectively lower tax rates. High corporate tax rates lead to greater benefits from debt financing, and hence high-tax-rate firms can carry more debt, other factors held constant, before the tax shield is offset by financial distress and agency costs.[10]

According to the trade-off models, each firm should set its target capital structure such that its costs and benefits of leverage are balanced at the margin, because such a structure will maximize its value. We would expect to find actual target structures that are consistent with the three points just noted. Furthermore, we would generally expect to find that firms within an industry have similar capital structures, because such firms have roughly the same types of assets, business risk, and profitability.

The empirical evidence

The trade-off models have intuitive appeal because they lead to the conclusion that both no debt and all debt are bad, while a "moderate" debt level is good. However, we must ask ourselves whether these models explain actual behavior. If they do not, then we must search for other explanations or else assume that managers, and hence investors, are acting irrationally, an assumption that we are unwilling to make.

The trade-off models do have some empirical support.[11] For example, firms that have primarily tangible assets tend to borrow more heavily than firms whose value stems from intangibles or growth opportunities or both. However, other empirical evidence refutes the trade-off models. First, several studies have examined models of financing behavior to see if firms' financing decisions reflect adjustment toward a target capital structure. These studies provide some evidence that this occurs, but the explanatory power of the models is very low, suggesting that trade-off models capture only a part of actual behavior. Second, no study has clearly demonstrated that a firm's tax rate has a predictable, material effect on its capital structure. In fact, firms used debt financing long before corporate income taxes even existed. Finally, actual debt ratios tend to vary widely across apparently similar firms, whereas the trade-off models suggest that the use of debt should be relatively consistent within industries.

All in all, empirical support for the trade-off models is not strong, which suggests that other factors not incorporated into these models are also at work. In other words, the trade-off models do not tell the full story.

Self-Test Questions:

What is a trade-off model of capital structure?

What are the implications of the trade-off models?

Does the empirical evidence support the trade-off models?

Asymmetric Information Model of Capital Structure

The asymmetric information model of capital structure traces its roots back to the work done in the 1960s by Gordon Donaldson.[12] Donaldson conducted an extensive survey of investor-owned corporations to find out how managers make financing decisions, and reached the following conclusions:

1. Firms prefer to finance with internally generated funds, that is, with retained earnings and depreciation cash flow.

2. Firms set target dividend payout ratios on the basis of their expected future investment opportunities and their expected

future cash flows. The target payout ratio is set at a level such that expected retentions plus depreciation cash flow will meet expected capital expenditure requirements.

3. Dividends are "sticky" in the short run—firms are reluctant to make major changes in the dollar dividend, and they are especially reluctant to cut the dividend. Thus, in any given year, depending on realized cash flows and actual investment opportunities, a firm may or may not have sufficient internally generated funds to cover its capital expenditures.

4. If the firm has more internal cash flow than is needed for capital investment, then it will invest the excess in marketable securities or else use the funds to retire debt.

5. If the firm has insufficient internal cash flow to finance its capital investments, then it will first draw down its marketable securities portfolio, then issue debt, then issue convertible bonds (bonds that can be exchanged in the future for common stock), and only as a last resort will it issue new common stock.

Thus, Donaldson observed a "pecking order" of financing, and not the balanced approach that is called for by the trade-off models. Indeed, the pecking order causes firms to move away from rather than toward a well-defined capital structure because equity funds are raised in two forms: retained earnings at the top of the pecking order and new common stock sales at the bottom.

Until recently, no theoretical model was available to explain this observed behavior of firms, so Donaldson's survey results were not given much credence by academics. Then, Stewart C. Myers proposed the *asymmetric information model* of capital structure.[13] The model is based on two assumptions: (1) managers know more about their firms' future prospects than do investors; and (2) managers are motivated to maximize the wealth of their firms' current shareholders. Although the first assumption is contrary to the strong form of the efficient markets hypothesis (EMH), few, if any, people believe that the strong form holds.

If managers think that their firm's stock is undervalued, they will be motivated to use debt financing, because selling stock at a "bargain" is detrimental to the firm's existing shareholders. However, if managers think that their firm's stock is overvalued, they will be motivated to issue new common stock. By issuing stock for more that it is actually worth, value is transferred from the buyers of the new stock to the existing shareholders. Thus, managers are motivated to issue new stock only when they believe that the stock is overvalued. Since investors are rational, they treat new common stock issues as "signals" that management considers the stock to be overvalued. Thus, investors revise downward their expectations for the firm and the stock price falls.[14]

Since new stock issues have an adverse effect on stock price, managers are reluctant to issue new stock. Although large amounts of new stock are issued each year, the vast majority is issued by small, rapidly growing companies that have large capital needs and hence little choice. Stock issues by mature companies are relatively rare. If external financing is required, debt is the first choice, and new common stock will be used only in unusual circumstances. Thus, the asymmetric information model leads managers to act in accordance with Donaldson's pecking order.

Because managers want to avoid new stock issues, especially when they might be least advantageous, it becomes prudent for firms to maintain a *reserve borrowing capacity* that can be used whenever capital investments require an unusually large amount of external capital. By maintaining a reserve borrowing capacity, and then tapping it when necessary, managers can avoid issuing new common stock under unfavorable conditions.

Note that the degree of information asymmetry and its impact on investors' perceptions differ substantially across firms. To illustrate, the degree of asymmetry is typically much greater in the drug industry than in the hospital industry because success in the drug industry depends on secretive proprietary research and development. Thus, managers in this industry hold significantly more information about their firms' prospects than do outside analysts and investors. Also, emerging firms with limited capital and good growth opportunities are recognized as having to use external financing, so new stock offerings by such firms are not viewed with as much concern by investors as are new offerings by mature firms with limited growth opportunities. Thus, although the asymmetric information theory is applicable to all investor-owned firms, its influence on managerial decisions varies from firm to firm and over time.

Self-Test Questions:

Briefly explain the asymmetric information model of capital structure.

What does the model suggest about capital structure decisions?

A Summary of the Capital Structure Models

The great contribution of the trade-off models of M-M, Miller, and their followers is that these models identify the specific benefits and costs of using debt—the tax effects, financial distress costs, and so on. Prior to these models, no capital structure theory existed, and we had no systematic way of analyzing the effects of debt financing.

The trade-off model is summarized in Figure 9.5. The top graph shows the relationships between the debt ratio and the cost of debt, cost of equity, and the WACC. Both k_s and $k_d(1 - T_c)$ rise steadily with increases in leverage, but the rate of increase accelerates at higher debt levels, reflecting agency costs and the increased probability of financial distress and its attendant costs. The WACC first declines, then hits a minimum at D/V^*, and then begins to rise. Note that the value of D in D/V^* in the upper graph is the same as D^*, the level of debt in the lower graph that maximizes the firm's value. Thus, a firm's WACC is minimized and its value is maximized at the same capital structure. Also note that the general shapes of the curves apply once we consider the effects of financial distress and agency cost regardless of whether we are using the M-M with corporate taxes model or the Miller model.

Unfortunately, it is extremely difficult for financial managers to actually quantify the costs and benefits of debt financing to their firms, so it is virtually impossible to pinpoint D/V^*, the capital structure that truly maximizes a firm's value. Most experts believe that such a structure exists for every taxable firm, but that it changes substantially over time as the nature of the firm and the capital markets changes. Most experts also believe that, as shown in the lower portion of Figure 9.5, the relationship between firm value and leverage is relatively flat; thus, relatively large deviations from the optimum can occur without materially affecting a firm's value.

Now consider the asymmetric information model. Because of asymmetric information, investors know less about a firm's prospects than do its managers. Further, managers try to maximize value for current stockholders, not new ones; so if the firm has excellent prospects, management will not want to issue new shares, but if things look bleak, then a new stock offering may be sold. Therefore, investors take a stock offering to be a signal of bad news, so stock prices tend to decline when new issues are announced. As a result, new equity financing can be very expensive, and this fact must be incorporated into the capital structure decision. Its effect is to motivate firms to maintain a reserve borrowing capacity, which permits future investment opportunities to be financed by debt when internal funds are insufficient.

By combining the two theories, we obtain this possible explanation for the capital structure decisions of taxable firms: (1) Debt financing

Figure 9.5   Summary of the Trade-Off Models

(a) Effects of Leverage on Capital Costs

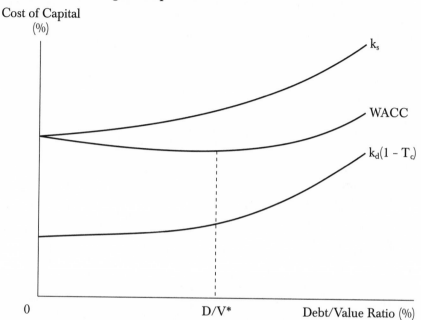

(b) Effect of Leverage on Firm Value

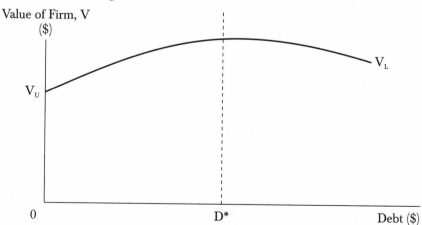

Source: E. F. Brigham and L. C. Gapenski. 1994. *Financial Management: Theory and Practice,* 7th ed. Fort Worth, TX: The Dryden Press.

provides benefits because of the tax deductibility of interest. Hence, firms should have some debt in their capital structures. (2) However, financial distress and agency costs place limits on debt usage—beyond some point, these costs offset the tax advantage of debt. (3) Finally, because of asymmetric information, firms maintain a reserve borrowing capacity to take advantage of good investment opportunities, and, at the same time, avoid having to issue stock at distressed prices.

Self-Test Questions:

Do the capital structure models provide managers with specific quantifiable guidance regarding optimal capital structures?

Summarize the information that capital structure models provide to decision makers.

Application of Capital Structure Theory to Not-for-Profit Firms

So far, the discussion of capital structure theory has focused on investor-owned firms. Do the models discussed earlier apply to not-for-profit firms? Although no rigorous research has been conducted into the optimal capital structures of not-for-profit firms, some loose analogies can be drawn. Although not-for-profit firms do not receive a direct tax subsidy when debt financing is used, they do have access to the tax-exempt debt market, which provides an indirect tax subsidy. (If not-for-profits had to issue taxable debt, their costs of debt would increase.) Thus, not-for-profit firms receive about the same benefits from the use of debt financing as do investor-owned firms.

What about the costs associated with debt financing? As discussed in Chapter 8, a not-for-profit firm's fund capital has an opportunity cost that is roughly equivalent to the cost of equity of a similar investor-owned firm. Thus, we would expect the opportunity cost of fund capital to rise as more and more debt financing is used, just as for an investor-owned firm. Furthermore, not-for-profit firms are subject to the same types of financial distress and agency costs that are borne by investor-owned firms, so these costs are equally applicable. Thus, we would expect the trade-off models to be roughly applicable to not-for-profit firms, and hence for such firms to have optimal capital structures defined, as least in theory, as a trade-off between the costs and benefits of debt financing. Note, however, that the asymmetric information model is not applicable to not-for-profit firms, because such firms do not issue common stock.

Although the trade-off models may be partially applicable for not-for-profit firms, a problem arises because for-profit firms have more-or-less unlimited access to equity capital. Thus, if they have more capital investment opportunities than they can finance with retained earnings and debt financing, investor-owned firms can always raise the needed funds by a new stock issue. (According to the asymmetric information theory, managers may not want to issue new stock, but the opportunity still exists.) Additionally, it is quite easy for investor-owned firms to alter their capital structures. If they are financially underleveraged (using too little debt), they can simply issue more debt and use the proceeds to repurchase stock. On the other hand, if they are financially overleveraged (using too much debt), they can issue additional shares and use the proceeds to refund debt.

Not-for-profit firms do not have access to the equity markets—their sole source of "equity" capital is through governmental grants, private contributions, and excess revenues (retained earnings). Managers of not-for-profit organizations do not have the same degree of flexibility in either capital investment or capital structure decisions as do their proprietary counterparts. Thus, it is often necessary for not-for-profit firms to (1) delay new projects, even profitable ones, because of funding insufficiencies and (2) use more than the theoretically optimal amount of debt because that is the only way that needed services can be financed. Although these actions may be required in certain situations, not-for-profit managers must recognize that such strategies increase costs. Project delays mean that needed services are not being provided on a timely basis. Using more debt than optimal pushes the firm beyond the point of the greatest net benefit of debt financing, and hence capital costs are increased above the minimum. If a not-for-profit firm is forced into a situation where it is using more than the optimal amount of debt financing, its managers should plan to reduce the firm's level of debt as soon as the situation permits.

The ability of a not-for-profit firm to garner governmental grants, attract private contributions, and generate excess revenues plays an important role in establishing its competitive position. A firm that has an adequate amount of fund capital can operate at its optimal capital structure, and thus minimize capital costs. If insufficient fund capital is available, too much financial leverage is then used, and the result is higher capital costs. Consider two not-for-profit hospitals that are similar in all respects, except that one has more fund capital and can operate at its optimal structure, while the other has insufficient fund capital and thus must use more debt financing than optimal. In effect, the hospital with insufficient fund capital must operate at an inefficient capital structure. The former has a significant competitive advantage because it can either offer more services at the same cost by using additional (nonoptimal) debt financing, or it can offer matching services at lower costs. Thus, sufficient fund capital provides the flexibility to offer all of the necessary services and still operate at the lowest capital cost structure. Like companies that have low operating cost structures, not-for-profit firms that have low capital cost structures—companies that are at their optimal capital structures—have an advantage over their competitors that have higher capital cost structures.

Any firm that is forced to use more than the optimal amount of debt financing is operating inefficiently, and hence has an economic incentive to obtain more fund capital. As in any competitive industry, not-for-profit health care managers have limited control over their firms' abilities to generate excess revenues. On the other hand, managers have much greater control over the amount of effort applied to public and private fund raising. Thus, not-for-profit firms that require fund capital to operate efficiently must emphasize fund raising. Years ago, public and private contributions were a critical source of funds for not-for-profit providers, but many firms deemphasized this source of capital during the cost-plus era of the 1970s and early 1980s. It might be time for many not-for-profit managers to reevaluate their fund-raising efforts.

Self-Test Questions:

Do the capital structure models apply to not-for-profit firms?

Why is capital structure important to not-for-profit firms?

Making the Capital Structure Decision

Since one cannot determine precisely the optimal capital structure, managers must apply judgment along with quantitative analysis. The judgmental analysis involves several different factors, and in one situation a particular factor might have great importance, while the same factor might be relatively unimportant in another situation. This section discusses some of the more important judgmental issues that should be taken into account.

Long-run viability

Managers of large firms, especially those providing vital health care services, have a responsibility to provide continuous service, so they must refrain from using leverage to the point where the firm's long-run viability is endangered.

Managerial conservatism

Well-diversified investors have eliminated most, if not all, of the diversifiable risk from their portfolios. Therefore, the typical investor can tolerate some chance of financial distress, because a loss on one stock will probably be offset by random gains on other stocks in the investor's portfolio. However, managers of investor-owned firms often view financial distress with more concern—they are typically not well diversified in their careers, and thus the present value of their expected earnings can be seriously affected by the onset of financial distress. Therefore, it is not difficult to imagine that managers might be more "conservative" in their use of leverage than the average stockholder would desire. If this is true, then managers would set somewhat lower target capital structures than the ones that maximize firm value.

For not-for-profit firms, one could argue that managerial conservatism is appropriate. Not-for-profit firms have no shareholders, and many of the stakeholders are typically not well diversified in regard to their relationships with the firm. Thus, these stakeholders have much more to lose if the firm fails than do well-diversified shareholders of investor-owned firms. However, the managers of not-for-profit firms can adopt a conservative approach to capital structure only if the firm has sufficient fund capital.

Lender and rating agency attitudes

Regardless of a manager's own analysis of the proper leverage for his or her firm, there is no question but that lenders' and rating agencies' attitudes are frequently important determinants of financial structures. In the majority of cases, corporate managers discuss the firm's financial structure with lenders and rating agencies, and give much weight to their advice. Typically, managers want to maintain some target debt rating, say, single-A. Also, if a particular firm's management is so confident of the future that it seeks to use leverage beyond the norms for its industry, its lenders may be unwilling to accept such debt increases, or may do so only at a high price.

Reserve borrowing capacity

Under the asymmetric information model, firms should maintain a reserve borrowing capacity that preserves the ability to issue debt at favorable terms. For example, suppose Merck had just successfully completed an R&D program on a new drug and its internal projections forecast much higher earnings in the future. However, the new earnings are not yet anticipated by investors, and hence are not reflected in the price of its stock. Merck's managers would not want to issue stock, they would prefer to finance with debt until the higher earnings materialized and were reflected in the stock price, at which time the firm could sell an issue of common stock, retire the debt, and return to its target capital structure. To maintain a reserve borrowing capacity, firms generally use less debt under "normal" conditions, and hence present a stronger financial picture than they otherwise would. This is not suboptimal from a long-run standpoint, although it might appear so if viewed strictly on a short-run basis.

Industry averages

Presumably managers act rationally, so the capital structures of other firms in the industry (particularly the industry leaders) should provide insights as to the optimal structure. In general, there is no reason to believe that the managers of one firm are better than the managers of any other firm. Thus, if one firm has a capital structure that is significantly different from other firms in its industry, the managers of that firm should identify the unique circumstances that contribute to the anomaly. If unique circumstances cannot be identified, then it is doubtful that the firm has identified the correct target structure.

Control of investor-owned corporations

The effect that its choice of securities has on a management's control position may also influence its capital structure decision. If a firm's management just barely has majority control (just over 50 percent of the stock), but it is not in a position to buy any more stock, debt may be the choice for new financings. On the other hand, a management group that is not concerned about voting control may decide to use equity rather than debt if the firm's financial situation is so weak that the use of debt might subject the company to serious risk of default.

Asset structure

Firms whose assets are suitable as security for loans tend to use debt rather heavily. Thus, hospitals tend to be highly leveraged, but companies involved in technological research employ relatively little debt. Also, if the firm's assets carry high business risk, then it will be less able to use financial leverage than a firm with low business risk. Accordingly, factors such as sales stability and operating leverage, which influence business risk, also influence firms' optimal capital structure.

Growth rate

Other factors the same, faster-growing firms must rely more heavily on external capital—slow growth can be financed with retained earnings, but rapid growth generally requires the use of external funds. As postulated in the information asymmetry theory, firms first turn to debt financing to meet external funding needs. Further, the flotation costs involved in selling common stock exceed those incurred when selling debt. Thus, rapidly growing firms tend to use somewhat more debt than do slower-growth companies.

Profitability

One often observes that firms with very high rates of return on investment use relatively little debt. This behavior is consistent with the asymmetric information theory, and the practical reason seems to be that highly profitable firms simply do not need to do much debt financing: their high rates of return enable them to do most of their financing with retained earnings.

Taxes

Interest is a deductible expense, while dividends are not deductible, so the higher a firm's corporate tax rate, the greater the advantage of using corporate debt.[15]

Self-Test Questions:

Is the capital structure decision mostly objective or subjective?

What are some of the factors that managers must consider when setting the optimal capital structure?

Variations in Capital Structures among Firms

As would be expected, wide variations in the use of financial leverage occur both across industries and among the individual firms in an industry. For example, in 1995, the average firm in the pharmaceutical industry used about 30 percent debt financing, while the average hospital used almost 50 percent. The drug industry used significantly less debt than the hospital industry because pharmaceutical firms have significantly more business risk, arising both from research and development uncertainties and high product liability exposure.

To illustrate variations within an industry, consider the hospital industry. The average debt ratio in 1995 was about 50 percent, but about 10 percent of the hospitals had less than 20 percent debt, while another 10 percent of the hospitals had over 80 percent debt. Clearly, there is a wide variation among hospitals, firms that are essentially in the same industry. Thus, factors unique to individual firms, including managerial attitudes, play an important role in setting actual capital structures.

Self-Test Questions:

Why does the average capital structure vary from industry to industry?

Do firms within the same industry have roughly the same capital structures?

An Approach to Setting the Target Capital Structure

Thus far, we have discussed several models of capital structure and a myriad of factors that influence the capital structure decisions of most firms. In this section, we describe a pragmatic approach to setting the target capital structure used at Ann Arbor Health Systems. The approach requires judgmental assumptions, but it also allows managers to see how alternative capital structures would affect future profitability, the firm's ability to meet its debt payments, and external financing requirements under a variety of assumptions.

The analysis uses a five-year forecasting model that is set up especially to test the effects of capital structure changes. Basically, the model generates forecasted data based on inputs supplied by Ann Arbor's managers. Each data item can be fixed, or it can be allowed to vary from year to year. The required data include the most recent balance sheet and income statement, plus a large number of inputs that represent either expectations or policy variables. For example, the input variables include items such as annual growth rates in volume and reimbursement, cost inflation rates, marginal component costs of capital, capital structure percentages, and dividend growth rates. The model uses the input data to forecast Ann Arbor's balance sheets and income statements for five years. Further, the model calculates and displays other applicable financial information for each of the forecast years, such as external financing requirements, return on equity (ROE), earnings per share (EPS), dividends per share (DPS), coverage ratios on debt, and weighted average cost of capital (WACC).

Ann Arbor's managers begin the process by entering base year values and data on expected volume and reimbursement growth rates, expected inflation rates, and so on. These inputs are used by the model to forecast operating income and asset requirements that, in general, will not depend on financing decisions. Next, the managers must consider the financing mix. The model permits as inputs both the debt/equity mix and the debt maturity mix. (By debt maturity, we mean the proportion of short-term versus long-term debt.) Furthermore, Ann Arbor's managers must estimate as best they can the effects of the capital structure on the component costs of capital, and then must enter these cost rate estimates. A higher debt ratio will lead to increases in the costs of all components, and vice versa if less debt is used. With all inputs entered, the model then completes the forecasted financial statements.

Next, the model's output must be reviewed and analyzed. Since the model focuses on the capital structure decision, Ann Arbor's managers pay particular attention to forecasted earnings, debt coverage ratios, and external funding requirements. Finally, the model is used to analyze alternative scenarios. This analysis takes two forms: (1) changing the financing inputs to get some idea of how the financing mix affects the key outputs and (2) changing the operating inputs to see how the basic business risk of the firm affects the key outputs under various financing strategies.

The model can generate the output "answers" quite easily, but it remains up to Ann Arbor's managers to assign input values, to interpret the output, and finally, to set the target capital structure. Reaching a decision is not easy, but a capital structure forecasting model such as the one Ann Arbor uses at least permits managers to analyze the effects of alternative courses of action, which is an essential element of good decision making.

It should be noted again that, although capital structure decisions do affect overall capital costs and the prices of investor-owned companies' stocks, those effects are relatively small in comparison to the effects of operating decisions. A company's ability to identify (or create) market opportunities, and to produce and sell products or services efficiently, is the primary determinant of success. Financial arrangements can facilitate or hamper operations, but the best of financial plans cannot overcome deficiencies in the operations area. These opinions are supported by empirical studies, which generally find a weak statistical relationship between capital structure and stock price. The opinions are also supported by Ann Arbor's computer model, which shows stock price to be affected significantly by changes in patient volume, reimbursement rates, fixed costs, and variable costs, but not to be affected much by changes in capital structure.

A similar model can be used by not-for-profit firms. The major difference is the binding constraint against new stock issues. Since a not-for-profit firm's new equity financing is constrained, growth may have to be curtailed due to lack of capital. Of course, the same situation could arise for investor-owned firms if the firm's managers are reluctant to issue new equity.

Self-Test Questions:

Briefly describe the elements of a financial forecasting model that could be used to help set the target capital structure.

How critical is the optimal capital structure to the financial performance of a firm?

Summary

This chapter presented a variety of topics related to capital structure decisions. The key concepts are listed next.

- The use of debt (or preferred stock) financing increases the *rate of return* to stockholders (owners), but it also increases their *risk*.

- *Business risk* is the inherent riskiness in a firm's operations if it uses no debt financing. *Financial risk* is the additional risk that is concentrated on the shareholders when debt financing is used.

- In 1958, Franco Modigliani and Merton Miller (M-M) startled the academic community by proving, under a restrictive set of assumptions including zero taxes, that *capital structure is irrelevant*—a firm's value is not affected by its financial mix.

- Modigliani and Miller later added *corporate taxes* to their model, leading to the conclusion that capital structure does matter, and that firms should use almost 100 percent debt financing in order to maximize value.

- The M-M model with corporate taxes illustrates that the benefits of debt financing stem solely from the *tax deductibility of interest payments.*
- Much later, Miller extended the model to include *personal taxes.* The introduction of personal taxes reduces, but does not eliminate, the benefits of debt financing. Thus, the *Miller model* also prescribes 100 percent debt financing.
- The addition of financial distress and agency costs to either the M-M corporate tax model or the Miller model results in a *trade-off model.* Here the marginal costs and benefits of debt financing are balanced against one another, and the result is an optimal capital structure that falls somewhere between zero and 100 percent debt.
- *Not-for-profit firms* face a set of benefits and costs associated with debt financing similar to those faced by investor-owned firms, so the trade-off model is at least partially applicable to such firms. However, the inability to issue stock may keep a not-for-profit firm's capital structure above the optimal point, at least temporarily.
- The *asymmetric information model,* which is based on the assumption that managers have better information than investors, postulates that there is a preferred order to financing: first retained earnings (and depreciation), then debt, and finally, as a last resort only, new common stock.
- The asymmetric information model prescribes that firms maintain a *reserve borrowing capacity* so that they can always issue debt on reasonable terms rather than being forced into a new equity issue at the wrong time.
- Unfortunately, capital structure theory does not provide neat, clean answers to the question of the optimal capital structure. Thus, many factors must be considered when actually choosing a firm's target capital structure, and the final decision will be based on both analysis and judgment.
- Firms generally have *computerized planning models* that are used for financial planning. These models, if built to include the effects of alternative capital structures, can be used to help set the optimal structure.

The capital structure decision is not an easy one, but it is an essential element of any business's long-term plan.

Notes

1. Leasing is discussed in detail in Chapter 16.
2. See F. Modigliani and M. H. Miller, "The Cost of Capital, Corporation Finance and the Theory of Investment," *American Economic Review* (June 1958: 261–97; "The Cost of Capital, Corporation Finance and the Theory of Investment: Reply," *American Economic Review* (September 1958): 655–69; "Taxes and the Cost of Capital: A Correction," *American Economic Review* (June 1963): 433–43; and "Reply," *American Economic Review* (June 1965): 524–27. In a 1979 survey of Financial Management Association members, the original M-M article was judged to have had the greatest impact on the field of finance of any work ever published. See P. L. Cooley and J. L. Heck, "Significant Contributions to Finance Literature," *Financial Management*, Tenth Anniversary Issue (1981): 23–33.
3. M-M actually developed three propositions, but the third one is not material to our discussion here.
4. *Arbitrage* means the simultaneous buying and selling of essentially identical assets at different prices. The buying increases the price of the undervalued asset, and the selling decreases the price of the overvalued asset. Arbitrage operations will continue until prices have been adjusted to the point where the arbitrager can no longer earn a profit. At this point, the market is in equilibrium.
5. For an illustration of M-M's arbitrage proof, see E. F. Brigham and L. C. Gapenski, *Intermediate Financial Management* (Fort Worth, TX: Dryden Press, 1996), chap. 11.
6. The annual interest expense associated with D dollars of debt financing is k_dD, and the resulting tax savings is Tk_dD. Since M-M assume that all cash flows are perpetuities, the present value of the tax savings stream is $Tk_dD/k_d = TD$.
7. Note that health care providers that receive capital pass-through payments for interest expense receive a third party payer subsidy for using debt financing that is similar to the tax subsidy. Thus, we could modify Equation 9.1a to reflect a higher value for V_L and Equation 9.1b to reflect a lower cost of equity if the firm receives interest pass-throughs. Rather than worry about the exact form of the modified equations, just recognize that firms that receive capital pass-through payments gain greater benefits from the use of financial leverage than firms that do not.
8. See M. H. Miller, "Debt and Taxes," *Journal of Finance* (May 1977): 261–75. The paper was first presented as the Presidential Address at the 1976 meeting of the American Finance Association.
9. For some examples, see R. A. Haugen and J. L. Pappas, "Equilibrium in the Pricing of Capital Assets, Risk-Bearing Debt Instruments, and the Question of Optimal Capital Structure," *Journal of Financial and Quantitative Analysis* (June 1971): 943–54; J. Stiglitz, "A Re-Examination of the Modigliani-Miller Theorem," *American Economic Review* (December 1969): 784–93; and M. E. Rubenstein, "A Mean-Variance Synthesis of Corporate Financial Theory," *Journal of Finance* (March 1973): 167–81.

10. Health care providers with large capital pass-through payments should also carry higher levels of debt, because the benefits associated with debt financing are enhanced by such payments.

11. For examples of the empirical research in this area, see R. Taggart, "A Model of Corporate Financing Decisions," *Journal of Finance* (December 1977): 1467–84; and P. Marsh, "The Choice between Equity and Debt: An Empirical Study," *Journal of Finance* (March 1982): 121–44.

12. See G. Donaldson, *Corporate Debt Capacity: A Study of Corporate Debt Policy and the Determination of Corporate Debt Capacity* (Boston: Harvard Graduate School of Business Administration, 1961).

13. See S. C. Myers, "The Capital Structure Puzzle," *Journal of Finance* (July 1984): 575–92. It is interesting to note that, like the Miller model, Myers' paper was presented as a Presidential Address to the American Finance Association.

14. Many studies support the contention that the announcement of a new stock issue results in a decrease in stock price. For example, one study found that stock prices decline about 3 percent following the announcement of a new stock issue. See P. Asquith and D. W. Mullins, Jr., "Equity Issues and Offering Dilution," *Journal of Financial Economics* (June 1986): 61–89.

15. The same logic applies to pass-through payments for interest expense. Health care providers that have higher effective pass-through rates should use more debt financing, all else the same, than those with lower pass-through rates.

Selected Additional References

Boles, K. E. 1986. "What Accounting Leaves Out of Hospital Financial Management." *Hospital and Health Services Administration* (March/April): 8–27.

Gapenski, L. C. 1993. "Hospital Capital Structure Decisions: Theory and Practice." *Health Services Management Research* (November): 237–47.

Harris, J. P., and V. E. Schimmel. 1987. "Market Value: An Underused Financial Planning Tool." *Healthcare Financial Management* (April): 40–46.

McCue, M. J., and Y. A. Ozcan. 1992. "Determinants of Capital Structure." *Hospital and Health Services Administration* (Fall): 333–46.

Valvona, J., and F. A. Sloan. 1988. "Hospital Profitability and Capital Structure: A Comparative Analysis." *Health Services Research* (August): 343–57.

Wedig, G. J., F. A. Sloan, M. Hassan, and M. A. Morrisey. 1988. "Capital Structure, Ownership, and Capital Payment Policy: The Case of Hospitals." *Journal of Finance* (March): 21–40.

Case 9

HealthPower Unlimited: Capital Structure Decisions

HealthPower Unlimited franchises "rent-a-nurse" businesses to independent operators throughout the United States. The concept of the business is the same as that for other temporary help services such as Manpower and Kelly Temporary Services, except that HealthPower Unlimited deals only with registered nurses. The rationale for the concept is as follows:

1. Many health care providers, especially hospitals, have difficulty hiring and retaining nurses, so there is almost always a demand for nursing professionals. Perhaps more importantly, providers are becoming very reluctant to build a large base of fixed costs, so any staffing requirements that are not certain to be permanent in nature are often filled by temporary workers. Finally, when vacancies occur among permanent workers, providers often need temporary nurses to carry the load until the vacancies are filled.

2. Although nursing salaries have increased substantially over the past ten years, a large number of nurses have quit the profession for a variety of reasons, including family responsibilities. Many of these nurses are willing to work occasionally, but not on a permanent basis.

3. Typically, the nurses who want to work on a selective basis are married and their health insurance is provided by their spouses. Also, these nurses do not require extensive fringe benefits such as pension plans or paid vacations, and since they are part-time workers, they are not eligible for unemployment insurance or workers' compensation. Thus, if the average fringe benefit

package paid for permanent nurses is 25 percent of salary, a temporary services company can, for example, offer a salary to its nurses 5 percent higher than can providers; "rent" the nurses out at 5 percent less than it costs providers to hire permanent nurses, including all fringe benefits; and pocket what remains of the 15 percent spread after administrative costs are paid.

Basically, the franchisee buys the exclusive right to use the Health-Power Unlimited name within a given territory, and also receives marketing and management support from HealthPower Unlimited, the franchisor. Additionally, franchisees can lease personal computers and other office equipment from HealthPower Unlimited under relatively favorable terms, since the firm purchases them in large quantities, and expendable office supplies can be purchased directly from HealthPower Unlimited at a substantial savings from retail prices.

To start operations, a franchisee recruits a pool of nurses from the local labor market. Then, when a client needs a temporary nurse, the local manager matches the client's specific needs with a qualified nurse from the pool. The bill for services is sent to the client by the franchisee based on the number of hours that the nurse works for the client (as verified by the client on a timecard). The client has no responsibility for the nurse's salary or fringe benefits—this is all handled by the HealthPower Unlimited franchisee.

HealthPower Unlimited was founded in 1980 by Dana Clark, a registered nurse from Houston who left the profession to get her MBA degree from the University of Texas. The company grew rapidly from its base in Houston, first by expanding operations into different cities across Texas, and then by franchising into other parts of the country. Dana was a devout believer in the virtues of equity financing. Although the company had issued debt periodically, especially to finance company-owned business expansion, Dana always used HealthPower Unlimited's cash flows to retire the debt as soon as possible. Recent growth has involved franchising, where the franchisee puts up the required capital, and hence there has been no need for outside capital for several years.

Dana believes that her firm's high-growth days are over. First, numerous companies that offer competing services have appeared on the scene. Second, the number of hospitals, which are her primary clients, has actually declined over the years since she founded the firm and, based on bed usage in major managed care markets in California, it appears that the hospital industry will continue to shrink. Finally, the nursing shortage of the 1980s has eased, and many formerly good customers are now able to meet almost all of their nursing needs by direct recruitment. Thus, Dana expects the firm's 1995 earnings before interest and taxes (EBIT) of $3,000,000 to grow very slowly, if at all, well into the future.

HealthPower Unlimited has 10 million shares of common stock outstanding, and they are traded in the over-the-counter market. The current share price is $1.20, so the total market value of the firm's equity is $12 million. The book value of equity is also $12 million, so the stock now sells at its book value. HealthPower Unlimited's federal-plus-state tax rate is 40 percent. Dana owns 20 percent of the outstanding stock, and others in the management group own an additional 10 percent.

Dana's financial manager, Bruce Vogel, has been preaching for years that HealthPower Unlimited should use debt in its capital structure. "After all," says Bruce, "everybody else uses debt, and some of our competitors use over 50 percent debt financing. Also, an underleveraged company is exposed to a hostile takeover, because raiders can use the firm's excess debt capacity to finance the bid." If HealthPower Unlimited were to recapitalize, the borrowed funds would be used to repurchase stock in the open market, since the funds are not needed for growth. Dana's reaction to Bruce's prodding is cautious, but she is willing to give Bruce the chance to prove his point.

Bruce has worked with Dana for the past six years, and he knows that the only way he can convince her that the firm should use debt financing is to conduct a comprehensive analysis. To begin, Bruce arranged for a joint meeting with an investment banker who specializes in corporate financing for service companies. After several hours, the pair agreed on the estimates for the relationships between the use of debt financing and HealthPower Unlimited's capital costs contained in Table 1. Table 1 also shows what HealthPower's debt rating might be at each debt level on the basis of rough guidance given by Standard & Poor's. Table 2 contains some industry average data for companies that franchise health care services.

Although HealthPower Unlimited's EBIT is expected to be $3 million in any future year, there is a great deal of uncertainty in the estimate, as indicated by the following probability distribution:

Probability	EBIT
0.25	$2,000,000
0.50	3,000,000
0.25	4,000,000

Table 1   Relationships Between the Level of Debt Financing and Capital Costs

Amount Borrowed	Cost of Debt	Cost of Equity	Debt Rating
$ 0	—	15.0%	—
2,500,000	10.0%	15.5	AAA
5,000,000	11.0	16.5	AA
7,500,000	13.0	18.0	A
10,000,000	16.0	20.0	BBB
12,500,000	20.0	25.0	BB

Table 2   Industry Average Data

Percentile	Book Value Debt Ratio
10th	32%
25th	46
Median	58
75th	71
90th	82

Notes:

1. The debt ratio is defined as Total debt/Total assets.
2. The average stock in the health care service franchising industry has a market-to-book ratio of 1.25.

On the basis of previous conversations, Bruce knows that Dana has two major concerns regarding the use of debt financing. First, she is concerned about the impact of debt financing on the firm's reported profitability; that is, the impact of debt financing on net income and return on equity (ROE) as reported in the firm's financial statements. Furthermore, any risk implications to stockholders must be identified. To help in this regard, Bruce plans to construct partial income statements (beginning with earnings before interest and taxes) for four levels of debt as measured by the book Total debt/Total assets ratio: zero, 25 percent, 50 percent, and 75 percent.

In addition to accounting effects, Dana is obviously concerned about the potential impact of debt financing on the firm's shareholders, specifically, what impact debt financing will have on stock price. To help address this issue, Bruce is aware of a technique that can be used to value zero-growth firms at different debt levels. In essence, the following equations are used:

$$S = [EBIT - k_d(D)](1 - T)/k_s. \tag{1}$$

$$V = S + D. \tag{2}$$

$$P = (V - D_0)/n_0. \tag{3}$$

$$n_1 = n_0 - D/P. \tag{4}$$

Here

S = market value of equity.

$EBIT$ = earnings before interest and taxes.

k_d = cost of debt.

D = market (and book) value of new debt.

D_0 = market value of old debt.

T = tax rate.

k_s = cost of equity.

V = total market value.

P = stock price after recapitalization.

n_0 = number of shares before recapitalization.

n_1 = number of shares after recapitalization.

Bruce is also concerned about potential changes in the health care industry, and how they might affect the basic business risk of HealthPower Unlimited. Table 3 contains leverage/cost estimates at alternative business risk levels.

Bruce knows that Dana is familiar with capital structure theory and will want to know the value of the firm according to the Modigliani-Miller model with corporate taxes and the Miller model. Since most of the other board members are not very familiar with capital structure decisions, it will be necessary to conduct a tutorial on the issues involved, including the difference between business and financial risk, the relationship between capital structure and EPS, and a host of additional qualitative factors that influence the decision.

Finally, George Watson, a member of the board, is particularly concerned about what would happen if the firm identified an optimal capital structure, but then moved to it in stages rather than in a single recapitalization. For example, suppose that the optimal capital structure was judged to be $5 million of debt. Is there any difference in the ending situation between (1) issuing $5 million of debt at once or (2) first issuing $2.5 million and then, some time later, issuing another $2.5 million?

Table 3   Level of Debt and Cost Estimates at Different Business
Risk Levels

Amount Borrowed	*Cost of Debt*	*Cost of Equity*
Significant Increase in Business Risk		
$ 0	—	16.0%
2,500,000	11.0%	17.0
5,000,000	13.0	19.0
7,500,000	16.0	22.0
10,000,000	20.0	26.0
12,500,000	25.0	31.0
Significant Decrease in Business Risk		
$ 0	—	14.0%
2,500,000	9.0%	14.3
5,000,000	9.5	15.0
7,500,000	10.5	16.0
10,000,000	12.5	17.5
12,500,000	15.5	20.0

Part V

Capital Allocation

10

The Basics of Capital Budgeting

In Chapters 8 and 9, we described how firms estimate their costs of capital and make capital structure decisions. Now we turn our attention to fixed asset acquisition decisions. Although some investment decisions, such as the decision to expand the operating hours of a walk-in clinic, involve only the expenditure of operating funds, most investment decisions entail the acquisition of new facilities or equipment. Thus, decisions of this type are often called *capital investment*, or *capital budgeting, decisions*. Capital budgeting decisions are of fundamental importance to the success or failure of any firm, for a firm's capital budgeting decisions, more than anything else, shape its future.

Our discussion of capital budgeting is divided into two chapters. First, in Chapter 10, we provide an overview of the capital budgeting process, discuss the key elements of cash flow estimation, and finally explain the basic techniques used to assess a project's profitability. Then in Chapter 11, we consider the very important topic of capital budgeting risk analysis.

Importance of Capital Budgeting

A number of factors combine to make capital budgeting decisions the most important ones that managers must make. First and most importantly, since the results of capital budgeting decisions generally affect the firm for an extended period, the impact of the decision is often not known for years. For example, the decision of a long-term care facility to add a new wing affects the costs and capacity of the facility for a prolonged period. If a firm invests too heavily in fixed assets, it will have too much capacity and its costs will necessarily be too high. On the other hand, a firm that invests too little in fixed assets may face two problems.

First, the firm's assets may not be technologically current. A hospital in this situation will lose patients to its more up-to-date competitors and, further, its patients may not be getting the benefit of the best health care diagnostics and treatments available. Second, if a firm has inadequate capacity, it may lose a portion of its market share to competitors. A hospital in this situation would have to incur heavy costs to regain its lost market share; these would include increased marketing expenses and aggressive price reductions to managed care organizations.

Another important aspect of capital budgeting is timing—capital assets must be placed "on line" at the time they are needed. A long-term care facility that plans a new wing only after patient demand clearly shows the need for one might find that the demand was met by competitors that expanded during the two years it took the slower facility to design, finance, and complete the project. Good capital budgeting requires that demand be forecasted, and that assets come on line to meet new demand as it arises.

Effective capital budgeting procedures improve both the timing of asset acquisitions and the cost and quality of the assets purchased. A firm that forecasts its needs for capital assets well in advance will have the opportunity to plan the purchases carefully, and thus will be able to negotiate the best assets at the best prices.

Finally, capital budgeting is important because asset expansion typically involves substantial expenditures, and because large amounts of funds are not usually at hand and must be raised externally. A firm with major capital expenditures should arrange its financing in advance to be sure of having the funds available at the time they are needed.

Self-Test Question:

Why are capital budgeting decisions so crucial to the success of a business?

Project Classifications

Analyzing capital expenditure proposals is not a costless operation: benefits can be gained from a careful analysis, but such efforts can be costly. For certain types of projects, a relatively detailed analysis may be warranted; for others, cost/benefit studies suggest that simpler procedures should be used. Accordingly, firms generally classify projects into categories, such as the following, and then analyze those in each category differently.

Category 1: Mandatory replacement. Category 1 consists of expenditures needed to replace worn-out or damaged equipment necessary to the operations of the business. In general, these expenditures are mandatory, so they are usually made without going through an elaborate decision process.

Category 2: Discretionary replacement. This category includes expenditures to replace serviceable but obsolete equipment. The purpose of these projects is to lower costs or provide more effective services. Since Category 2 projects are not mandatory, a more detailed analysis is generally required to support the expenditure than that needed for Category 1 projects.

Category 3: Expansion of existing products, services, or markets. Expenditures to increase capacity, or to expand within markets currently being served, are included here. These decisions are more complex, so still more detailed analysis is required, and the final decision is made at a higher level within the organization.

Category 4: Expansion into new products, services, or markets. These are projects necessary to provide new products or services, or to expand into geographical areas not currently being served. Such projects involve strategic decisions that could change the fundamental nature of the business, and they normally require the expenditure of large sums of money over long periods. Invariably, a particularly detailed analysis is required, and final decisions are generally made by the board of directors as part of the strategic plan.

Category 5: Safety/Environmental projects. This category consists of expenditures necessary to comply with government orders, labor agreements, accreditation requirements, and so on. Unless the expenditures are large, Category 5 expenditures are treated like Category 1 expenditures.

Category 6: Other. This category is a catch-all for projects that do not fit neatly into one of the other categories. The primary determinant in evaluating Category 6 projects is their size.

Self-Test Question:

Briefly explain how capital project classifications are used in the capital budgeting process.

The Role of Financial Analysis in
Health Care Investment Decisions

For investor-owned firms, with shareholder wealth maximization as the primary goal, the role of financial analysis in investment decisions is clear. Those projects that are profitable contribute to shareholder wealth, so it is important to identify such projects. However, as we pointed out in Chapter 2, most hospitals, and many other health care providers, are not-for-profit firms that do not have shareholders. In such firms, the appropriate goal is providing quality, cost-effective service to the communities served. (One could make a strong argument that this should also be the goal of investor-owned firms in the health care industry, especially providers.) In this situation, capital budgeting decisions must consider many factors besides a project's financial implications. For example, noneconomic factors such as the needs of the medical staff and the good of the community must also be taken into account and, in some instances, these factors will outweigh financial considerations.

Nevertheless, good decision making, and hence the future viability of the organization, requires that the financial impact of capital investments be fully recognized. If a firm takes on several highly unprofitable projects that meet nonfinancial goals but are not offset by profitable projects, the firm's financial condition will deteriorate. If this situation persists over time, the firm will eventually lose its financial viability and may even be forced into bankruptcy and closure. Since bankrupt firms obviously cannot meet a community's needs, a project's potential impact on the firm's financial condition must be considered, even by managers of not-for-profit firms. Managers may make a conscious decision to accept a project with a poor financial prognosis because of its nonfinancial virtues, but it is important that managers know the financial impact up front, rather than being surprised when the project drains the firm's financial resources. Financial analysis provides managers with the relevant information about a project's financial impact, and hence helps managers make better decisions, including those decisions based primarily on medical staff or community needs.

Self-Test Question:

What is the role of financial analysis in capital budgeting decision making within health care firms?

Overview of Capital Budgeting Financial Analysis

The financial analysis of capital investment proposals typically involves these five steps:

1. The capital outlay, or cost, of the project must be estimated.

2. Then, the operating and terminal cash flows of the project must be forecasted. Steps 1 and 2 constitute the cash flow estimation phase, which is discussed in the next section.

3. Next, the riskiness of the estimated cash flows must be assessed. Risk assessment will be discussed in Chapter 11.

4. Then, given the riskiness of the project, the project's cost of capital is estimated. As we discussed in Chapter 8, the firm's overall cost of capital reflects the aggregate risk and debt capacity of the firm's assets, that is, the riskiness and optimal capital structure inherent in the firm's "average project." If the project being evaluated does not have average risk and debt capacity, the firm's cost of capital must be adjusted to reflect these differentials.

5. Finally, the profitability of the project is assessed. Several measures can be used for this purpose; we will discuss three commonly used measures in this chapter.

Self-Test Question:

List the five steps in capital budgeting financial analysis.

Cash Flow Estimation

The most important, but also the most difficult, step in evaluating capital investment proposals is cash flow estimation: the investment outlays, the annual net operating flows expected when the project goes into operation, and the cash flows associated with project termination. Many variables are involved in cash flow forecasting, and many individuals and departments participate in the process. It is difficult to make accurate projections of the costs and revenues associated with a large, complex project, so forecast errors can be quite large. Thus, it is essential that risk analyses be performed on prospective projects. One manager with a good sense of humor developed the following five principles of capital budgeting cash flow estimation:

1. It is very difficult to forecast cash flows, especially those that occur in the future.
2. Those who live by the crystal ball soon learn how to eat ground glass.
3. The moment you forecast cash flows, you know you are wrong— you just don't know by how much and in what direction.
4. If you are right, never let your bosses forget.
5. An expert is someone who has been right at least once.

It is difficult to overstate either the difficulty or the importance of cash flow forecasts. However, if the principles discussed in the next sections are observed, errors that often arise in the process can be minimized.

Identifying the relevant cash flows

The relevant cash flows to consider when evaluating a new capital investment are the project's *incremental cash flows*, which are defined as the difference in the firm's cash flows in each period if the project is undertaken versus the firm's cash flows if the project is not undertaken:

$$\text{Incremental } CF_t = CF_{t(Firm with project)}$$
$$- CF_{t(Firm without project)}.$$

Here the subscript t specifies a time period, normally years, so CF_0 is the cash flow during Year 0, which is generally assumed to end today, CF_1 is the cash flow during the first year, CF_2 is the cash flow during Year 2, and so on. In practice, the early cash flows, and Year 0 in particular, are usually cash outflows, the costs associated with getting the project "up and running." Then, as the project begins to generate revenues, the cash flows normally turn positive.

Cash flow versus accounting income

Accounting income statements are in some respects a mix of apples and oranges. For example, accountants deduct labor costs, which are cash outflows, from revenues, which may not be entirely cash. (For health care providers, most of the collections are from third party payers, and payment may not be received until several months after the service is provided.) At the same time, the income statement does not recognize capital outlays, which are cash flows, but it does deduct depreciation expense, which is not a cash flow. In capital investment decisions, it is critical that the decision be based on the actual dollars that flow into and out of the firm, because a firm's true profitability, and hence its ability to provide health care services, depends on its cash flows, and not on income as reported in accordance with generally accepted accounting principles. Note, however, that accounting items can influence cash flows, because items like depreciation can affect tax or reimbursement cash flows.

Cash flow timing

Financial analysts must be careful to account properly for the timing of cash flows. Accounting income statements are for periods such as years or quarters, so they do not reflect exactly when, during the period, revenues and expenses occur. In theory, capital budgeting cash flows should be analyzed exactly as they occur. Of course, there must be a compromise between accuracy and simplicity. A time line with daily cash flows would in theory provide the most accuracy, but daily cash flow estimates would be costly to construct, unwieldy to use, and probably no more accurate than annual cash flow estimates. Thus, in most cases, analysts simply assume that all cash flows occur at the end of every year. However, for some projects, it may be useful to assume that cash flows occur every six months, or even to forecast quarterly or monthly cash flows.

Project life

One of the first decisions that must be made in forecasting a project's cash flows is the life of the project—do we need to forecast cash flows for 20 years, or is 5 years sufficient? Many projects, such as a new hospital wing or an ambulatory care clinic, potentially have very long lives, perhaps 50 years or more. In theory, a cash flow forecast should extend for the full life of a project; yet most managers would have very little confidence in any cash flow forecasts beyond the near term. Thus, most organizations set an arbitrary limit on the project life assumed in capital budgeting analyses, often five or ten years. If the forecasted life is less than the arbitrary limit, the forecasted life is used to develop the cash flows, but if the forecasted life exceeds the limit, project life is truncated and the operating cash flows beyond the limit are ignored in the analysis.

Although cash flow truncation is a practical solution to a difficult problem, it does create another problem: the value inherent in the cash flows beyond the truncation point is lost to the project. This problem can be addressed either objectively or subjectively. The standard procedure at some organizations is to estimate the project's *terminal value,* which is the estimated value of the cash flows beyond the truncation point. Often, the terminal value is estimated as the liquidation value of the project at that point in time. If the terminal value is too difficult to estimate, the fact that some portion of the project's cash flow value is being ignored should, at a minimum, be subjectively recognized by decision makers. The saving grace in all of this is that cash flows well into the future typically contribute a relatively small amount to a project's profitability. For example, a $100,000 terminal value projected ten years in the future contributes only about $38,500 to the project's value when the cost of capital is 10 percent.

Sunk costs

A *sunk cost* refers to an outlay that has already occurred (or has been irrevocably committed), so it is an outlay that is unaffected by the current decision to accept or reject the project. To illustrate, suppose that in 1996 Bayside Memorial Hospital is evaluating the purchase of a lithotripter system. To help in the decision, the hospital hired and paid $10,000 to a consultant in 1995 to conduct a marketing study. Is this 1995 cash flow relevant to the 1996 capital investment decision? The answer is no. The $10,000 is a sunk cost; Bayside cannot recover it whether or not the lithotripter is purchased. Sometimes a project appears to be unprofitable when all of the associated costs, including sunk costs, are considered. However, on an *incremental* basis, the project may be profitable and should be undertaken. Thus, the correct treatment of sunk costs may be critical to the decision.

Assume for a moment that Bayside goes ahead with the lithotripter project. Then, in 1998, when conducting a periodic analysis of the *historical* profitability of the project, the $10,000 cost of the consultant's report would be included, because it was part of the total cash flows attributable to the project. However, when making the 1996 decision regarding project acceptance, the $10,000 is *nonincremental,* and hence not relevant to the decision.

Opportunity costs

All relevant *opportunity costs* must be included in a capital investment analysis. To illustrate, one opportunity cost involves the use of the capital.

If the firm uses its capital to invest in Project A, it cannot use the capital to invest in Project B, and so on. The opportunity cost associated with capital use is accounted for in the project's cost of capital, which is used to discount the project's expected cash flows and represents the return that the firm could earn by investing in alternative investments of similar risk.

There are many types of opportunity costs. For another example, assume that Bayside's lithotripter would be installed in a freestanding facility, and that the hospital currently owns the land on which the facility would be constructed. In fact, the hospital purchased the land ten years ago at a cost of $50,000, but the current market value of the property is $130,000, net of legal and real estate fees. When evaluating the lithotripter, should the value of the land be disregarded because no cash outlay is necessary? The answer is no, because there is an opportunity cost inherent in the use of the property. Using the property for the lithotripter facility deprives Bayside of its use for anything else. The property might be used for a walk-in clinic or ambulatory surgery center or parking garage rather than sold, but the best measure of its value to Bayside, and hence the opportunity cost inherent in its use, is the cash flow that could be realized from selling the property. By considering the property's current market value, Bayside is letting market forces assign the value for the land's best alternative use. Thus, the lithotripter project should have a $130,000 opportunity cost charged against it. Note that the opportunity cost is the property's $130,000 net market value, irrespective of whether the property was acquired for $50,000 or $200,000.

Effect on the firm's other projects

Capital budgeting analyses must consider the effect of the project under consideration on the firm's other projects. When the effect is negative, it is often called *cannibalization*. To illustrate, assume that some of the patients that are expected to use Bayside's new lithotripter would have been treated surgically at Bayside, so these surgical revenues will be lost if the lithotripter facility goes into operation. Thus, the incremental revenues to Bayside are the revenues attributable to the lithotripter, less the revenues lost from forgone surgery services.

On the other hand, new patients who use the lithotripter may utilize other services provided by the hospital. In this situation, the incremental cash flows generated by the lithotripter patients' utilization of other services should be credited to the lithotripter project. If possible, both positive and negative effects on other projects should be quantified, but at a minimum they should be noted so that the final decision maker will be aware of their existence.

Shipping and installation costs

When a firm acquires fixed assets, it often incurs substantial costs for shipping and installing the equipment. These charges are added to the invoice price of the equipment to determine the overall cost of the project. Also, the full cost of the equipment, including shipping and installation charges, is used as the basis for calculating depreciation charges. Thus, if Bayside Memorial Hospital purchases intensive care monitoring equipment that costs $200,000, but another $20,000 is required for shipping and installation, then the full cost of the equipment would be $220,000, and this amount would be the starting point for all depreciation calculations.

Changes in net working capital

Normally, expansion projects require additional inventories, and expanded sales also lead to additional accounts receivable. The increase in these current assets must be financed, just as an increase in fixed assets must be financed. However, accounts payable and accruals will probably also increase as a result of the expansion, and these current liability funds will reduce the net cash needed to finance the increase in inventories and receivables. The difference between the increase in current assets and the increase in current liabilities that result from a new project is called a change in *net working capital*. If this change is positive, that is, if the increase in current assets exceeds the increase in current liabilities, then this amount is as much a cash cost to the project as is the cost of the asset itself. Such projects must be charged an additional amount above the cost of the new asset to reflect the net financing needed for the current asset accounts. Similarly, if the change in net working capital is negative, the project is generating a positive working capital cash flow, because the increase in liabilities exceeds the project's current asset requirements and this cash flow partially offsets the cost of the asset being acquired.

As the project approaches termination, inventories will be sold off and not replaced, and receivables will be converted to cash without new receivables being created. In effect, the firm will recover its investment in net working capital when the project is terminated. This will result in a cash flow that is equal but opposite in sign to the change in net working capital cash flow that arises at the beginning of a project.

For health care providers, where inventories often represent a very small part of the investment in new projects, the change in net working capital can often be ignored without materially affecting the results of the analysis. However, when a project results in a large change in net working capital, failure to consider the net investment in current assets will result in an overstatement of the project's profitability.

Inflation effects

Because inflation is a fact of life, and because inflation effects can have a considerable influence on a project's profitability, it must be considered in any sound capital budgeting analysis. As we discussed in Chapter 8, a firm's cost of capital is a weighted average of its costs of debt and equity. These costs are estimated on the basis of investors' required rates of return, and investors incorporate an inflation premium into their required returns. For example, a debt investor might require a 5 percent return on a ten-year bond in the absence of inflation. However, if inflation is expected to average 6 percent over the coming ten years, then the investor would require an 11 percent return. Thus, investors add an inflation premium to their required rates of return to help protect them against the loss of purchasing power that stems from inflation.

Since inflation effects are already imbedded in the firm's cost of capital, and since the cost of capital will be used to discount the cash flows in our profitability measures, it is necessary to ensure that inflation effects are also built into the project's estimated cash flows. If cash flow estimates do not include inflation effects (*real* cash flows), and then a discount rate is used that does include inflation effects (*nominal* discount rate), then the profitability of the project will be understated.

The most effective way to deal with inflation is to build inflation effects into each cash flow element using the best available information about how each element will be affected. Since it is impossible to estimate future inflation rates with much precision, errors are bound to be made. Often, inflation is assumed to be neutral; that is, it is assumed to affect revenues and costs (except depreciation) equally. However, situations can arise where costs may be rising faster than charges, or vice versa. When such situations are expected to occur, then different inflation rates should be applied to each cash flow element. For example, charges net of bad debt losses and discounts may be expected to increase at a 4 percent rate, while labor costs are expected to increase at an 8 percent rate. Inflation adds to the uncertainty, or riskiness, of capital budgeting, as well as to its complexity. Fortunately, computers and spreadsheet programs are available to help with inflation analysis, so the mechanics of inflation adjustments are not difficult.

Cash flow estimation bias

As stated previously, cash flow estimation is the most critical, and the most difficult, part of the capital budgeting process. Cash flow components such as volume and charges often must be forecasted many years into the future, and estimation errors are bound to occur, some of which can be quite large.[1] However, large firms evaluate and accept many projects every year, and as long as cash flow estimates are unbiased and the errors are random, the estimation errors will tend to offset one another. That is, some cash flow estim. will be too high and some will be too low, but in the aggregate for all projects, the realized cash flows will be very close to the estimates; hence, realized profitability will be close to that expected.

Unfortunately, there are strong indications that capital budgeting cash flow forecasts are not unbiased; rather, managers tend to be overly optimistic in their forecasts and, as a result, revenues tend to be overstated and costs tend to be understated.[2] The result is an upward bias in estimated profitability. This bias may result because managers are often rewarded on the basis of the size of their divisions or departments, so they have an incentive to maximize the number of projects accepted rather than the profitability of the projects. Or managers may be emotionally attached to their projects and become unable to assess a project's potential objectively.

Top management can use two procedures to identify cash flow estimation bias. First, if a project is judged to be highly profitable, this question should be asked: "What is the underlying cause of this project's high profitability?" If the firm has some underlying advantage, such as a monopoly position in a managed care market, or a superior reputation in providing a specific service such as organ transplants, then there may be a logical rationale supporting the high profitability. If no such unique factor can be identified, then senior management should be concerned about the possibility of estimation bias. Even when these unique factors exist, it is likely that the project's profitability, at some point in the future, will be eroded by competitive pressure from firms seeking to capture some of this high profitability.

Second, the post-audit process, which we discuss later in this chapter, will help to identify divisions and departments that habitually overstate or understate project profitability. (It is difficult to identify projects whose cash flows are understated, because many of those projects will be rejected and hence no cash flow comparisons can be made. Perhaps the best indicator of underestimation bias is when competing firms undertake projects of the type that are being rejected.) Many firms are now identifying managers and divisions that typically submit biased cash flow estimates, and are compensating for this bias in the decision process by reducing cash inflows that are thought to be too rosy, or by increasing the cost of capital to such projects.

Strategic value

In the previous section, we discussed the problem of cash flow estimation bias, which can result in overstating a project's profitability. Another problem that can occur in cash flow estimation is underestimating a project's true profitability by not recognizing its *strategic value*, which is the value of future investment opportunities that can be undertaken only if the project currently under consideration is accepted.

To illustrate this concept, consider a hospital management company that is analyzing a management contract for a hospital in Hungary, its first move into Eastern Europe. On a stand-alone basis this project might be unprofitable, but the project might provide entry into the Eastern European market, which would unlock the door to a whole range of highly profitable new projects. Or consider Bayside Memorial Hospital's decision to start a kidney transplant program. The financial analysis of this project showed the program to be unprofitable, but Bayside's managers considered kidney transplants to be the first step in an aggressive transplant program that would not only be profitable in itself, but would enhance the hospital's reputation for technological and clinical excellence, and thus would contribute to the hospital's overall profitability.

In theory, the best approach to dealing with strategic value is to forecast the cash flows from the follow-on projects, estimate their probabilities of occurrence, and then add the expected cash flows from the follow-on projects to the cash flows of the project under consideration. In practice, this is usually impossible to do—either the follow-on cash flows are too nebulous to forecast or the potential follow-on projects are too numerous to quantify.[3] At a minimum, decision makers must recognize that some projects have strategic value, and this value should be qualitatively considered when making capital budgeting decisions.

Self-Test Question:

Briefly discuss the following concepts associated with cash flow estimation:

1. Incremental cash flow
2. Cash flow versus accounting income
3. Cash flow timing
4. Project life
5. Sunk costs
6. Opportunity costs
7. Effects on other projects
8. Shipping and installation costs
9. Changes in net working capital
10. Inflation effects
11. Cash flow estimation bias
12. Strategic value.

Cash Flow Estimation Example

Up to this point, we have discussed several critical aspects of cash flow estimation. In this section, we present an example that illustrates some of the concepts already covered and introduces several others that are important to good cash flow estimation.

The basic data

Consider the situation faced by Bayside Memorial Hospital, a not-for-profit hospital, in its evaluation of a new magnetic resonance imaging (MRI) system. The system costs $1,500,000, and the hospital would have to spend another $1,000,000 for site preparation and installation. Since the system would be installed in the hospital, the space to be used has a very low, or zero, market value to outsiders, and thus no opportunity cost has been assigned to account for the value of the space.

The MRI site is estimated to generate weekly usage (volume) of 40 scans, and each scan would, on average, cost the hospital $15 in supplies. The site is expected to operate 50 weeks a year, with the remaining 2 weeks devoted to maintenance. The estimated average charge per scan is $500, but 25 percent of this amount, on average, is expected to be lost to

Table 10.1   Bayside Memorial Hospital: MRI Site Revenue
Analysis

Payer	Number of Scans per Week	Charge per Scan	Total Charges	Basis of Payment	Net Payment per Scan	Total Payments
Medicare	10	$500	$ 5,000	Fixed fee	$370	$ 3,700
Medicaid	5	500	2,500	Fixed fee	350	1,750
Private insurance	9	500	4,500	Full charge	500	4,500
Blue Cross	5	500	2,500	Percent of charge	420	2,100
Managed care	7	500	3,500	Percent of charge	390	2,730
Self-pay	4	500	2,000	Full charge	55	220
Total	40		$20,000			$15,000
Average			$ 500			$ 375

indigent patients, contractual allowances, and bad debt losses. Bayside's managers developed the project's forecasted revenues by conducting the revenue analysis contained in Table 10.1.

The MRI site would require two technicians, resulting in an incremental increase in annual labor costs of $50,000, including fringe benefits. Cash overhead costs would increase by $10,000 annually if the MRI site is activated. The equipment would require maintenance, which would be furnished by the manufacturer for an annual fee of $150,000, payable at the end of each year of operation. For book purposes, the MRI site will be depreciated by the straight line method over a five-year life.

The MRI site is expected to be in operation for five years, at which time the hospital's master plan calls for a brand-new imaging facility. The hospital plans to sell the MRI system at that time for an estimated $750,000 salvage value, net of removal costs. The inflation rate is estimated to average 5 percent over the period, and this rate is expected to affect all revenues and costs except depreciation. Bayside's managers initially assume that projects under evaluation have average risk, and thus the hospital's current 10 percent cost of capital is the appropriate project cost of capital. Later, in Chapter 11, a risk assessment of the project may indicate that a different cost of capital is appropriate.

Although the MRI project is expected to take away some patients from the hospital's other imaging systems, the new MRI patients are

expected to generate revenues for some of the hospital's other departments. On net, the two effects are expected to balance out; that is, the
cash flow loss from other imaging systems is expected to be offset by the
cash flow gain from other services utilized by the new MRI patients.

Cash flow analysis

The first step in the financial analysis is to estimate the MRI site's net
cash flows. This analysis is presented in Table 10.2.[4] Here are the key
points of the analysis by line number:

Line 1. Line 1 contains the estimated cost of the MRI system. In general,
capital budgeting analyses assume that the first cash flow, normally an
outflow, occurs today, or at the end of Year 0. Note that expenses, or cash
outflows, are shown in parentheses.

Line 2. The related construction expense, $1,000,000, is also assumed
to occur at Year 0.

Line 3. Gross revenues = (Weekly throughout) (Weeks of operation)
(Charge per scan) = (40) (50) ($500) = $1,000,000 in the first year. The
5 percent inflation rate is applied to all charges and costs that would
likely be affected by inflation, so the gross revenue amount shown on
Line 3 increases by 5 percent over time. Although most of the operating
revenues and costs would occur more or less evenly over the year, it is
very difficult to forecast exactly when most of the flows would occur.
Furthermore, there is significant potential for large errors in cash flow
estimation. For these reasons, operating cash flows are often assumed to
occur at the end of each year. Also, we assume that the MRI system could
be placed in operation quickly. If this were not the case, then the first
year's operating flows would be reduced. In some situations, it might
take several years from the first investment cash flow to the point when
the project is operational and begins to generate operating cash inflows.

Line 4. Deductions from charges are estimated to average 25 percent
of gross revenues, so in Year 1, 0.25($1,000,000) = $250,000 of gross
revenues would be uncollected. This amount increases each year by the
5 percent inflation rate.

Line 5. Line 5 contains the net operating revenues in each year, Line 3
− Line 4.

Table 10.2   Bayside Memorial Hospital: MRI Site Cash Flow Analysis

				Cash Revenues and Costs			
		0	*1*	*2*	*3*	*4*	*5*
1. System cost		($1,500,000)					
2. Related expenses		(1,000,000)					
3. Gross revenues			$1,000,000	$1,050,000	$1,102,500	$1,157,625	$1,215,506
4. Less: Deductions			250,000	262,500	275,625	289,406	303,877
5. Net revenues			$ 750,000	$ 787,500	$ 826,875	$ 868,219	$ 911,630
6. Less: Labor costs			50,000	52,500	55,125	57,881	60,775
7. Maintenance costs			150,000	157,500	165,375	173,644	182,326
8. Supplies			30,000	31,500	33,075	34,729	36,465
9. Incremental overhead			10,000	10,500	11,025	11,576	12,155
10. Depreciation			350,000	350,000	350,000	350,000	350,000
11. Operating income			$ 160,000	$ 185,500	$ 212,275	$ 240,389	$ 269,908
12. Taxes			0	0	0	0	0
13. Net operating income			$ 160,000	$ 185,500	$ 212,275	$ 240,389	$ 269,908
14. Plus: Depreciation			350,000	350,000	350,000	350,000	350,000
15. Plus: Net salvage value							750,000
16. Net cash flow		($2,500,000)	$ 510,000	$ 535,500	$ 562,275	$ 590,389	$1,369,908

Note: Totals are rounded.

Line 6. Labor costs are forecasted to be $50,000 during the first year, but increase over time at the 5 percent inflation rate.

Line 7. Maintenance fees must be paid to the manufacturer at the end of each year of operation. These fees are assumed to increase at the 5 percent inflation rate.

Line 8. Each scan uses $15 of supplies, so supply costs in the first year total 40(50)($15) = $30,000, and they are expected to increase each year by the inflation rate.

Line 9. If the project is accepted, overhead cash costs will increase by $10,000 in the first year. Note that the $10,000 are cash costs that are related directly to the acceptance of the MRI project. Existing overhead costs that are arbitrarily allocated to the MRI site are not incremental cash flows, and thus should not be included in the analysis. Overhead costs are also assumed to increase over time at the inflation rate.

Line 10. Depreciation in each year is calculated by the straight-line method, assuming a five-year depreciable life. The depreciable basis is equal to the capitalized cost of the project, which includes the cost of the asset and related construction, less the estimated salvage value. Thus, the depreciable basis is ($1,500,000 + $1,000,000) − $750,000 = $1,750,000. Then, the straight-line depreciation in each year of the project's five-year depreciable life is (1/5)($1,750,000) = $350,000. Note that depreciation is based solely on acquisition costs, so it is unaffected by inflation. Also, note that the Table 10.2 cash flows are presented in a generic format that can be used by both investor-owned and not-for-profit hospitals. Depreciation expense is not a cash flow, but an accounting convention that recognizes the reduction in value of fixed assets caused by wear and tear and obsolescence. Since Bayside Memorial Hospital is tax exempt, and hence depreciation will not affect taxes, and since depreciation is added back to the cash flows on Line 14, depreciation could be totally omitted from the cash flow analysis.

Line 11. Line 11 shows the project's operating income in each year, which is merely the net revenues less all operating expenses.

Line 12. Line 12 contains zeros, because Bayside is not-for-profit and hence does not pay taxes.

Line 13. Bayside pays no taxes, so the project's net operating income equals its operating income.

Line 14. Since depreciation, a noncash expense, was included on Line 10, it must be added back to the project's net operating income in each year to obtain each year's net cash flow.

Line 15. Finally, the project is expected to be terminated after five years, at which time the MRI system would be sold for an estimated $750,000. This salvage value cash flow is shown as an inflow at the end of Year 5 on Line 15.

Line 16. The project's net cash flows are shown on Line 16. The project requires a $2,500,000 investment at Year 0, but then generates cash inflows over its five-year operating life.

Note that the Table 10.2 cash flows do not include any allowance for interest expense. On average, Bayside hospital will finance new projects in accordance with its target capital structure, which consists of 50 percent debt financing and 50 percent equity (fund) financing. The costs associated with this financing mix, including interest costs, are incorporated into the firm's weighted average cost of capital of 10.0 percent. Since the cost of debt financing is included in the discount rate that will be applied to the cash flows, recognition of interest expense in the cash flows would be double counting.

Taxable organizations

The Table 10.2 cash flow analysis can be easily modified to reflect tax implications if the analyzing firm is taxable. To illustrate, assume that the MRI project is being evaluated by Ann Arbor Health Systems, an investor-owned hospital chain. Furthermore, assume that all of the project data present earlier apply to Ann Arbor, except that (1) the MRI falls into the MACRS 5-year class for tax depreciation and (2) the firm has a 40 percent tax rate. Table 10.3 contains Ann Arbor's cash flow analysis. Note the following differences.

Line 10. First, depreciation expense must be modified to reflect tax depreciation rather than book depreciation. As we discussed in Chapter 2, tax depreciation is calculated using the Modified Accelerated Cost

Table 10.3   Ann Arbor Health Systems: MRI Site Cash Flow Analysis

			Cash Revenues and Costs			
	0	1	2	3	4	5
1. System cost	($1,500,000)					
2. Related expenses	(1,000,000)					
3. Gross revenues		$1,000,000	$1,050,000	$1,102,500	$1,157,625	$1,215,506
4. Less: Deductions		250,000	262,500	275,625	289,406	303,877
5. Net revenues		$ 750,000	$ 787,500	$ 826,875	$ 868,219	$ 911,630
6. Less: Labor costs		50,000	52,500	55,125	57,881	60,775
7. Maintenance costs		150,000	157,500	165,375	173,644	182,326
8. Supplies		30,000	31,500	33,075	34,729	36,465
9. Incremental overhead		10,000	10,500	11,025	11,576	12,155
10. Depreciation		500,000	800,000	475,000	300,000	275,000
11. Operating income		$ 10,000	($ 264,500)	$ 87,275	$ 290,389	$ 344,908
12. Taxes		4,000	(105,800)	34,910	116,156	137,963
13. Net operating income		$ 6,000	($ 158,700)	$ 52,365	$ 174,233	$ 206,945
14. Plus: Depreciation		500,000	800,000	475,000	300,000	275,000
15. Plus: Net salvage value						510,000
16. Net cash flow	($2,500,000)	$ 506,000	$ 641,300	$ 527,365	$ 474,233	$ 991,945

Note: Totals are rounded.

Recovery System (MACRS). Table 2.9 in Chapter 2 gives the MACRS depreciation factors for several different class lives. To determine the MACRS depreciation allowance in any year, multiply the asset's depreciable basis, without considering its estimated salvage value, by the appropriate depreciation factor. In the MRI illustration, the depreciable basis is $2,500,000, and since the MRI system falls into the MACRS five-year class, the MACRS factors are 0.20, 0.32, 0.19, 0.12, 0.11, and 0.06, in Years 1 to 6, respectively. Thus, the tax depreciation in Year 1 is 0.20($2,500,000) = $500,000; in Year 2 the depreciation is 0.32($2,500,000) = $800,000; and so on.

Line 12. Taxable firms must reduce the operating income on Line 11 by the amount of taxes. Taxes, which appear on Line 12, are computed by multiplying the Line 12 pretax operating income by the firm's marginal tax rate. For example, the project's taxes for Year 1 are 0.40($10,000) = $4,000. Note that the taxes shown for Year 2 are a negative $105,800. In this year, the project is expected to lose $264,500, and hence Ann Arbor's taxable income (assuming its existing projects are profitable) will be reduced by this amount if the project is undertaken. This reduction in taxable income would lower the firm's tax bill by T(Taxable income reduction) = 0.40($264,500) = $105,800.[5]

Line 14. The MACRS depreciation is added back in Line 14.

Line 15. Investor-owned firms will normally incur a tax liability on the sale of a capital asset at the end of the project's life. According to the IRS, the value of the MRI system at the end of Year 5 is the *tax book value*, which is the depreciation that remains on the tax books. In the illustration, five years worth of depreciation would be taken, so only one year of depreciation remains. The MACRS factor for Year 6 is 0.06, so by the end of Year 5, Ann Arbor has expensed 0.94 of the MRI's depreciable basis and the remaining tax book value is 0.06($2,500,000) = $150,000. Thus, according to the IRS, the value of the MRI system is $150,000. When Ann Arbor sells the system for its estimated salvage value of $750,000, it realizes a "profit" of $750,000 − $150,000 = $600,000, and it must repay the IRS an amount equal to 0.4($600,000) = $240,000. The $240,000 tax bill recognizes that Ann Arbor took too much depreciation on the MRI system, so it represents a recapture of the excess tax benefit taken over the five-year life of the system. The $240,000 in taxes reduces the cash received from the sale of the MRI equipment, so the salvage value net of taxes is $750,000 − $240,000 = $510,000.

As can be seen by comparing Line 16 in Tables 10.1 and 10.2, all else the same, the taxes paid by investor-owned firms tend to reduce a project's net operating cash flows and net salvage value, and hence reduce the project's profitability.

Replacement analysis

Bayside Hospital's MRI project was used to illustrate how the cash flows from an *expansion project* are analyzed. All firms, including Bayside Memorial Hospital, also make *replacement decisions*, in which a new asset is being considered to replace an existing asset that could, if not replaced, continue in operation. The cash flow analysis for a replacement decision is somewhat more complex than for an expansion decision because the cash flows from the existing asset must be considered.

Again, the key to cash flow estimation is to focus on the incremental cash flows. If the new asset is acquired, the existing asset can be sold, so the current market value of the existing asset is a cash inflow in the analysis. When considering the operating flows, the incremental flows are the cash flows expected from the replacement asset less the flows that the existing asset produces. By applying the incremental cash flow concept, the correct cash flows can be estimated for replacement decisions.[6]

Self-Test Questions:

Briefly describe how a project cash flow analysis is constructed.

Is it necessary to include depreciation expense in a cash flow analysis by a not-for-profit provider? Explain.

What are the key differences in cash flow analyses performed by investor-owned and not-for-profit organizations?

How do expansion and replacement project analyses differ?

Breakeven Analysis

Breakeven analysis is used to gain insights into the potential profitability and risk of a project. Furthermore, as illustrated in Case 10, breakeven analysis is often useful in evaluating projects that do not require an initial capital investment, such as expanding the hours of operation of a clinic. Although breakeven analysis can be applied in many different ways, we will focus here on two types of breakeven: (1) usage (volume) breakeven and (2) time breakeven.

Usage (volume) breakeven

To illustrate usage breakeven, first consider how it can be applied to operating cash flows. Specifically, let's examine operating breakeven in Year 1. From Table 10.2, we know that 40 scans a week would produce a net cash flow in Year 1 of $510,000. But a logical question to ask would be how many scans per week would be necessary to reach operating breakeven in Year 1? That is, how many scans per week are required to generate a positive net cash flow in Year 1? With the basic analysis performed using a spreadsheet program, it is very easy to do breakeven analysis. Table 10.4 contains the Year 1 net cash flow at different usage levels and, as indicated by the data, the project breaks even in Year 1 if the hospital performs 12 scans per week.

Usage breakeven can also be applied to the entire project. Here we want to know the answer to this question: What weekly usage would allow the hospital to recover all of the costs associated with the project, including capital costs? Again, if the analysis is modeled on a spreadsheet, answers to these types of questions are easy to develop. As we discuss in a later section, total breakeven occurs for the project when its net present value (NPV) equals zero (or just turns positive). In Bayside's MRI project, this occurs at a weekly usage of 39 scans, so the project in its entirety just breaks even when the hospital averages 39 scans per week over the five-year forecasted life of the project. Such information is clearly useful to Bayside's managers. If they feel strongly that usage will exceed 39 scans per week, then it is highly likely that the project will

Table 10.4 Bayside Memorial Hospital: MRI Site Year 1
Breakeven Analysis

Number of Scans per Week	Year 1 Net Cash Flow
0	($210,000)
5	(120,000)
10	(30,000)
11	(12,000)
12	6,000
13	24,000
14	42,000
15	60,000
20	150,000
30	330,000
40	510,000

be profitable. Conversely, if they believe that usage will be less than the breakeven level, then the project will probably be unprofitable. Also, if, as in this situation, the projected volume is just above breakeven, a small forecasting error can result in a project that is profitable on paper but unprofitable if undertaken.

Time breakeven (payback)

The *payback*, or *payback period*, measures time breakeven. Payback is defined as the expected number of years required to recover the investment in the project. To illustrate, consider the net cash flows for the MRI project contained in Table 10.2. The best way to determine the project's payback is to construct the project's cumulative cash flows as shown in Table 10.5. The $2,500,000 investment in the MRI site would be recovered some time during Year 5. If the project's cash flows are assumed to come in evenly during the year, then breakeven would occur $301,836/$1,369,908 = 0.22 of the way through Year 5, so the payback is 4.22 years.

Payback is a breakeven measure—if cash flows come in at the expected rate until payback, then the project will break even in the sense that the initial investment will be recovered. Thus, the shorter the payback, the more quickly the funds invested in the project will become available for other purposes, and hence the more liquid the project. Also, cash flows expected in the distant future are generally regarded as being riskier than near-term cash flows. Therefore, payback is often used as a rough measure of a project's riskiness. Note, though, that payback does not consider the opportunity cost of the capital employed in the project; that is, it does not consider the project's cost of capital.[7]

Self-Test Questions:

Why is breakeven information valuable to decision makers?

Describe several types of breakeven analysis.

Table 10.5   Bayside Memorial Hospital: MRI Site Cumulative Cash Flow

Year	Annual Cash Flows	Cumulative Cash Flows
0	($2,500,000)	($2,500,000)
1	510,000	(1,990,000)
2	535,500	(1,454,500)
3	562,275	(892,225)
4	590,389	(301,836)
5	1,369,908	1,068,072

Profitability Analysis

Up to this point, the chapter has focused on cash flow estimation and breakeven analysis. Perhaps the most important element in a project's financial analysis is its expected profitability. In general, the expected profitability of capital investments can be measured either in dollars or in percentage rate of return. In the next sections, we present one dollar measure, net present value, and two rate of return measures, internal rate of return and modified internal rate of return.

Net present value (NPV)

Net present value (NPV) is a profitability measure that uses the discounted cash flow (DCF) techniques discussed in Chapter 4, so it is often referred to as a *DCF measure*. To apply the NPV method, we proceed as follows:

1. Find the present (Time 0) value of each net cash flow, including both inflows and outflows, discounted at the project's cost of capital.
2. Sum the present values. This sum is defined as the project's net present value.
3. If the NPV is positive, the project is profitable, and the higher the NPV the more profitable the project. If the NPV is zero, the project just breaks even in profitability; if the NPV is negative, the project is unprofitable.

With a project cost of capital of 10 percent, the NPV of Bayside's MRI project is calculated as follows:

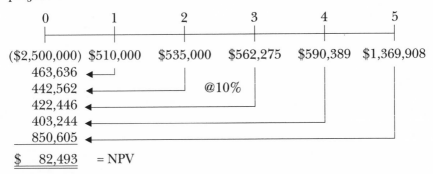

Financial calculators and spreadsheets have NPV functions that easily perform the mathematics given the cash flows and cost of capital.

The rationale behind the NPV method is straightforward. An NPV of zero signifies that the project's cash inflows are just sufficient to (1) return the capital invested in the project and (2) provide the required rate of return on that invested capital. If a project has a positive NPV, then it is generating excess cash flows, and these excess cash flows are available to management to reinvest in the firm and, for investor-owned firms, to pay dividends. For investor-owned firms, NPV is a direct measure of the contribution of the project to shareholder wealth. If a project has a negative NPV, its cash inflows are insufficient to compensate the firm for the capital invested, so the project is unprofitable and acceptance would cause the financial condition of the firm to deteriorate.

The NPV of the MRI project is $82,493, so on a present value basis the project is projected to generate a cash flow excess of over $80,000. Thus, the project is profitable, and its acceptance would have a positive effect on Bayside's financial condition.

Internal rate of return (IRR)

Whereas NPV measures a project's dollar profitability, *internal rate of return (IRR)* measures a project's percentage profitability or its expected rate of return. Mathematically, the IRR is defined as that discount rate that equates the present value of the project's expected cash inflows to the present value of the project's expected cash outflows, so the IRR is simply that discount rate that forces the NPV of the project to equal zero. Financial calculators and spreadsheets have IRR functions that calculate IRRs very rapidly. Simply input the project's cash flows, and the computer or calculator computes the IRR.

For Bayside's MRI project, the IRR is that rate that causes the sum of the present values of the cash inflows to equal the $2,500,000 cost of the project:

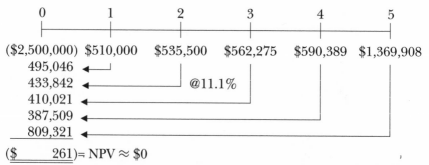

When all of the MRI project's cash flows are discounted at 11.1 percent, the NPV of the project is approximately zero. Thus, the MRI project's IRR is 11.1 percent. Put another way, the project is expected to generate an 11.1 percent rate of return on its $2,500,000 investment.

If the IRR exceeds the project's cost of capital, a surplus remains after recovering the invested capital and paying for its use, and this surplus accrues to the firm's stockholders (in Bayside's case, to its stakeholders). On the other hand, if the IRR is less than the project's cost of capital, then taking on the project imposes a cost on the firm's stockholders (or stakeholders). The MRI project's 11.1 percent IRR exceeds the project's 10.0 percent cost of capital. Thus, as measured by the IRR, the MRI project is profitable, and its acceptance would enhance Bayside's financial condition.

Comparison of the NPV and IRR methods

Consider a project with a zero NPV. In this situation, the project's IRR must equal its cost of capital. The project has zero profitability, and acceptance would neither enhance nor diminish the firm's financial condition. In order to have a positive NPV, the project's IRR must be greater than its cost of capital, and a negative NPV signifies a project with an IRR less than its cost of capital. Thus, projects that are deemed profitable by the NPV method will also be deemed profitable by the IRR method. In the MRI example, the project would have a positive NPV for all costs of capital less than 11.1 percent. If the cost of capital was greater than 11.1 percent, the project would have a negative NPV. In effect, the NPV and IRR are perfect substitutes for one another in measuring whether a project is profitable or not.[8]

Modified internal rate of return (MIRR)

In general, academics prefer the NPV profitability measure. This preference stems from two factors: (1) NPV measures profitability in dollars, which is a direct measure of the contribution of the project to the financial strength of the firm. (2) Both the NPV and the IRR, since they are discounted cash flow techniques, require an assumption about the rate at which project cash flows can be reinvested, and the NPV method has the better assumption.

To further explain the second point, consider the MRI project's Year 2 net cash flow of $535,500, as shown in Table 10.2. In effect, the discounting process inherent in the NPV and IRR methods automatically assigns a reinvestment rate to this cash flow. That is, both the NPV and IRR methods assume that Bayside has the opportunity to reinvest the $535,500 Year 2 cash flow in other projects, and each method automatically assigns a reinvestment rate to this flow for Years 3, 4, and 5. The NPV method assumes reinvestment at the project's cost of capital, 10 percent, while the IRR method assumes reinvestment at the IRR rate, 11.1 percent. Which is the better assumption—reinvestment at the cost of capital or reinvestment at the IRR rate? In general, firms will take on all projects that exceed their cost of capital. Thus, at the margin, the returns expected from capital reinvested within the firm are more likely to be at, or close to, the cost of capital than at the project's IRR, especially for projects with exceptionally high or low IRRs. Furthermore, firms can obtain outside capital at a cost roughly equal to the firm's cost of capital, so project cash flows can be replaced by capital having this cost. Thus, in general, reinvestment at the cost of capital is a better assumption than reinvestment at the IRR rate, so NPV is a better measure of profitability than IRR.[9]

Even though academics strongly favor the NPV method, practicing managers prefer the IRR method by a margin of three to one. Apparently, managers find it intuitively more appealing to analyze investments in terms of percentage rates of return than dollars of NPV. Thus, an alternative rate of return measure has been developed that eliminates the primary problem with IRR. This method is the *modified IRR (MIRR)*, and it is calculated as follows:

1. Discount all of the project's net cash outflows back to Year 0 at the project's cost of capital.

2. Compound all of the project's net cash inflows forward to Year n, the last (terminal) year of the project, at the project's cost of capital. This value is called the *inflow terminal value*.

3. The discount rate that forces the present value of the inflow terminal value to equal the present value of costs is defined as the MIRR.

Applying these steps to Bayside's MRI project produces a MIRR of about 10.7 percent:

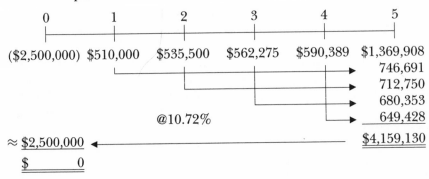

The MIRR method, by compounding the cash inflows forward at 10 percent, forces the reinvestment rate to equal 10 percent, the project's cost of capital. Note that the MIRR for the MRI project is less than the project's IRR, because the cash inflows are reinvested at only 10 percent rather than the project's 11.1 percent IRR. In general, the MIRR is less than the IRR when the IRR is greater than the cost of capital, but greater than the IRR when the IRR is less than the cost of capital. In effect, the IRR overstates the profitability of profitable projects and understates the profitability of unprofitable projects. By forcing the correct reinvestment rate, the MIRR method provides decision makers with a better measure of a project's percentage rate of return profitability than does the IRR.

Self-Test Questions:

Briefly describe net present value (NPV), internal rate of return (IRR), and modified IRR (MIRR).

Explain the rationale behind each method.

Why is MIRR a better rate of return profitability measure than IRR?

Some Final Thoughts on Breakeven and Profitability Analysis

We have presented several approaches to breakeven analysis and three profitability measures. In the course of our discussion, we purposely compared the methods against one another to highlight their relative strengths and weaknesses, but in the process we may have created the impression that firms would use only one method in the decision process. Today, virtually all capital budgeting decisions of financial consequence are analyzed by computer, and hence it is easy to calculate and list numerous breakeven measures along with NPV, IRR, and MIRR. Since each measure contributes slightly different information about the financial consequences of a project, it would be foolish for decision makers to focus on a single financial measure. Thus, we believe that a thorough financial analysis of a new project includes numerous financial measures, and that capital budgeting decisions are enhanced if all the information inherent in all of the measures is considered.

Self-Test Question:

Should capital budgeting analyses look at only one breakeven or profitability measure? Explain.

Evaluating Projects with Unequal Lives

Occasionally, firms must choose between two mutually exclusive projects that have unequal lives. (Two projects are *mutually exclusive* when acceptance of one implies rejection of the other.) When this situation arises, if the shorter-life project will be replicated, then an adjustment to the normal capital budgeting process is necessary. We now discuss two procedures—the replacement chain method and the equivalent annual annuity method—both to illustrate the problem and to show how to deal with it.

Suppose that American Dental Equipment Corporation is planning to modernize its production facilities, and as part of the process, it is considering either a conveyor system (Project C) or forklift trucks (Project F) for moving materials from the parts department to the main assembly line. Table 10.6 shows both the expected net cash flows and the NPVs for these two mutually exclusive alternatives. We see that Project C, when discounted at the company's 11.5 percent cost of capital, has the higher NPV and thus appears to be the more profitable project.

Replacement chain (common life) analysis

Although the analysis in Table 10.6 suggests that Project C is the more profitable project, the analysis is incomplete and this conclusion is actually incorrect. If the company chooses Project F, it will have the opportunity to make a similar investment in three years, and if cost and revenue conditions continue at the Table 10.6 levels, this second, or replication, investment will also be profitable. However, if the company chooses Project C, it will not have this second investment opportunity. Therefore, to make a proper comparison between the three-year and six-year projects, we could apply the *replacement chain (common life)* approach;

Table 10.6   Expected Net Cash Flows for Projects C and F

Year	Project C	Project F
0	($40,000)	($20,000)
1	8,000	7,000
2	14,000	13,000
3	13,000	12,000
4	12,000	—
5	11,000	—
6	10,000	—
NPV @ 11.5%	$ 7,165	$ 5,391

that is, we could find the extended NPV of Project F over a six-year period by assuming that the project is replicated, and then compare this extended NPV with the NPV of Project C over the same period.

The NPV for Project C, as calculated in Table 10.6, is already over the six-year common life. For Project F, however, we must take three additional steps: (1) determine the NPV of the replication project three years hence, (2) discount this NPV back to the present, and (3) sum the two components to obtain the project's extended NPV. If we assume that the replication project will have the same cash flows as the original project, then Project F's extended NPV is $9,280:

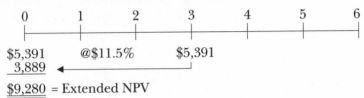

Since Project F's six-year (extended) NPV is greater than Project C's six-year NPV, Project F is more profitable when the opportunity to replicate the project is considered.

Note that the time-line analysis above uses NPVs to summarize Project F's estimated cash flows. An alternative approach to the analysis is to place the individual cash flows on the time line:

```
      0        1         2          3          4          5          6
      |        |         |          |          |          |          |
 ($20,000)  $7,000   $13,000    $12,000
                                (20,000)    $7,000    $13,000    $12,000
                                ($8,000)
```

NPV @ 11.5% ≈ $9,280.

Clearly, the former method is simpler. However, if the cash flows for the replicated project are not the same as the cash flows for the initial project, then the more complex individual cash flow method must be used. By showing each cash flow, the analysis can accommodate changes in project cash flows that occur as the project is replicated.

Equivalent annual annuity approach

Although the preceding example illustrates why an extended analysis is necessary if two mutually exclusive projects with different lives are being analyzed, the analysis is generally more complex in practice. For example, one project might have a six-year life versus a ten-year life for the other. This would require a replacement chain analysis over 30 years, the lowest common multiple of the two lives. In such a situation, it is simpler to use the *equivalent annual annuity (EAA)* approach.

The EAA approach involves three steps:

1. Find each project's NPV over its original life. In Table 10.6, we see that $NPV_C = \$7,165$ and $NPV_F = \$5,391$.

2. For each project, find the annuity (constant value) cash flow over the project's original life that has the same present value as the project's NPV. This cash flow is called the *equivalent annual annuity*. Here is the concept on a time line for Project F:

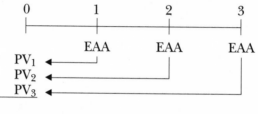

$\underline{\$5,391}$ = NPV_F

To find the value of EAA_F on a financial calculator, enter 5,391 (or $-5,391$) as the PV, i = 11.5, and n = 3. Then, solve for PMT = 2,225. Thus, the equivalent annual annuity for Project F is $2,225. This annuity stream over the original life of the project, three years, when discounted at the project cost of capital, 11.5 percent, has a present value equal to Project F's NPV, $5,391. The EAA for Project C is found in a like manner, and it is $1,718. Thus, Project C has an NPV which is equivalent to an annuity of $1,718 per year for six years, while Project F's NPV is equivalent to an annuity of $2,225 for three years.

3. Now, when projects are replicated, assuming that the cash flows remain the same, they earn the same NPV over and over, which is equivalent to replicating the project's EAA over time. Thus, over any common life, whether it be 6 years or 30 years, the project with the higher EAA will have the higher NPV, because its equivalent cash flow will be higher in every year. Since Project F has the higher EAA, under the assumption of constant cash flow replication, it is more profitable than Project C.

The EAA method is generally easier to apply, but the replacement chain method is often easier to explain to decision makers. Still, the two methods always lead to the same results if consistent assumptions are used. When should managers worry about unequal life analysis? As a general rule, the unequal life issue does not arise for independent projects; it is only an issue when mutually exclusive projects are being analyzed. However, even for mutually exclusive projects, it is not always appropriate to extend the analysis to a common life. This should only be done if there is a high probability that the projects will actually be replicated beyond their original lives.

There are several weaknesses inherent in the types of analysis just described. (1) If inflation is expected, then replacement cost will probably be higher than the initial cost, both sales price and operating costs will probably rise, and hence the static conditions built into the example will not be appropriate. (2) Future replacements may use different technologies, which might also change the project's cash flows. (3) It is difficult enough to estimate the lives of most projects, so estimating the lives of a future series of projects is often just speculation.

In view of these problems, no experienced manager would be too concerned about comparing mutually exclusive projects with lives of, say, eight years and ten years. Given all of the uncertainties in the estimation process, such projects could, for all practical purposes, be assumed to have the same life. Still, it is important to recognize that a problem does exist if mutually exclusive projects that will be replicated have substantially different lives. When the managers of Ann Arbor Health Systems encounter such problems, they build expected inflation or possible efficiency gains, or both, directly into the cash flow estimates, and then use the replacement chain approach to estimate the projects' extended NPVs. The cash flow estimation is more complicated than in our example, but the concepts involved are exactly the same.

Self-Test Questions:

Is it always necessary to adjust project cash flows to account for unequal lives?

Briefly describe the two methods for adjusting for unequal lives.

Abandonment Value

Customarily, projects are analyzed as though the firm will operate the project over its full *physical*, or *engineering, life*. However, this may not be the best course of action financially—it may be best to abandon a project prior to the end of its potential life, and this possibility can materially affect a project's estimated profitability. To illustrate the concept of *abandonment value* and its effects on capital budgeting decisions, consider the cash flows associated with Bayside Memorial Hospital's proposal to establish a taxable food services division. The project's cash flows are contained in Table 10.7. For simplicity, we have shortened the physical life of the project to three years. The project's investment and operating cash flows are shown in the middle column, while the right-hand column contains the project's *abandonment values*. Abandonment values are equivalent to net salvage values, except that they have been estimated for each year of the project's physical life.

Using a 10 percent cost of capital, the NPV over the project's three-year physical life, with zero abandonment value, is −$11,743. Thus, the project is unprofitable when the single alternative of a three-year life with a zero salvage value is considered. However, what would its NPV be if the project were abandoned after two years? In this situation, Bayside would receive operating cash flows for two years, plus the $190,000 abandonment value at the end of Year 2, and the project's NPV would be $13,802. Thus, the project is profitable if Bayside operates it for only two years and then sells it. To complete the abandonment analysis, note that if the project were abandoned after one year, its NPV would be −$25,455.

The *economic life* of the project, which is the life that produces the highest NPV, is two years. As a general rule, if profitability were the sole criterion in capital budgeting decisions, a project should be abandoned when the net abandonment value is greater than the present value of all cash flows beyond the abandonment point, discounted to the abandonment point. For example, if Bayside were to operate the division for one year, the abandonment value at that point is $300,000, but the present value at Year 1 of the cash flows beyond Year 1 would be $187,500/$(1.10)^1$ + $190,000/$(1.10)^1$ = $343,182, assuming abandonment at the end of Year 2. Thus, the Year 1 abandonment value is less than the Year 1 present value of continuing the project, so the project should not be abandoned

Table 10.7   Food Service Division's Projected Cash Flows

Year	Initial Investment and Operating Cash Flows	End of Year Net Abandonment Value
0	($480,000)	($480,000)
1	200,000	300,000
2	187,500	190,000
3	175,000	0

at this point. However, a similar analysis at the end of Year 2 would show that the abandonment value is greater than the discounted value of future cash flows, so abandonment at Year 2 would produce the greater profitability. This is, of course, the same conclusion that we reached when calculating the NPVs of each possible project life. In essence, the abandonment decision examines the incremental cash flows to the firm at the abandonment point—the abandonment cash flows versus the cash flows associated with continuing the project—to determine the most profitable course of action.

Two very different types of abandonment can occur: (1) sale by the original owner of a still valuable asset to some other party who can operate the asset more efficiently, and (2) abandonment of an asset because the asset is losing money. The first type of situation is illustrated by Bayside Memorial Hospital's sale of its two walk-in clinics to a physician group. Although the clinics were profitable to Bayside, the physician group could presumably operate them more efficiently, and hence were willing to pay Bayside a premium over the value the clinics would have if they remained under hospital control. The second type of abandonment is illustrated by Northeast Medical's decision to discontinue its HMO operation in Boston. Although Northeast's GoodHealth plan had proved profitable in several areas, competition in the Boston market proved destructive, so the company made the decision to cut its losses.

Self-Test Questions:

Define economic life, as opposed to physical life.

Should projects be viewed as having one, fixed life, or should they be considered as having alternative lives?

Capital Budgeting by Not-for-Profit Firms

Although the capital budgeting techniques discussed up to this point are appropriate for use by both investor-owned and not-for-profit firms, a not-for-profit firm has the additional consideration of meeting its charitable mission. In this section, we discuss two models that extend the capital budgeting decision to not-for-profit firms.

Net present social value (NPSV) model[10]

Except for our discussion of strategic value, the financial analysis techniques discussed thus far have focused exclusively on the cash flow implications of a proposed project. Some health care firms, particularly not-for-profit firms, have the goal of producing social services along with commercial services. For these firms, the proper analysis of proposed projects must systematically consider the social value of a project along with its pure financial, or cash flow, value.

When social value is considered, the total net present value (TNPV) of a project can be expressed as follows:

$$TNPV = NPV + NPSV. \tag{10.1}$$

Here, NPV represents the conventional NPV of the project's cash flow stream and NPSV is the net present social value of the project. The second term on the right-hand side of Equation 10.1 clearly differentiates capital budgeting in not-for-profit firms from that in investor-owned firms. NPSV represents managers' assessment of the social value of the project as opposed to its pure financial value as measured by NPV.

In evaluating each project, a project is acceptable if its TNPV is greater than or equal to zero, because that means that the sum of the project's financial and social values is at least zero. In other words, when both facets of value are considered, the project has positive, or at least nonnegative, worth. Probably not all projects will have social value, but if a project does, it is considered formally in this decision model. Note, however, that no project should be accepted if its NPSV is negative, even if its TNPV is positive. Also, to ensure the financial viability of the firm, the sum of the NPVs of all projects initiated in a planning period plus the value of the unrestricted contributions received must equal or exceed zero. If this restriction were not imposed, social value could displace financial value over time, and a firm cannot continue to provide social value unless it has financial integrity.

NPSV can be defined as follows:

$$NPSV = \sum_{t=1}^{n} \frac{\text{Social value}_t}{(1 + k_s)^t}. \tag{10.2}$$

where the social value of a project in each Year t is discounted back to Year 0 and then summed. In essence, the suppliers of fund capital to a not-for-profit firm never receive a cash return on their investment. Instead, they receive a return on their investment in the form of social dividends. These dividends take the form of services with social value to the community such as charity care, medical research and education, and a myriad of other services that, for one reason or another, do not pay their own way. Services provided to patients at a price equal to or greater than the full cost of production do not create social value. Similarly, if governmental entities purchase care directly for beneficiaries of a program or in support of research, the resulting social value is created by that governmental entity, and not by the provider of the services.

In estimating a project's NPSV, that is, in evaluating Equation 10.2, it is necessary to (1) estimate the social value of the services provided by the project in each year and (2) determine the discount rate to apply to those services. First, let's examine the social value of the services provided by a project. When a project produces services to individuals who are willing and able to pay for those services, the value of those services is captured by the amount that they actually pay. Thus, the value of the services provided to those who cannot pay, or to those who cannot pay the full amount, can be estimated by the average net price paid by those individuals who are able to pay.

This approach to valuing social services has intuitive appeal, but there are several points that merit further discussion.

1. Price is a fair measure of value only if the payer has the capacity to judge the true value of the service provided. Many observers of the health care industry would argue that information asymmetries between the provider and the purchaser inhibit the ability of the purchaser to judge true value.

2. The fact that most payments for health care services are made by third party payers may result in price distortions. For example, insurers might be willing to pay more for services than an individual would pay in the absence of insurance, or the existence of monopsony power by Medicare might result in a net price that is less than individuals would be willing to pay.

3. The amount that an individual is willing to pay may be more or less than the amount a contributor or other fund supplier would be willing to pay.

4. Finally, there is a great deal of controversy over the true value of treatment in many situations. If we are entitled to whatever health care is available, regardless of cost, and if we are not required to personally pay for the care, even though society as a whole must cover the bill, then we may demand a level of care that is of questionable value. For example, should $500,000 be spent to keep a comatose 92-year-old person alive for 11 more days? If the true value of such an expenditure is zero,

it makes little sense to assign a $500,000 value just because that is its cost.

In spite of the potential problems, it still seems reasonable to assign a social value to many, but not all, health care services on the basis of the price that others are willing to pay for those services.

The second element required to estimate the NPSV of a project is the discount rate to apply to the annual social value stream. Like the required rate of return on equity for not-for-profit firms, there has been considerable controversy over the proper discount rate to apply to future social values. However, it is clear that contributors of fund capital can capture social value in two ways. First, as is commonly done, contributions can be made directly to not-for-profit organizations. Second, contributors can always invest the funds in a portfolio of securities, and then use the proceeds to purchase the health care services directly. In the second situation, there would be no tax consequences on the portfolio's return because the contributed proceeds would qualify for tax exemption, but the contributor would lose the tax exemption on the full amount of the funds placed in the portfolio. Since the second alternative exists, providers should require a return on their social value stream that approximates the return available on the equity investment in for-profit firms offering the same services.

The net present social value model formalizes the capital budgeting decision process applicable to not-for-profit health care firms. Although few organizations attempt to quantify NPSV, not-for-profit firms should at a minimum subjectively consider the social value inherent in projects under consideration.

A more pragmatic approach

Managers of not-for-profit firms, as well as many managers of investor-owned firms, recognize that considerations other than financial should be considered in any capital budgeting analysis. The net present social value model examines only one other factor, and it is difficult to implement in practice. Thus, many firms use a quasi-subjective approach to capital budgeting decisions that attempts to capture both financial and nonfinancial factors. Table 10.8, the project scoring matrix used by Peachtree Health Systems, an Atlanta-based not-for-profit hospital system, illustrates one such approach.

Peachtree ranks projects on three dimensions: stakeholder factors, operational factors, and financial factors. Within each dimension, multiple factors are examined and assigned scores ranging from two points

Table 10.8 Peachtree Health Systems: Project Scoring Matrix

Criteria	Relative Score			
	2	1	0	−1
Stakeholder Factors				
Physicians	Strongly support	Support	Neutral	Opposed
Employees	Helps morale a lot	Helps morale a little	No effect	Hurts morale
Visitors	Greatly enhances visit	Enhances visit	No effect	Hurts image
Social value	High	Moderate	None	Negative
Operational Factors				
Outcomes	Greatly improves	Improves	No effect	Hurts outcomes
Length of stay	Documented decrease	Anecdotal decrease	No effect	Increases
Technology	Breakthrough	Improves current	Adds to current	Removes technology
Productivity	Large decrease in FTEs	Decrease in FTEs	No change in FTEs	Adds FTEs
Financial Factors				
Life cycle	Innovation	Growth	Stabilization	Decline
Payback	Less than 2 years	2–4 years	4–6 years	Over 6 years
IRR	Over 20%	15–20%	10–15%	Less than 10%
Correlation	Negative	Uncorrelated	Somewhat positive	Highly positive

Stakeholder Factor score _____

Service Factor score _____

Financial Factor score _____

Total score ══════

for very favorable impact to minus one point for negative impact. The scores within each dimension are added to obtain scores for stakeholder, operational, and financial factors, and then the dimension scores are aggregated to obtain a total score for the project. The total score gives Peachtree's decision makers a feel for the relative values of projects under consideration when all factors, including financial, are taken into account.

Of course, Peachtree's managers recognize that the scoring system is completely arbitrary, so a project with a score of, say, 10 is not really twice as good as a project scoring 5. Nevertheless, Peachtree's project scoring matrix forces its managers to address multiple issues when making capital budgeting decisions. Although Peachtree's approach should not be used at other organizations without modification for firm- and industry-unique circumstances, it does provide some insights into how a firm-unique matrix might be developed.

Self-Test Questions:

Describe the net present social value model of capital budgeting.

Describe the construction and use of a project scoring matrix.

The Post-Audit

Capital budgeting is not a static process. First, if there is a long lag between a project's acceptance and its implementation, any new information concerning either capital costs or the project's cash flows should be analyzed before the final go-ahead is given. Second, the performance of each project should be monitored throughout the project's life. This process is called the *post-audit*, and it involves (1) comparing actual results with those projected by the project's sponsors, (2) explaining why differences occur, and (3) analyzing potential changes to the project's operations, including replacement or abandonment.

The post-audit has several purposes, including the following:

1. *Improve forecasts.* When decision makers systematically compare their projections to actual outcomes, there is a tendency for estimates to improve. Conscious or unconscious biases that occur can be identified and, one hopes, eliminated; new forecasting methods are sought as the need for them becomes apparent; and managers tend to do everything better, including forecasting, if they know that their actions are being monitored.

2. *Develop historical risk data.* Post-audits permit managers to develop historical data on new project analyses regarding risk and expected rates of return. These data can then be used to make judgments about the relative risk of future projects as they are evaluated.

3. *Improve operations.* Businesses are run by managers, and they can perform at higher or lower levels of efficiency. When a forecast is made, say, by the surgery department, the department director and medical staff are, in a sense, putting their reputations on the line. If costs are above predicted levels and usage is below expectations, the people involved will strive, within ethical bounds, to improve the situation and to bring results into line with forecasts. As one hospital CEO put it: "You academics worry only about making good decisions. In the health care industry, we also have to worry about making decisions good."

4. *Reduce losses.* Post-audits monitor the performance of projects over time, so the first indication that abandonment or replacement should be considered often arises when the post-audit indicates that a project is performing poorly.

Self-Test Questions:

What is a post-audit?

Why are post-audits important to the efficiency of a business?

Summary

This chapter discussed the basic capital budgeting process, and the key concepts are listed next:

- *Capital budgeting* is the process of analyzing potential expenditures on fixed assets and deciding whether the firm should undertake those investments.

- A *financial analysis* requires the firm to (1) estimate the investment outlay on the project, (2) estimate the expected cash inflows from the project and assess the riskiness of those flows, (3) determine the appropriate cost of capital at which to discount those flows, and (4) determine the project's profitability and breakeven characteristics.

- The most important, but also the most difficult, step in analyzing a project is estimating the *incremental cash flows* that the project will generate.

- In determining incremental cash flows, *opportunity costs* (the cash flows forgone by using an asset) must be considered, but *sunk costs* (cash outlays that cannot be recouped) are not included. Further, any impact of the project on the firm's *other cash flows* must be included in the analysis.

- *Tax laws* generally affect investor-owned firms in three ways: (1) taxes reduce a project's operating cash flows, (2) tax laws prescribe the depreciation expense that can be taken in any year, and (3) taxes affect a project's salvage value cash flow.

- Capital projects often require an investment in *net working capital* in addition to the investment in fixed assets. Such increases represent a cash outlay that, if material, must be included in the analysis. This investment is recovered when the project is terminated.

- *Cash flow estimation bias* can result if managers are overly optimistic in their forecasts. Estimation bias should be identified and dealt with in the decision process.

- A project may have some *strategic value* that is not accounted for in the estimated cash flows. At a minimum, strategic value should be noted and considered qualitatively in the analysis.

- The *effects of inflation* must be considered in project analyses. The best procedure is to build inflation effects directly into the component cash flow estimates.

- *Breakeven analysis* provides decision makers with insights concerning a project's profitability, liquidity, and risk. Intertemporal (time) breakeven is measured by the *payback period*.

- The *net present value (NPV)*, which is simply the sum of the present values of all of the project's net cash flows when discounted at the project's cost of capital, measures a project's dollar profitability. An NPV greater than $0 indicates that the project is profitable, and the higher the NPV, the more profitable the project.

- The *internal rate of return (IRR)*, which is that discount rate that forces a project's NPV to equal zero, measures a project's percentage rate of return profitability. If a project's IRR is greater than its cost of capital, the project is profitable, and the higher the IRR, the more profitable the project.

- The NPV and IRR profitability measures provide identical indications of profitability; that is, a project that is judged to be profitable by its NPV will also be profitable by its IRR. However, when mutually exclusive projects are being evaluated, NPV might rank a different project higher than IRR. This difference can occur because the two measures have different *reinvestment rate assumptions*: IRR assumes that cash flows can be reinvested at the project's IRR, while NPV assumes that cash flows can be reinvested at the project's cost of capital.

- The *modified internal rate of return (MIRR)*, which forces a project's cash flows to be reinvested at the project's cost of capital, is a better measure of a project's percentage rate of return than the IRR.

- If mutually exclusive projects have *unequal lives*, it may be necessary to adjust the analysis to place the projects on an equal life basis. This can be done using either the *replacement chain* approach or the *equivalent annual annuity (EAA)* approach.

- A project's profitability may be enhanced if it can be *abandoned* before the end of its physical life.

- The *net present social value (NPSV) model* formalizes the capital budgeting decision process for not-for-profit firms.

- Firms often use *project scoring matrixes* to subjectively incorporate a large number of factors, including financial and nonfinancial, into the capital budgeting decision process.

- The *post-audit* is a key element in capital budgeting. By comparing actual results with predicted results, decision makers can improve both their operations and their cash flow estimation process.

Notes

1. For a discussion of the cash flow estimation practices of some large firms, as well as some estimates of the inaccuracies involved, see R. A. Pohlman, E. S. Santiago, and F. L. Markel, "Cash Flow Estimation Practices of Large Firms," *Financial Management* (Summer 1988), 71–79.

2. For more on cash flow estimation bias, see S. W. Pruitt and L. J. Gitman, "Capital Budgeting Forecast Biases: Evidence from the *Fortune* 500," *Financial Management* (Spring 1987), 46–51.

3. In most situations, the strategic value of a project stems from managerial *options* brought about by the project that may or may not be undertaken. One way to assess the value of these options is to use option pricing techniques that were first developed to value stock options, which confer on their holders the right, but not the obligation, to buy (or sell) a particular stock at a specified price. The Spring 1987 edition of the *Midland Corporate Finance Journal* contains several articles related to the use of stock option concepts in capital budgeting analyses. For an overview, see S. C. Myers, "Finance Theory and Financial Strategy," 6–13.

4. If Bayside's third party payers reimbursed the hospital for capital expenses (capital pass-through), such reimbursements would be incorporated into

the analysis. In general, under these circumstances, capital pass-through would (1) lower the cost of debt component of the project's cost of capital and (2) create a reimbursement cash inflow tied to the project's depreciation schedule.

5. If Ann Arbor did not have taxable income to offset in Year 2, and had had no taxable income to offset in the three previous years, then the loss would have to be carried forward, and hence the tax benefit would not be immediately realized. In this situation, the tax shield value of the loss would be reduced, because it would be pushed into the future rather than recognized immediately.

6. For a more complete discussion of replacement analysis, see E. F. Brigham and L. C. Gapenski, *Intermediate Financial Management* (Fort Worth, TX: Dryden Press, 1996), chap. 8.

7. Another measure, the *discounted payback*, is similar to the straight payback, except that the cash flows in each year are discounted to Year 0 by the project's cost of capital prior to calculating the payback. Thus, the discounted payback solves the straight payback's problem of not considering the project's cost of capital in the payback calculation.

8. However, when mutually exclusive projects are being analyzed (two or more projects are being investigated, but only one can be chosen), the NPV and IRR rankings can conflict. That is, Project A could have the higher NPV, but Project B could have the higher IRR. In such situations, the NPV method is generally considered to be the best measure of profitability. See E. F. Brigham and L. C. Gapenski, *Intermediate Financial Management* (Fort Worth, TX: Dryden Press, 1996), chap. 7.

9. One could argue that not-for-profit firms do not have unlimited access to capital, and thus such firms cannot replace project cash flows with external capital. Furthermore, not-for-profit firms usually do not have sufficient capital to accept all projects that have positive NPVs, so the return on a not-for-profit firm's marginal project may not equal the firm's cost of capital. Nevertheless, for not-for-profit firms, the average aggregate return on projects will usually be close to the firm's cost of capital, so the cost of capital is still a better reinvestment rate than the project's IRR, especially when projects with exceptionally high or low IRRs are being evaluated.

10. This section is drawn primarily from an article by J. R. C. Wheeler and J. P. Clement. See "Capital Expenditure Decisions and the Role of the Not-for-Profit Hospital: An Application of the Social Goods Model," *Medical Care Review* (Winter 1990), 467–86.

Selected Additional References

Allen, R. J. 1989. "Proper Planning Reduces Risk in New Technology Acquisitions." *Healthcare Financial Management* (December): 48–56.

Bergman, J. T., and B. J. McIntyre. 1989. "Valuation Analysis." *Topics in Health Care Financing* (Summer): 32–40.

Campbell, C. 1994. "Hospital Plant and Equipment Replacement Decisions: A Survey of Hospital Financial Managers." *Hospital and Health Services Administration* (Winter): 538–56.

Chow, C. W., and A. H. McNamee. 1991. "Watch for Pitfalls of Discounted Cash Flow Techniques." *Healthcare Financial Management* (April): 34–43.

Chow, C. W., K. M. Haddad, and A. Wong-Boren. 1991. "Improving Subjective Decision Making in Health Care Administration," *Hospital and Health Services Administration* (Summer): 191–210.

Carroll, J. J., and G. D. Newbold. 1986. "Inflation, Risk, Replacement, Closure: Concerns in Capital Budgeting." *Healthcare Financial Management* (December): 64–68.

———. 1986. "NPV versus IRR: With Capital Budgeting, Which Do You Choose?" *Healthcare Financial Management* (November): 62–68.

Cleverley, W. O., and J. G. Felkner. 1984. "The Association of Capital Budgeting Techniques with Hospital Financial Performance." *Health Care Management Review* (Summer): 45–55.

Gapenski, L. C. 1989. "A Better Approach to Internal Rate of Return." *Healthcare Financial Management* (April): 93–99.

———. 1989."Analysis Provides Test for Profitability of New Services." *Healthcare Financial Management* (November): 48–58.

———. 1993. "Capital Investment Analysis: Three Methods." *Healthcare Financial Management* (August): 60–66.

Gordon, D. C., and D. F. Londal. 1989. "Guidelines to Capital Investment." *Topics in Health Care Financing* (Summer): 9–17.

Horowitz, J. L., and P. F. Straley. 1988. "Developing Investment Criteria: There Is More To It Than Financial Criteria Alone." *Topics in Health Care Financing* (Fall): 23–31.

Horowitz, J. L. 1993. "Contribution Margin Analysis: A Case Study." *Healthcare Financial Management* (June): 129–33.

Kamath, R. R., and J. Elmer. 1989. "Capital Investment Decisions in Hospitals: Survey Results." *Health Care Management Review* (Spring): 45–56.

Kennedy, W. F., and D. A. Plath. 1994. "A Return-Based Alternative to IRR Evaluations." *Healthcare Financial Management* (March): 38–49.

Manecke, S. R. 1993. "Practice Acquisition: Buy or Build." *Healthcare Financial Management* (December): 33–41.

Mellen, C. M. 1992. "Valuing a Long-Term Care Facility." *Healthcare Financial Management* (October): 20–25.

Meyer, A. D. 1985. "Hospital Capital Budgeting: Fusion of Rationality, Politics and Ceremony." *Health Care Management Review* (Spring): 17–27.

Ryan, J. B., M. E. Ward, and D. S. Kolb. 1990. "Capital Management Balances Charitable, Financial Goals." *Healthcare Financial Management* (March): 32–40.

Ryan, J. B., and M. E. Ward (eds.). 1992. "Capital Management." Fall issue of *Topics in Health Care Financing*.

Schramm, C. J., and G. D. Pillari. 1987. "Investing in the Wrong Future for Hospitals." *Health Care Management Review* (Fall): 31–37.

Straley, P. F., and C. R. Swaim. 1993. "Financial Analysis of Medical Office Buildings." *Topics in Health Care Financing* (Spring): 76–85.

Watts, D., D. L. Finney, and B. Louie. 1993. "Integrating Technology Assessment into the Capital Budgeting Process." *Healthcare Financial Management* (February): 21–29.

Wedig, G. J., M. Hassan, and F. A. Sloan. 1989. "Hospital Investment Decisions and the Cost of Capital." *Journal of Business:* 517–37.

Case 10

Bay City Medical Center: Breakeven Analysis

Bay City Medical Center (BCMC), an acute care hospital with 300 beds and 160 staff physicians, is one of 75 hospitals owned and operated by Health Services of America, a for-profit, publicly owned company. The hospital operates an emergency room within the hospital complex and a stand-alone walk-in clinic located about two miles from the hospital across the street from the area's largest shopping mall. Although there are two other acute care hospitals serving the same general population, BCMC historically has been highly profitable due to its well-appointed facilities, fine medical staff, reputation for quality care, and the amount of individual attention given to its patients.

In spite of its overall financial soundness, Carol Rigal, BCMC's CEO, is concerned about the hospital's walk-in clinic. About ten years ago, all three area hospitals jumped onto the walk-in clinic bandwagon, and in a short time there were five clinics scattered around the city. Now, only three are left, and none of them appears to be a big money maker. Rigal wonders if BCMC should continue to operate its clinic or close it down. The clinic is currently handling a patient load of 45 visits per day, but it has the physical capacity to handle many more visits, up to 85 a day. Rigal's decision has been complicated by the fact that John Samuelson, BCMC's marketing director, has been pushing to embark on a new marketing program for the clinic. He believes that an expanded marketing effort aimed at local businesses would bring in a sufficient number of new patients to make the clinic a financial success.

Rigal has asked Marcia Miller, BCMC's CFO, to look into the whole matter of the walk-in clinic. In their meeting, Rigal stated that she visualizes three potential outcomes for the clinic: (1) the clinic could be closed; (2) the clinic could continue to operate as is, that is, without expanding its marketing program; or (3) the clinic could continue to operate, but with the expanded marketing effort. As a starting point for the analysis, Miller has collected the most recent historical financial and operating data for the clinic, which is summarized in Table 1. In assessing the historical data, Miller noted that one competing clinic had just closed its doors in December 1996. Further, a review of several years of financial data revealed that the BCMC clinic does not have a pronounced seasonal usage or cost pattern.

Next, Miller met several times with the clinic's administrator, Mark Crenshaw. The primary purpose of the meetings was to estimate the additional costs that would have to be borne if clinic usage rose above the current January/February average level of 45 visits per day. Any incremental usage would require additional expenditures for administrative and medical supplies, estimated to be $4.00 per patient visit for medical supplies, such as tongue blades and rubber gloves, and $1.00 per patient visit for administrative supplies, such as file folders and clinical record sheets.

Because of the relatively low usage level, the clinic has purposely been staffed at the bare minimum. In fact, some clinic employees have started to grumble about not being able to do their jobs well due to patient overload. Thus, any increase in patient load would require immediate administrative and medical staff increases. Further, at an increase of 11 visits, the clinic would have to replace a part-time receptionist/record keeper with a full-time employee. At an additional 21 visits per day, another part-time nurse and physician would have to be added to the clinic's staff, and another part-time clerk would have to be hired if patient visits increased by 31 per day. These incremental costs are summarized in Table 2.

Miller also learned that the building is leased on a long-term basis, but the lease payment is adjusted every January 1 to reflect current interest rates, as measured by the one-year constant maturity T-bill index. BCMC could cancel the lease, but the lease contract calls for a cancellation penalty of three months rent, or $37,500 at current interest rates. In addition, Miller was startled to read in the morning paper that Baptist Hospital, BCMC's major competitor, had just bought the city's largest primary care group practice, and Baptist's CEO was quoted as saying that more group practice acquisitions are planned.

Finally, Miller met with BCMC's marketing director and clinic administrator to learn more about the proposed expansion of the clinic's marketing program. The primary focus of the new marketing program would be on occupational health services (OHS). Basically, OHS involves

Table 1   Clinic Historical Financial Data

| | CY 1996 | Jan 1997 | Feb 1997 | Monthly Averages | | Total |
				1996	Jan/Feb 1997	
Number of visits	14,522	1,365	1,335	1,210	1,350	1,230
Gross revenue	$578,237	$58,231	$57,996	$48,186	$58,114	$49,605
Allowance percentage	5.1%	5.5%	5.6%	5.1%	5.6%	5.2%
Net revenue	$548,747	$55,028	$54,748	$44,729	$54,888	$47,037
Salaries and wages	$154,250	$13,540	$13,544	$12,854	$13,542	$12,952
Physician fees	192,000	18,000	18,000	16,000	18,000	16,286
Malpractice insurance	31,440	3,215	3,215	2,620	3,215	2,705
Travel and education	5,365	538	665	447	602	469
General insurance	8,112	843	843	676	843	700
Subscriptions	189	0	0	16	0	14
Electricity	11,820	1,124	1,029	985	1,077	998
Water	1,260	135	142	105	139	110
Equipment rental	1,260	105	105	105	105	105
Building lease	155,745	12,500	12,500	12,979	12,500	12,910
Other operating expenses	103,779	8,152	7,923	8,648	8,038	8,561
Total operating expenses	$665,220	$58,152	$57,966	$55,435	$58,059	$55,810
Net profit (loss)	($116,473)	($3,124)	($3,218)	($9,706)	($3,171)	($8,773)
Gross margin (%)	-21.2%	-5.7%	-5.9%	-21.2%	-5.8%	-18.7%

Table 2   Monthly Incremental Cost Data

		Number of Additional Visits per Day			
	0	1–10	11–20	21–30	31–40
Variable Costs					
Medical supplies			$4.00 per visit		
Administrative supplies			$1.00 per visit		
Total monthly variable costs			$5.00 per visit		
Semifixed Costs					
Salaries and wages		$1,000	$2,000	$ 3,000	$ 4,000
Physician fees		5,000	5,000	10,000	10,000
Total monthly semifixed costs	$0	$6,000	$7,000	$13,000	$14,000
Fixed Costs					
Marketing secretarial salary	$1,500	$1,500	$1,500	$ 1,500	$ 1,500
Advertising expenses	500	500	500	500	500
Total monthly fixed costs	$2,000	$2,000	$2,000	$ 2,000	$ 2,000

providing medical care to local businesses, including (1) physical examinations; (2) treatment of illnesses that occur during working hours; and (3) treatment of work-related injuries, especially those covered by workers' compensation. Although some of the clinic's current business is OHS-related, Samuelson believes that a strong marketing effort coupled with specialized OHS record keeping could bring additional patients to the clinic. The proposed marketing expansion requires a secretary to run the clinic's OHS program. Additionally, the new marketing program would incur advertising costs for newspaper, radio, and TV adds, as well as for brochures and handouts. The incremental costs of the expanded marketing program are also summarized in Table 2.

With this information in hand, and a spreadsheet on the screen, Miller began to construct a model that would provide Rigal with information that would help her make a rational, informed decision. At first, Miller planned to conduct a standard capital budgeting NPV/IRR analysis. Then she realized that the expanded marketing program requires no actual capital investment. However, she also realized that no valid data were available on the incremental increase in visits that would be generated by the expanded marketing program. Finally, she remembered that Rigal requested that the analysis consider the inherent profitability of the clinic without the expanded marketing program.

With these points in mind, Miller thought that a breakeven analysis would be very useful in making the final decision. Specifically, she wanted to find the projected profitability of BCMC's walk-in clinic if usage were to continue at its current level; the number of additional visits per day that would be required to break even without the new marketing program; and the number of additional visits per day that would be required to break even assuming that the marketing program were expanded. Additionally, it would be useful to know the incremental value of the marketing program, that is, the number of additional daily visits that the new program would have to bring in to make it worthwhile.

In earlier conversations, Carol Rigal also had wondered if the clinic could "inflate" its way to profitability. That is, if usage remained at its current level, could the clinic be expected to become profitable in, say, five years, solely due to inflationary increases in revenues? All-in-all, Miller must consider all relevant factors, both quantitative and qualitative, and come up with a reasonable recommendation.

11

Capital Budgeting Risk Analysis

In Chapter 10, we discussed the basics of capital budgeting, including cash flow estimation, breakeven measures, and profitability measures. In this chapter, we discuss capital budgeting risk analysis, which includes three elements: (1) defining the type of risk relevant to the project, (2) measuring the project's risk, and (3) incorporating that risk assessment into the capital budgeting decision process. Although risk analysis is a key element in all financial decisions, the importance of capital investment decisions to a health care organization's success or failure makes risk analysis vital in such decisions.

We know that the higher the risk associated with an investment, the higher its required rate of return. This principle is just as valid for health care organizations making capital expenditure decisions as it is for individuals making personal investment decisions. Thus, the ultimate goal in project risk analysis is to ensure that the cost of capital used in a project's profitability analysis properly reflects the riskiness of that project. In Chapter 8, we discussed how to estimate a firm's overall, or corporate, cost of capital. This value reflects the cost of capital to the organization based on its aggregate risk, that is, based on the riskiness of the firm's "average project." In project risk analysis, we assess a project's risk relative to the firm's average project—does the project have average risk, below-average risk, or above-average risk? Then we modify the corporate cost of capital to reflect the project's differential risk. High-risk projects are assigned a project cost of capital that is higher than the overall cost of capital, average risk projects are evaluated at the cost of capital, and low-risk projects are assigned a discount rate that is less than the firm's cost of capital.

Types of Project Risk

As discussed in Chapter 5, three separate and distinct types of financial risk can be defined: (1) stand-alone risk, which views the risk of a project as if it were held in isolation and hence ignores portfolio effects both within the firm and among equity investors; (2) corporate risk, which views the risk of a project within the context of the firm's portfolio of projects; and (3) market risk, which views a project's risk from the perspective of a shareholder who holds a well-diversified portfolio of stocks.[1] The type of risk that is most relevant to a particular capital budgeting decision depends on the number of projects that the firm holds and the form of ownership.

Stand-alone risk

Conceptually, *stand-alone risk* is only relevant in one situation: when a not-for-profit firm (which has no shareholders) is evaluating its first project. In this situation, the project will be operated in isolation, and no portfolio diversification is present: the firm does not have a collection (portfolio) of different projects, nor does the firm have stockholders who hold portfolios of stocks of different companies. Although stand-alone risk is generally not relevant in real world decision making, the other types of risk, which are more relevant, are very difficult, if not impossible, to measure. Thus, in practice, most project risk analyses measure stand-alone risk, and then subjective adjustments are applied to convert the project's assessed stand-alone risk to either corporate risk or market risk.

Stand-alone risk is present in a project whenever there is some chance of a return that is less than the expected return. In effect, a project is risky whenever its cash flows are not known with certainty. Furthermore, the greater the probability of a return far below the expected return, the greater the risk. In this context, stand-alone risk can be measured by the *standard deviation* of the project's profitability, as measured typically by net present value (NPV) or internal rate of return (IRR). Since standard deviation measures the dispersion of a distribution about its expected value, the larger the standard deviation, the greater the dispersion, and hence the greater the probability of the project's profitability (NPV or IRR) being far below that expected.

In comparing the stand-alone risk of one project to another, or comparing a project's stand-alone risk to that of the firm in the aggregate, it is often useful to use *coefficient of variation (CV)* as the risk measure. Remember that CV, which measures risk per unit of return, is the standard deviation divided by the expected value. By standardizing the risk measure, CV is a better measure of relative risk when projects being compared have widely differing profitabilities (NPVs or IRRs).

Corporate, or within-firm, risk

The previous section discussed stand-alone risk, which is measured by a project's standard deviation or coefficient of variation of profitability, and which is relevant only when a not-for-profit firm is considering its first project. In reality, firms usually offer a myriad of different products or services, and thus can be thought of as having a large number (hundreds or even thousands) of individual projects. For example, MinuteMan Healthcare, a New England HMO, offers health care services to a large number of diverse employee groups in numerous service areas, and each different group could be considered to be a separate project. In this situation, the stand-alone risk of a project under consideration by MinuteMan is not relevant, because the project will not be held in isolation. The relevant risk of a new project to MinuteMan is its contribution to the HMO's overall risk, or the impact of the project on the variability of the overall profitability of the firm. This type of risk, which is relevant when the project is part of a not-for-profit firm's portfolio of projects, is called *corporate risk*.

Conceptually, a project's corporate risk is measured by its corporate beta coefficient, which reflects the volatility of the project's profitability relative to that of the firm as a whole, which has a corporate beta of 1.0. A project with a high corporate beta, say, 1.5, has returns that are more volatile than the firm's average project, and hence has high corporate risk. Similarly, a project with a low corporate beta, say, 0.5, has returns that are less volatile than the aggregate firm, and hence has low corporate risk. Note that a project's corporate risk depends on the context (the firm's other projects), so a project may have high corporate risk to one firm, but low corporate risk to another, particularly when the two firms operate in widely different business lines.

Market risk

Market risk is generally viewed as the relevant risk for project risk assessment by investor-owned firms. The goal of shareholder wealth maximization implies that a project's returns, as well as its risk, should be defined and measured from the shareholders' perspective. The riskiness of an individual project, as seen by a well-diversified shareholder, is not the riskiness of the project as if it were owned and operated in isolation (its stand-alone risk), nor is it the contribution of the project to the riskiness of the firm (its corporate risk). Most shareholders hold a large diversified portfolio of stocks of many firms, which can be thought of as a very large diversified portfolio of individual projects. Thus, the risk of any single project as seen by a firm's stockholders is its contribution to the riskiness of a well-diversified stock portfolio, which is measured by the project's market beta.

A project's market beta measures the volatility of the project's returns relative to the returns on a well-diversified portfolio of stocks. To managers of investor-owned firms, a project's market risk relative to the market risk of the firm's other projects is measured by comparing the project's market beta to the firm's market beta. A project with a market beta higher than the firm's market beta has higher-than-average market risk, where average is defined as the market risk of the firm's stock. Note that a project's absolute market risk, as measured by its market beta, is the same to all firms (assuming the cash flows are the same to all firms), but the market risk of a project relative to the firm's other projects depends on the aggregate market risk of the firm.

Self-Test Questions:

What are the three types of project risk?

How is each type measured, both in absolute and relative terms?

Relationships among Stand-Alone, Corporate, and Market Risk

Once one understands the three different types of project risk, and the situations in which each is relevant, it is tempting to say that (1) stand-alone risk is almost never important, (2) not-for-profit firms should focus on a project's corporate risk, and (3) investor-owned firms should focus on a project's market risk. Unfortunately, things aren't quite that simple.

First, it is almost impossible in practice to quantify a project's corporate or market risk because it is extremely difficult (some practitioners would say impossible) to estimate the prospective returns distributions for given economic states for either the project, the firm as a whole, or for the market. If these distributions cannot be estimated, then it is impossible to precisely quantify a project's corporate or market risk.

Fortunately, as we shall demonstrate in the next section, it is possible to get a rough idea of the relative stand-alone risk of a project. Thus, managers can make statements such as Project A has above-average risk, Project B has below-average risk, or Project C has average risk, all in the stand-alone sense. Once a project's stand-alone risk has been assessed, the primary factor in converting stand-alone risk to either corporate or market risk is correlation. If a project's returns are expected to be highly positively correlated with the firm's returns, then high stand-alone risk translates to high corporate risk. Similarly, if the firm's returns are expected to be highly correlated with the stock market's returns, then high corporate risk translates to high market risk. The same analogies hold when the project is judged to have average or low stand-alone risk.

Most projects will be in a firm's primary line of business, and hence will be in the same line of business as the firm's average project. Since all projects in the same line of business are generally influenced by the same economic factors, such projects' returns are usually highly correlated. When this situation exists, a project's stand-alone risk is a good proxy for its corporate risk. Furthermore, most projects' returns are also positively correlated with the returns on other assets in the economy: most assets have high returns when the economy is strong, and low returns when the economy is weak. When this situation holds, a project's stand-alone risk is a good proxy for its market risk.

Thus, for most projects, the stand-alone risk assessment also gives good insights into a project's corporate and market risk. The only exception is when a project's returns are expected to be independent of or negatively correlated to the firm's average project. In these situations, considerable judgment is required, because the stand-alone risk assessment will overstate the project's corporate risk. Similarly, if a project's returns are expected to be independent of or negatively correlated to the market's returns, the project's stand-alone risk overstates its market risk.

A second risk assessment problem arises with investor-owned health care firms. Finance theory specifies that investor-owned firms should focus on market risk when making capital budgeting decisions. However, most health care firms, even proprietary ones, have corporate goals that focus on the provision of quality health care services in addition to shareholder wealth maximization. Furthermore, a proprietary health care firm's stability and financial condition, which primarily depends on corporate risk, is important to all of the firm's other stakeholders—to its managers, physicians, patients, community, and so on. Some financial theorists even argue that stockholders, including those that are well diversified, consider factors other than market risk when setting required returns. Considering all this, it may be reasonable for managers of proprietary health care firms to be just as concerned about corporate risk as are managers of not-for-profit firms. Fortunately, in most real world situations, a project's risk in the corporate sense will be the same as its risk in the market sense.[2]

Self-Test Questions:

How are stand-alone, corporate, and market risk related?

Should investor-owned firms focus exclusively on a project's market risk?

Project Risk Analysis Illustration

To illustrate project risk analysis, consider Bayside Memorial Hospital's evaluation of a new magnetic resonance imaging (MRI) system presented in Chapter 10. Table 11.1 contains the project's cash flow analysis. If all of the project's component cash flows were known with certainty, say, fixed by contract, the projected net cash flows would be known with certainty, and hence the project would have no risk. However, in most project analyses, future cash flows are uncertain, so risk is present.

The starting point for analyzing a project's stand-alone risk involves estimating the uncertainty inherent in the project's cash flows. Most of the individual cash flows in Table 11.1 are subject to uncertainty. For example, volume was projected at 40 scans per week. However, volume would almost certainly be higher or lower than the 40 scan forecast. In effect, the volume estimate is really an expected value taken from some probability distribution of potential usage, as are many of the other values listed in Table 11.1. The distributions could be relatively "tight," reflecting small standard deviations and low risk, or they could be relatively "flat," denoting a great deal of uncertainty about the variable in question, and hence a high degree of risk.

The nature of the component cash flow distributions, and their correlations with one another, determine the nature of the project's profitability distribution, and thus the project's stand-alone risk. In the following sections, we discuss four techniques for assessing a project's stand-alone risk: (1) sensitivity analysis, (2) scenario analysis, (3) Monte Carlo simulation, and (4) decision tree analysis.

Sensitivity Analysis

Intuitively, we know that many of the variables which determine a project's cash flows are subject to some type of a probability distribution

Table 11.1 Bayside Memorial Hospital: MRI Site Cash Flow Analysis

			Cash Revenues and Costs			
	0	1	2	3	4	5
1. System cost	($1,500,000)					
2. Related expenses	(1,000,000)					
3. Gross revenues		$1,000,000	$1,050,000	$1,102,500	$1,157,625	$1,215,506
4. Less: Deductions		250,000	262,500	275,625	289,406	303,877
5. Net revenues		$ 750,000	$ 787,500	$ 826,875	$ 868,219	$ 911,630
6. Less: Labor costs		50,000	52,500	55,125	57,881	60,775
7. Maintenance costs		150,000	157,500	165,375	173,644	182,326
8. Supplies		30,000	31,500	33,075	34,729	36,465
9. Incremental overhead		10,000	10,500	11,025	11,576	12,155
10. Depreciation		350,000	350,000	350,000	350,000	350,000
11. Operating income		$ 160,000	$ 185,500	$ 212,275	$ 240,389	$ 269,908
12. Taxes		0	0	0	0	0
13. Net operating income		$ 160,000	$ 185,500	$ 212,275	$ 240,389	$ 269,908
14. Plus: Depreciation		350,000	350,000	350,000	350,000	350,000
15. Plus: Net salvage value						750,000
16. Net cash flow	($2,500,000)	$ 510,000	$ 535,500	$ 562,275	$ 590,389	$1,369,908

Net present value (NPV) = $82,493.
Internal rate of return (IRR) = 11.1%.
Modified IRR (MIRR) = 10.7%.

rather than known with certainty. We also know that if a key input variable such as volume changes, so will the project's profitability. *Sensitivity analysis* is a technique that indicates exactly how much a project's profitability (NPV, IRR, or MIRR) will change in response to a given change in a single input variable, other things held constant.

Sensitivity analysis begins with a *base case* analysis developed using *expected values* for all uncertain variables. To illustrate, assume that Bayside's managers believe that all of the MRI project's component cash flows are known with certainty except for weekly volume, salvage value, and cost of capital. The expected values for these variables (volume = 40, salvage value = $750,000, cost of capital = 10%) were used in Table 11.1 to obtain the base case NPV of $82,493. Sensitivity analysis is designed to provide decision makers the answers to such questions as these: What if volume is less than the expected level? What if salvage value is more than expected? What if the cost of capital is higher than expected?

In a sensitivity analysis, each uncertain variable is usually changed by a fixed percentage amount above and below its expected value, holding all other variables constant at their expected values. The resulting NPVs (or IRRs or MIRRs) are recorded and plotted. Table 11.2 presents the sensitivity analyses for the MRI project considering three uncertain variables: volume, salvage value, and cost of capital. Figure 11.1 plots the results on a single graph.

The slopes of the lines in Figure 11.1 show how sensitive the MRI project's NPV is to changes in each of the uncertain input variables: the steeper the slope, the more sensitive NPV is to a change in the variable. Note that spreadsheet models are ideally suited for performing sensitivity analysis, because such models automatically recalculate NPV when an input value is changed.[3]

Table 11.2   MRI Project Sensitivity Analysis

Change from Base Level	*Net Present Value (NPV)*		
	Volume	*Salvage Value*	*Cost of Capital*
−30%	($814,053)	($ 57,215)	$330,476
−20	(515,193)	(10,646)	243,969
−10	(216,350)	35,923	161,382
0	82,493	82,493	82,493
+10	381,335	129,062	7,095
+20	680,178	175,631	(65,004)
+30	979,020	222,200	(133,985)

Figure 11.1   Sensitivity Analysis Graphs

Net Present Value
(thousands of dollars)

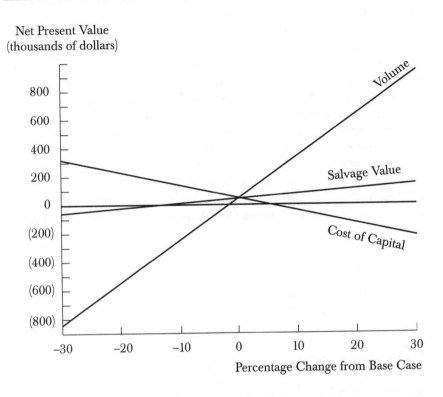

Percentage Change from Base Case

We see that the MRI project's NPV is very sensitive to volume and mildly sensitive to changes in the cost of capital and salvage value. Note that the cost of capital sensitivity plot has a negative slope, because increases in the cost of capital have a negative impact on NPV. If we were comparing two projects, the one with the steeper sensitivity lines would be regarded as riskier because a relatively small error in estimating a variable, for example volume, would produce a large error in the project's projected NPV.

Although sensitivity analysis is widely used in project risk analysis, it does have severe limitations. Suppose that Bayside Memorial Hospital had a contract with a Blue Cross HMO that guaranteed a minimum MRI usage at a fixed reimbursement rate. In that situation, the project might not be very risky at all, in spite of the fact that the sensitivity analysis showed NPV to be highly sensitive to changes in volume. In general, a project's stand-alone risk depends on both the sensitivity of its profitability to changes in key input variables and the ranges of likely values of these variables. Because sensitivity analysis considers only the first factor, it can give misleading results. Furthermore, sensitivity analysis does not consider any interactions among the uncertain input variables—it considers each variable independently of the others.

Despite the shortcomings of sensitivity analysis as a risk measure, it does provide decision makers with valuable information. First, it provides profitability breakeven information for the uncertain variables. For example, Table 11.1 tells us quickly that just a 10 percent decrease in expected volume, which would be 36 scans per week, makes the project unprofitable, whereas the project remains profitable if salvage value falls by 10 percent. Second, sensitivity analysis tells decision makers which input variables are most critical to the project's profitability. In our MRI example, volume is clearly the key input variable (of the three we examined), so Bayside's analysts should ensure that the volume estimate is the best possible.

Self-Test Questions:

Briefly describe sensitivity analysis.

What are its strengths and weaknesses?

Scenario Analysis

Scenario analysis is a stand-alone risk analysis technique that considers (1) the sensitivity of NPV to changes in key variables, (2) the likely range of variable values, and (3) the interactions among variables. To conduct a scenario analysis, the managers pick a "bad" set of circumstances (low volume, low salvage value, and so on), an average or "most likely" set, and a "good set." The resulting input values are then used to create a probability distribution of NPV.

To illustrate scenario analysis, assume that Bayside's managers regard a drop in weekly volume below 30 scans as very unlikely, and a volume value above 50 as also improbable. On the other hand, salvage value could be as low as $500,000 or as high as $1,000,000. The most likely values are 40 scans per week for volume and $750,000 for salvage value. Thus, volume of 30 and a $500,000 salvage value define the lower bound, or *worst case* (pessimistic) scenario, while volume of 50 and a salvage value of $1,000,000 define the upper bound, or *best case* (optimistic) scenario.

Bayside can now use the worst, most likely, and best case values for the input variables to obtain the corresponding NPVs. We performed the analysis using a spreadsheet model, and Table 11.3 summarizes the results. We see that the most likely case results in a positive NPV; the worst case produces a negative NPV; and the best case results in a very large positive NPV. We can now use these results to determine the expected NPV, standard deviation of NPV, and coefficient of variation of NPV. For this, we need an estimate of the probabilities of occurrence of the three scenarios. Suppose Bayside's managers estimate that there is a 20 percent chance of the worst case occurring, a 60 percent chance of the most likely case, and a 20 percent chance of the best case. Of course, it is very difficult to estimate scenario probabilities accurately.

Table 11.3 contains a discrete distribution of returns, so we can find the expected NPV as follows:

$$\begin{aligned} \textit{Expected NPV} &= 0.20(-\$819,844) + 0.60(\$82,493) \\ &\quad + 0.20(\$984,829) \\ &= \$82,493. \end{aligned}$$

Note that the expected NPV in the scenario analysis is the same as the base case NPV, $82,493. The consistency of results occurs because the expected values of the uncertain variables in the scenario analysis—40 scans for volume and $750,000 for salvage value—are the same as the expected values used in the Table 11.1 base case analysis. If inconsistencies exist between the expected NPVs in the base case and scenario analyses, then the two analyses have inconsistent input assumptions. Such inconsistencies should be identified and removed to ensure that common assumptions are used throughout the analysis.

Table 11.3 MRI Project Scenario Analysis

Scenario	Probability of Outcome	Volume	Salvage Value	NPV
Worst case	0.20	30	$ 500,000	($819,844)
Most likely case	0.60	40	750,000	82,493
Best case	0.20	50	1,000,000	984,829
Expected value		40	$ 750,000	$ 82,493
Standard deviation				$570,688
Coefficient of variation				6.9

The standard deviation of NPV, as shown below, is $570,688:

$$\sigma_{NPV} = [0.20(-\$819,844 - \$82,493)^2 + 0.60(\$82,493 \\ - \$82,493)^2 + 0.20(\$984,829 - \$82,493)^2]^{\frac{1}{2}} \\ = \$570,688,$$

and the MRI project's coefficient of variation (CV) of NPV is 6.9:

$$CV = \frac{\sigma}{Expected\ NPV} = \frac{\$570,688}{\$82,493} = 6.9.$$

The MRI project's standard deviation and coefficient of variation measure its stand-alone risk. Suppose, when a similar scenario analysis is applied to Bayside's aggregate cash flows, or average project, it has a coefficient of variation of NPV in the range of 1.5 to 2.5. Then, on the basis of its stand-alone risk, Bayside's managers would conclude that the MRI project is riskier than the firm's average project, so it would be classified as a high-risk project.

Scenario analysis can also be used in a less mathematical way. The worst case NPV, a loss of about $800,000 for the MRI project, represents an estimate of the worst possible financial consequences of the project. If Bayside can absorb such a loss without much impact on its financial condition, then the project does not represent a significant financial danger to the hospital. Conversely, if such a loss would mean financial ruin for the hospital, its managers might be unwilling to undertake the project, regardless of its profitability under the most likely and best case scenarios.

While scenario analysis provides useful information about a project's stand-alone risk, it is limited in two ways. First, it only considers a few discrete states of the economy, and hence profitability outcomes (NPVs or IRRs or MIRRs), for the project. In reality, there are an almost infinite number of possibilities. Although the illustrative scenario analysis contained only three scenarios, it could be expanded to include more states of the economy, say five or seven. However, there is a practical limit on how many scenarios can be included in a scenario analysis.

Second, scenario analysis—at least as normally conducted—implies a very definite relationship among the uncertain variables. That is, our analysis assumed that the worst value for volume (30 scans per week) would occur at the same time as the worst value for salvage value ($500,000), because the worst case scenario was defined by combining the worst possible value of each uncertain variable. Although this relationship (all worst values occurring together) may hold in some situations, in others it may not hold. For example, if volume is low, maybe the MRI will have less wear and tear, and hence be worth more after five years of use. Then the worst value for volume should be coupled with the best salvage value. Conversely, poor volume may be symptomatic of poor medical acceptance of the MRI, and hence lead to limited demand for used equipment and a low salvage value. Scenario analysis tends to create extreme profitability values for the worst and best cases because it automatically combines all worst and best input values, even if these values actually have only a remote chance of occurring together. The next section describes a method of assessing a project's stand-alone risk that deals with these two problems.

Self-Test Questions:

Briefly describe scenario analysis.

What are the strengths and weaknesses of scenario analysis?

Monte Carlo Simulation

Monte Carlo simulation, so named because it grew out of work on the mathematics of casino gambling, describes uncertainty in terms of continuous probability distributions rather than just a few discrete values, and hence it provides a better view of a project's risk than does scenario analysis. Although the use of Monte Carlo simulation in capital investment decisions was first proposed over 25 years ago, it has not been used extensively in practice, primarily because it required a mainframe computer along with relatively powerful financial planning or statistical software. Recently, however, Monte Carlo simulation software has become available for personal computers as an add-in to spreadsheet software. Since more and more financial analysis is being done with spreadsheets, Monte Carlo simulation is now accessible to virtually all health care organizations.

The first step in a Monte Carlo simulation is to create a model that calculates the project's net cash flows and profitability measures, just as we have done for Bayside's MRI project. The relatively certain variables are estimated as single, or point, values in the model, while continuous probability distributions are used to specify the uncertain cash flow variables. Once the model has been created, the simulation software automatically executes the following steps:

1. The Monte Carlo program chooses a single random value for each uncertain variable on the basis of its specified probability distribution.

2. The value selected for each uncertain variable, along with the point values for the relatively certain variables, are combined in the model to estimate the net cash flow for each year.

3. Using the net cash flow data, the model calculates the project's profitability, say, as measured by NPV. A single completion of Steps 1, 2, and 3 constitutes one iteration, or "run," in the Monte Carlo simulation.

4. The Monte Carlo software repeats the above steps many times, say 5,000, resulting in 5,000 NPVs (or IRRs or MIRRs).

The ultimate result of the simulation is an NPV (or IRR or MIRR) probability distribution based on 5,000 individual "scenarios," and hence which encompasses all of the likely financial outcomes. Monte Carlo software usually displays the results of the simulation in both tabular and graphical forms, and automatically calculates summary statistical data such as expected value, standard deviation, and skewness.

To illustrate Monte Carlo simulation, again consider Bayside Hospital's MRI project. As in the scenario analysis, we have simplified the illustration by specifying the distributions for only two key variables, weekly volume and salvage value. Weekly volume is not expected to vary by more than ±10 scans from its expected value of 40 scans. Since this is a symmetrical situation, the normal distribution can be used to represent the uncertainty inherent in volume. In a normal distribution, the expected value plus or minus three standard deviations will encompass almost the entire distribution. Thus, a normal distribution with an expected value of 40 scans and a standard deviation of $10/3 = 3.33$ scans is a reasonable description of the uncertainty inherent in weekly volume.

We chose a triangular distribution for salvage value because it specifically fixes the upper and lower bounds, whereas the tails of a normal distribution are, in theory, limitless. The triangular distribution is also used extensively when the input distribution is nonsymmetrical because it can easily accommodate skewness. We specified salvage value uncertainty with a triangular distribution with a lower limit of $500,000, a most likely value of $750,000, and an upper limit of $1,000,000.

We used the basic MRI model containing these two continuous distributions, plus a Monte Carlo add-in program, to conduct a simulation with 5,000 iterations. The output is summarized in Table 11.4, and the resulting probability distribution of NPV is plotted in Figure 11.2. The mean, or expected, NPV, $82,498, is about the same as the base case NPV and expected NPV indicated in the scenario analysis, $82,493. In theory, all three results should be the same, because the expected values for all input variables are the same in the three analyses. However, there is some randomness in the Monte Carlo simulation, and this leads to an expected NPV that is slightly different from the others. The more iterations that are run, the more likely the Monte Carlo NPV will be the same as the base case NPV.

The standard deviation and coefficient of variation of NPV are lower in the simulation analysis, because the NPV distribution in the

Table 11.4   Simulation Results Summary

Expected NPV	$82,498
Minimum NPV	($951,760)
Maximum NPV	$970,191
Probability of a positive NPV	62.8%
Standard deviation	$256,212
Coefficient of variation	3.1
Skewness	0.002

Figure 11.2   Monte Carlo Simulation: NPV Probability Distribution

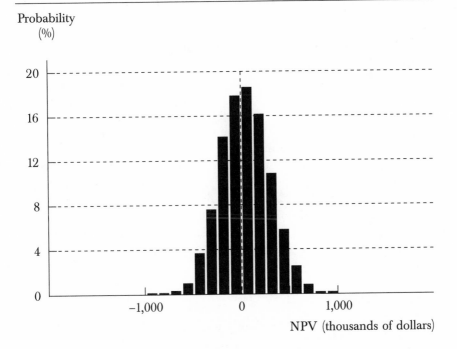

Probability (%)

NPV (thousands of dollars)

simulation contains values within the entire range of possible outcomes, while the NPV distribution in the scenario analysis contains only the most likely value and the best and worst case extremes.

In this illustration, volume uncertainty was restricted to a single year, the first year of operating the MRI site. That is, the value chosen by the Monte Carlo software for volume in Year 1, say 40 scans, was used as the volume input for the remaining four years in that iteration of the simulation analysis. As an alternative, the normal distribution for Year 1 could be applied to each year separately, and hence specify individual volumes for each year. Then, the Monte Carlo software might choose 35 as the value for Year 1, 43 as the Year 2 input, 32 for Year 3, and so on. But does this seem realistic? Probably not—a high usage in the first year presumably means strong acceptance of MR imaging, and hence high usage in the remaining years. Similarly, low usage in the first year probably portends low usage in future years.

Note that the volume and salvage value variables were treated as independent in the simulation; that is, the value chosen from the salvage value distribution was not related to the value chosen from the volume distribution. Thus, in any run, a low volume could be coupled with a high salvage value, and vice versa. If Bayside's managers believed that high usage at the hospital indicates a strong national demand for MRI systems, then they might specify a positive correlation between these variables. This would tend to increase the riskiness of the project, since low volume could not be offset by a high salvage value. Conversely, if the salvage value is more a function of the technological advances that occur over the next five years than local usage, then it might be best to specify the variables as being independent, as was done. Mechanically, it is easy to incorporate into a simulation model both the probability distributions for uncertain variables as well as the correlations among variables and in a single variable over time. However, it is much more difficult to realistically specify what those distributions and correlations should be.

As in scenario analysis, the project's simulation results must be compared with a similar analysis of the firm's average project. If Bayside's average project has a Monte Carlo simulation coefficient of variation of NPV of 0.5 to 1.0, then, on the basis of the Monte Carlo simulation, the MRI project would be judged to have above-average (high) stand-alone risk.

Self-Test Questions:

Briefly describe Monte Carlo simulation.

What are its strengths and weaknesses?

Decision Tree Analysis and Abandonment

Up to this point, we have focused primarily on techniques for estimating a project's risk. Although this is an integral part of capital budgeting, managers are at least as concerned (or maybe more concerned) about managing risk than they are about measuring it. One way of managing risk is to structure large projects as a series of decision points over time. This provides managers the opportunity to reevaluate decisions as additional information becomes available, and possibly to *cancel* (or once production begins, to *abandon*) the project if events take a turn for the worse.

Decision tree analysis

Projects that are structured as a series of decision points over time are evaluated using *decision trees*. For example, suppose Medical Equipment International (MEI) is considering the production of a totally new and innovative intensive care monitoring system. The net investment for this project is broken down into three stages, as set forth in Figure 11.3. If the go-ahead is given, at Stage 1 (Year 0), which is sometime in the near future, the firm will conduct a $500,000 study of the market potential for the new monitoring system. This study will take about one year. If the results are unfavorable, the project will be canceled, but if the results are favorable, MEI will (at Year 1) spend $1,000,000 to design and fabricate several prototype systems. These systems will then be tested at two hospitals and the reactions of the hospital medical staffs will determine whether MEI should proceed with the project.

If reaction at the test hospitals is positive, MEI will establish a production line for the monitoring systems at one of its plants at a net cost of $10,000,000. If this stage is reached, then MEI's managers estimate that the project will generate net cash flows over the following four years that depend on the vitality of the hospital industry at that time and overall acceptance of the system.

A decision tree such as the one in Figure 11.3 is often used to analyze such multistage, or sequential, decisions. Here, for simplicity, we assume that one year goes by between decisions. Each circle represents a decision point, or stage. The dollar value to the left of each decision point represents the net investment required to go forward at that decision point, and the cash flows under the $t = 3$ to $t = 6$ headings represent the cash inflows if the project is carried to completion. Each diagonal line, which represents the beginning of a branch of the decision tree, has an estimated probability for moving along that branch based on

Figure 11.3 Decision Tree Analysis (thousands of dollars)

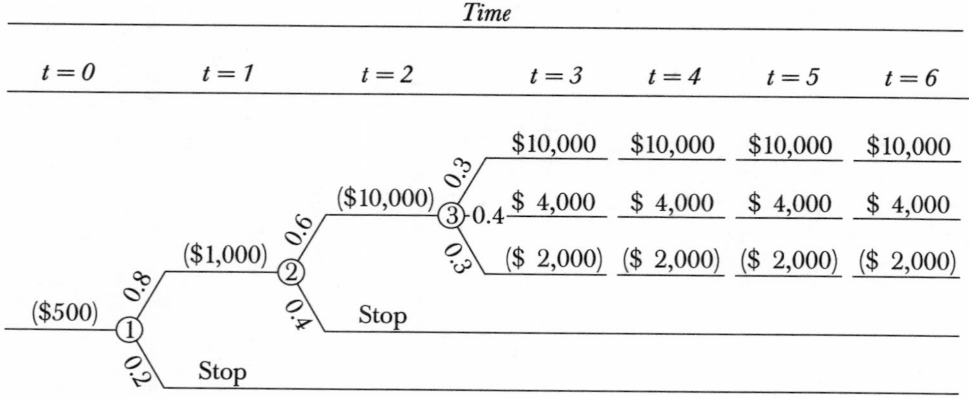
Time
t = 0
t = 1
t = 2
t = 3
t = 4
t = 5
t = 6
($500)
1
0.8
0.2
Stop
($1,000)
2
0.6
0.4
Stop
($10,000)
3
0.3
0.4
0.3
$10,000 $10,000 $10,000 $10,000
$ 4,000 $ 4,000 $ 4,000 $ 4,000
($ 2,000) ($ 2,000) ($ 2,000) ($ 2,000)

Joint Probability	NPV	Product: Prob. × NPV
0.144	$15,250	$2,196
0.192	436	84
0.144	(14,379)	(2,071)
0.320	(1,397)	(447)
0.200	(500)	(100)
1.000	Expected NPV =	($ 338)
	σ_{NPV} =	$7,991

information available to MEI's managers today. For example, management estimates that there is a probability of 0.8 that the initial study will produce favorable results, leading to the expenditure of $1,000,000 at Stage 2, and a 0.2 probability that the initial study will produce negative results, leading to cancellation after Stage 1.

The joint probabilities shown in Figure 11.3 give the probability of occurrence of each final outcome; that is, the probability of moving completely along each branch. Each joint probability is obtained by multiplying together all of the probabilities along a particular branch. For example, the probability that MEI will, if Stage 1 is undertaken, move through Stages 2 and 3, and that a strong demand will produce $10,000,000 in net cash flows in each of the next four years, is $(0.8)(0.6)(0.3) = 0.144 = 14.4\%$.

The NPV of each final outcome is also given in Figure 11.3. MEI has a cost of capital of 11.5 percent, and its management assumes initially that all projects have average risk. The NPV of the top (most favorable) outcome is about $15,250 (in thousands of dollars):

$$NPV = -\$500 - \frac{\$1,000}{(1.115)^1} - \frac{\$10,000}{(1.115)^2} + \frac{\$10,000}{(1.115)^3} + \frac{\$10,000}{(1.115)^4}$$
$$+ \frac{\$10,000}{(1.115)^5} + \frac{\$10,000}{(1.115)^6}$$
$$= \$15,250.$$

Other NPVs were calculated similarly.

The last column in Figure 11.3 gives the product of the NPV for each branch times the joint probability of that branch occurring, and the sum of the NPV products is the expected NPV of the project. Based on the expectations set forth in Figure 11.3, and assuming a cost of capital of 11.5 percent, the monitoring equipment project's expected NPV is −$338,000.

Since the expected NPV is negative, it would appear that this project is unprofitable, and hence should be rejected by MEI unless other considerations prevail. However, this initial judgment may not be correct. MEI must now consider whether this project is more, less, or about as risky as the firm's average project. The expected NPV is a negative $338,000, and the standard deviation of NPV is $7,991,000, so the coefficient of variation of NPV is quite large. This suggests that the project is highly risky in terms of stand-alone risk. Note also that there is a $0.144 + 0.320 + 0.200 = 0.664 = 66.4\%$ probability of incurring a loss. Based on all of this, the project appears to be unacceptable financially unless (1) it can be abandoned after production begins if demand is poor, or (2) it has some strategic value that is not inherent in the NPV analysis.

Abandonment

We discussed *abandonment* in Chapter 10, in connection with estimating a project's economic life. The possibility of abandonment can affect a project's risk as well as its expected profitability. Suppose that MEI is not contractually bound to continue the project once production has begun. Thus, if sales are poor during Year 3 ($t = 3$) and MEI experiences a cash flow loss of $2,000,000, and similar results are expected for the remaining three years, MEI can abandon the project at the end of Year 3 rather than continue to suffer losses. In this situation, low first-year sales signify that the monitoring equipment is not selling well so future sales will also be poor, and MEI has the opportunity to act on this new information once it becomes available.

The ability to abandon the project changes the branch of the decision tree in Figure 11.3 that contains the series of $2,000,000 losses. It now looks like this (in thousands of dollars):

	Joint Probability	NPV	Product: Prob. × NPV
③ 0.3 ($2,000) ④ Stop	0.144	(10,883)	(1,567)

Changing this branch to reflect the abandonment alternative eliminates the $2,000,000 cash losses in Years 4, 5, and 6, and thus causes the NPV for the branch to be higher (although still negative). This increases the project's expected NPV from −$338,000 to about $166,000, and also lowers the project's standard deviation from $7,991,000 to $7,157,000. Thus, abandonment possibilities changed the project's expected NPV from negative to positive, and also lowered its stand-alone risk as measured by either the standard deviation or coefficient of variation of NPV.

Here are some additional points to note concerning decision tree analysis and abandonment:

1. Managers can reduce project risk if they can structure the decision process to include several decision points rather than just one. If MEI were to make a total commitment to the monitoring equipment project at $t = 0$, signing contracts that would in effect

require completion of the project, it might save some money and accelerate the project, but doing so would substantially increase the project's riskiness.

2. Once production (or service) begins, the ability of the firm to abandon a project can dramatically reduce the project's risk.

3. The cost of abandonment is generally reduced if the firm has alternative uses for the project's assets. If MEI can convert the abandoned monitoring equipment production line to a different, more productive use, the cost of abandonment will be reduced, so the attractiveness of the monitoring equipment project will be enhanced.

Finally, note that capital budgeting is a dynamic process. Virtually all inputs to a capital budgeting decision change over time, and firms must periodically review both their expenditure plans and their ongoing projects. In the MEI example, conditions might change between Decision Points 1 and 2, and if so, this new information should be used to develop revised probability and cash flow estimates. If a capital budgeting decision can be structured with multiple decision points, including abandonment, and if the firm's managers have the fortitude to admit it when a project is not working out as initially planned, then risks can be reduced and expected profitability can be increased.

Self-Test Questions:

How can the possibility of abandonment affect a project's profitability and stand-alone risk?

What are the costs and benefits of structuring large capital budgeting decisions in stages rather than as a single decision?

Incorporating Risk into the Decision Process

Thus far, we have seen that capital budgeting decisions can affect a firm's market risk, its corporate risk, or both. We have also seen that it is exceedingly difficult to quantify either type of risk. It may be possible to reach the general conclusion that one project is more or less risky than another, or to compare the riskiness of a project with the firm as a whole, but it is difficult to develop a really good measure of project risk. This lack of precision in measuring project risk adds to the difficulties involved in incorporating differential risk into capital budgeting decisions.

There are two methods for incorporating project risk into the capital budgeting decision process: the certainty equivalent method, in which a project's expected cash flows are adjusted to reflect project risk, and the risk-adjusted discount rate method, in which differential risk is dealt with by changing the cost of capital. Although the risk-adjusted discount rate method is used by most businesses, the certainty equivalent method has some advantages, plus it raises some interesting issues related to the risk-adjustment process.

The certainty equivalent method

The *certainty equivalent (CE) method* follows directly from the concept of utility theory. Under the CE approach, the decision maker must first evaluate a cash flow's risk, and then specify how much money, with certainty, would be required to be indifferent between the riskless sum and the risky cash flow's expected value. To illustrate, suppose a rich eccentric offered someone the following two choices:

1. Flip a coin. If a head comes up, the person receives $1 million, but if a tail comes up, the person gets nothing. The expected value of the gamble is $(0.5)($1,000,000) + (0.5)($0) = $500,000$, but the actual outcome will be either $0 or $1 million, so the gamble is quite risky.

2. Do not flip the coin and simply pocket $400,000 in cash.

If the person is indifferent to the two alternatives, then $400,000 is defined to be his or her *certainty equivalent* for this particular risky expected $500,000 cash flow. The certain (riskless) $400,000 provides that individual with the same utility as the risky $500,000 expected return.

Now ask yourself this question: In the example, exactly how much cash-in-hand would it take to make you indifferent between a certain sum and the risky $500,000 from the coin flip? If you are risk averse, the certainty equivalent will be some amount less than the $500,000 expected value, and the greater your degree of risk aversion, the lower the certainty equivalent amount.

The CE concept can be applied to capital budgeting decisions, at least in theory, in the following way.

1. Convert each net cash flow of a project to its certainty equivalent value. Here, the riskiness of each cash flow is assessed, and a certainty equivalent cash flow is chosen on the basis of that risk. The greater the risk, the greater the difference between the

expected value and the certainty equivalent value. (Note that if a cash outflow is being adjusted, the certainty equivalent value is higher than the expected value.)

2. Once each cash flow is expressed as a certainty equivalent, discount the project's certainty equivalent cash flows by the risk-free rate to obtain the project's differential risk-adjusted NPV.[4] The risk-free rate is used as the discount rate because certainty equivalent cash flows are analogous to risk-free cash flows.

3. As before, a positive risk-adjusted NPV indicates that the project is profitable even after adjusting for differential project risk.

The CE method is simple and neat. Furthermore, it can easily handle differential risk among the individual net cash flows. For example, the final year's certainty equivalent cash flow might be adjusted downward an additional amount to account for salvage value risk if that risk is considered to be greater than the risk inherent in the operating cash flows. Unfortunately, there is no practical way to estimate a risky cash flow's certainty equivalent. There are no benchmarks available to help make the estimation, so each individual will have his or her own estimate, and these can vary significantly. Also, the risk assessment process, which measures the stand-alone risk of a project in its entirety, cannot identify the riskiness of individual cash flows, so there is no basis for adjusting each cash flow for its own unique risk.

The risk-adjusted discount rate method

In the *risk-adjusted discount rate (RADR) method,* expected cash flows are used in the valuation process, and the risk adjustment is made to the discount rate. All average-risk projects are discounted at the firm's overall cost of capital, which represents the opportunity cost of capital for average-risk projects; high-risk projects are assigned a higher cost of capital; and low-risk projects are discounted at a lower cost of capital.

The advantage of the RADR method is that the process has a starting benchmark, the firm's cost of capital. This discount rate reflects the riskiness of the firm's overall cash flows. Also, the risk assessment techniques commonly used identify a project's aggregate risk—the combined risk of all of the cash flows—and the RADR applies a single adjustment to the cost of capital rather than attempting to adjust individual cash flows. However, there is typically no theoretical basis for setting the size of the RADR adjustment, so that is usually a matter of judgment.

The RADR method has one additional disadvantage. Risk-adjusted discount rates combine the factor that accounts for time value, the risk-free rate, and the adjustment for risk, the risk premium: Cost of capital = Discount rate = Risk-free rate + Risk premium. The CE approach, on the other hand, keeps risk adjustment and time value separate; time value in the denominator and risk in the numerator. By lumping together risk and time value, the RADR method compounds the risk premium over time—just as interest compounds over time, so does the risk premium. This compounding of the risk premium means that the RADR method automatically assigns more risk to cash flows that occur in the distant future, and the farther into the future, the greater the implied risk. Since the CE method assigns risk to each cash flow individually, it does not impose any assumptions regarding the relationship between risk and time.

Consciously or unconsciously, the RADR method as it is normally used (with a constant discount rate applied to all cash flows of a project) implies that risk increases with time. This imposes a greater burden on long-term projects, so short-payoff projects will tend to look better financially than long-payoff projects. For most projects, the assumption of increasing risk over time is probably reasonable because cash flows are more difficult to forecast the farther one moves into the future. However, decision makers should be aware that the RADR approach automatically penalizes distant cash flows, and an additional explicit penalty based solely on cash flow timing is probably not warranted unless some specific additional risk can be identified.

Incorporating risk in practice

In most cases, it is impossible to assess quantitatively a project's corporate or market risk, and, like Bayside's MRI project, managers are left with only an assessment of the project's stand-alone risk. However, like the MRI project, most projects being evaluated are in the same line of business as the firm's other projects, and the profitability of most firms is highly correlated with the national economy. Thus, stand-alone, corporate, and market risk are usually highly correlated. This suggests that managers can get a feel for the relative risk of most projects on the basis of the scenario, simulation, and/or decision tree analyses conducted to assess the project's stand-alone risk. In Bayside's case, its managers conclude that the MRI project has above-average risk, and hence the project is categorized as a high-risk project.

The firm's overall cost of capital provides the basis for estimating a project's differential risk-adjusted discount rate: average-risk projects are discounted at the firm's cost of capital, high-risk projects are discounted at a higher cost of capital, and low-risk projects are discounted at a rate below the firm's cost of capital. Unfortunately, there is no good way of specifying exactly how much higher or lower these discounts rates should be; given the present state of the art, risk adjustments are necessarily judgmental, and somewhat arbitrary. Bayside Hospital's standard procedure is to add four percentage points to its 10 percent overall cost of capital when evaluating high-risk projects, and to subtract three percentage points when evaluating low-risk projects. Thus, to estimate the high-risk MRI project's differential risk-adjusted NPV, the project's expected cash flows shown in Table 11.1 are discounted at 10% + 4% = 14%. This rate is called the *project's cost of capital*, as opposed to the firm's cost of capital, since it reflects the risk characteristics of a specific project, rather than the aggregate risk characteristics of the firm (or average project). The resultant NPV is −$200,017, so the project becomes unprofitable when the analysis is adjusted to reflect its high risk. Bayside might still decide to go ahead with the MRI project, but at least the hospital's managers know that the project's expected profitability is not sufficient to make up for its riskiness.

Self-Test Questions:

What are the differences between the certainty equivalent (CE) and risk-adjusted discount rate (RADR) methods for risk incorporation?

What assumptions about time and risk are inherent in the RADR method?

Explain how most firms incorporate differential risk in the capital budgeting decision process.

Incorporating Debt Capacity Differentials into the Decision Process

Just as different firms have different optimal capital structures, so do individual projects. Within any firm, the overall optimal capital structure, which is reflected by the weights used in the firm's weighted average (overall) cost of capital, represents an aggregation of the optimal capital structures of the firm's individual projects. However, some projects probably support only a little debt, while other projects support a high level of debt. The optimal proportion of debt in a project's (or firm's) optimal capital structure is called the project's (or firm's) *debt capacity*.

One mistake that is often made when considering a project's debt capacity is to look at how the project is actually financed. For example, even though Bayside Memorial Hospital may be able to obtain a secured loan for the entire cost of the MRI equipment, the MRI project does not have a debt capacity of 100 percent. The willingness of lenders to furnish 100 percent debt capital for the MRI project is based more on Bayside's overall creditworthiness than it is on the financial merits of the MRI project, since all of the hospital's operating cash flow, less interest payments on embedded debt, is available to pay the lender. Think of it this way: would lenders provide 100 percent financing if Bayside were a start-up firm with the MRI project as its sole source of income?

The logical question that arises here is whether or not debt capacity differences should be taken into consideration in the capital budgeting process. In theory, if there are meaningful debt capacity differences between a project and the firm, capital structure differentials, as well as risk differentials, should be taken into account in the capital budgeting process. For example, an academic health center might be evaluating two projects: one involves research and development (R&D) of a new surgical procedure and the other involves building a primary care clinic in a local residential area. The R&D project would have relatively low debt capacity because it is a high business risk project with no assets suitable as loan collateral. Conversely, the clinic project would have relatively high debt capacity because it has low business risk and involves real estate suitable as collateral.

Incorporating capital structure differentials is mechanically easy. Merely change the weights used to compute the firm's weighted average cost of capital to reflect project debt capacity, as opposed to using the standard weights that reflect the firm's aggregate debt capacity. Projects with higher-than-average debt capacity would use a relatively high value for the weight of debt and a relatively low value for the weight of equity, and vice versa. However, in making debt capacity adjustments, a problem arises. We know from Chapter 9 that increased debt usage raises capital costs, so both the cost of debt and the cost of equity increase as more and more debt financing is used. This dependency of capital costs on capital structure means that as the weights are changed in the weighted average cost of capital calculation, so should the component costs change. However, it is very difficult, if not impossible, to estimate individual project costs of debt and equity that correspond to the project's optimal capital structure. Thus, capital structure adjustments quickly become a somewhat futile guessing game, so most firms do not make such adjustments unless there are specific benchmark values that can be used for both a project's unique debt capacity and the corresponding capital costs.[5]

Self-Test Question:

Discuss the pros and cons of incorporating debt capacity differences in the capital budgeting decision process.

Subsidiary Costs of Capital

Even though it is not common to make capital structure adjustments for individual projects, firms often make both capital structure and risk adjustments when developing subsidiary costs of capital. To illustrate, a for-profit health care system might have one subsidiary that invests primarily in real estate for medical uses, and another subsidiary that runs an HMO. Clearly, each subsidiary has its own unique business risk and optimal capital structure. The low-risk, high debt capacity real estate subsidiary might have an overall cost of capital of 10 percent, while the high-risk, low debt capacity HMO subsidiary might have a cost of capital of 14 percent. The health system, which consists of 50 percent real estate assets and 50 percent HMO assets would have a cost of capital of 12 percent.

If all capital budgeting decisions within the system were made on the basis of the system's 12 percent cost of capital, the process would be biased in favor of the higher-risk HMO subsidiary. The cost of capital would be too low for the HMO subsidiary and too high for the real estate subsidiary. Over time, this cost of capital bias would result in too many HMO projects being accepted and too few real estate projects, which would skew the business line mix toward HMO assets and hence increase the overall riskiness of the firm. Of course, the answer to this problem is to use subsidiary costs of capital, rather than the overall corporate cost of capital, in the capital budgeting decision process.

Unlike individual project costs of capital, subsidiary costs of capital often can be estimated with some confidence because it is usually possible to identify publicly traded firms that are predominantly in the same line of business as the subsidiary. For example, the cost of capital for the HMO subsidiary could be estimated by looking at the debt and equity costs of the major for-profit HMOs, such as United Healthcare and U.S Healthcare. With such market data at hand, it is relatively easy to develop subsidiary costs of capital. As a final check, the weighted average of the subsidiary costs of capital should equal the firm's overall cost of capital estimate.

Although the process is not exact, many firms use a two-step procedure to develop capital budgeting discount rates. (1) Subsidiary costs of capital are established for each of the major subsidiaries on the basis of its estimated riskiness and debt capacity. (2) Within each subsidiary, all projects are classified into three categories—high risk, average risk, and low risk—and then the subsidiary's cost of capital is adjusted to reflect the riskiness of each project. This procedure is far from precise, but it does at least recognize that different subsidiaries have different debt capacities and riskiness, and that different projects within each subsidiary can have different riskiness.

The final result of the risk assessment and incorporation process is a project discount rate, and hence NPV, that incorporates to the extent possible the project's debt capacity and riskiness. However, managers also must consider other possible risk factors that may not have been included in the quantitative analysis. For example, could the MRI project that we considered earlier significantly increase Bayside's liability exposure? Conversely, does the project have any strategic value or social value or abandonment possibilities that could affect its profitability and riskiness? Such additional factors must be considered, at least subjectively, before a final decision can be made. Typically, if the project involves new products or services and is large relative to the firm's average project, then the additional subjective factors will be very important to the final decision: one large mistake can bankrupt a firm, and "bet the company" decisions are not made lightly. On the other hand, the decision on a small replacement project would be made mostly on the basis of the numerical analysis.

Ultimately, capital budgeting decisions require an analysis of a mix of objective and subjective factors such as risk, debt capacity, profitability, medical staff needs, and social value. The process is not precise, and often there is a temptation to ignore one or more important factors because they are so nebulous and difficult to measure. Despite the imprecision and subjectiveness, a project's risk, as well as its other attributes, should be assessed and incorporated into the capital budgeting decision process.

Self-Test Questions:

Should all subsidiaries of a firm use the firm's overall cost of capital in making capital budgeting decisions?

Describe a typical capital budgeting decision process.

Risky Cash Outflows

Some projects are evaluated on the basis of minimizing the present value of future costs rather than on the basis of the projects' NPVs. This is done because (1) it is often impossible to allocate revenues to a particular project and (2) it is easier to focus on comparative costs when two projects will produce the same revenue stream. For example, suppose that Bayside Memorial Hospital must choose one of two ways for disposing of its medical wastes. There is no question about the need for the project, and the hospital's revenue stream is unaffected by which method is chosen. In this case, the decision will be based on the present value of expected future costs—the method with the lower present value of costs will be chosen.

Table 11.5 contains the projected costs associated with each method. The in-house system would require a large expenditure at Year 0 to upgrade the hospital's current disposal system, but the operating costs are relatively low. Conversely, if Bayside contracts for disposal services with an outside contractor, it will only have to pay $25,000 up front to initiate the contract. However, the annual contract fee would be $200,000 a year.[6]

If both methods were judged to have average risk, then Bayside's overall cost of capital, 10 percent, would be applied to the cash flows to obtain the present value (PV) of costs for each method. Since the PV of

Table 11.5   Bayside Memorial Hospital: Waste Disposal Cash Flows

Year	In-House System	Outside Contract
0	($500,000)	($ 25,000)
1	(75,000)	(200,000)
2	(75,000)	(200,000)
3	(75,000)	(200,000)
4	(75,000)	(200,000)
5	(75,000)	(200,000)
PV of Costs at $k =$		
10%	($784,309)	($783,157)
14%	—	($711,616)
6%	—	($867,473)

costs for the in-house system is $784,309, and for the contract method the PV of costs is $783,157, on a financial basis, Bayside's managers are basically indifferent as to which method should be chosen.

However, Bayside's managers believe that the contract method is much riskier than the in-house method. The cost of modifying the current system is known almost to the dollar, and operating costs can be predicted fairly well. Further, with the in-house system, operating costs are under the control of Bayside's management. Conversely, once Bayside relies on the contractor for waste disposal, the hospital is more or less stuck with continuing the contract, because it will not have the in-house capability. Since the contractor is only willing to quote a price for the first year, maybe this bid was "low-balled" to get the contract, with the expectation of large price increases in future years. Since the two methods have about the same PV of costs when both are considered to have average risk, which method should be chosen if the contract method is judged to have high risk? Clearly, if the costs are the same, the lower-risk project should be chosen.

Now, let's try to incorporate our intuitive differential risk assessment into the quantitative analysis. Conventional wisdom is to increase the project cost of capital for high-risk projects, so we would discount the contract cash flows using a project cost of capital of 14 percent, the rate that Bayside applies to high-risk projects. But, at a 14 percent discount rate, the contract method has a PV of costs of only $711,616, which is about $70,000 lower than that for the in-house method. If we upped the discount rate to 20 percent on the contract method, it would appear to be $161,000 cheaper than the in-house method. Thus, the riskier the contract method is judged to be, the better it looks!

Something is obviously wrong. If we want to penalize a cash outflow for higher-than-average risk, then that outflow must have a *higher* present value, not a *lower* present value. *Therefore, a cash outflow that has higher-than-average risk must be evaluated with a lower-than-average cost of capital.* Recognizing this, Bayside's managers actually applied a 10% − 4% = 6% discount rate to the high-risk contract method's cash flows. This produced a PV of costs for the contract method of $867,473, which is about $83,000 more than the PV of costs for the average-risk in-house method.

The appropriate risk adjustment for cash outflows is also applicable to other situations. For example, the City of Detroit offered Ann Arbor Health Systems the opportunity to use a city-owned building in one of the city's blighted areas for a walk-in clinic. The city offered to pay to refurbish the building, and all revenues made by the clinic would have accrued to Ann Arbor. However, after ten years, Ann Arbor would have had to buy the building from the city at the then current market value.

The value estimate that Ann Arbor used in its analysis was $2,000,000, but the realized cost could be much greater, or much less, depending on the economic condition of the neighborhood at that time. The rest of the project's cash flows were of average risk, but this single outflow had high risk, so Ann Arbor lowered the discount rate that it applied to this one cash flow.

Self-Test Question:

Is there any difference between the risk adjustments applied to cash inflows and cash outflows? Explain.

Capital Rationing

Standard capital budgeting procedures assume that firms can raise virtually unlimited amounts of capital to meet capital budgeting needs. Presumably, as long as the firm is investing the funds in profitable (positive NPV) projects, it should be able to raise the debt and equity needed to fund the projects. Of course, we also assume that the firm raises the capital roughly in accordance with its target capital structure.

This picture of a firm's capital financing/capital investment process is probably appropriate for most investor-owned firms. However, not-for-profit firms do not have unlimited access to capital. Their equity (fund) capital is limited to retentions, contributions, and grants, and their debt capital is limited to the amount supported by the equity (fund) capital base. Thus, it is likely that not-for-profit firms will face periods in which the capital needed for investment in new projects will exceed the amount of capital available. This situation is called *capital rationing*.

If capital rationing exists, and hence the firm has more acceptable projects than capital, then, from a financial perspective, the firm should accept that set of capital projects that maximizes aggregate NPV and still meets the capital constraint. This approach could be called "getting the most bang from the buck," and it picks those projects that have the most positive impact on the firm's financial condition. In the health care setting, priority may be assigned to some low or even negative NPV projects. This is fine as long as these projects are offset by the selection of profitable projects, which would prevent the low-profitability, priority projects from eroding the firm's financial condition.

Self-Test Questions:

What is capital rationing?

From a financial perspective, how are projects chosen when capital rationing exists?

Some Final Views on Project Risk Analysis

From our discussion of project risk assessment and incorporation, it should be apparent that project risk analysis is far from precise. The first problem encountered is that three types of project risk can be considered. Should health care managers place most emphasis on a project's stand-alone, corporate, or market risk? To answer this question, consider the following two points.

First, stand-alone risk is truly relevant only to a not-for-profit start-up firm that is evaluating its first project. Thus, in most situations, a project's riskiness is measured better by its corporate or market risk, which takes into account portfolio effects. Second, well-diversified stockholders should be concerned primarily with market risk, and managers of investor-owned firms should give strong weight to shareholders' best interests. However, stockholders are also concerned about costs related to financial distress, and these costs are captured by corporate risk, not market risk. Furthermore, managers, especially of health care firms, should be concerned about the firm's other stakeholders (current and prospective patients, bondholders, medical staff, employees, suppliers, and so on). This implies that corporate risk should be taken into account even by managers of investor-owned firms.

In most cases, it is impossible to assess quantitatively a project's corporate or market risk, and managers are often left with only an assessment of a project's stand-alone risk. However, the project under consideration usually will be in the same line of business as the firm's (or division's) other projects. Further, most firms' profitability is highly correlated with the national economy. Thus, stand-alone, corporate, and market risk usually are highly correlated, and hence a project's stand-alone risk often is a good measure of both its corporate and its market risk. This suggests that managers can get a feel for the relative risk of most projects from conducting scenario, simulation, and/or decision tree analyses.

The firm's overall cost of capital provides the starting point for estimating a project's risk-adjusted discount rate. If all projects had equal risk and equal debt capacity, then all projects would be evaluated at the corporate cost of capital. However, larger firms typically have several divisions that vary in risk and debt capacity, and projects within divisions can have risk and debt capacity differences.

The first step in developing a project's cost of capital calls for adjusting the firm's cost of capital to reflect divisional risk and debt capacity. Divisions with above-average risk or below-average debt capacity would have a divisional cost of capital above the corporate cost of capital, while divisions with below-average risk or above-average debt capacity would have a lower than average cost of capital. (Of course, the combined divisional costs of capital must equal the firm's overall cost of capital.) A project is then assigned to a risk category on the basis of its own risk relative to the division's average risk. If a project is riskier than average for its division, then its risk-adjusted discount rate is set above the divisional cost of capital, and the opposite holds true if the project has below-average risk. (Remember that the risk adjustment process is reversed if the adjustment is being made to cash outflows.) Also, adjustments should be made when projects have debt capacities which differ widely from the divisional average. The most difficult part of this process is judging how large the divisional and project adjustments should be. If it is possible to estimate the division's or project's market beta, then the CAPM can be used to help estimate the size of the risk adjustments. However, in many situations the adjustments are judgmental, and often a range of two to five percentage points is used.

The result is a project cost of capital and NPV that incorporates, to the extent possible, at least one dimension of the project's relative risk and its relative debt capacity. Managers must also consider other possible risk factors that may not have been included in the analysis. For example, if the project could lead to litigation against the firm, then the project has additional risk that should be taken into account—a number of drug and asbestos companies have learned this, to their regret. Conversely, if a project can easily be abandoned, or if the assets can easily be converted to other productive uses within the firm, then the project may be less risky than it appears in a conventional analysis. Such additional risk factors must be considered, at least subjectively, in making the final decision. Typically, if the project involves new products or services and is large relative to the firm's average project, then these additional risk factors will be very important to the final decision. On the other hand, if the project being considered is a small replacement project, then the decision would be made almost exclusively on the basis of a straight numerical analysis.

Ultimately, capital budgeting decisions, especially in the health care industry, require a mix of objective and subjective factors that will determine a project's risk, debt capacity, profitability, and ultimate acceptability. The process is not precise, and often there is a temptation to ignore risk considerations because they are so nebulous. Nevertheless, despite the imprecision and subjectiveness, a project's risk should be assessed and incorporated into the decision process.[7]

Self-Test Question:

Summarize the major considerations in project risk assessment and incorporation.

Summary

This chapter discussed project risk definition, assessment, and incorporation, and the key concepts are listed next:

- Three separate and distinct *types of project risk* can be defined: (1) stand-alone risk, (2) corporate risk, and (3) market risk.

- A project's *stand-alone risk* is the risk the project would have if it were the sole project of a not-for-profit firm. It is measured by the variability of profitability, generally by the *standard deviation* or *coefficient of variation* of NPV. Stand-alone risk is often used as a proxy for both corporate and market risk because (1) corporate and market risk are often impossible to measure and (2) the three types of risk are usually highly correlated.

- *Corporate risk* reflects the contribution of a project to the overall riskiness of the firm. It is measured conceptually by the project's *corporate beta*. Corporate risk ignores stockholder diversification, so it is the relevant risk for not-for-profit firms.

- *Market risk* reflects the contribution of a project to the overall riskiness of the stockholders' well-diversified portfolios. It is measured conceptually by the project's *market beta*. In theory, market risk is the relevant risk for investor-owned firms, but many people argue that corporate risk is also relevant to stockholders, and it is certainly relevant to a firm's other stakeholders.

- Four techniques can be used to *assess a project's stand-alone risk*: (1) sensitivity analysis, (2) scenario analysis, (3) Monte Carlo simulation, and (4) decision trees.

- *Sensitivity analysis* shows how much a project's profitability, say as measured by NPV, changes in response to a given change in an input variable such as volume, other things held constant.

- *Scenario analysis* defines a project's best, most likely, and worst cases, and then uses these data to measure its stand-alone risk.

- Whereas scenario analysis focuses on only a few possible outcomes, *Monte Carlo simulation* uses continuous distributions to reflect the uncertainty inherent in a project's component cash flows. The result is a probability distribution of NPV (or IRR), which provides a great deal of information about the project's riskiness.

- Projects that require capital outlays in stages over time are often evaluated using *decision trees*. Here, the branches of the tree represent different outcomes and, when subjective probabilities are assigned, the tree provides the profitability distribution for the project.

- The ability to *abandon* a project once operations have begun can increase the project's return and decrease its riskiness.

- Projects are generally classified as *high risk, average risk,* or *low risk* on the basis of their stand-alone risk assessment. High-risk projects are evaluated at a discount rate greater than the firm's overall cost of capital, average-risk projects are evaluated at the firm's cost of capital, and low-risk projects are evaluated at a rate less than the corporate cost of capital.

- When evaluating *risky cash outflows*, the risk adjustment process is reversed; that is, lower rates are used to discount more risky cash flows.

- Ultimately, capital budgeting decisions require an analysis of a mix of objective and subjective factors such as risk, debt capacity, profitability, medical staff needs, and service to the community. The process is not precise, but good managers do their best to ensure that none of the relevant factors are ignored.

Notes

1. If you do not have a good understanding of the three types of risk relevant to capital budgeting decisions, now is a good time to review the pertinent sections of Chapter 5.
2. For an algebraic representation of the relationships among stand-alone, corporate, and market risk, see L. C. Gapenski, "Project Risk Definition and Measurement in a Not-For-Profit Setting," *Health Services Management Research* (November 1992): 216–24.
3. Note also that spreadsheet programs have Data Table functions that automatically perform sensitivity analyses—once the table is roughed in, the spreadsheet calculates and records the NPV (or other profitability measure) values.
4. Note that the risk-free rate does not incorporate the tax advantages of debt financing, so such benefits to taxable firms should be incorporated in the cash flows when the certainty equivalent method is used.

5. One example where debt capacity adjustments are often made involves *project financing*. In project financing, lenders provide debt capital on the basis of the cash flows of the project because they may have limited, or no, recourse against the firm's other cash flows. In this situation, there is a readily identifiable cost of debt and debt capacity for the project.
6. For simplicity, we have ignored inflation effects.
7. Risk incorporation is much more important than debt capacity considerations, because a project's cost of capital is affected to a much greater degree by differential risk than by differential debt capacity.

Selected Additional References

Allen, R. J. 1989. "Proper Planning Reduces Risk in New Technology Acquisitions." *Healthcare Financial Management* (December): 48–56.

Ang, J. S., and W. G. Lewellen. 1982. "Risk Adjustment in Capital Investment Project Evaluations." *Financial Management* (Summer): 5–14.

Capettini, R., C. W. Chow, and J. E. Williamson. 1990. "Breakdown Approach Helps Managers Select Projects." *Healthcare Financial Management* (November): 48–56.

Gapenski, L. C. 1992. "Accuracy of Investment Risk Models Varies." *Healthcare Financial Management* (April): 40–52.

———. 1992. "Project Risk Definition and Measurement in a Not-for-Profit Setting." *Health Services Management Research* (November): 216–24.

———. 1990. "Using Monte Carlo Simulation to Help Make Better Capital Investment Decisions." *Hospital and Health Services Administration* (Summer): 207–19.

Gup, B. E., and S. W. Norwood III. 1981. "Divisional Cost of Capital: A Practical Approach." *Financial Management* (Spring): 20–24.

Hastie, K. L. 1974. "One Businessman's View of Capital Budgeting." *Financial Management* (Winter): 36–43.

Hertz, D. B. 1964. "Risk Analysis in Capital Investments." *Harvard Business Review* (January-February): 96–106.

Lewellen, W. G., and M. S. Long. 1972. "Simulation versus Single-Value Estimates in Capital Expenditure Analysis." *Decision Sciences* (October): 19–33.

Ryan, J. B., and J. L. Gocke. 1988. "Incorporating Risk into the Investment Decision." *Topics in Health Care Financing* (Fall): 49–65.

Ryan, J. B., and M. E. Ward (eds.). 1992. "Capital Management." Fall issue of *Topics in Health Care Financing*.

Weaver, S. C., P. J. Clemmens III, J. A. Gunn, and B. D. Danneburg. 1989. "Divisional Hurdle Rates and the Cost of Capital." *Financial Management* (Spring): 18–25.

Case 11A

Valley Forge Hospital: Project Analysis

Valley Forge Hospital is a 250-bed, investor-owned hospital located in Valley Forge, Pennsylvania, a Philadelphia suburb. The hospital was founded in 1946 by Richard Kelly Biddle, a prominent Philadelphia physician, upon his return from service in World War II. Biddle relinquished control to the hospital in 1967, while it was still a small hospital in a relatively rural setting. However, in the 1970s and 1980s, the Philadelphia suburbs boomed, and Valley Forge was no exception. Its position on Philadelphia's prestigious Main Line, and the movement of both people and businesses from the inner city to the suburbs, assured Valley Forge of high economic growth. Today, under a succession of excellent chief executive officers, Valley Forge Hospital is acknowledged to be one of the leading health care providers in the Philadelphia metropolitan area.

Valley Forge's management is currently evaluating a proposed ambulatory (outpatient) surgery center. Over 80 percent of all outpatient surgery is performed by specialists in gastroenterology, gynecology, ophthalmology, otolaryngology, orthopedics, plastic surgery, and urology. Ambulatory surgery requires an average of about one and one-half hours, with minor procedures taking about one hour and major procedures taking about two or more hours. About 60 percent of the procedures are performed under general anesthesia, 30 percent under local anesthesia, and 10 percent under regional or spinal anesthesia. In general, operating rooms are built in pairs so one patient can be prepped while the surgeon is completing a procedure in the other room.

The outpatient surgery market has experienced significant growth in recent years. In 1990, about 2.5 million procedures were performed, but by 1996 over 4 million procedures were being performed annually. This growth has been fueled by three main factors. First, rapid advancements in technology have enabled many procedures that were historically performed in inpatient surgical suites to be switched to outpatient settings. This shift has been due mainly to advances in laser, laproscopic, endoscopic, and arthroscopic technologies. Second, Medicare has been aggressive in approving new outpatient surgery techniques, so the number of Medicare patients utilizing outpatient surgery services has grown substantially. Finally, patients prefer outpatient surgeries because they are more convenient, and third party payers prefer them because they are less costly. All of these factors have led to a situation where the number of inpatient surgeries has remained flat over the last few years while the number of outpatient procedures has been growing at about 10 percent annually. Rapid growth in the number of outpatient surgeries has been accompanied by a corresponding growth in the number of outpatient facilities nationwide, so competition in many areas is becoming intense.

Valley Forge currently owns a parcel of land adjacent to the hospital that is suitable for the center. It bought the land five years ago for $150,000, and last year the hospital spent $25,000 to clear the land and put in sewer and utility lines. If sold in today's market, the land would bring in $200,000, net of all fees, commissions, and taxes. Land prices have been extremely volatile in the western suburbs, so the hospital's standard procedure is to assume a salvage value equal to the current value of the land. Of course, land is not depreciated for either book or tax purposes.

The building and equipment, which will house and equip four operating rooms, would cost $4,000,000. For ease, assume that both the building and the equipment fall into the MACRS five-year class for tax depreciation purposes. (In reality, the building would have to be depreciated over a much longer period than the equipment.) The project will probably have a long life, but Valley Forge typically assumes a five-year life in its capital budgeting analyses, and then captures the value of the cash flows beyond Year 5 by estimating a terminal, or salvage, value for the project. The salvage value, which is the market value of the building and equipment if sold in five years, is estimated at $2 million before taxes, excluding the land value. (Note that taxes must be paid on the difference between an asset's salvage value and its tax book value at termination. For example, if an asset has been depreciated down to $50, and then sold for $120, the firm owes taxes on the $70 excess in salvage value over tax book value.)

The expected patient load at the center is 12 procedures a day. The average hospital charge per procedure is $1,050, but charity care, bad debts, managed care plan discounts, and other allowances are expected to total 25 percent of charges. The center will be open 5 days a week, 50 weeks a year, for a total of 250 days a year. As detailed in Table 1, labor costs to run the center are estimated at $483,600 per year, including fringe benefits. Utilities, including hazardous waste disposal, would add another $50,000 in annual costs.

If the surgery center is built, the hospital's cash overhead costs would increase by $50,000 annually, primarily for housekeeping and buildings and grounds maintenance. In addition, the center would be allocated $25,000 of Valley Forge's current $2,800,000 in administrative overhead costs. On average, each procedure would require $200 in expendable medical supplies, including anesthetics. Although the hospital's inventories and receivables would rise slightly if the center is constructed, its accruals and payables would also increase. The overall change in net working capital is expected to be small, and hence not material to the decision. The hospital's marginal federal-plus-state tax rate is 40 percent.

One of the most difficult factors to deal with in project analysis is inflation. Input costs, as well as charges, in the health care industry have been rising at a rate well in excess of inflation. Furthermore, inflationary pressures have been highly variable. Because of the difficulties involved

Table 1   Projected Surgery Center Staffing Requirements

Position	Annual Salary	FTEs	Total Salary
Executive director	$50,000	1	$ 50,000
Director of nursing	35,000	1	35,000
Accounting clerk	25,000	1	25,000
Collections clerk	20,000	1	20,000
Scheduling clerk	17,000	1	17,000
Registered nurses	26,000	8	208,000
Nursing assistants	15,000	2	30,000
Transcriptionists	18,000	1	18,000
Total			$403,000
Plus 20 percent fringe benefit allowance			80,600
Total salaries and benefits			$483,600

in forecasting inflation rates, Valley Forge begins each analysis by assuming that both costs, except for depreciation, and charges will increase at a constant rate. Under current conditions, this rate is assumed to be 5 percent.

When the project was mentioned briefly at the last meeting of the hospital's board of directors, several questions were raised. In particular, one director wanted to make sure that a complete risk analysis, including sensitivity and scenario analyses, and possibly even Monte Carlo simulation, was performed prior to presenting the proposal to the board. Recently, the board was forced to close a day care center that appeared to be profitable when analyzed two years ago, but which actually turned out to be a big money loser. They do not want a repeat of that occurrence.

Also, Ruth Coleman, one of Valley Forge's directors, stated that she thought the hospital was putting too much faith in the numbers. "After all," she pointed out, "That is what got us into trouble on the day care center. We need to start worrying more about how projects fit into our strategic vision and how they impact the mix of services that we offer."

To develop the data needed for the risk analysis, Jules Bergman, the hospital's director of capital budgeting, met with the surgery, marketing, and facilities department heads. After several sessions, they concluded that four input variables were very uncertain: number of procedures per day, average charge per procedure, uncollectible percentage, and building/equipment salvage value. Currently, there were no outpatient surgery centers in Valley Forge's immediate service area, but if another hospital or other provider were to enter the ambulatory surgery market, the number of procedures per day could be as low as eight. Conversely, if acceptance were strong and no competing centers were built, the number of procedures could be as high as 16 per day, compared to a most likely value of 12.

The average charge, with a most likely value of $1,050, is a function of the types of procedures performed. If surgery severity were high, that is, if there were a higher number of complicated procedures performed than anticipated, then the average charge could be as high as $1,250. Conversely, if the severity were lower than expected, the average charge could be as low as $850. If there were no increase in managed care plan market power, and if the hospital could do a good job of controlling bad debt losses, the uncollectible percentage could be as low as 20 percent, compared to the most likely value of 25 percent. Conversely, heavy penetration by managed care plans could drive the uncollectible percentage to as high as 30 percent. Finally, if real estate and medical equipment values stayed strong, the building/equipment salvage value could be as high as $3 million, but if the market weakened, the salvage value could be as low as $1 million, compared to a mostly likely value of $2 million.

Bergman also discussed the probabilities of the various scenarios with the medical and marketing staffs, but after considerable debate, no consensus could be reached. To add to the confusion, one member of the medical staff, who had just returned from a Harvard executive program on financial management, questioned why the scenario analysis had to be confined to just three scenarios. "Why not five or seven?" he queried. Additionally, he said that the executive program had taught him a good way to assess the impact of inflation on project profitability; create and analyze an inflation impact table such as the one shown in Table 2.

Bergman also discussed with Mark Hauser, Valley Forge's chief financial officer, both the risk inherent in the hospital's average project and how the firm typically adjusts for risk. Hauser told Bergman that, based on historical scenario analysis data using worst case, most likely, and best case values, Suburban's average project has a coefficient of variation of NPV in the range of 1.0 to 1.5, and that the hospital typically adds or subtracts four percentage points to its 10 percent overall cost of capital to adjust for differential project risk. However, Hauser was quick to admit that the risk adjustment factor is arbitrary, and that it could just as easily be two percentage points or six percentage points.

Assume that you have been hired by Valley Forge as a financial consultant. Your task is to conduct a complete project analysis on the ambulatory surgery center and to present your findings and recommendations to the hospital's board of directors.

Table 2   Inflation Impact Table

| | | \multicolumn{7}{c}{*Level of Charge Inflation*} |
		0%	2.5%	5.0%	7.5%	10.0%	12.5%	15.0%
	0%	NPV	NPV	NPV	NPV	NPV	NPV	NPV
Level	2.5%	NPV	NPV	NPV	NPV	NPV	NPV	NPV
of	5.0%	NPV	NPV	NPV	NPV	NPV	NPV	NPV
Cost	7.5%	NPV	NPV	NPV	NPV	NPV	NPV	NPV
Inflation	10.0%	NPV	NPV	NPV	NPV	NPV	NPV	NPV
	12.5%	NPV	NPV	NPV	NPV	NPV	NPV	NPV
	15.0%	NPV	NPV	NPV	NPV	NPV	NPV	NPV

Case 11B

Pacific Laboratories: Staged Entry Analysis

Pacific Laboratories, a for-profit pharmaceutical firm headquartered in Los Angeles, was founded in 1970 by three physician-scientists: Karen Arndt, Mark Collier, and Robert Stringer. The company's initial strategy was to develop and market a line of prescription drugs, specializing in drugs that treat hypertension, arrythmia, and other cardiovascular conditions. The company grew rapidly, with several highly successful drugs introduced in the late 1970s and early 1980s, including Cardizol and Cardipace.

Pacific's products are regarded as being effective, safe, and of high quality, and hence the firm has an excellent reputation in the prescription drug industry. Furthermore, the firm is highly profitable and well-regarded by industry analysts at major brokerage firms. However, deteriorating sales and margins of two of the company's early successes have raised early warning signs that the firm is contracting the dreaded "off-patent syndrome." The symptoms of this sometimes fatal pharmaceutical company malady are a feverish burst of earnings from one or more blockbuster drugs, followed by the chill of sliding profits as generic drug competitors move in. Prescription drugs generally have 17 years of patent protection, during which time profits can be astronomical for blockbuster drugs. However, sales often drop 30–40 percent in the first year after a patent expires. Furthermore, it is not uncommon to lose 60 percent of market share within three years of loss of patent protection.

With its research and development (R&D) effort showing few signs of developing any prescription drug winners in the foreseeable future, something needs to be done to offset the effect of expiring patents. Pacific's board is currently considering the strategic options available, including (1) refocusing its R&D effort, (2) seeking to be acquired by a larger pharmaceutical company, (3) merging with another similar-sized firm with complementary strengths, and (4) moving into the over-the-counter (nonprescription) drug business. Pacific considered creating a nonprescription drug business line several times in the past, but its technological, marketing, and distribution advantages have always been in prescription drugs. Furthermore, intense competition in the over-the-counter business makes it difficult to achieve the profit margins necessary to make the investment worthwhile. However, industry developments in the 1990s, including the rapid growth in foreign over-the-counter sales and the political pressure in the United States to curb prescription drug prices, prompted the decision to reconsider this alternative. Also, newly developed production technology, as well as some existing over-capacity, could be used in the over-the-counter line, which could lead to economies that would lower production costs from previous estimates.

Pacific's officers are examining two proposals related to nonprescription drugs. Proposal A involves a single, large investment that would give the company all of the research, production, and marketing capacity needed for a major move into the nonprescription drug market. Proposal B, on the other hand, involves a more deliberate, two-stage sequence. Stage 1 of Proposal B calls for the construction of a relatively unsophisticated, no-frills manufacturing plant that has limited capacity and that would not capture all of the available production efficiencies. Stage 2 calls for the development of a major facility that would house the entire over-the-counter division—research and development, manufacturing, marketing, and general management.

Proposal A, which has an operational life of at least 15 years, requires a much larger capital investment than Stage 1 of Proposal B. However, Proposal B is more costly than Proposal A in total, even when time value is considered, because Proposal A's short project schedule leads to greater efficiencies in contracting, construction, and production, and hence to lower costs. Although the analysis of Proposal A has not been completed, initial work indicates that Proposal A will probably have an expected NPV of about $10 million. Its riskiness has not yet been assessed. However, several board members are concerned about the wisdom of making a very large investment in a business line that is new to the firm. Other board members, though, see no difference between prescription and nonprescription drugs, and one board member was even heard to mutter "drugs is drugs."

The primary task at hand now is to evaluate Proposal B. To date, the company has spent $7 million in research and development, including marketing studies, on over-the-counter drugs. Of this amount, $2 million has been expensed for tax purposes, while the remaining $5 million has been capitalized and will be amortized over the five-year operating life of Stage 1. According to a specific IRS ruling requested by Pacific, if the over-the-counter drug project is not undertaken, the $5 million can be immediately expensed.

If it decides to build the plant, Pacific would require a 20-acre site. For convenience in laying out the cash flows, assume that land acquisition would occur at Time 0. The firm currently owns a suitable tract of land that cost $500,000 several years ago, but it could be sold now for $1 million, net of realty fees and taxes.

The first nine months of Year 1 would be spent obtaining federal, state, and local approvals for the project, but these costs are not material to the decision. Plant construction would take place during the last quarter of Year 1 and all during Year 2 at a cost of $8 million. For planning purposes, assume that the entire expenditure would occur at the end of Year 1. The building falls into the MACRS 31.5-year class, and Pacific could begin to depreciate it during Year 4, the year the plant would go into service. Although its depreciable life is 31.5 years, the plant would actually be used for only five years, starting at the beginning of Year 4, with operating cash flows (assumed to be end-of-year) occurring from Year 4 to Year 8. It is estimated that the land would have a market value of $2 million at the end of Year 8 while the building would have a market value of $6 million.

The required production equipment would be obtained and installed during Year 3 at a cost of $12 million. (For analysis purposes, assume that payment would be made at the end of Year 2.) The equipment falls into the MACRS seven-year class, and like the building, tax depreciation would begin when the plant begins operations in Year 4. At the end of five years of wear and tear and technological obsolescence, the equipment would be worth very little—the best estimate is only $1 million. Table 1 contains the project's tax depreciation schedules.

If Pacific goes ahead with Stage 1, the initial investment in net working capital would equal 30 percent of estimated first year dollar sales. (Assume that the investment would be made at the end of Year 3.) Additions to net working capital in each subsequent year would be 30 percent of the dollar sales increase expected in the following year. For example, any additional net working capital required to support the

Table 1   MACRS Depreciation Rates

MACRS Class	Recovery Year				
	1	*2*	*3*	*4*	*5*
7-year	14.3%	24.5%	17.5%	12.5%	8.9%
31.5-year	3.2	3.2	3.2	3.2	3.2

Notes:

1. For ease, these allowances were rounded to the nearest one-tenth of a percent. In actual applications, the allowances would not be rounded.
2. Since the plant is entering service on January 1, a full year's depreciation can be taken on the building in the first year. In most situations, the first year's depreciation allowance on the building would be reduced because the allowance is based on the month that the property is placed in service. The first year's depreciation on the equipment follows the half-year convention regardless of the time, during the year, that the equipment is placed into service.

projected increase in Year 5 sales over Year 4 sales would be paid for at the end of Year 4.

Pacific's marketing department has projected two sales scenarios for Stage 1. If public acceptance is poor, sales are forecasted to be 15 million units (bottles) for Year 4. However, if public acceptance is good, sales are expected to be 20 million units. At this point, the best guess is that there is 50 percent chance of poor acceptance and 50 percent chance of good acceptance. Sales price is expected to average $5 per unit regardless of the demand scenario.

The production department has estimated variable manufacturing costs at 70 percent of sales, while fixed costs are expected to be $17.5 million annually, excluding depreciation, regardless of demand in Stage 1. Fixed costs other than depreciation are forecasted to increase after Year 4 at the expected rate of inflation, 4 percent. Unit sales, however, are expected to increase at an annual rate of 10 percent as the products gain more and more market recognition and acceptance. Sales price, on the other hand, is expected to remain flat due to heavy competition in the nonprescription drug market. Variable costs, since they are tied to unit sales, will increase at the same 10 percent rate as dollar sales.

Stage 2 would begin at the end of Year 6 when Pacific would spend $50.8 million on additional land and buildings. Capital investment would continue for two more years, and the cash inflows (assumed to be end-of-year) would begin the year following the shutdown of the Stage 1 plant. The Stage 2 flows are forecasted as follows:

	Net Cash Flow		
End of Year	*High Demand*	*Medium Demand*	*Low Demand*
6	($50,800,000)	($50,800,000)	($50,800,000)
7	(4,600,000)	(4,600,000)	(4,600,000)
8	(1,600,000)	(1,600,000)	(1,600,000)
9	25,000,000	15,000,000	5,000,000
10	30,000,000	16,000,000	5,000,000
11	35,000,000	17,000,000	5,000,000
12	200,000,000	100,000,000	50,000,000

Regardless of the demand scenario for Stage 2, the entire amount of net working capital from Stage 1 would be transferred to Stage 2 in Year 8 if it is undertaken. This required transfer is not included in the above cash flows, but any additional working capital requirements beyond Year 8 are included. Stage 2 is projected to last beyond Year 12, but cash flow estimation is so difficult when looking that far ahead that Pacific assigned a terminal value at the end of Year 12 that incorporates the anticipated value of all cash flows beyond that point, including any recovery of net working capital.

The Stage 2 demand scenarios are related to the public's response to the over-the-counter drugs experienced in Stage 1. If acceptance is poor in Stage 1, there is a 10 percent probability that demand will be high during Stage 2, a 30 percent probability that demand will be medium, and a 60 percent chance that demand will be low. However, if acceptance during Stage 1 is good, there is a 60 percent probability that demand will be high during Stage 2, a 30 percent probability that demand will be medium, and a 10 percent chance that demand will be low. Of course, these expectations may change over time as new information becomes available.

Pacific's current federal-plus-state tax rate is 40 percent, and this rate is projected to remain roughly constant into the future. The firm's weighted average cost of capital is 11.0 percent, but Pacific adjusts this amount up or down by 2 percentage points to adjust for project risk. The firm's average project is quite risky, in keeping with the characteristics of the pharmaceutical industry. Pacific defines low-risk projects as those having a coefficient of variation (CV) of NPV less than 2.0; average-risk projects have CVs in the range of 2.0–5.0; and high-risk projects have CVs over 5.0.

One of the most important advantages of staged entry is that new information will become available throughout the investment period. Pacific's managers recognize this feature, and believe that they will have a better estimate of the Stage 2 probabilities and cash flows prior to making the Year 6 investment. Furthermore, there is some possibility that the project could be abandoned at the end of Year 9 if the low demand scenario materializes. If the project is abandoned at that point, the best estimate for the Year 9 cash flow is $75 million, which includes both recovery of net working capital and salvage value. The uncertainty about whether abandonment would occur or not lies in the politics rather than the economics of the decision. In the past, there has been little inclination for Pacific's managers to admit mistakes and cut losses, so there is some doubt whether the abandonment decision would be made, even if it is the financially right thing to do at the time.

Assume that you have been hired as a consultant to analyze the situation regarding nonprescription drugs and to make a recommendation to Pacific's board of directors regarding the best course of action. In addition to a detailed analysis of Proposal B, you have been asked to compare qualitatively the relative merits of the two proposals.

Case 11C

Motor City Health System: Make or Buy Analysis

Motor City Health System is a large not-for-profit health care holding company that operates both for-profit and not-for-profit subsidiaries in Detroit and Southeast Michigan. The not-for-profit subsidiaries consist of four acute care hospitals—Metropolitan Memorial, River Rouge, Dearborn, and Livonia General—and one service company (MCSERVICES). MCSERVICES provides various services, such as food, laundry, and waste disposal, to the four hospitals. The single for-profit subsidiary (MCPROP-ERTIES) operates several for-profit businesses, but its primary business line is real estate development, particularly medical office buildings.

Motor City's chief executive officer, Richard Brooks, has been thinking about the firm's printing situation for some time. Motor City has a printshop that currently operates under MCSERVICES and provides some of the printing required by the hospitals, but it does not have the capabilities to do all of the work required. As shown in Table 1, Motor City currently (1996) spends about $830,000 a year on commercial contract printing, some of which could be done in-house if Motor City expands its printing operation. Of the $830,000, about $132,000 represents graphics printing (annual report, brochures, and other promotional material). Most of the graphics printing could be moved in-house, but about 10 percent of the work, for example, the four-color annual report, would have to continue to be done by outside vendors.

Conversely, only about 15 percent of the almost $700,000 in forms printing, or just over $100,000, could be moved in-house. This is because most forms printing requires very specialized equipment, and it is just not cost-effective for firms, except for very large ones, to print their own forms in-house. Motor City's vendor print contracts (both graphics and forms) increased in dollar volume by about 7 percent (2 percent volume

Table 1   Printing Currently Done by Outside Vendors

	Fiscal Year	
	1995	*1996*
Graphics Printing		
Mercury	$ 85,002.31	$ 7,727.86
Universal Color Graphics	16,982.44	12,588.00
Southern Louisiana Press	9,300.00	24,446.00
Southland	5,628.50	711.94
Pickett	3,526.14	2,337.10
Sir Speedy	1,962.58	8,939.50
Factors	85.46	0.00
C & S Printing	1,161.00	0.00
New Orleans Printing Service	0.00	75,292.83
Total graphics printing	$123,648.43	$132,043.23
90% to be brought in-house	$111,283.59	$118,838.91
Forms Printing		
Continuous	$223,826.43	$239,493.82
Stock tab	77,150.41	82,550.50
Labels	68,032.88	65,965.88
Carbon snap	97,563.27	106,283.44
Envelopes	61,096.52	62,435.89
Lab mount	5,095.35	5,126.33
Flat ½ side	42,266.69	40,986.45
Special	39,910.37	46,295.47
Oversize	1,458.19	0.00
Special service	1,190.00	2,743.98
Card stock	21,237.40	23,479.11
NCR flat	21,017.01	22,798.19
Total forms printing	$659,844.52	$698,159.06
15% to be brought in-house	$ 98,976.68	$104,723.86

increase and 5 percent inflationary price increase) from 1995 to 1996, and this trend is expected to continue into the foreseeable future.

In fiscal year 1996, Motor City's in-house printshop handled $42,837 in hospital billings. (To avoid any potential problems with MCSERVICES's not-for-profit status, the printshop only performs work for Motor City's not-for-profit hospitals.) The printshop bills for materials only, but since materials costs represent, on average, 30 percent of commercial vendors' total billings, the printshop currently does about $42,837/0.30 = $142,790 in annual work on a commercial billing basis. The equipment in the printshop has a current market value of $200,000, and the printshop generates about $20,000 in annual depreciation expense when calculated according to Internal Revenue Service (IRS) rules.

To move 90 percent of the vendor graphics printing and 15 percent of the vendor forms printing in-house, Motor City would have to invest in additional equipment. The capital investment necessary for expansion can vary significantly depending on whether new or used equipment is purchased, the type of main press selected, and whether only essential or "nice-to-have" equipment is purchased. Table 2 summarizes the equipment capital investment requirements. The main press is the largest single piece of equipment. Although a new press would cost about $100,000, a used two-color press in good condition that meets all of the requirements is available locally for $65,000. Note that the old equipment would be retained if the printshop is expanded. Also, the new equipment would generate tax depreciation of about $25,000 per year and the delivery van would cost $2,000 a year to operate (in 1996 dollars).

The printshop is currently located in leased space adjacent to Metropolitan Memorial, the largest of the four hospitals. The cost of

Table 2   Equipment Capital Investment Requirements

Item	Estimated Cost
Two-color press	$ 65,000.00
Two-color press (small), Model 9860	26,000.00
10-hole drill press	7,800.00
Futura F-20 folder system	13,000.00
Collator-stitcher, 12-bin	28,000.00
Bookmaker, Michael 1000E	5,300.00
Camera with processor	14,000.00
Paper plate, AB Dick 148	11,500.00
Three knife trimmer	12,000.00
Infrared dryer systems (2)	5,000.00
Delivery van	20,000.00
Miscellaneous items	5,000.00
Total capital investment	$212,600.00

this site is $2.85 per square foot per year. The printshop occupies 2,500 square feet, and hence current building costs are $7,125 in annual lease payments plus an additional $200 monthly in utilities and insurance. Unfortunately, this site cannot be expanded, and hence new space is required for the expanded facility. Suitable space in a good location can be leased for $3.75 per square foot. Since the new printshop would require 3,500 square feet, the lease cost would be $13,125. (Assume lease payments occur at the beginning of each year.) In addition, the new space would require $50,000 in initial remodeling and $300 per month in utilities and insurance (in 1996 dollars). Note that all leases are negotiated for a five-year period, so lease payments are not affected by inflation.

The expanded printshop would require an increase in labor costs. These costs are summarized in Table 3. Labor costs to run the current printshop amount to $50,000 annually, and all current printshop personnel would be retained if the expansion takes place.

After discussing the printshop situation with his CFO, Charlene Garcia, Richard Brooks defined three possible printshop alternatives:

1. Close the printshop completely and use outside vendors for *all* printing.

2. Expand the printshop as envisioned. Essentially, this means expanding the printshop and performing all feasible work in-house. Under this proposal, the printshop would remain under MCSERVICES, Motor City's not-for-profit service subsidiary. Thus, there would be no tax consequences.

3. Expand the printshop as in Alternative 2. However, all printing

Table 3   Incremental Labor Costs (1995 Dollars)

Number	*Position*	*Annual Salary*
1	Lead printer ($10.26 per hour)	$21,340.80
1	Printer ($9.00 per hour)	18,720.00
1	Delivery person ($7.00 per hour)	14,560.00
2	Clerical assistants ($4.92 per hour)	20,467.20
	Projected raw labor expense	$75,088.00
	Plus: 20 percent fringe benefits	15,017.60
	Total annual incremental labor costs	$90,015.60

activities would be transferred to MCPROPERTIES, Motor City's for-profit subsidiary. In this situation, capital expenses such as depreciation and lease payments would be tax deductible. The primary motivation behind this alternative is to permit the printshop to enter the for-profit commercial printing business.

Motor City's overall cost of capital is estimated to be 9.0 percent, but the company also computes the weighted average cost of capital (WACC) for each subsidiary. MCSERVICES, the not-for-profit service subsidiary has access to municipal debt which currently yields about 7.0 percent. Its target capital structure consists of 60 percent debt and 40 percent equity (fund) financing. Since MCSERVICES has a captive business relationship with Motor City's four hospitals, it has relatively low business risk. Consequently, it has a relatively low 13.0 percent cost of equity.

MCPROPERTIES, the for-profit subsidiary, cannot issue municipal debt. The bulk of its debt consists of mortgage loans provided by banks and insurance companies. Mortgage debt, which is secured by pledged property, has a relatively low interest rate for taxable debt. Currently, this rate is 9.0 percent. The subsidiary's combined federal-plus-state tax rate is 40 percent. Since MCPROPERTIES competes with other property development companies, its inherent business risk is high, and hence it has a relatively high cost of equity, 17.0 percent. However, its ability to use property as collateral for its debt financing gives it a relatively high debt capacity, about 75 percent.

Motor City's capital budgeting policy guidelines call for all cash flow analyses to be restricted to a five-year horizon with zero end-of-project salvage values. The rationale is that it is just too difficult to estimate cash flows any further into the future. It is now December 1996, and the printshop analysis is due in one week. Thus, for ease, assume that all capital investment cash flows, as well as lease payments for 1996, occur at the beginning of 1997 (the end of 1996). Then, the five years of operating flows occur from 1997 through 2001. Also, it is Motor City's capital budgeting policy to assume that all costs and prices that are not fixed by contract will increase at a 5.0 percent annual rate. Thus, any 1996 dollar costs must be increased by 5 percent annually beginning in 1997, and any 1996 volume amounts must be increased by 2 percent annually beginning in 1997.

In regard to the feasibility of expanding the printing business should it be placed into the MCPROPERTIES subsidiary, Ms. Garcia discussed the profitability of commercial printing businesses with Mark

Stanton, president of the Michigan Printers Association, the state trade organization. Mr. Stanton pointed out that the average printer in the United States has a before-tax profit margin of 5.3 percent, while the average in Michigan is just over 4 percent. Return on assets in the industry is 7.5 percent nationwide and 5.1 percent locally.

If the printshop is moved into MCPROPERTIES, it would go after printing business external to Motor City. Estimates are far from precise, but new business in 1997 could bring in $10,000 in additional pre-tax earnings (in 1997 dollars). This amount could double in 1998 (in 1998 dollars), given more time to advertise and build customer relationships. Although very uncertain, the pre-tax earnings stemming from external business is expected to increase by 5 percent per year after 1998, including both volume growth and price inflation.

Finally, George Jamal, Motor City's purchasing manager, has questioned the company's policy regarding external printing contracts. What is the company's current policy, and might a change in policy have a bearing on the decision at hand? The discount rate to use in the analysis has also been an issue under discussion. Charlene Garcia believes that the discount rate should reflect the divisional placement of the printshop, but other staffers have disagreed with this view.

Assume that you are the administrative resident at Motor City Health System and you have been given the task of analyzing the print shop situation and developing a recommended course of action. In assigning the project, your preceptor indicated that a risk analysis was appropriate. When asked for more guidance, his response was this: "You know more about this sort of thing than I do; just do it!"

Part VI

Analysis and Forecasting

12

Financial and Operating Analyses

$\mathbf{F}$inancial and operating analyses are of vital concern to health care managers, security analysts, investors, and lenders, all of whom use them for a variety of purposes. *Financial analysis* focuses on the data contained in a firm's financial statements, such as revenues, operating costs, accounts receivable, and retained earnings. *Operating analysis,* on the other hand, focuses on operating factors such as occupancy (census), patient mix, length of stay, and productivity. Both types of analysis are used to assess a firm's strengths and weaknesses, which reflect the results of past managerial decisions. Note, however, that the really interesting question is where the firm will go in the future. Therefore, managers invariably use the types of analysis discussed in this chapter as a springboard to predicting and planning for the future—the subject of the next chapter.

Financial Reporting in the Health Care Industry

Financial reporting in all industries follows standards set forth by the accounting profession called *generally accepted accounting principles (GAAP).*[1] The two primary bodies that promulgate standards for the health care industry are the *Financial Accounting Standards Board (FASB),* which deals with issues pertaining to private organizations, and the *Government Accounting Standards Board (GASB),* which deals with issues related to governmental entities. Generally, the principles promulgated by FASB and GASB relate to issues relevant to a broad range of industries, while industry-specific issues are resolved by the various industry committees of the American Institute of Certified Public Accountants (AICPA).

Financial statements

An organization's *annual report* provides a verbal description of the firm's operating results during the past year and a discussion of developments that will affect its future operations. More important, the report usually contains several *financial statements*, including three basic financial statements—the *income statement,* the *balance sheet,* and the *statement of cash flows.* Taken together, these statements give an accounting picture of the firm's operations and its financial position. Detailed data are provided for the two or three most recent years, and brief historical summaries of key operating statistics for the past five or ten years are often included.[2]

Income statement

Table 12.1 contains the 1994 and 1995 income statements (also called statements of revenues and expenses) for Bayside Memorial Hospital, a 650-bed, not-for-profit, acute care hospital.[3] Bayside had an excess of revenues over expenses (or net income) of $8,572,000 in 1995. Of course, being not-for-profit, the hospital paid no dividends, so it retained all of its $8,572,000 in net income. Also of interest is Bayside's cash flow. A firm's net cash flow from operating and nonoperating sources is approximately equal to its net income plus any noncash expenses. In 1995, Bayside's cash flow was $8,572,000 net income plus $4,130,000 depreciation expense, for a total net cash flow of $12,702,000. Depreciation does not really *provide* funds; it is simply a noncash charge which is added back to net income to obtain an estimate of the firm's net cash flow from operating and nonoperating sources. Later in this section, we will discuss the statement of cash flows, which provides a better insight into Bayside's cash flows.

Note that the income statement reports on transactions *over a period of time*—for example, during Fiscal Year 1995. (Note that Bayside's fiscal year coincides with the calendar year.) The balance sheet, which we discuss next, may be thought of as a snapshot of the firm's asset and liability position *at a single point in time*—for example, on December 31, 1995.

Balance sheet

Table 12.2 contains Bayside's 1994 and 1995 balance sheets. Although the assets are all stated in terms of dollars, only cash represents actual money. We see that Bayside could—if it liquidated any securities held—write checks at the end of 1995 for a total of $6,263,000 (versus current

Table 12.1 Bayside Memorial Hospital: Income Statements for Years Ended December 31 (thousands of dollars)

	1995	1994
Net patient services revenue	$108,600	$ 97,393
Other operating revenue	6,205	9,364
Total operating revenue	$114,805	$106,757
Operating expenses:		
Nursing services	$ 58,285	$ 56,752
Dietary services	5,424	4,718
General services	13,198	11,655
Adminstrative services	11,427	11,585
Employee health and welfare	10,250	10,705
Provision for uncollectibles	3,328	3,469
Provision for malpractice	1,320	1,204
Depreciation	4,130	4,025
Interest expense	1,542	1,521
Total operating expenses	$108,904	$105,634
Income from operations	$ 5,901	$ 1,123
Contributions and grants	$ 2,253	$ 874
Investment income	418	398
Nonoperating gain (loss)	$ 2,671	$ 1,272
Excess of revenues over expenses	$ 8,572	$ 2,395

liabilities of $13,332,000 due during 1996). The noncash current assets will presumably be converted to cash within a year, but they do not represent cash on hand.

The claims against assets are of two types—liabilities, or money the company owes, and fund capital.[4] Fund capital is a residual, so for 1995:

Assets	—	Liabilities	=	Fund capital
$151,278,000	—	$13,332,000 + $30,582,000	=	$107,364,000.

Liabilities consist of $13,332,000 of current liabilities plus $30,582,000 of long-term liabilities. If assets decline in value—suppose some of Bayside's fixed assets were sold at less than book value—liabilities remain constant, so the value of the fund capital declines.

A firm's fund (equity) account is built up over time by retentions (retained earnings). Note that in 1995 Bayside reported on its income

Table 12.2   Bayside Memorial Hospital: Balance Sheets for December 31 (thousands of dollars)

	1995	*1994*
Cash and securities	$ 6,263	$ 5,095
Accounts receivable	21,840	20,738
Inventories	3,177	2,982
Total current assets	$ 31,280	$ 28,815
Gross plant and equipment	$145,158	$140,865
Accumulated depreciation	25,160	21,030
Net plant and equipment	$119,998	$119,835
Total assets	$151,278	$148,650
Accounts payable	$ 4,707	$ 5,145
Accrued expenses	5,650	5,421
Notes payable	825	4,237
Current portion of long-term debt	2,150	2,000
Total current liabilities	$ 13,332	$ 16,803
Long-term debt	$ 28,750	$ 30,900
Capital lease obligations	1,832	2,155
Total long-term liabilities	$ 30,582	$ 33,055
Fund balance	$107,364	$ 98,792
Total liabilities and funds	$151,278	$148,650

statement an $8,572,000 excess of earnings over expenses. Since none of this amount can be paid out in dividends, the entire excess is retained in the firm. Barring any asset sales or revaluations, Bayside's fund account should increase from year to year by the amount of net income (excess of revenues over expenses). Thus,

1995 Fund balance	=	1994 Fund balance	+	1995 Net income
$107,364,000	=	$98,792,000	+	$8,572,000.

Note that accumulated depreciation reported on the balance sheet is a *contra asset* account. That is, it is subtracted from gross fixed assets, so the larger a firm's accumulated depreciation, all else the same, the smaller its total assets. However, as noted earlier, the larger the amount of depreciation in any year, the greater the firm's cash flow, because depreciation is a noncash expense. Accumulated depreciation on the balance sheet increases each year by the amount of depreciation expense reported on the income statement. For example,

1995 Accumulated depreciation		1994 Accumulated depreciation		1995 Depreciation expense
$25,160,000	=	$21,030,000	+	$4,130,000.

Statement of cash flows

Twenty years ago, most annual reports contained a statement called the "sources and uses of funds statement." The purpose of the statement was to report where the firm had obtained funds during the past year and how it had used them. For example, had the firm obtained most of its funds from such sources as bank loans and bond issues, or as retained earnings? Had it used those funds to retire debt, to build new facilities, to build up inventories, or to pay dividends? One could look at the statement and see the total sources and total uses (which were equal), and how funds were obtained and used, but there was no summary figure that could be used to judge whether the company ended the year in a stronger or weaker financial position.

After several format revisions, organizations now report fund flows in the *statement of cash flows,* which is usually organized into three sections: (1) cash flow from operations, (2) cash flow from investing activities, and (3) cash flow from financing activities. Health care providers often add a fourth section, nonoperating cash flow. Accountants adopted the new format because it provides information in the way most useful for financial analysis.

Table 12.3 contains Bayside's statement of cash flows, which focuses on the sources and uses of overall cash flow for 1995. The top part shows cash generated by and used in operations: for Bayside, operations provided $8,525,000 in net cash flow. Note that the income statement reported income from operations plus depreciation of $5,901,000 + $4,130,000 = $10,031,000, but as part of its operations Bayside invested $1,735,000 in current assets and generated $229,000 in spontaneous liabilities, for net cash from operations of $10,031,000 −$1,735,000 + $229,000 = $8,525,000.

The next section of the statement of cash flows, "Cash Flow from Investing Activities," shows that Bayside spent $4,293,000 on capital expenditures in 1995. Bayside's financing activities as shown in the third section highlight the fact that Bayside used cash generated from

Table 12.3   Bayside Memorial Hospital: Statement of Cash Flows, 1995 (thousands of dollars)

Cash Flow from Operations	
Total operating revenue	$114,805
Total cash operating expenses	(104,774)
Change in accounts receivable	(1,102)
Change in inventories	(195)
Change in accounts payable	(438)
Change in accruals	229
Net cash flow from operations	$ 8,525
Cash Flow from Investing Activities	
Investment in plant and equipment	$ 4,293
Cash Flow from Financing Activities	
Repayment of long-term (LT) debt	($ 2,150)
Repayment of notes payable	(3,412)
Capital lease principal repayment	(323)
Change in current portion of LT debt	150
Net cash flow from financing	($ 5,735)
Nonoperating Cash Flow	
Contributions and grants	$ 2,253
Investment income	418
Nonoperating cash flow	$ 2,671
Net increase (decrease) in cash	$ 1,168
Beginning cash and securities	$ 5,095
Ending cash and securities	$ 6,263

operations (and from nonoperating gains) to pay off debt during 1995. On net, Bayside made $5,735,000 of principal payments to creditors during 1995. Finally, the hospital generated $2,671,000 in nonoperating cash flow during the year.

When all of these items are totaled, we see that Bayside had a $1,168,000 net cash inflow during 1995, and the very bottom of Table 12.3 reconciles the 1995 net cash flow with the 1995 ending cash balance. Bayside's statement of cash flows shows nothing unusual or alarming. It does show that Bayside's operations are inherently profitable, at least in 1995. Had the statement showed an operating cash drain, then we would have had something to worry about, because such a drain, if it continued, could bleed the hospital to death.

Managers, security analysts, loan officers, and corporate raiders all pay close attention to the statement of cash flows. Finance is, after all, a cash flow-oriented discipline, and this statement gives a good picture of the annual cash flows generated by the business. For example, a bank loan officer could examine Table 12.3 (or, better yet, a series of such tables going back for perhaps the last five years and projected out several years into the future) to get an idea of whether or not the hospital could generate the necessary cash to pay off a requested loan. If projected cash flows appear sufficient, then the loan will be granted. If the cash flows are questionable, then the banker will pay close attention to the balance sheet, attempting to determine whether, if the firm were forced into bankruptcy and liquidation, the asset sale would bring in enough cash to satisfy the loan.

Notes to the financial statements

Information that can significantly affect a firm's financial condition is often contained in the notes to its financial statements. For health care providers, these notes contain information on the firm's pension plan, its malpractice insurance, its noncapitalized lease agreements, the amount of charity care it provides, its accounting policies, and so forth. For example, the more important notes to Bayside's 1995 financial statements contained the following information:

1. Inventories are valued at the lower of cost or market, with costs determined by the last-in, first-out (LIFO) method.

2. Accounts receivable were reduced by $3.986 million in 1995 and by $3.458 million in 1994 to allow for doubtful accounts.

3. Noncancelable operating lease commitments are estimated at $858,000 for 1996, $842,000 for 1997, and $671,000 for 1998.

4. The hospital's pension costs were $1.325 million in 1995 and $1.214 million in 1994. As of December 31, 1995, the hospital had a $20.985 million actuarial present value of vested pension benefits and plan assets with a market value of $22.568 million, resulting in a pension plan excess of $1.580 million. (For simplicity, we excluded this amount from the balance sheet. Typically, any pension fund excess would be reported on the balance sheet as other assets. Annual pension expense is reported on the income statement in the employee health and welfare category.)

5. Patient service revenue is reported net of provisions for charity care of $3.256 million in 1995 and $2.985 million in 1994. The amount of charity care provided is measured at the hospital's established rates. The hospital has agreements with third party payers that provide for payments to the hospital at amounts different from its established rates.

6. The hospital is self-insured for the purpose of protecting itself against professional and patient care claims. Professional insurance consultants have been retained to determine funding requirements. The amounts funded have been placed in a self-insurance trust account that is administered by a trustee. (The insurance trust account would normally be listed on the balance sheet as assets whose use is limited. Again, for simplicity, we have omitted that account from Bayside's illustrative balance sheet.)

7. The hospital is an income beneficiary of the Robert A. Mitchell Charitable Trust. Because the assets of the trust are not controlled by the hospital, they are not included on the hospital's balance sheet. On December 31, 1995, the market value of the trust assets allocated to the hospital totaled $2.086 million. Income distributed to the hospital amounted to $168,000 in 1995 and $155,000 in 1994.

Clearly, the information contained in the notes to the financial statements has a bearing on Bayside's financial position, and it should be considered, either directly or indirectly, in any financial analysis. Indeed, professional analysts occasionally use the footnote information to recast financial statements before they even begin an analysis, and to these analysts the notes are especially vital.

Self-Test Questions:

What organizations govern financial reporting requirements in the health care industry?

Briefly describe these three basic financial statements: (1) income statement, (2) balance sheet, and (3) statement of cash flows.

What type of information is provided by each type of statement?

What is the difference between net income and cash flow, and which is more meaningful to a firm's financial condition?

What types of information are contained in the notes to a firm's financial statements?

Financial Statement Analysis

Financial statement analysis involves a number of techniques that extract information contained in a firm's financial statements and combine it in a form that facilitates making judgments about the firm's financial condition. In the next sections, we discuss four common analytical techniques—Du Pont analysis, ratio analysis, common size analysis, and percentage change analysis—along with some problems inherent in such analyses.

Du Pont Analysis

Du Pont analysis provides a "quick and dirty" view of a firm's financial condition. The name reflects the fact that this type of analysis was developed by the Du Pont Company. In essence, Du Pont analysis combines some basic *financial ratios* in a way that provides valuable insights into a firm's financial condition. The analysis focuses on one of the most important measures of a firm's profitability, *return on equity (ROE)*, which is defined as Net income/Total equity (fund capital). Then, Du Pont analysis decomposes ROE into the product of three other ratios, each of which has an important economic interpretation. The result is the *Du Pont equation*:

$$\text{ROE} = \text{Profit margin} \times \begin{matrix}\text{Total asset}\\ \text{runover}\end{matrix} \times \begin{matrix}\text{Equity}\\ \text{multiplier}\end{matrix}$$

$$\frac{\text{Net income}}{\text{Total equity}} = \frac{\text{Net income}}{\text{Revenues}} \times \frac{\text{Revenues}}{\text{Total assets}} \times \frac{\text{Total assets}}{\text{Total equity}}.$$

We will use Bayside's 1995 data to illustrate the Du Pont equation:

$$\frac{\$8,572}{\$107,364} = \frac{\$8,572}{\$114,805} \times \frac{\$114,805}{\$151,278} \times \frac{\$151,278}{\$107,364}$$

$$7.98\% = 7.47\% \times 0.76 \times 1.41.$$

Note that the product of the first two terms on the right-hand side of the Du Pont equation is *return on assets (ROA)*, which is defined as Net income/Total assets. Bayside's 1995 *profit margin* was 7.47 percent, so the hospital made 7.47 cents profit on each dollar of total revenue. Furthermore, assets were "turned over" 0.76 times during the year, so Bayside earned a return of $7.47\%(0.76) = 5.68\%$ on its assets.[5]

If Bayside used only equity (fund) financing, its 5.68 percent ROA would equal its ROE. However, almost 30 percent of the firm's capital was supplied by creditors. Since the 5.68 percent ROA all goes into fund capital, which comprises only 30 percent of total capital, Bayside's ROE is higher than 5.68 percent. Specifically, ROA must be multiplied by the *equity multiplier*, which shows the total assets working for each dollar of common equity (fund capital), to obtain the ROE of 7.98 percent. This 7.98 percent ROE could, of course, be calculated directly: ROE = Net income/Total equity = $8,572/$107,364 = 7.98%. However, the Du Pont equation shows how profit margin (which measures expense control), turnover (which measures asset utilization), and financial leverage (which measures debt utilization) interact to determine ROE.

Bayside's managers use the Du Pont equation to analyze ways of improving the hospital's performance. To influence the profit margin (expense control), Bayside's marketing staff can study the effects of raising charges (or lowering them to increase volume), of moving into new services or markets with higher margins, of entering into new contracts with managed care organizations, and so on; and cost accountants can study the expense items and, working with department heads and clinical staff, seek ways to reduce costs. Looking at total asset turnover (asset utilization), Bayside's analysts, working with both clinical and marketing staffs, can investigate ways of reducing investments in various types of assets. Finally, Bayside's financial staff can analyze the effects of alternative financing strategies on the equity multiplier (debt utilization), seeking to hold down interest expenses and the risks of debt while still using debt to increase ROE.

The Du Pont equation provides a useful comparison between a firm's performance as measured by ROE and the performance of an average hospital:[6]

Bayside Hospital: ROE = 7.5% × 0.76 × 1.41 ≈ 8.0%

Industry average: ROE = 4.9% × 0.79 × 1.98 ≈ 7.7%.

We see (1) that Bayside has a significantly higher profit margin, and thus better control over expenses; (2) that the average hospital has about the same total asset turnover, and thus Bayside is getting average utilization from its assets; but (3) that the average hospital has offset some of Bayside's advantage in expense control by using more financial leverage, although Bayside's lower use of debt financing decreases its risk. The result here is that Bayside gets slightly more return on its fund capital than the average hospital does.

One potential problem with Du Pont analysis applied to not-for-profit organizations, especially hospitals, is that a large portion of a hospital's net income (excess of revenues over expenses) may come from nonoperating gains rather than from operations. If such nonoperating gains are highly variable and unpredictable, as they often are, then return on equity as defined above may be a poor measure of the hospital's inherent profitability. This difficulty can be overcome by recasting the Du Pont equation using operating income rather than net income:

$$\begin{array}{ccccccc}
\text{Operating} & = & \text{Operating} & \times & \text{Total asset} & \times & \text{Equity} \\
\text{ROE} & & \text{margin} & & \text{turnover} & & \text{multiplier}
\end{array}$$

$$\frac{\text{Op income}}{\text{Total equity}} = \frac{\text{Op income}}{\text{Revenues}} \times \frac{\text{Revenues}}{\text{Total assets}} \times \frac{\text{Total assets}}{\text{Total equity}}.$$

$$\frac{\$5,901}{\$107,364} = \frac{\$5,901}{\$114,805} \times \frac{\$114,805}{\$151,278} \times \frac{\$151,278}{\$107,364}$$

$$5.50\% = 5.14\% \times 0.76 \times 1.41.$$

Now we can compare the operating income form of the Du Pont equation with the industry average:

Bayside Hospital: ROE $= 5.1\% \times 0.76 \times 1.41 \approx 5.5\%$.

Industry average: ROE $= 2.2\% \times 0.79 \times 1.98 \approx 3.4\%$.

We see that the same general relationships hold as discussed before, so Bayside's nonoperating gain does not affect our earlier conclusions.

Finally, note that the operating income form of the Du Pont equation can be expanded to include the effect of nonoperating gains and losses as follows:

$$\begin{array}{ccccccccc}
\text{Return on} & = & \text{Operating} & \times & \text{Total asset} & \times & \text{Equity} & \times & \text{Nonoperating} \\
\text{Equity} & & \text{margin} & & \text{turnover} & & \text{multiplier} & & \text{gain multiplier}
\end{array}$$

$$\frac{\text{Net income}}{\text{Total equity}} = \frac{\text{Op income}}{\text{Revenues}} \times \frac{\text{Revenues}}{\text{Total assets}} \times \frac{\text{Total assets}}{\text{Total equity}} \times \frac{1}{1 - \text{Nonoperating gain ratio}}$$

$$\frac{\$8,572}{\$107,364} = \frac{\$5,901}{\$114,805} \times \frac{\$114,805}{\$151,278} \times \frac{\$151,278}{\$107,364} \times \frac{1}{1 - 0.312}$$

$$7.98\% = 5.14\% \times 0.76 \times 1.41 \times 1.45.$$

Here the nonoperating gain ratio is defined as Nonoperating gain (or loss)/Net income $= \$2,671/\$8,572 = 0.312$.[7] The expanded form of the Du Pont equation is especially useful for not-for-profit entities, particularly hospitals, but the basic format presented at the beginning of this section is typically used in other situations.

Self-Test Questions:

Explain how the Du Pont equation combines several ratios to obtain an overview of a firm's financial condition.

Why are there several different forms of the Du Pont equation?

Ratio Analysis

Financial statements report both on a firm's position at a point in time and on its operations over some past period. However, the real value of financial statements lies in the fact that they can be used to help predict a firm's future financial condition. From a creditor's (or a stockholder's) standpoint, predicting the future is what financial statement analysis is all about, while from management's standpoint, financial statement analysis is useful both as a way to anticipate future conditions and, more importantly, as a starting point for planning actions that will influence the future course of events.

A full analysis of the firm's financial ratios is generally the second step in a financial analysis, after the overview provided by a Du Pont analysis. Ratios are designed to show relationships between financial statement accounts. For example, Hospital A might have debt of $5,248,760 and interest charges of $419,900, while Hospital B might have debt of $52,647,980 and interest charges of $3,948,600. The true burden of these debts, and each hospital's ability to pay the interest and principal due on them, can be ascertained by comparing each firm's debt to its assets, and the interest it pays versus the income it has available for payment of interest. Such comparisons are made by *ratio analysis.*

Unfortunately, an almost unlimited number of financial ratios can be constructed, and the choice of ratios depends in large part on the purpose of the analysis. Generally, ratios are grouped into categories to make them easier to interpret. In the paragraphs that follow, we will calculate some typical 1995 financial ratios for Bayside Memorial Hospital and compare the ratios with hospital industry averages.[8] Note that all dollar amounts in the ratio calculations are in thousands.

Profitability ratios

Profitability is the net result of a large number of policies and decisions, so *profitability ratios* show the combined effects of liquidity, asset management, and debt management on operating results. Note that several of the profitability ratios were discussed earlier in the section on Du Pont analysis.

Profit, or total, margin

The *profit margin*, often called the *total margin,* is computed by dividing net income (excess of revenues over expenses) by revenues, and it gives the profit per dollar of sales:

$$\text{Profit margin} = \frac{\text{Net income}}{\text{Revenues}} = \frac{\$8,572}{\$114,805} = 7.5\%.$$

Industry average $= 4.9\%.$

Thus, the hospital makes 7.5 cents on every dollar of revenue. Bayside's profit margin is substantially above the industry average of 4.9 percent, indicating either that its charges are relatively high, its allowances are relatively low, its costs are relatively low, it has relatively high nonoperating gains, or some combination of these factors.

Operating margin

The *operating margin* is computed by dividing operating income (excess of revenues over expenses) by revenues, and it gives the profit per dollar of sales:

$$\text{Operating margin} = \frac{\text{Operating income}}{\text{Revenues}} = \frac{\$5,901}{\$114,805} = 5.1\%.$$

Industry average $= 2.2\%.$

Bayside's operating margin is substantially above the industry average of 2.2 percent, indicating that its charges are relatively high, its allowances are relatively low, and/or its costs are relatively low. Note that operating margin removes the influence of nonoperating gains and losses.

Basic earning power (BEP)

The ratio of operating earnings before interest and taxes (EBIT) to total assets measures the firm's *basic earning power (BEP)*:

$$\text{Basic earning power} = \frac{\text{Operating EBIT}}{\text{Total assets}} = \frac{\$5,901 + \$1,542}{\$151,278}$$

$$= 4.9\%.$$

Industry average $= 3.4\%.$

Note that the BEP ratio removes the influence of interest (capital structure), taxes (ownership), and nonoperating gains and losses. Thus, BEP is the best measure of the basic profitability of a firm's assets, and it is a good ratio to use when comparing investor-owned and not-for-profit organizations. Bayside's 4.9 percent BEP is well above the 3.4 percent average for the industry. This rate indicates that Bayside is better able to generate income from its assets than is the average hospital.

Return on assets (ROA)

The ratio of net income to total assets measures the *return on assets (ROA)*:

$$\text{Return on assets} = \frac{\text{Net income}}{\text{Total assets}} = \frac{\$8,572}{\$151,278} = 5.7\%.$$
$$\text{Industry average} = 3.9\%.$$

Bayside's 5.7 percent ROA is well above the 3.9 percent average for the industry. As we saw in the Du Pont analysis, Bayside's high ROA is due to its high profit margin.

Return on equity (ROE)

The ratio of net income to total equity (fund capital) measures the *return on equity (ROE)*:

$$\text{Return on equity} = \frac{\text{Net income}}{\text{Total equity}} = \frac{\$8,572}{\$107,364} = 8.0\%.$$
$$\text{Industry average} = 7.7\%.$$

Bayside's 8.0 percent ROE is slightly above the 7.7 percent industry average. In our Du Pont analysis, we discussed the components of ROE and how they interact.

For investor-owned firms, ROE should focus on the return to *common stockholders,* so any preferred stock financing should be treated as debt. ROE measures the return to the owners of the firm, and preferred stockholder claims are more like creditor's claims than owner's claims. Also, note that ROA and ROE could be calculated on the basis of operating income rather than net income to remove the impact of nonoperating gains and losses.

Liquidity ratios

One of the first concerns of most managers, and the major concern of a firm's creditors, is the firm's liquidity. Will the firm be able to meet its obligations in a timely manner as they become due? Bayside has debts totaling over $13 million (its current liabilities) that must be paid off within the coming year. Will Bayside have trouble satisfying those obligations? A full liquidity analysis requires the use of a cash budget, which we will discuss in Chapter 14. However, by relating the amount of cash and other current assets to current obligations, ratio analysis provides a quick, easy-to-use, approximate measure of liquidity.

Current ratio

The *current ratio* is computed by dividing current assets by current liabilities:

$$\text{Current ratio} = \frac{\text{Current assets}}{\text{Current liabilities}} = \frac{\$31,280}{\$13,332} = 2.3, \text{ or } 2.3 \text{ times.}$$

Industry average = 2.0.

Current assets normally include cash, marketable securities, accounts receivable, and inventories, plus other current assets. Current liabilities consist of accounts payable, short-term notes payable, current maturities of long-term debt, accrued income taxes (for investor-owned firms), and other accrued expenses (principally wages).

If a company is getting into financial difficulty, it will begin paying its bills (accounts payable) more slowly, building up bank loans, and so on. If these current liabilities rise faster than current assets, then the current ratio will fall, and this could spell trouble. Since the current ratio is an indicator of the extent to which the claims of short-term creditors are covered by assets that are expected to be converted to cash in a period roughly corresponding to the maturity of the claims, it is one commonly used measure of short-term liquidity.

Bayside's current ratio is slightly above the average for the industry. It appears that Bayside is about in line with most other hospitals. Since current assets are scheduled to be converted to cash in the near future, it is highly probable that they could be liquidated at close to their stated value. With a current ratio of 2.3, Bayside could liquidate current assets at only 43 percent of book value and still pay off current creditors in full.[9]

Although industry average figures are discussed later in some detail, it should be stated at this point that an industry average is not a magic number that all firms should strive to maintain; in fact, some very well managed firms will be above the average, while other good firms will be below it. However, if a firm's ratios are far removed from the average for its industry, its managers should be concerned about why this variance occurs.

Quick ratio

The *quick ratio* is calculated by deducting inventories from current assets and dividing the remainder by current liabilities:

$$\text{Quick ratio} = \frac{\text{Current assets} - \text{Inventories}}{\text{Current liabilities}} = \frac{\$31,280 - \$3,177}{\$13,332}$$
$$= 2.1.$$

Industry average $= 1.8$.

Inventories are typically the least liquid of a firm's current assets, and hence they are the assets on which losses are most likely to occur in the event of liquidation. Therefore, a measure of the firm's ability to pay off short-term obligations without relying on the sale of inventories often is important.[10]

The industry average quick ratio is 1.8, so Bayside's 2.1 ratio compares favorably with other hospitals. If receivables can be collected, Bayside can pay off its current liabilities even if it cannot sell its inventory. Since hospitals typically have small inventories, the quick ratio does not provide much more information about a hospital's liquidity than does the current ratio. However, other health care firms, such as drug and medical equipment manufacturers, have relatively large inventories, and the quick ratio is more meaningful in those industries.

Days cash on hand

The current and quick ratios attempt to measure liquidity on the basis of balance sheet accounts (stocks) as opposed to income statement items (flows). However, the true measure of a firm's liquidity is whether it can meet its payments as they become due, and so liquidity is more related to flows than to stocks. The *days cash on hand ratio* combines stocks with flows:

$$\text{Days cash on hand} = \frac{\text{Cash} + \text{Marketable securities}}{(\text{Operating expense} - \text{Depreciation})/365}$$
$$= \frac{\$6,623}{(\$108,904 - \$4,130)/365} = \frac{\$6,263}{\$287.05}$$
$$= 21.8 \text{ days.}$$

Industry average $= 19.6$ days.

Note that the denominator of the equation represents average daily *cash* expenses, and the numerator is the cash and securities that are available to make those payments. Since Bayside's days cash on hand is somewhat better than the industry average, this measure confirms that Bayside's liquidity position is somewhat better than that of the average hospital.

Debt management (capital structure) ratios

The extent to which a firm uses debt financing, or *financial leverage,* has three important implications. (1) By raising funds through debt, owners of for-profit firms can maintain control of the firm with a limited investment. For not-for-profit firms, debt financing allows the organization to provide more services than it could if it were solely financed with fund capital. (2) Creditors look to owner-supplied funds (or fund capital) to provide a margin of safety; if the owners (noncreditor stakeholders) have provided only a small proportion of total financing, then the risks of the enterprise are borne mainly by its creditors. (3) If the firm earns more on investments financed with borrowed funds than it pays in interest, then the return on the owners' (or fund) capital is magnified, or "leveraged."

When analysts examine a company's financial statements, they develop two different types of debt management ratios. (1) They use balance sheet data to determine the extent to which borrowed funds have been used to finance assets. These ratios are called *capitalization ratios.* (2) They use income statement data to determine the extent to which fixed financial charges are covered by operating profits. These ratios are called *coverage ratios.* The two sets of ratios are complementary, and most analysts use both types.

Total debt to total assets (debt ratio)

The ratio of total debt to total assets, generally called the *debt ratio,* measures the percentage of total funds provided by creditors:

$$\text{Debt ratio} = \frac{\text{Total debt}}{\text{Total assets}} = \frac{\$43,914}{\$151,278} = 0.0290, \text{ or } 29.0\%.$$

Industry average $= 48.8\%$.

Debt is defined here to include both current liabilities and long-term debt. Creditors prefer low debt ratios, since the lower the ratio, the greater the cushion against creditors' losses in the event of liquidation. Owners of for-profit firms, on the other hand, may seek high leverage either to magnify earnings or because selling new stock would mean giving up some degree of control. In not-for-profit firms, managers may seek high leverage to offer more services.

Bayside's debt ratio is 29.0 percent; this means that its creditors have supplied somewhat less than one-third of the firm's total financing.

Since the average debt ratio for the hospital industry is almost 50 percent, Bayside uses significantly less debt than the average hospital. Bayside's managers recognize this, and they have set their target capital structure at 50 percent debt, but high profitability and a recent shortage of good capital investment opportunities have held the hospital's debt ratio down. Once the projects are identified, Bayside would find it relatively easy to borrow additional funds.

Debt to equity ratio

Another commonly used capitalization ratio is the *debt to equity ratio*. The debt to asset and debt to equity ratios are transformations of each other, and hence provide the same information:

$$\text{Debt to equity ratio} = \frac{\text{Total debt}}{\text{Total equity}} = \frac{\$43,914}{\$107,364}$$
$$= 0.409, \text{ or } 40.9\%.$$

Industry average $= 95.3\%$.

Thus, Bayside's creditors have contributed 40.9 cents for each dollar of equity (fund) capital, while the industry average is 95.3 cents per dollar. Both the debt to assets and debt to equity ratios increase as a firm of a given size uses a greater proportion of debt, but the debt to assets ratio rises linearly and approaches a limit of 100 percent, while the debt to equity ratio rises exponentially and approaches infinity. Bank analysts often prefer the debt to equity ratio because it indicates explicitly the dollars of creditors' capital per dollar of owners' capital used to finance the company's assets.

Note that yet another capitalization ratio often used is the *equity ratio*, which is the complement of the debt ratio: Total equity (fund capital)/Total assets = 1 − Debt ratio. Since Bayside's debt ratio is 29.0 percent, its equity ratio is 71.0 percent.

Times-interest-earned ratio

The *times-interest-earned (TIE) ratio* is determined by dividing operating earnings before interest and taxes (EBIT) by the interest charges:

$$\text{TIE ratio} = \frac{\text{Operating EBIT}}{\text{Interest expense}} = \frac{\$7,443}{\$1,542} = 4.8 \text{ times.}$$

Industry average $= 3.1$.

The TIE ratio measures the extent to which *operating income* can decline before the firm's earnings are less then its annual interest costs. Failure to pay interest can bring legal action by the firm's creditors, possibly resulting in bankruptcy. Note that earnings *before* interest and taxes is used in the numerator. Because interest is a deductible expense, the ability of investor-owned firms to pay current interest is not affected by taxes.

Bayside's interest is covered 4.8 times. Since the industry average is 3.1 times, the company is covering its interest charges by a relatively high margin of safety. Thus, the TIE ratio reinforces our conclusion based on the debt ratio, namely, that the company could easily expand its use of debt financing. Note that the TIE could be redefined to include nonoperating gains and loses. To do this, the amount of nonoperating gain or loss would be added to the numerator of the TIE equation.

Note also that coverage ratios are often better measures of a firm's debt utilization than capitalization ratios, because coverage ratios discriminate between low interest rate debt and high interest rate debt. For example, one hospital might have $10 million of 4 percent debt on its balance sheet, while another might have $10 million of 8 percent debt. If both hospitals have the same total assets, both have the same debt ratio, but the hospital with the 4 percent debt is clearly in sounder financial position. If capitalization ratios are recast on a market value basis, they will provide better information than the typical book value ratios: market value ratios will show the hospital with the 8 percent debt as having a greater amount of debt.

Fixed-charge-coverage ratio

The *fixed-charge-coverage (FCC) ratio* is similar to the times-interest-earned ratio, but it is more inclusive in that it recognizes that firms incur fixed long-term obligations other than interest payments under lease and debt contracts. Leasing has become widespread in recent years, making this ratio preferable to the times-interest-earned ratio for many purposes. Furthermore, many debt contracts require that principal payments be made over the life of the loan, rather than only at maturity. Fixed charges are defined as interest plus annual long-term lease payments plus debt principal repayments, and the fixed charge coverage ratio is defined as:

$$\text{FCC ratio} = \frac{\text{EBIT} + \text{Lease payments}}{\text{Interest expense} + \text{Lease payments} + \text{Debt principal}/(1 - T)}$$

$$= \frac{\$7,443 + \$1,368}{\$1,542 + \$1,368 + \$2,000/(1 - 0)} = 1.8 \text{ times.}$$

Industry average $= 1.4$.

Here we assume that Bayside had $1,368,000 of lease payments and $2,000,000 of debt principal repayments in 1995. Note that, for investor-owned firms, the debt principal repayments, since they are paid with after-tax dollars, must be "grossed up" by dividing by $1 - T$. This gives the amount of pre-tax dollars that are required to cover the principal repayments.

Bayside's fixed charges are covered 2.3 times, as compared to the industry average of 1.4 times. This indicates that the hospital has a lower fixed charge financial burden than the average hospital.

Cash flow coverage ratio

So far we have ignored the fact that accounting income, whether it be operating income or net income, does not measure the actual cash flow available to meet fixed charge payments. This deficiency is corrected in the *cash flow coverage ratio*, which shows the margin by which operating cash flows cover fixed financial requirements:

$$\text{FCC ratio} = \frac{\text{EBIT} + \text{Lease payments} + \text{Depreciation expense}}{\text{Interest expense} + \text{Lease payments} + \text{Debt principal}/(1 - T)}$$

$$= \frac{\$7,443 + \$1,368 + \$4,130}{\$1,542 + \$1,368 + \$2,000/(1 - 0)} = 2.6 \text{ times.}$$

Industry average $= 2.1$.

Again, Bayside exceeds industry standards.

Asset management (activity) ratios

The next group of ratios, the *asset management ratios*, is designed to measure how effectively the firm is managing its assets. These ratios help to answer this question: Does the total amount of each type of asset as reported on the balance sheet seem reasonable, too high, or too low in view of current and projected operating levels? Bayside and other hospitals must borrow or raise fund (equity) capital to acquire assets. If they have too many assets, then their interest expenses will be too high and their profits will be depressed. On the other hand, if assets are too low, then profitable sales may be lost or vital services not offered.

Inventory turnover ratio

The *inventory turnover ratio*, also called the *inventory utilization ratio*, is defined as sales divided by inventories:

$$\text{Inventory turnover} = \frac{\text{Revenues}}{\text{Inventory}} = \frac{\$114,805}{\$3,177} = 36.1 \text{ times.}$$

Industry average $= 34.5$.

As a rough approximation, each item of Bayside's inventory is used and restocked, or "turned over," 36.1 times per year.

Bayside's turnover of 36.1 times compares favorably with an industry average of 34.5 times. This suggests that the hospital does not hold excessive stocks of inventory. Excess stocks are, of course, unproductive, yet they must be financed in the same way as productive assets. Inventory turnover is not as critical to hospitals as it is to other businesses—say, for instance, a medical equipment manufacturer. If a medical equipment manufacturer had an inventory turnover well below the industry average, we would wonder whether the firm was holding damaged or technologically obsolete items not actually worth their stated book values.

Two problems arise in calculating and analyzing inventory turnover. First, sales are stated at market prices, so if inventories are carried at cost, as they generally are, then the calculated turnover overstates the true turnover ratio. Therefore, it would be more appropriate to use cost of goods sold in place of sales in the numerator of the formula. However, most established compilers of financial ratio statistics use the ratio of sales to inventories carried at cost, so to develop a figure that can be compared with those published by Dun & Bradstreet and similar organizations, it is necessary to measure inventory utilization with sales in the numerator, as we do here.

The second problem lies in the fact that sales occur over the entire year, whereas the inventory figure is for one point in time, the end of the fiscal year. This makes it better to use an average inventory measure. Preferably, the average inventory value would be calculated by summing the monthly figures during the year and dividing by 12. If monthly data are not available, one can add the beginning and ending figures and divide by 2; this will adjust for growth but not for seasonal effects. If it was determined that the firm's business is highly seasonal, or if there has been a strong upward or downward sales trend during the year, it becomes essential to make some such adjustment. To maintain comparability with industry averages, however, we did not use an average inventory figure.

Current asset turnover ratio

The *current asset turnover ratio* measures how well a firm uses its current assets:

$$\text{Current asset turnover} = \frac{\text{Revenues}}{\text{Current assets}} = \frac{\$114,805}{\$31,280} = 3.7 \text{ times.}$$

Industry average $= 3.3.$

When we say turnover, or utilization, we mean how well the firm can turn those assets into revenues. The higher the utilization ratio, the more efficient the firm is at using those assets. Bayside generates $3.70 in total revenue for each $1.00 of current assets. This compares favorably with the industry average, so Bayside is able to get more revenue "bang" from its current asset "buck" than can the average hospital.

Fixed asset turnover ratio

The *fixed asset turnover ratio*, also called the *fixed asset utilization ratio*, measures the utilization of plant and equipment, and it is the ratio of revenues to fixed assets:

$$\text{Fixed asset turnover} = \frac{\text{Revenues}}{\text{Net fixed assets}} = \frac{\$114,805}{\$119,998}$$
$$= 0.96 \text{ times.}$$

Industry average $= 1.5$.

Bayside's ratio of 0.96 compares poorly with the industry average of 1.5 times, indicating that the hospital is not using its fixed assets as productively as the average hospital.

However, a major potential problem exists with the use of the fixed asset turnover ratio for comparative purposes. Recall that all assets except cash and accounts receivable reflect historical costs rather than current value. Inflation and depreciation have caused the value of many assets that were purchased in the past to be seriously understated. Therefore, if we were comparing an old hospital that had acquired much of its plant and equipment years ago to a new hospital that had acquired its fixed assets only recently, then the old hospital would probably report a higher turnover. This would be more reflective of the inability of financial statements to deal with inflation than of any inefficiency on the part of the new hospital. The accounting profession is trying to devise ways of making financial statements more reflective of current rather than historical values. If balance sheets were stated on a current (market) value basis, this would eliminate the problem of comparisons, but at the moment the problem still exists. Since financial analysts typically do not have the data necessary to make adjustments, they simply recognize that a problem exists and deal with it judgmentally.[11]

Total asset turnover ratio

The *total asset turnover ratio* measures the turnover, or utilization, of all of the firm's assets; it is calculated by dividing sales by total assets:

$$\text{Total asset turnover } = \frac{\text{Revenues}}{\text{Total assets}} = \frac{\$114,805}{\$151,278} = 0.76 \text{ times.}$$

Industry average $= 0.79$.

Bayside's ratio is just below the industry average, indicating that any deficiency in fixed asset utilization is almost offset by Bayside's superior current asset utilization.

Average collection period

The *average collection period (ACP)* is used to appraise accounts receivable, and it is computed by dividing average daily sales into accounts receivable to find the number of days' sales tied up in receivables. Note that this ratio is often called *days sales outstanding (DSO)* or *days in accounts receivable.* Thus, the ACP represents the average length of time that the firm must wait after making a sale (or providing a service) before receiving cash:[12]

$$\text{Average collection period } = \frac{\text{Accounts receivable}}{\text{Sales}/365} = \frac{\$21,840}{\$314.53}$$
$$= 69 \text{ days.}$$

Industry average $= 77$ days.

Bayside is doing a better job than the average hospital in collecting its receivables.

In many industries, the ACP can also be evaluated by comparison with the terms on which the firm sells its goods. For example, a medical supplier may sell on terms that call for payment within 60 days. If this company had a 69-day ACP, this would indicate that customers, on average, are not paying their bills on time. Indeed, since some customers undoubtedly pay in less than 60 days, others must be paying very late to push the firm's ACP out to 69 days. If the trend in the collection period over the past few years has been rising, but the credit policy has not changed, this would be even stronger evidence that steps should be taken to expedite the collection of accounts receivable.

Average payment period

Whereas the average collection period measures a firm's receivables management, the *average payment period (APP)*, or *days in accounts payable,* measures a firm's payables management. The APP is computed by dividing average daily credit purchases into accounts payable to find the number of days' credit available from accounts payable. Thus, the APP represents the average length of time the firm waits after making a purchase before paying for the purchase:[13]

$$\text{Average payment period} = \frac{\text{Accounts payable}}{\text{Credit purchases}/365} = \frac{\$4,707}{\$90.52}$$
$$= 52 \text{ days.}$$

Industry average $= 58$ days.

Here we assumed that Bayside purchases $33,039,800 of supplies annually on credit. It is difficult to assess whether Bayside's management of payables is good or bad: the higher the APP, the more credit that a firm is extracting from its suppliers, but, if this credit is costly trade credit as opposed to free trade credit, the firm may be better off with a lower APP. We will have much more to say about the cost of trade credit in Chapter 14.

Other ratios

The final group of ratios examines other facets of a firm's financial condition. For investor-owned firms, at least those whose stock is publicly traded, some ratios can be developed that relate the firm's stock price to its earnings and book value per share. These *market value ratios* give management an indication of what investors think of the company's past performance and future prospects. If the firm's liquidity, asset management, debt management, and profitability ratios are all good, then its market value ratios will be high and its stock price will probably be as high as can be expected.

Average age of plant

The *average age of plant* gives a rough measure of the average age (in years) of a firm's fixed assets:

$$\text{Average age of plant} = \frac{\text{Accumulated depreciation}}{\text{Depreciation expense}} = \frac{\$25,160}{\$4,140}$$
$$= 6.1 \text{ years.}$$

Industry average $= 7.5$ years.

Bayside's physical assets are newer than those of the average hospital. Thus, Bayside is offering more up-to-date facilities than average, and hence it will probably have fewer capital expenditures in the near future. On the other hand, Bayside's net fixed asset valuation will be relatively high, biasing the hospital's fixed asset turnover ratio downward.

Price/Earnings ratio

For investor-owned firms, the *price/earnings (P/E) ratio* shows how much investors are willing to pay per dollar of reported profits. Suppose the stock of General Medical Systems, an investor-owned hospital company, sells for $28.50, while the firm had 1995 earnings per share (EPS) of $2.20. Then, its P/E ratio would be 13.0:

$$\text{P/E ratio} = \frac{\text{Price per share}}{\text{Earnings per share}} = \frac{\$28.50}{\$2.20} = 13 \text{ times.}$$

Industry average $= 15$.

P/E ratios are higher for firms with high growth prospects, other things held constant, but they are lower for riskier firms. General's P/E ratio is slightly below the average of other investor-owned hospitals, which suggests that the company is regarded as being somewhat riskier than most, as having poorer growth prospects, or both.

Market/Book ratio

The ratio of a stock's market price to its book value gives another indication of how investors regard the company. Companies with relatively high rates of return on equity generally sell at higher multiples of book value then those with low returns. General's book value per share is $16.00, so dividing the price per share by the book value gives a *market/book (M/B) ratio* of 1.8 times:

$$\text{M/B ratio} = \frac{\text{Price per share}}{\text{Book value per share}} = \frac{\$28.50}{\$16.00} = 1.8 \text{ times.}$$

Industry average $= 2.1$.

Note that General reported $80 million in total equity on its 1995 balance sheet, and the firm had 5 million shares outstanding, for a book value per share of $80/5 = $16.00. Investors are willing to pay slightly less for each dollar of General's book value than for that of an average investor-owned hospital company.

Comparative and trend analysis

In our discussion of Bayside's ratios, and in our Du Pont analysis, we focused on *comparative analysis;* that is, we compared Bayside's ratios with the average ratios for its industry. Another useful ratio analysis tool is *trend analysis,* in which we analyze the trend of a single ratio over time.

Trend analysis gives clues about whether a firm's financial situation is improving, holding constant, or deteriorating.

It is easy to combine comparative and trend analyses in a single graph such as the one shown in Figure 12.1. Here we plotted Bayside's ROE and the industry average ROE over the past five years. The graph shows that Bayside's ROE has been declining faster than the industry average from 1991 through 1994, but that it rose above the industry in 1995. Other ratios could be analyzed similarly.

Self-Test Questions:

What is the purpose of ratio analysis?

What are two ratios that measure profitability? That measure liquidity? That measure debt management? That measure asset management? That measure market value?

How can comparative and trend analyses be used to help interpret ratio results?

Common Size Analysis

In *common size analysis*, all income statement items are divided by revenues, and all balance sheet items are divided by total assets. Thus, a common size income statement shows each item as a percentage of revenues, and a common size balance sheet shows each account as a percentage of total assets. The significant advantage of common size statements is that they facilitate comparisons of income statements and balance sheets over time and across companies because they compensate for scale differentials.

Table 12.4 contains Bayside's common size income statement for 1995, along with the composite statement for the hospital industry. A higher percentage of Bayside's operating revenue comes from patient services than is true of the average hospital, and Bayside overall is doing a better job of controlling expenses. Further, Bayside appears to have been more aggressive in its fund-raising efforts than the industry average. The net result is a higher profit margin.

Table 12.5 contains Bayside's common size balance sheet for 1995, along with industry average data. Three striking differences are revealed: (1) Bayside's current assets are significantly lower than the industry average, (2) its net plant and equipment are significantly higher, and (3) Bayside uses far less debt financing than the average hospital.

Figure 12.1   Bayside Memorial Hospital: ROE Analysis, 1991–1995

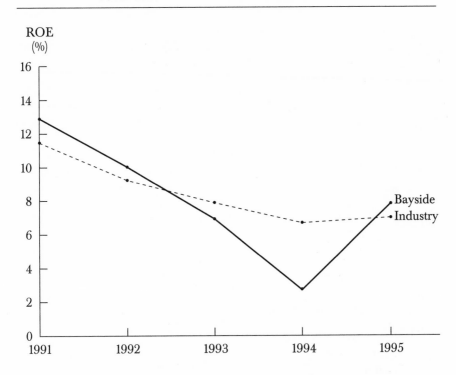

	Return on Equity (ROE)	
Year	*Bayside*	*Industry*
1991	12.5%	11.7%
1992	10.0	9.8
1993	6.7	7.6
1994	2.4	6.9
1995	8.0	7.8

Self-Test Questions:

How are common size statements created?

What advantage do common size statements have over regular statements when conducting a financial analysis?

Table 12.4 Bayside Memorial Hospital: Common Size Income Statement, 1995

	Bayside	Industry Average
Net patient services revenue	94.6%	90.4%
Other operating revenue	5.4	9.6
Total operating revenue	100.0%	100.0%
Operating expenses:		
Nursing services	50.8%	51.0%
Dietary services	4.7	4.5
General services	11.5	11.3
Administrative services	10.0	10.8
Employee health and welfare	8.9	9.6
Provision for uncollectibles	2.9	3.0
Provision for malpractice	1.1	1.0
Depreciation	3.6	4.1
Interest expense	1.3	2.2
Total operating expenses	94.9%	97.5%
Income from operations	5.1%	2.5%
Contributions and grants	2.0%	1.8%
Investment income	0.4	0.6
Nonoperating gain (loss)	2.4%	2.4%
Excess of revenues over expenses	7.5%	4.9%

Percentage Change Analysis

Another frequently used technique when analyzing financial statements is percentage change analysis. Here, the percentage changes in the individual accounts on the balance sheet and items on the income statement over some time period are calculated and compared. In this format, it is easy to see which items are growing faster or slower than others, and hence to see which of them are under control and which are out of control.

The conclusions reached in a percentage change analysis, as well as in a common size analysis, generally parallel those derived from ratio

Table 12.5   Bayside Memorial Hospital: Common Size Balance
Sheet, 1995

	Bayside	Industry Average
Cash and securities	4.1%	5.7%
Accounts receivable	14.4	17.2
Inventories	2.1	2.5
Total current assets	20.7%	25.4%
Gross plant and equipment	96.0%	90.1%
Accumulated depreciation	16.6	15.5
Net plant and equipment	79.3%	74.6%
Total assets	100.0%	100.0%
Accounts payable	3.1%	3.9%
Accrued expenses	3.7	4.1
Notes payable	0.5	3.2
Current portion of long-term debt	1.4	2.1
Total current liabilities	8.8%	13.3%
Long-term debt	19.0%	36.5%
Capital lease obligations	1.2	0.9
Total long-term liabilities	20.2%	37.4%
Fund balance	71.0%	49.3%
Total liabilities and funds	100.0%	100.0%

analysis. However, occasionally a serious deficiency is highlighted by only
one of the three analytical techniques, while the other two techniques
fail to bring the deficiency to light. Thus, a thorough financial statement
analysis will begin with a Du Pont analysis for an overview, and will then
include ratio, common size, and percentage change analyses.

Self-Test Questions:

What is a percentage change analysis?

Why is it useful?

Which analytical techniques should be used in a complete financial
statement analysis?

MVA And EVA

Two financial analysis measures being used with increasing frequency focus directly on management's success or failure in maximizing shareholder wealth: they are Market Value Added (MVA) and Economic Value Added (EVA). These measures are especially useful in investor-owned businesses because of their direct link with the primary goal of the firm. However, the second measure, Economic Value Added, can be used also in not-for-profit firms, so this section has relevance to both forms of ownership.

Market Value Added (MVA)

The primary goal of any investor-owned firm should be shareholder wealth maximization. This goal obviously benefits shareholders, and it also ensures that scarce resources are allocated as efficiently as possible. Note, however, that managerial zeal to enhance shareholder wealth does not mean that other stakeholders, including creditors, employees, patients, and so on, should be treated unfairly, for such actions will ultimately be detrimental to shareholders.

Although the fundamental goal of shareholder wealth maximization is widely accepted, managers must recognize that it is not the same thing as maximizing the firm's total market value. A firm's total market value can be increased by raising and investing as much capital as possible, which increases the size of the firm and hence often benefits managers. However, this strategy rarely is in the best interests of shareholders, because it ignores the fact that shareholders have opportunity costs, and hence must earn some minimum rate of return on their investment. Shareholders' wealth is maximized by pursuing the strategy of maximizing the *difference* between the firm's total market value and the amount of capital that investors have supplied to the firm. This difference is called *Market Value Added (MVA)*:

MVA = Total market value − Total capital supplied

Here, total market value is the sum of the book value of debt and the market value of equity, while total capital supplied is the sum of the book values of debt and equity. The book value of debt is used in the calculation of total market value because (1) the purpose of the analysis is to focus on the addition to shareholders' wealth; (2) it very difficult, if not impossible, to determine the market value of most corporate debt issues because they are not actively traded; (3) debt market values are usually relatively close to book values; and (4) in general, the market value of a firm's debt is more closely tied to interest rate movements than to managerial actions that affect shareholder wealth. In essence, the assumption is made that the market value of debt equals its book value. Note that, with book value of debt in both terms on the right-hand side of the equation, MVA can also be defined more simply as follows:

MVA = Market value of equity − Book value of equity

To illustrate the MVA concept, consider Columbia/HCA Health-care. In 1994, its total market value was $15.8 billion, while its investors had supplied only $9.4 billion. Thus, Columbia/HCA's MVA was $15.8 − $9.4 = $6.4 billion. This $6.4 billion represents the difference between the funds, including retained earnings, that Columbia/HCA's equity investors have put into the corporation since its founding and the value of the cash they could get by selling the business. By maximizing this spread, management maximizes the wealth of its equity investors relative to other uses of their capital.

While the managers of Columbia/HCA have done a spectacular job of maximizing shareholder wealth, National Medical Enterprises (NME) managers have done poorly. In 1994, NME's total market value was $4.0 billion, which, on the surface, looks like its managers are doing a good job—$4.0 billion is a lot of money. However, equity investors have supplied NME with $4.1 billion of capital, so NME's MVA was a negative $100 million. In effect, NME is left with only $0.98 of equity value for every dollar shareholders put up, whereas Columbia/HCA has turned $1 of equity investment into $1.68 of wealth.

There is a direct tie between MVA and the net present value (NPV) capital budgeting rule. To illustrate, consider a company that decides to retain $10 million in earnings for investment in a project, but the market expects a present value of future cash flows from the project of only $8 million. Even though the project will cause the total market value of the company to be $8 million greater than if the earnings had been paid out as dividends, shareholders will have $2 million less wealth. This loss occurs because shareholders have been deprived of the opportunity to invest the $10 million in alternative investments (including cash) that would have a market value of at least $10 million. With $10 million added to the capital invested in the company, but only $8 million added to the company's total market value, the firm's MVA would fall by $2 million and thereby register the erosion in shareholder wealth. Note, though, that the project would have an NPV of negative $2 million. Since NPV measures the amount that a project can be expected to add (or subtract) from MVA, by following the NPV rule managers should, at a minimum, be able to avoid creating negative MVA. Of course, those companies with high MVAs, like Columbia/HCA, have done a very good job of ferreting out high-NPV projects, which then produced their high MVAs.

Clearly, the MVA concept is applicable only to investor-owned firms, because it focuses on how well managers have done in creating value for shareholders. However, the next measure, EVA, applies to both investor-owned and not-for-profit firms.

Economic Value Added (EVA)

Whereas MVA measures the combined effect of managerial actions to enhance shareholder wealth since the inception of the company, *Economic Value Added (EVA)* focuses on managerial effectiveness in a given year. The basic formula for EVA is this:

$$\text{EVA} = \text{Operating profit} - (\text{Total capital supplied} \times \text{Cost of capital})$$

Here, operating profit is revenues minus all operating costs, including taxes but excluding interest expense; total capital supplied is the sum of the book values of debt and equity, and cost of capital is the overall corporate cost of capital. Unlike MVA, EVA does not focus directly on market values, and hence EVA can be applied to not-for-profit firms.[14]

To illustrate the EVA concept, consider Birmingham Health Providers, a medical group practice. The group had $1 million in operating profits in 1995 generated from $5 million of investor-supplied debt and equity capital. Also, the firm's weighted average cost of capital was 10 percent. (The group uses 50 percent debt financing with an after-tax cost of 6 percent and 50 percent equity financing with a cost of 14 percent.) With these assumptions, Birmingham Health Providers' 1995 EVA was $500,000:

$$\text{EVA} = \$1 - \$5(0.10) = \$1 - \$0.5 = \$0.5 \text{ million}$$

EVA is an estimate of a business's true economic profit for the year, and it differs substantially from accounting profitability measures. EVA represents the residual income that remains after **all** costs have been recognized, including the opportunity cost of the employed capital. Accounting profit, on the other hand, is formulated without imposing a charge for equity capital. EVA depends on both operating efficiency and balance sheet management: without operating efficiency profits will be low, and without efficient balance sheet management there will be too many assets and, hence, too much capital, which results in higher-than-necessary capital costs.

For not-for-profit firms, fund capital is a scarce resource that must be managed well to ensure the financial viability of the firm, and hence its ability to continue to perform its stated mission. EVA lets managers know how well they are doing in managing this scarce resource, for the higher the EVA in any year, the better job managers are doing in using fund capital to create additional value. Of course, EVA measures only economic value, so any social value created by the fund capital is ignored and, hence, must be subjectively considered.

Note that EVA (but not MVA) can be applied to divisions as well as to entire companies, and that the charge for capital should reflect the riskiness of the business unit, whether it be the whole company or an operating division. Note also that the specific calculation of EVA for a company or division is much more complex than presented here because many accounting issues, such as inventory valuation, depreciation, amortization of research and development costs, and the like, must be addressed properly when estimating a firm's operating profit.[15]

EVA is a link in the economic value creation chain that begins with the NPV of an individual project and ends with the firm's MVA (or implied MVA in the case of not-for-profit firms). Each project's expected economic profitability, which is initially measured by its NPV, contributes to the firm's EVA for any given year. Furthermore, MVA is the present value of the EVAs that the firm is expected to produce in the future. Thus, the creation of good investment opportunities (high-NPV projects) creates the expectation of high future EVAs, which investors recognize by bidding up the price of the firm's stock, which in turn creates a large MVA.

Although EVA is currently a hot topic, the underlying concept is not new—managers have known for quite a while that companies need to earn more than the cost of capital. However, this basic premise is often lost because of a misguided focus on accounting profitability, which accounts for the cost of debt but does not account for the even higher cost of equity.

Self-Test Questions:

What is Market Value Added (MVA), and how is it measured?

What is Economic Value Added (EVA), and how is it measured?

Can MVA and EVA be applied to not-for-profit firms?

Why is EVA a better measure of managerial performance than are accounting measures such as earnings per share and return on equity?

Operating Analysis

Operating analysis goes one step beyond financial statement analysis in that operating analysis examines operating variables with the goal of explaining a firm's financial condition. Like ratio analysis, operating analysis variables are typically grouped into major categories to make interpretation easier. For hospitals, the categories are (1) profit indicators, (2) net price indicators, (3) volume indicators, (4) length of stay indicators, (5) service intensity indicators, (6) efficiency indicators, and (7) unit cost indicators. Because of space constraints, we cannot discuss operating analysis in detail here. However, to give you a flavor, we will define and illustrate eight commonly used hospital operating analysis ratios.

Net price per discharge

Net price per discharge measures the average revenue collected on each inpatient discharge. In 1995, Bayside collected $97,740,000 from inpatient services and discharged 25,281 patients:

$$\text{Net price per discharge} = \frac{\text{Net inpatient revenue}}{\text{Total discharges}}$$

$$= \frac{\$97,740,000}{25,281} = \$3,866.$$

Industry average $= \$3,880.$

Bayside collects about the same amount per discharge as the average hospital. However, if Bayside's case mix, which measures the average intensity of services provided, is higher than average, then perhaps its net price per discharge should be higher than average.

Net price per visit

Net price per visit measures the amount collected per outpatient visit. For 1995, Bayside collected $10,860,000 from 67,453 outpatient visits:

$$\text{Net price per visit} = \frac{\text{Net outpatient revenue}}{\text{Total outpatient visits}} = \frac{\$10,860,000}{67,453}$$

$$= \$161.$$

Industry average $= \$147.$

Bayside realizes more revenue per outpatient visit than the average hospital.

Medicare payment percentage

Medicare payment percentage measures the exposure of a hospital to Medicare patients, and hence to payments set by political, rather than economic, processes:

$$\text{Medicare payment percentage} = \frac{\text{Medicare discharges}}{\text{Total discharges}}$$

$$= \frac{12,105}{25,281} = 47.9\%.$$

Industry average $= 35.9\%$.

Bayside has a much higher percentage of Medicare patients than the average hospital. To the extent that Medicare payments are less than payments from most other third party payers, a higher Medicare payment percentage puts pressure on operating revenues. Similar operating ratios could be constructed for Medicaid patients, bad debt and charity care patients, and so on.

Outpatient revenue percentage

The *outpatient revenue percentage* measures the mix between outpatient and inpatient revenues:

$$\text{Outpatient revenue percentage} = \frac{\text{Net outpatient revenue}}{\text{Net total revenue}}$$

$$= \frac{\$10,860,000}{\$108,600,000} = 10.0\%.$$

Industry average $= 22.1\%$.

Bayside has a much smaller outpatient program, relative to its size, than the average hospital. During the 1980s, hospitals, on average, significantly expanded their outpatient programs based on the belief that such services were more profitable because Medicare still pays for outpatient services on a charge basis. However, the claims of increased profitability were never proved, and in the near future Medicare is expected to change to a prospective payment system for outpatient services.

Occupancy rate

Occupancy rate measures the extent of utilization of a hospital's beds, and hence fixed assets. Since overhead costs are incurred on all assets, whether used or not, higher occupancy spreads fixed costs over more patients, and hence increases per patient profitability. Since Bayside had 180,079 inpatient days in 1995, its occupancy percentage is 75.9 percent:

$$\text{Occupancy percentage} = \frac{\text{Inpatient days}}{\text{Number of staffed beds} \times 365}$$

$$= \frac{180,079}{650 \times 365} = 75.9\%.$$

Industry average $= 68.5\%$.

Bayside has a higher occupancy rate, and hence is using its fixed assets more productively that the average hospital. Note that this conclusion is contrary to our financial analysis interpretation of Bayside's 1995 fixed asset turnover ratio. While that ratio is affected by inflation and accounting convention, the occupancy percentage is not.

Average length of stay (ALOS)

The *average length of stay (ALOS)* is the number of days that an average inpatient is hospitalized with each admission.

$$\text{ALOS} = \frac{\text{Inpatient days}}{\text{Total discharges}} = \frac{180,079}{25,281} = 7.1 \text{ days}.$$

Industry average $= 6.4$ days.

Bayside keeps its patients in the hospital slightly longer, on average, than the average hospital. (Bayside has a *case-mix index* of 1.28 compared with an average for the industry of 1.19. The case-mix index is a weighted average of DRG weights, so the higher the index, the more intense the services provided. Thus, Bayside's patients, on average, require more intensive treatment than patients in the average hospital.)

Cost per discharge

So far, our operating analysis has focused on revenue and volume measures. *Cost per discharge* measures the dollar amount of resources, on average, expended on each discharge. Since Bayside's inpatient operating expenses for 1995 were $94,865,000, its cost per discharge is $3,752:

$$\text{Cost per discharge} = \frac{\text{Inpatient operating expenses}}{\text{Total discharges}}$$

$$= \frac{\$94,865,000}{25,281} = \$3,752.$$

Industry average $= \$3,818$.

Even though Bayside's price per discharge is slightly below average, its cost per discharge is even more so. Thus, Bayside's average margin on each discharge is more than that for the hospital industry. Note that another operating ratio of interest is the cost per visit ratio, which measures the cost per outpatient visit.

FTEs per occupied bed

The number of *full-time equivalent employees (FTEs)* per occupied bed is a measure of work force productivity—the lower this figure, the more productive the hospital's work force.

$$\text{FTEs per occupied bed} = \frac{\text{Inpatient } FTEs}{\text{Average daily census}} = \frac{2,005}{0.759 \times 650}$$
$$= 4.06.$$

Industry average $= 4.34.$

Note that we calculated the average daily census (the number of patients hospitalized on an average day) by multiplying Bayside's occupancy rate times the number of staffed beds. The FTEs per occupied bed ratio indicates that Bayside is using its human resources more efficiently than the average hospital does. Other operating ratios that would be of interest here are outpatient work force per visit and salary per FTE.

As you can see from the eight operating ratios presented here, operating analysis goes beyond financial analysis in an attempt to identify the operating strengths and weaknesses that underlie a firm's financial condition. Although we have illustrated operating analysis using the hospital industry, the concepts can be applied to any industry, although the ratios selected would differ. Also, operating ratios are interpreted in the same way as financial ratios, that is, by using comparative and trend analysis.

Self-Test Questions:

What is the difference between financial and operating analyses?

Why is operating analysis important?

Describe four ratios commonly used in operating analysis.

Financial Control Systems

Thus far we have discussed financial statement analysis on an overall corporate basis. Such a consolidated analysis is useful for managers of stand-alone health care businesses. However, managers in large corporations or systems use the procedures described in this chapter primarily on a divisional, or business line, basis. In a health care system, each provider would be a separate profit or cost center, depending on the reimbursement methodology, and the techniques described earlier would be applied to each line of business. If the divisions are all performing well, then the overall system will also look good. If not, then top management should see to it that corrective actions are taken.

Such a *financial control system*, used with good judgment, is essential for the proper management of any corporation with multiple divisions. An extended discussion of financial controls would go beyond the scope of this book, but we should point out a few problems with such systems. (1) Different divisions may have assets of different ages. This will affect depreciation and hence reported profits, and also the investment base and hence ROA and ROE. (2) Frequently, one division sells to another, and the transfer price used in such intercorporate sales will have a major effect on the divisions' relative profitability. (3) The allocation of corporate overheads will affect relative profitability. (4) Certain types of investments may have no payoff for a number of years, and if divisional managers are rewarded only on the basis of short-term results, this may bias decisions against long-run projects. (5) Certain divisions may be riskier than others, so different profitability standards must be applied. (6) Certain divisions may have more debt capacity than others, yet borrowing is generally done at the corporate level; this must be taken into account.

These are just a few of the problems that arise when one attempts to utilize a system of divisional financial controls. Some top managers, when faced with these problems, have just given up and let their division managers operate autonomously. However, this is a sure path to corporate destruction. Well-run corporations recognize and deal with these problems.

Self-Test Questions:

Why are financial control systems so important to corporate success?

How should control systems be established in corporations with multiple lines of business?

Problems in Financial and Operating Analyses

In our discussion of ratio analysis, we mentioned some of the problems one encounters in financial statement analysis. In this section, we discuss some of the additional problems and limitations that affect both financial and operating analyses.

Development of comparative data

Many large firms operate a number of different divisions in quite different industries, and in such cases it is difficult to develop meaningful industry averages. This tends to make financial statement analysis more useful for small firms with single product lines than for large, multiproduct companies.

Additionally, most firms want to be better than average (although half will be above and half will be below the median), so merely attaining average performance is not necessarily good. Compilers of industry data, such as Dun & Bradstreet, Robert Morris Associates, and the Center for Healthcare Industry Performance Studies (CHIPS), generally report industry ratios in quartiles or other percentiles. For example, CHIPS recently reported that 10 percent of hospitals have a current ratio over 1.1, 25 percent are above 1.5, the median is 2.0, 75 percent are above 2.6, and 10 percent have current ratios higher than 3.6. This presentation gives managers an idea of the distribution of ratios within an industry, and hence they can make better judgments about how their firms compare with the top firms in the industry.

Also, it is beneficial for managers to compare their firms not only with the industry average, but also with their leading competitors. Thus, when Bayside's managers conduct a complete financial and operating analysis, they compare Bayside's ratios with their three leading competitors, as well as with industry averages. In the end, however, it is extremely important that senior managers establish their own standards of performance, and ensure that all other managers are aware of those standards and are taking actions on a daily basis to achieve them.

Interpretation of results

It is often difficult to generalize about whether a particular ratio is "good" or "bad." For example, a high quick ratio may show a strong liquidity position, which is good, or an excessive amount of cash, which is bad because cash is a nonearning asset. Similarly, a high asset turnover ratio may denote either a firm that uses its assets efficiently or one that is undercapitalized and simply cannot afford to buy enough assets. Also, firms often have some ratios that look "good" and others that look "bad," making it difficult to tell whether the firm is, on balance, in a strong or a weak financial position. For this reason, ratio analysis is normally used as an input to judgmental decisions.

Various systems have been developed that attempt to reduce the information contained in a financial analysis to a single value, and hence make interpretation much easier. One method applied is multiple discriminant analysis, which attempts to divide companies into two groups on the basis of their probabilities of going bankrupt. Another method merely combines ratios selected judgmentally into a composite index, which is then compared to the industry average index. Needless to say, it is very difficult to distill the wide variety of information contained in a ratio analysis into a single measure of financial condition.[16]

Differences in accounting treatment

Different accounting practices can distort ratio comparisons. For example, firms can use different accounting conventions to value cost of goods sold and ending inventories. During inflationary periods these differences can lead to ratio distortions. Other accounting practices, such as those related to leases, can also create distortions.

Effects of inflation

The high inflation rates of the late 1970s and early 1980s drew increased attention to the need to assess both the impact of inflation on businesses and the success of management in coping with it. Numerous reporting methods have been proposed to adjust accounting statements for inflation, but no consensus has been reached either on how to do this or even on the practical usefulness of the resulting data. Nevertheless, accounting standards encourage, but do not require, businesses to disclose supplementary data to reflect the effects of general inflation.

Financial statement effects

Traditionally, financial statements have been prepared on the basis of historical costs, that is, the actual number of dollars paid for each asset purchased. However, inflation has caused the purchasing power of dollars to erode over time: in 1995 it required over $4.00 to purchase the same amount of goods that $1.00 would purchase in 1965. As a result of inflation, financial statements can be badly distorted. To illustrate, a $2,000,000 expenditure on land for a hospital in 1995 might be equivalent to a $300,000 purchase in 1950, so combining 1995 and

1950 dollars is much like adding apples and oranges. (Remember that land is not depreciated, so it remains on the balance sheet at its original cost until sold.) Nevertheless, this is done when the typical balance sheet is constructed.

To reflect the effects of inflation, and thus to express operating results in dollars of comparable purchasing power, companies are encouraged to report "income from continuing operations," calculated as if all of the depreciable assets of the company had been purchased with current-year dollars, and consequently its depreciation were based on higher-valued assets. Such an adjustment comes closer to showing what profits might be in the long run, when the old, undervalued assets have been replaced with new, inflated-value assets, and depreciation is correspondingly higher.

Companies are also encouraged to present a supplementary five-year comparison of selected financial data in current dollars. Operating revenues, net income, and cash dividends per common share are typically restated in constant dollars. This allows investors to see what portion of growth stems from inflation effects, as opposed to true economic growth.

Ratio analysis effects

If a ratio analysis is based on "regular" financial statements, unadjusted for inflation, then distortions can creep in. Obviously, there will be a tendency for the value of the fixed assets to be understated, and inventories will also be understated if the firm uses last-in first-out (LIFO) accounting. At the same time, increasing rates of inflation will lead to increases in interest rates that will, in turn, cause the value of the outstanding long-term debt to decline. Further, profits will vary from year to year as the inflation rate changes, and these variations will be especially severe if inventory is charged to cost of goods sold based on the first-in first-out (FIFO) method.

These factors tend to make ratio comparisons over time for a given company, and across companies at any point in time, less reliable than would be the case in the absence of inflation. This is especially true if a company changes its accounting procedures (say, from straight-line to accelerated depreciation or from FIFO to LIFO), or if various companies in a given industry use different accounting data. However, analysts ought to recognize that there are weaknesses in ratio analysis, and they should apply judgment in interpreting the data.

Self-Test Question:

Briefly describe some of the problems encountered when performing financial and operating analyses.

Summary

The primary purposes of this chapter were (1) to describe the basic financial statements and (2) to discuss techniques used by managers to analyze them. The key concepts covered are listed next.

- The three basic statements contained in the annual report are the *balance sheet,* the *income statement,* and the *statement of cash flows.*

- *Financial analysis,* which is designed to identify a firm's financial condition, focuses on the firm's financial statements. *Operating analysis* gives insights into *why* a firm is in a strong, or weak, financial condition.

- The *Du Pont equation* is designed to show how the profit margin, the total asset turnover ratio, and the use of debt interact to determine the rate of return on equity. It provides a good overview of a firm's financial condition.

- *Ratio analysis* is designed to reveal the relative strengths and weaknesses of a company as compared to other companies in the same industry, and to show whether the firm's position has been improving or deteriorating over time.

- *Liquidity ratios* indicate the firm's ability to meet its short-term obligations.

- *Asset management ratios* measure how effectively a firm is managing its assets.

- *Debt management ratios* reveal (1) the extent to which the firm is financed with debt and (2) the extent to which operating cash flows cover debt service and other fixed charge requirements.

- *Profitability ratios* show the combined effects of liquidity, asset management, and debt management on operating results.

- Ratios are analyzed using *comparative analysis,* in which a firm's ratios are compared with industry averages (or those of another firm), and *trend analysis,* in which a firm's ratios are examined over time.

- In a *common size analysis,* a firm's income statement and balance sheet are expressed in percentages. This facilitates comparisons between firms of different sizes and for a single firm over time.

- *Market Value Added (MVA)* and *Economic Value Added (EVA)* are two measures of firm performance that focus directly on management's ability to enhance shareholder wealth.

- Like ratio analysis, operating analysis variables are typically grouped into major categories to make interpretation easier. For example, hospital operating ratios are grouped into seven categories: (1) *profit indicators*, (2) *net price indicators*, (3) *volume indicators*, (4) *length of stay indicators*, (5) *service intensity indicators*, (6) *efficiency indicators*, and (7) *unit cost indicators*.

- Financial and operating analyses are not without problems. Some of the major difficulties are (1) *development of comparative data*, (2) *interpretation of results*, and (3) *inflation effects*.

Financial and operating analyses have limitations, but used with care and judgment, they can provide a sound picture of a firm's financial condition as well as identify those operating factors than contribute to that condition.

Notes

1. For more information on the various organizations involved in setting accounting principles for the health care industry, see W. Grossman and W. Warshauer, Jr., "An Overview of the Standard Setting Process," *Topics in Health Care Financing* (Summer 1990): 1–8.
2. Some firms also provide quarterly reports, but these are much less comprehensive than the annual reports. In addition, larger investor-owned firms must file even more detailed statements, giving the particulars of each major division or subsidiary, with the Securities and Exchange Commission (SEC). These reports, called *10-K Reports*, are made available to stockholders upon request to a company's secretary. Finally, many larger firms also publish *statistical supplements*, which give financial statement data and key ratios going back about ten years. Like the 10-K, statistical supplements may be obtained from the corporate secretary.
3. At the time we were writing this chapter, the American Institute of Certified Public Accountants (AICPA) was circulating for public comment a revised version of its accounting and auditing guide for health care providers titled *Audits of Providers of Health Care Services*. This guide may mandate some changes to the financial statements presented in this chapter. For more information, see W. R. Titera, "AICPA Seeks Comments on Proposed Accounting Changes," *Healthcare Financial Management* (August 1995): 72–81.
4. One could divide liabilities into (1) interest-bearing debt owed to specific firms or individuals and (2) non-interest-bearing debt owed to suppliers, employees, and in the case of taxable firms, governments. We do not make this distinction, so the terms *debt* and *liabilities* are used synonymously. Also,

note that an investor-owned firm would show common equity rather than fund capital on its balance sheet.

5. The return on assets calculation can be easily checked by using the basic definition of ROA:

$$ROA = \frac{\text{Net income}}{\text{Total assets}} = \frac{\$8,572}{\$151,278} \approx 5.68\%.$$

6. Throughout the remainder of the chapter, we will use illustrative industry averages that do not necessarily represent actual data. Thus, our industry averages should not be used for actual "real world" analyses.

7. If the nonoperating cash flow is a loss, then the term farthest to the right in the expanded Du Pont equation is less than 1.0, and hence the operating return on equity is reduced by the nonoperating cash flow.

8. The Center for Healthcare Industry Performance Studies (CHIPS) publishes an annual almanac that provides hospital industry data on 34 financial ratios and 42 operating ratios. The ratios are reported in several groupings, such as by hospital size and geographic location. See W. O. Cleverley, *Almanac of Hospital Financial and Operating Indicators* (Columbus, Ohio: CHIPS, published annually).

9. $1/2.3 = 0.43$, or 43 percent. Note that $0.43(\$31,280,000) \approx \$13,332,000$, the amount of current liabilities.

10. Another liquidity ratio sometimes used is the *acid test ratio*, which is defined as cash plus marketable securities all divided by current liabilities. Clearly, this ratio is even more restrictive than the quick ratio in defining liquidity.

11. See FASB Statement 33, *Financial Reporting and Changing Prices* (September 1979), for a discussion of the effects of inflation on financial statements and what the accounting profession is trying to do to provide better and more useful balance sheets and income statements. Also, we discuss the impact of inflation on financial statements in more depth later in the chapter. Finally, we will find later when we perform an operating analysis that Bayside has a higher than average occupancy rate, which would tend to refute any conclusions based solely on the fixed asset turnover ratio.

12. Because information on credit sales is generally unavailable, total sales must be used. Since all firms may not have the same percentage of credit sales, there is a chance that the days sales outstanding will be somewhat in error. Also, it would be better to use *average* receivables in the formula, either an average of the monthly figures or (Beginning + Ending)/2.

13. Because information on credit purchases is generally unavailable, total purchases is sometimes used, but even this information is often not available to analysts outside of the firm. Also, as with the ACP, it would be better to use *average* payables than to rely on the balance amount at any single point in time. Finally, note that the following ratio, which measures the average payment period on all expenses, is frequently used:

$$\text{Average payment period} = \frac{\text{Accounts payable} + \text{Accruals}}{(\text{Operating expenses} - \text{Depreciation})/365}$$

14. For an excellent example of the application of EVA in setting managerial compensation within not-for-profit firms, see W. O. Cleverley and R. K. Harvey, "Economic Value Added—A Framework for Health Care Executive Compensation," *Hospital and Health Services Administration* (Summer 1993): 215–28.

15. The EVA calculation was first developed in detail by the consulting firm of Stern Stewart and Company. For a more complete discussion, see G. B. Stewart, III, *The Quest for Value* (New York, HarperBusiness, 1991).

16. For a general discussion of multiple discriminant analysis, see E. F. Brigham and L. C. Gapenski, *Intermediate Financial Management* (Fort Worth, TX: Dryden Press, 1996), chap. 26. See W. O. Cleverley, "Predicting Hospital Failure with the Financial Flexibility Index," *Healthcare Financial Management* (May 1985): 29–37, for a discussion of his financial flexibility index.

Selected Additional References

Bazzoli, G. J., and W. O. Cleverley. 1994. "Hospital Bankruptcies: An Exploration of Potential Causes and Consequences." *Health Care Management Review* (Summer): 41–51.

Beaver, W. H., and J. E. Horngren. 1991. "Ten Commandants of Financial Statement Analysis," *Financial Analysts Journal* (January-February): 9.

Bitter, M. E., and J. Cassidy. 1992. "Perceptions of New AICPA Audit Guide." *Healthcare Financial Management* (November): 38–48.

Boles, K. E. 1992. "Insolvency in Managed Care Organizations: Financial Indicators." *Topics in Health Care Financing* (Winter): 40–57.

Cleverley, W. O., and R. K. Harvey. 1992. "Is There a Link Between Hospital Profit and Quality?" *Healthcare Financial Management* (September): 40–45.

———. 1990. "Profitability: Comparing Hospital Results with Other Industries." *Healthcare Financial Management* (March): 42–52.

———. 1985. "Predicting Hospital Failure with the Financial Flexibility Index." *Healthcare Financial Management* (May): 36–43.

———. 1990. "ROI: Its Role in Voluntary Hospital Planning." *Hospital and Health Services Administration* (Spring): 71–82.

———. 1994. "Trends in the Hospital Financial Picture." *Healthcare Financial Management* (February): 56–63.

———. 1995. "Understanding Your Hospital's True Financial Position and Changing It." *Health Care Management Review* (Spring): 62–73.

Coyne, J. S. 1990. "Analyzing the Financial Performance of Hospital-Based Managed Care Programs: The Case of Humana." *Journal of Health Administration Education* (Fall): 571–642.

———. 1985. "Measuring Hospital Performance in Multi-Institutional Organizations Using Financial Ratios." *Health Care Management Review* (Fall): 35–42.

Donnelly, J. T. 1993. "RBRVS as a Financial Assessment Tool." *Healthcare Financial Management* (February): 45–51.

Duis, T. E. 1993. "The Need for Consistency in Healthcare Reporting." *Healthcare Financial Management* (July): 40–44.

————. "Unravelling the Confusion Caused by GASB, FASB Accounting Rules." *Healthcare Financial Management* (November): 66–69.

Eastaugh, S. R. 1992. "Hospital Strategy and Financial Performance." *Health Care Management Review* (Summer): 19–32.

Finkler, S. A. 1982. "Ratio Analysis: Use with Caution." *Health Care Management Review* (Spring): 65–72.

Gapenski, L. C., W. B.Vogel, and B. Langland-Orban. 1993. "The Determinants of Hospital Profitability." *Hospital & Health Services Administration* (Spring 1993): 63–80.

Harkey, J., and R. Vraciu. 1992. "Quality of Health Care and Financial Performance: Is There a Link?" *Health Care Management Review* (Fall): 55–61.

Lynn, M. L., and P. Wertheim. 1993. "Key Financial Ratios Can Foretell Hospital Closures," *Healthcare Financial Management* (November): 66–70.

McCue, M. J. 1991. "The Use of Cash Flow to Analyze Financial Distress in California Hospitals." *Hospital & Health Services Administration* (Summer): 223–41.

Pelfrey, S. 1990. "How Proposed FASB Standards Would Affect Hospitals." *Healthcare Financial Management* (February): 54–67.

Prince, T. R. 1991. "Assessing Financial Outcomes of Not-for-Profit Community Hospitals." *Hospital & Healthcare Administration* (Fall): 331–49.

Robbins, W. A., and R. Turpin. 1993. "Accounting Practice Diversity in the Healthcare Industry." *Healthcare Financial Management* (May): 111–14.

Sherman, B. 1990. "How Investors Evaluate the Creditworthiness of Hospitals." *Healthcare Financial Management* (March): 25–31.

Sylvestre, J., and F. R. Urbancic. "Effective Methods for Cash Flow Analysis." *Healthcare Financial Management* (July): 62–72.

Titera, W. R. 1993. "FASB Proposes Changes in Not-for-Profit Reporting." *Healthcare Financial Management* (April): 39–49.

Vogel, W. B., B. Langland-Orban, and L. C. Gapenski. 1993. "Factors Influencing High and Low Profitability among Hospitals." *Health Care Management Review* (Spring): 15–26.

Case 12

St. Margaret's Hospital (A): Financial and Operating Analyses

St. Margaret's Hospital is a 210-bed, not-for-profit, acute care hospital with a long-standing reputation for quality service to a growing community. The hospital is affiliated with the Coalition of Catholic Hospitals. St. Margaret's competes with five other hospitals in its metropolitan statistical area (MSA), three that are not-for-profit and two for-profit. Competition among the hospitals has been keen, but friendly. However, Columbia/HCA Healthcare recently purchased one of the for-profit hospitals, which has resulted in some anxiety among the managers of the other hospitals. Relevant financial and operating data for St. Margaret's are contained in Tables 1 through 4, and selected industry data are contained in Tables 5 and 6. In addition, the following data were extracted from the notes section to St. Margaret's 1996 Annual Report.

1. A significant portion of the hospital's net patient revenue was generated by patients who are covered either by Medicare, Medicaid, or other government programs, or by various private plans, including managed care plans, that have contracts with the hospital that specify discounts from charges. Normal billings for services to covered patients are included in gross revenues, but then provisions are made to reduce such billings to their estimated final settlements for income statement reporting. The gross revenue breakdown is given below (in millions of dollars):

	1992	*1993*	*1994*	*1995*	*1996*
Gross patient revenue					
Inpatient	$25.161	$25.275	$26.117	$29.148	$33.216
Outpatient	4.748	5.969	6.535	9.130	11.912
Gross patient revenue	$29.909	$31.244	$32.652	$38.278	$45.128
Revenue deductions					
Contractual allowances	$ 2.489	$ 2.053	$ 1.729	$ 5.196	$ 7.516
Bad debts/charity care	1.759	1.955	2.127	2.506	3.030
Total deductions	$ 4.248	$ 4.008	$ 3.856	$ 7.702	$10.546
Net patient revenue	$25.661	$27.236	$28.796	$30.576	$34.582

2. Inventories are stated at the lower of cost, determined on a first-in first-out basis, or market value.

3. The breakdown of operating expenses between inpatient and outpatient activities for 1992 through 1996 is as follows (in millions of dollars):

	1992	*1993*	*1994*	*1995*	*1996*
Inpatient operating costs	$18.635	$19.221	$20.573	$22.229	$24.771
Outpatient operating costs	5.261	6.062	6.831	8.098	9.187
Total operating costs	$23.896	$25.283	$27.404	$30.327	$33.958

4. St. Margaret's has a contributory money accumulation (defined contribution) pension plan covering substantially all of its employees. Participants can contribute up to 20 percent of earnings to the pension plan. The hospital matches on a dollar-for-dollar basis employee contributions of up to 2 percent of wages, and it pays 50 cents on the dollar for contributions over 2 percent and up to 4 percent. Because the plan is a defined contribution plan (as opposed to a defined benefit plan), there are no unfunded pension liabilities. Pension expense was approximately $154,000 in 1995 and $181,000 in 1996.

5. The hospital is a member of the State Hospital Trust Fund under which it purchases professional liability insurance coverage for individual claims up to $1 million (subject to a deductible of $100,000 per claim). St. Margaret's is self-insured for amounts above $1 million but less than $5 million. Any liability award in excess of $5 million is covered by a commercial liability policy. For example, the policy would pay $2 million on a $7 million award. The hospital is currently

involved in eight suits involving claims of various amounts that could ultimately be tried before juries. Although it is impossible to determine the exact potential liability in these claims, management does not believe that the settlement of these cases could have a material effect on the hospital's financial position.

Assume that you have just joined the staff of St. Margaret's Hospital as assistant administrator. On your first day on the job, the administrator, Sister Mary Frances, stated that the best way to get to know the financial and operating condition of the hospital is to do a thorough financial and operating analysis, and thus she assigned you the task. Although you also believe that a financial and operating analysis is a good way to start, you wonder whether she has any ulterior motives. Perhaps the hospital is having problems, and she thinks that you can spot them. Or, perhaps, she wants to test your analytical skills—she is from the "old school" of hospital management and has been looking for someone to bring modern management methods to the hospital.

In any event, she has already scheduled a financial/operating analysis presentation for the next board of trustees meeting as a way for you to meet the board members. To help you structure your presentation, Sister Mary Frances suggests that you make the following points:

1. Discuss the hospital's statements of cash flows.

2. Present an overview of the hospital's financial position using the Du Pont equation as a guide.

3. Use ratio, common size, and percentage growth analyses to identify the hospital's financial strengths and weaknesses.

4. Use operating analysis to identify the operational factors that explain the hospital's current financial condition.

5. Summarize your evaluation of St. Margaret's financial condition. *Don't just rehash the numbers.* Rather, present your view of the potential underlying economic and managerial factors that might have caused any problems that surfaced in the financial and operating analyses.

6. Finally, make any recommendations that you believe St. Margaret's should follow to ensure future financial soundness.

Table 1 Statements of Revenues and Expenses (millions of dollars)

	1992	1993	1994	1995	1996
Operating Revenue					
Net patient revenue	$25.661	$27.236	$28.796	$30.576	$34.582
Other operating revenue	0.452	0.381	0.397	0.440	0.321
Total revenue	$26.113	$27.617	$29.193	$31.016	$34.903
Operating Expenses					
Salaries and wages	$10.829	$11.135	$12.245	$12.468	$13.994
Fringe benefits	1.496	1.731	1.830	2.408	2.568
Interest expense	1.341	1.305	1.181	1.598	1.776
Depreciation	1.708	1.977	2.350	2.658	2.778
Professional liability	0.102	0.157	0.140	0.201	0.218
Other	8.420	8.978	9.658	10.994	12.624
Total operating expense	$23.896	$25.283	$27.404	$30.327	$33.958
Income from operations	$ 2.217	$ 2.334	$ 1.789	$ 0.689	$ 0.945
Nonoperating Gains (Losses)					
Contributions	$ 0.023	$ 0.021	$ 0.005	$ 0.042	$ 0.002
Investment income	0.830	0.859	0.835	1.371	1.511
Total nonoperating gain	$ 0.853	$ 0.880	$ 0.840	$ 1.413	$ 1.513
Excess of revenues over expenses	$ 3.070	$ 3.214	$ 2.629	$ 2.102	$ 2.458

Table 2 Balance Sheets (millions of dollars)

	1992	1993	1994	1995	1996
Assets					
Cash and investments	$ 3.513	$ 5.799	$ 4.673	$ 5.069	$ 2.795
Accounts receivable (net)	5.915	4.832	4.359	5.674	7.413
Inventories	0.338	0.403	0.432	0.523	0.601
Other current assets	0.693	0.294	0.308	0.703	0.923
Total current assets	$10.459	$11.328	$ 9.772	$11.969	$11.732
Gross plant and equipment	$37.999	$42.005	$47.786	$55.333	$59.552
Accumulated depreciation	8.831	10.092	11.820	14.338	17.009
Net plant and equipment	$29.168	$31.913	$35.966	$40.995	$42.543
Total assets	$39.627	$43.241	$45.738	$52.964	$54.275
Liabilities and Fund Balance					
Accounts payable	$ 1.068	$ 1.273	$ 0.928	$ 1.253	$ 1.760
Accruals	1.085	1.311	1.804	1.823	1.473
Current portion of long-term debt	0.136	0.290	0.110	1.341	1.465
Total current liabilities	$ 2.289	$ 2.874	$ 2.842	$ 4.417	$ 4.698
Long-term debt	15.959	15.775	15.673	19.222	17.795
Fund balance	21.379	24.592	27.223	29.325	31.782
Total liabilities and funds	$39.627	$43.241	$45.738	$52.964	$54.275

Table 3   Cash Flow Statements (millions of dollars)

	1993	1994	1995	1996
Cash Flow from Operations				
Income from operations	$2.334	$1.789	$0.689	$0.945
Noncash expenses	1.952	2.326	2.633	2.756
Decrease (increase) in net working capital (except cash)	2.026	0.423	(0.202)	(1.733)
Net cash flow from operations	$6.312	$4.538	$3.120	$1.968
Cash Flow from Investing Activities				
Fixed asset acquisitions	($4.722)	($6.403)	($7.687)	($4.327)
Cash Flow from Financing Activities				
Long-term debt	($0.184)	($0.102)	$3.550	($1.428)
Nonoperating Cash Flow				
Nonoperating gains	$0.880	$0.840	$1.413	$1.513
Net increase (decrease) in cash	$2.286	($1.127)	$0.395	($2.273)
Beginning cash and investments	$3.513	$5.799	$4.673	$5.069
Ending cash and investments	$5.799	$4.672	$5.068	$2.796

Note: Some of the data in the statement of cash flows are slightly different than would be calculated from the income statement and balance sheet due to accounting complexities not shown.

Table 4   Selected Operating Data

	1992	1993	1994	1995	1996
Medicare discharges	3,008	2,960	2,721	2,860	2,741
Total discharges	9,680	9,311	8,784	8,318	8.576
Outpatient visits	30,754	31,960	32,285	32,878	36,796
Licensed beds	210	210	210	210	210
Staffed beds	192	196	193	197	178
Patient days	45,296	45,983	44,085	42,434	40,062
Case-mix index	0.9531	0.9274	0.9269	1.0493	1.0861
Full-time equivalents	604.5	618.1	610.8	625.8	619.3

Table 5 Selected Industry Financial Data

	1996 Industry Data (200–299 Beds)		
	+Quartile	*Median*	*− Quartile*
Profitability Ratios			
Deductible ratio*	0.34	0.26	0.18
Profit (total) margin	6.50%	3.10%	0.00%
Operating margin	4.30%	1.40%	−1.30%
Nonoperating revenue ratio	63.40%	32.70%	0.20%
Basic earning power	5.10%	2.90%	0.20%
Return on assets	5.80%	3.10%	0.40%
Return on equity	11.50%	6.50%	1.20%
Liquidity Ratios			
Current ratio	2.53	1.99	1.48
Quick ratio	2.21	1.72	1.31
Days cash on hand	32.35	15.89	6.24
Debt Management Ratios			
Debt ratio	62.90%	48.40%	35.20%
Long-term debt to equity	127.00%	64.70%	26.90%
Times interest earned	4.29	2.23	1.14
Fixed charge coverage	2.18	1.35	1.02
Cash flow coverage	5.32	3.22	1.76
Asset Management Ratios			
Inventory turnover	98.68	63.95	43.99
Current asset turnover	3.94	3.38	2.88
Fixed asset turnover	2.20	1.76	1.49
Total asset turnover	1.04	0.89	0.75
Average collection period	87.53	75.67	63.33
Average payment period	71.24	56.52	45.84
Other Ratios:			
Average age of plant (years)	8.86	7.39	6.14

Note: The industry data shown here are for illustration purposes only and should not be used outside this case.

*Deductions/Gross patient revenue.

Table 6   Selected Industry Operating Data

	1996 Industry Data (200–299 Beds)		
	+Quartile	Median	− Quartile
Profit Indicators			
Profit per discharge*	$89.04	($21.30)	($120.08)
Profit per visit†	$6.22	$0.66	($7.01)
Net Price Indicators			
Net price per discharge	$4,091	$3,411	$2,815
Net price per visit	$201	$139	$98
Medicare payment percentage	43.47%	36.60%	31.25%
Bad debt/Charity percentage‡	7.89%	4.76%	2.97%
Contractual allowance percentage§	25.27%	20.02%	12.12%
Outpatient revenue percentage	25.26%	21.03%	17.44%
Volume Indicators			
Occupancy rate	67.12%	58.10%	47.84%
Average daily census‖	173.23	144.73	114.39
Length of Stay Indicators			
Average length of stay (days)	6.80	6.07	5.41
Adjusted length of stay**	6.48	5.36	4.52
Intensity of Service Indicators			
Cost per discharge	$3,937	$3,392	$2,972
Adjusted cost per discharge††	$3,417	$2,924	$2,572
Cost per visit‡‡	$202.23	$141.97	$111.53
Case-mix index	1.2795	1.1756	1.0259
Efficiency Indicators			
FTEs per occupied bed	4.59	4.15	3.77
Outpatient manhours per visit§§	4.68	5.84	8.66
Unit Cost Indicators			
Salary per FTE‖‖	$24,447	$22,517	$20,347
Employee benefits percentage***	19.58%	17.04%	15.18%
Liability costs per discharge†††	$80.94	$42.05	$18.31

Note: The industry data shown here are for illustrative purposes only and should not be used outside this case.

  * (Net inpatient revenue − Inpatient cost)/Total discharges.

 ** Average length of stay/Case-mix index.

*** Fringe benefit costs/Total salaries.

  † (Net outpatient revenue − Outpatient cost)/Total visits.

†† Cost per discharge/Case-mix index.

††† Inpatient professional liability costs/Total discharges.

 ‡ (Bad debt + Charity care)/Gross patient revenue.

‡‡ Total outpatient expenses/Total outpatient visits.

 § Contractual allowances/Gross patient revenue.

§§ (Outpatient FTEs × 2,080)/Total visits.

‖ Patient days/365.

‖‖ Total salaries/FTEs.

13

Financial Forecasting

In the last chapter, we saw how managers can analyze financial statements to identify a firm's strengths and weaknesses. Now we consider the actions a firm can take to exploit its strengths and to overcome its weaknesses. As we shall see, managers are vitally concerned with *projected*, or *pro forma*, *financial statements*, and with the effects of alternative policies on these statements. An analysis of such effects is the key ingredient of financial planning. However, a good financial plan cannot, by itself, ensure that the firm's goals will be met; the plan must be backed up by a financial control system for monitoring the situation, both to make sure that the plan is carried out properly and to facilitate rapid adjustments if economic and operating conditions change from those built into the plan.

Strategic Plans

Financial plans are developed within the framework of the firm's overall strategic and operating plans. Thus, we begin our discussion with an overview of the strategic planning process.

Corporate mission

The long-run strategic plan should begin with a statement of the *corporate mission*, which defines the overall purpose of the firm. The mission can be defined either specifically or in general terms. For example, an investor-owned medical equipment manufacturer might state that its corporate mission is "to increase the intrinsic value of the firm's common stock." Another might say that its mission is "to maximize the growth rate in earnings and dividends per share while avoiding excessive risk." Yet another might state that its principal goal is "to provide our customers with state-of-the-art diagnostic systems at the lowest attainable cost, which in our opinion will also maximize benefits to our employees and stockholders."

Corporate missions for not-for-profit firms are normally stated in different terms, but the reality of competition in the health care industry forces all corporate missions, regardless of ownership, to be compatible with financial viability. To illustrate a not-for-profit corporate mission, consider the following mission statement of Bayside Memorial Hospital, a 650-bed, not-for-profit, acute care hospital:

> Bayside Memorial Hospital, along with its medical staff, is a recognized, innovative health care leader dedicated to meeting the needs of the community. We strive to be the best comprehensive health care provider in our service area through our commitment to excellence.

This mission statement provides Bayside's managers with an overall framework for establishing the hospital's goals and objectives.

Corporate goals

The corporate mission contains the general philosophy and approach of the business, but it does not provide managers with specific operational goals. *Corporate goals* set forth specific goals that management strives to attain. Corporate goals are generally qualitative in nature, such as "keeping the firm's research and development efforts at the cutting edge of the industry." Multiple goals are established, and they should be changed over time as conditions change. Further, a firm's corporate goals should be challenging, yet realistically attainable.

Bayside Memorial Hospital divides its corporate goals into five areas as follows:

1. *Quality and Customer Satisfaction*

    1.1 To make quality performance the goal of each employee.

    1.2 To be recognized by our patients as the provider of choice in our market area.

    1.3 To identify and resolve as rapidly as possible areas of patient dissatisfaction.

2. *Medical Staff Relations*

    2.1 To identify and develop timely channels of communication among all members of the medical staff, management, and board of directors.

2.2 To respond in a timely manner to all medical staff concerns brought to the attention of management.

2.3 To make Bayside Memorial Hospital a more desirable location to practice medicine.

2.4 To develop strategies to enhance the mutual commitment of the medical staff, administration, and board of directors for the benefit of the hospital's stakeholders.

2.5 To provide the highest-quality, most cost-effective medical care through a collaborative effort of the medical staff, administration, and board of directors.

3. *Human Resources Management*

3.1 To be recognized as the customer service leader in our market area.

3.2 To develop and manage human resources to make Bayside Memorial Hospital the most attractive location to work in our market area.

4. *Financial Performance*

4.1 To maintain a financial condition that permits us to be highly competitive in our market area.

4.2 To develop the systems necessary to identify inpatient and outpatient costs by unit of service.

5. *Health Systems Management*

5.1 To be a leader in applied technology based on patient needs.

5.2 To establish new services and programs in response to patient needs.

Of course, these goals occasionally conflict and, when they do, Bayside's senior managers have to make judgments regarding which objective takes precedence.

Corporate objectives

Once a firm has defined its mission and goals, it must develop objectives designed to help it achieve its stated goals. *Corporate objectives* are generally quantitative in nature, such as specifying a target market share, a target ROE, a target earnings per share growth rate, or a target EVA (economic value added). Furthermore, the extent to which corporate objectives are met is commonly used as a basis for managers' compensation. To illustrate some corporate objectives, consider Bayside's objectives for meeting Goal 4.1 above, to maintain a competitive financial position:

4.1.1   To maintain or exceed the hospital's current 7.5 percent profit margin.

4.1.2   Over time, to increase the firm's debt ratio to 50 percent. However, this objective will not be attained by accepting new projects that will lower the hospital's profit margin.

4.1.3   To maintain the hospital's liquidity as measured by the current ratio in the range of 2.0 to 2.5.

4.1.4   Over time, to increase fixed asset utilization as measured by the fixed asset turnover ratio to 1.3.

Corporate objectives give managers a precise target to shoot for. But the objectives must support the firm's mission and goals, and must be chosen carefully to be challenging yet attainable.

Self-Test Questions:

Briefly describe the nature and use of the following corporate planning tools:

1. Mission
2. Goals
3. Objectives.

Why do financial planners need to be familiar with the company's overall strategic plan?

Operating Plans

Operating plans can be developed for any time horizon, but most companies use a five-year horizon, and thus the term *five-year plan* has become common. In a five-year plan, the plans are most detailed for the first year, with each succeeding year's plan becoming less specific. The operating plan is intended to provide detailed implementation guidance to meet corporate objectives. The five-year plan explains in considerable detail who is responsible for what particular function and when specific tasks are to be accomplished.

Table 13.1 contains Bayside Memorial Hospital's annual planning schedule. This schedule illustrates the fact that for most organizations, the planning process is essentially continuous. Next, Table 13.2 outlines the key elements of the hospital's five-year plan, with an expanded section for finance. A full outline would require several pages, but Table 13.2 does at least provide insights into the format and content of a five-year plan. It should be noted that for Bayside, much of the planning function takes place at the department level, with technical assistance from the marketing, planning, and financial staffs. Larger firms, with divisions, would begin the planning process at the division level. Thus, each division has its own mission and goals, as well as objectives designed to support its goals, and these plans are then consolidated to form the corporate plan.

Self-Test Questions:

What is the purpose of a firm's operating plan?

What is the most common time horizon for operating plans?

Briefly describe the contents of a typical operating plan.

The Financial Plan

The financial planning process can be broken down into five steps:

1. Set up a system of projected financial statements that can be used to analyze the effects of planned operations on the firm's financial condition. This system can also be used to monitor operations after the plan has been finalized and put into effect. Rapid awareness of deviations from plans is essential to a good control system, and such a system in turn is essential to corporate success in a changing world.

2. Determine the specific financial requirements needed to support the company's five-year plan. This includes funds for plant and equipment as well as for inventory and receivables buildups, for R&D programs, and for major marketing campaigns.

3. Forecast the financing sources to be used over the next five years. This involves estimating the funds that will be generated internally, as well as those that must be obtained from external sources. Any constraints on planned operations imposed

Table 13.1   Bayside Memorial Hospital: Annual Planning
Schedule

Months	Action
April–May	Marketing department analyzes national and local economic factors likely to influence Bayside's patient volume and reimbursement rates. At this time, a preliminary volume forecast is prepared for each service line.
June–July	Operating departments prepare new project (capital budgeting) requirements as well as operating cost estimates based on the preliminary volume forecast.
August–September	Financial analysts evaluate proposed capital expenditures and department operating plans. Preliminary forecasted financial statements and cash budgets are prepared with emphasis on Bayside's sources and uses of funds and forecasted financial condition.
October–November	All previous input is reviewed and the hospital's five-year plan is drafted by the planning, financial, and departmental staffs. Any new information developed during the planning process "feeds back" into earlier actions.
December	The five-year plan is approved by the hospital's executive committee, and then submitted to the board of directors for final approval.

by financial limitations should be incorporated into the plan; examples include restrictions in debt covenants that limit the debt ratio, the current ratio, and coverage ratios.

4. Establish and maintain a system of controls governing the allocation and use of funds within the firm. Essentially, this involves making sure that the basic plan is carried out properly.

5. Develop procedures for adjusting the basic plan if the forecasted economic conditions on which the plan was based do not materialize. For example, if Bayside's forecast on Medicare and Medicaid reimbursement used to develop the five-year plan proves to be too high or too low, the correct amounts must be recognized and reflected in operational and financial plans as rapidly as possible. Thus, Step 5 is really a "feedback loop" that triggers modifications to the plan.

Table 13.2 Bayside Memorial Hospital: Five-Year Plan Outline

Chapter 1 Corporate mission and goals
Chapter 2 Corporate objectives
Chapter 3 Projected business environment
Chapter 4 Corporate strategies
Chapter 5 Summary of projected business results
Chapter 6 Service line plans
     A. Marketing
     B. Operations
     C. Finance
        1. Working capital
          a. Overall working capital policy
          b. Cash and marketable securities management
          c. Inventory management
          d. Credit policy and receivables management
        2. Financial forecast
          a. Capital budget
          b. Cash budget
          c. Pro forma financial statements
          d. External financing requirements
          e. Financial condition analysis
        3. Accounting plan
        4. Control plan
     D. Administration and human resources
     E. New service lines

The principal components of the *financial plan* are (1) an analysis of the firm's current financial condition, (2) a revenue forecast (for health care providers, a volume and reimbursement forecast), (3) the capital budget, (4) the cash budget, (5) a set of pro forma (or projected) financial statements, (6) the external financing plan, and (7) an analysis of the firm's projected financial condition. In previous chapters, we discussed the capital budget and financial statement analysis. In the remainder of this chapter, we focus on some of the plan's other elements—the revenue forecast, pro forma financial statements, and the external financing plan. Then, in Chapter 14, we will discuss cash budgeting.

Self-Test Questions:

What are the five steps of the financial planning process?

What are the principal components of the financial plan?

Revenue Forecasts

The *revenue forecast* generally starts with a review of revenues over the past five to ten years, expressed in a graph such as that in Figure 13.1. The first part of the graph shows actual total operating revenues for Bayside Memorial Hospital from 1991 through 1995. Over these five years (four growth periods), total operating revenues grew from $91,477,000 to $114,805,000, or at a compound annual growth rate of 5.8 percent. Alternatively, a time-series regression can be applied to total operating revenues. We used a spreadsheet to perform a log-linear regression on all five years of sales data, with a resulting annual growth rate of 6.2 percent.[1] However, Bayside's revenue growth rate accelerated in the second half of the historical period, primarily as a result of new capacity that came on line in late 1992. The increase in the number of beds, plus a new, aggressive marketing program resulted in an annual growth rate of 8.6 percent during the past three years.

On the basis of the recent trend in revenues, on new service introductions, and on the managers' forecasts of local competition and third party payer trends, Bayside's planning group projects a 10 percent growth rate during 1996, to a total operating revenue level of $126,286,000. That forecast was developed as follows:

1. To begin, demand for services was divided into four major groups: (1) inpatient, (2) outpatient, (3) ancillary, and (4) other services. Demand trends in each of these areas over the past ten years were plotted, and a "first approximation" demand forecast, assuming a continuation of past trends, was made.

2. Next, the level of population growth and disease trends were forecasted: for example, what will be the growth in the over-65 population in the hospital's service area, and what will be the growth in the number of AIDS cases? These forecasts were used to develop demand by major diagnoses, and to differentiate demand between normal services and critical care services.

3. Bayside's managers next looked at its competitive environment. Consideration was given to such factors as the hospital's inpatient and outpatient capacities, its competitors' capacities, and new services or service improvements that either Bayside or its competitors might institute.

4. Bayside's managers then considered (a) its pricing strategy for managed care plans, (b) its pricing strategy for private pay patients, (c) trends in third party payer reimbursement, and

Figure 13.1   Bayside Memorial Hospital: Historical and Projected
Revenues (thousands of dollars)

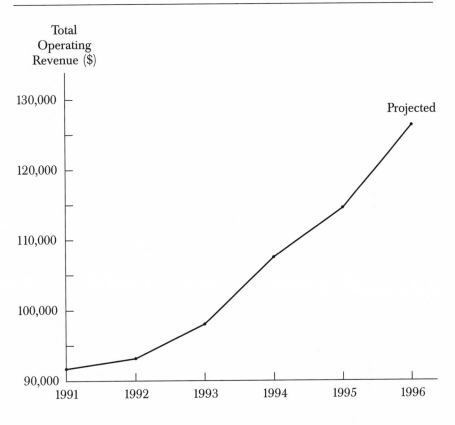

Year	Total Operating Revenue
1991	$ 91,477
1992	92,568
1993	97,351
1994	106,757
1995	114,805
1996 (Projected)	126,286

(d) price changes related to its other income, such as lease rates
to its tenant physicians. Some of the pricing strategy may have an
impact on demand for services: for example, does the hospital
have plans to raise outpatient charges to boost profit margins or

to lower charges to gain market share and utilize excess capacity? If such actions are expected to affect demand forecasts, then these forecasts must be revised.

5. Marketing campaigns and contracts (or loss of contracts) with managed care plans also affect demand, so probable developments in these areas were factored in. This facet of the forecast is particularly important to Bayside, which is in the process of buying physicians' group practices and creating an integrated delivery system. The success or failure of this venture could have a significant impact on future volume, and hence on operating revenues.

6. Forecasts were made for each service group, both in the aggregate—for example, inpatient operating revenue—and on an individual diagnosis basis. The individual diagnosis forecasts were summed and then compared with the aggregate service group forecasts. Differences were reconciled, and the result was a revenue forecast for the hospital as a whole but with breakdowns by major groups and for individual diagnoses.

If the hospital's volume forecast is off, the consequences can be serious. First, if the market for any particular service expands more than Bayside has expected and planned for, then the hospital will not be able to meet its patients' needs. Potential customers will end up going elsewhere, and Bayside will lose market share and perhaps miss a major opportunity. On the other hand, if its projections are overly optimistic, Bayside could end up with too much capacity, which means excess equipment, inventory, and staff. This would mean low turnover ratios, high costs for labor and depreciation, and possibly layoffs. All of this would result in low profitability, which could degrade the hospital's ability to compete in the future. If Bayside had financed the unneeded expansion primarily with debt, its problems would, of course, be compounded. Thus, an accurate volume forecast is critical to the well-being of any health care provider.

Note that a volume forecast (or virtually any forecast) is actually the *expected value of a probability distribution* of possible levels of volume. Because any forecast is subject to a greater or lesser degree of uncertainty, for financial planning purposes we are often just as interested in the degree of uncertainty inherent in the forecast (its standard deviation) as we are in the expected value.

In closing this section, we would like to reiterate one important point. Operating revenue forecasts are composed of two elements: demand forecasts and price (reimbursement) forecasts. Thus, revenue changes are composed of two elements: changes in volume and changes in reimbursement. Whereas volume changes tend to have a large impact on plant and staffing requirements, reimbursement changes generally do not have as much of an effect on operating decisions. Thus, it is important for managers to recognize whether revenue changes are due to changes in volume, which indicates that the firm is experiencing real changes in output, or to reimbursement effects, which may have no impact on volume.

Self-Test Questions:

Discuss some factors that must be considered when developing an operating revenue forecast.

Why is it necessary for planners to distinguish between volume changes and reimbursement changes?

Percentage of Sales Forecasting

Financial forecasting involves projecting financial statements, which are often called *pro forma financial statements*, or just *pro formas*, on the basis of a set of assumed operating conditions. In this section, we present the *percentage of sales* method, a simple technique with limited value in practice, but one that provides an excellent introduction to the forecasting process. The procedure is based on two assumptions: (1) that most income statement items and balance sheet accounts are tied directly to sales and (2) that the current levels of most income statement items and balance sheet accounts are optimal for the current level of sales. We will illustrate the percentage of sales method with Bayside Memorial Hospital, whose 1995 financial statements are given in Column 1 of Tables 13.3 and 13.4. We will explain the other columns of these tables as we discuss the percentage of sales method.

To begin the process, we will assume (contrary to fact) that Bayside operated its fixed assets at full capacity to support the $114,805,000 in total operating revenues in 1995; that is, the hospital had no excess beds or outpatient facilities.[2] Since we are assuming no excess capacity, if volume is to increase in 1996, Bayside will need to increase its fixed assets.

If, as projected, Bayside's total operating revenues increase to $126,286,000 in 1996, what will its pro forma 1996 income statement, balance sheet, and statement of cash flows look like, and how much external financing will the hospital require during 1996? The first step in using the percentage of sales method to forecast the firm's financial statements is to isolate those income statement items and balance sheet

Table 13.3   Bayside Memorial Hospital: Historical and Projected
Income Statements (thousands of dollars)

	1995 (1)	% of Sales (2)	1996 Projections	
			First Pass (3)	Second Pass (4)
Net patient services revenue	$108,600	94.60	$119,467	$119,467
Other operating revenue	6,205	5.40	6,819	6,819
Total operating revenue	$114,805	100.00	$126,286	$126,286
Operating expenses:				
Nursing services	$ 58,285	50.77	$ 64,114	$ 64,114
Dietary services	5,424	4.72	5,966	5,966
General services	13,198	11.50	14,518	14,518
Administrative services	11,427	9.95	12,570	12,570
Employee health and welfare	10,250	8.93	11,275	11,275
Provision for uncollectibles	3,328	2.90	3,661	3,661
Provision for malpractice	1,320	1.15	1,452	1,452
Depreciation	4,130	3.60	4,543	4,543
Interest expense	1,542	NA	1,542	1,769
Total operating expenses	$108,904	NA	$119,640	$119,868
Income from operations	$ 5,901	NA	$ 6,645	$ 6,418
Contributions and grants	$ 2,253	NA	$ 2,253	$ 2,253
Investment income	418	NA	418	418
Nonoperating gain (loss)	$ 2,671	NA	$ 2,671	$ 2,671
Excess of revenues over expenses	$ 8,572	NA	$ 9,316	$ 9,089

accounts that vary directly with revenues. Regarding the income statement, increased revenues are expected to bring direct increases in all of the variables except interest expense. That is, operating costs and administrative expenses are assumed to be tied directly to revenues, but interest expense is a function of financing decisions. Furthermore, we assume that Bayside's nonoperating cash flow will remain at its 1995 level, although any other assumption could be made.

We construct the first-pass forecasted, or pro forma, 1996 income statement as follows:

1. Find the 1995 percentage of sales for those items that are expected to increase proportionally with revenues. For exam-

Table 13.4 Bayside Memorial Hospital: Historical and Projected
Balance Sheets (thousands of dollars)

| | 1995 (1) | % of Sales (2) | 1996 Projections | |
			First Pass (3)	Second Pass (4)
Cash and securities	$ 6,263	5.46%	$ 6,889	
Accounts receivable	21,840	19.02	24,024	
Inventories	3,177	2.77	3,495	
Total current assets	$ 31,280	NA	$ 34,408	
Gross plant and equipment	$145,158	126.44	$159,674	
Accumulated depreciation	25,160	NA	29,703	
Net plant and equipment	$119,998	NA	$129,971	
Total assets	$151,278	NA	$164,379	$164,379
Accounts payable	$ 4,707	4.10%	$ 5,178	$ 5,178
Accrued expenses	5,650	4.92	6,215	6,215
Notes payable	825	NA	825	1,512
Current portion of long-term debt	2,150	NA	2,150	2,150
Total current liabilities	$ 13,332	NA	$ 14,368	$ 15,055
Long-term debt	$ 28,750	NA	$ 28,750	$ 30,812
Capital lease obligations	1,832	NA	1,832	1,832
Total long-term liabilities	$ 30,582	NA	$ 30,582	$ 32,654
Fund balance	$107,364	NA	$116,680	$116,453
Total liabilities and funds	$151,278	NA	$161,630	$164,152

ple, nursing services expenses were $58,285,000 in 1995, and these services supported $114,805,000 in total operating revenue. Thus, as a percentage of sales, nursing services represent $58,285/$114,805 = 0.5077 = 50.77%.[3] The percentage of sales amounts are shown in Column 2 of Table 13.3. Those items calculated within the forecasted income statement, such as total operating costs, as well as those items not expected to increase proportionally with revenues, such as contributions and grants, have an NA (for not applicable) in Column 2.

2. Forecast the first-pass 1996 pro forma amounts by multiplying the percentage of sales amounts in Column 2 by forecasted 1996

total operating revenue. To illustrate, the 1996 forecast for nursing services expenses is 0.5077($126,286,000) = $64,114,000.[4] As an alternative, the items that are expected to increase proportionally with revenues can be forecasted by increasing them at the forecasted revenue growth rate. For example, the 1996 forecast for nursing services expenses could be calculated as $58,285,000(1.10) = $64,114,000.

3. Some items marked NA, such as interest expense and contributions and grants, are carried over into 1996 at their 1995 values. We know that the interest expense in 1996 will likely be larger than in 1995 if Bayside will have to borrow additional funds, but we cannot predict the amount of interest increase until the first-pass financial statements have been completed. The remaining income statement items marked NA, such as total operating costs, are calculated by merely adding or subtracting other forecasted items.

4. When the first-pass income statement is completed (Column 3 in Table 13.3), we see that the projected net income (excess of revenues over expenses) is $9,316,000. Note that a 10 percent increase in net income would be $8,572,000(1.10) = $9,429,000. The forecasted amount is somewhat less than a 10 percent increase because the nonoperating gain was held to its 1995 level.

Turning to the balance sheet, since we assumed that Bayside was operating at full capacity in 1995, fixed assets as well as current assets must increase if sales are to rise. Thus, most asset accounts must increase if the higher level of sales is to be attained. More cash will be needed for transactions, receivables will be higher, additional inventory must be stocked, and new plant must be added.[5]

If Bayside's assets are to increase, its liabilities and/or equity must likewise rise—the balance sheet must balance, and an increase in assets must be financed in some manner. Accounts payable and accrued expenses will rise *spontaneously* with revenues; as revenues increase, so will purchases, and larger purchases will result in higher levels of accounts payable. Thus, if revenues double, accounts payable will also double. Similarly, a higher level of operations will require more labor, so accrued wages will increase. (If Bayside were an investor-owned hospital, an increase in profits would also lead to higher accrued taxes.) Bayside's fund balance should also increase, but not in direct proportion to the increase in revenues. Neither notes payable, current portion of long-term debt, long-term debt, nor capital lease obligations will rise spontaneously with revenues; higher revenues do not automatically trigger increases in these accounts. Thus, the 1995 values for these accounts will be used in 1996.

To construct the first-pass pro forma balance sheet contained in Column 3 in Table 13.4, we proceed as follows:

1. All balance sheet accounts that are expected to increase spontaneously with revenues are forecast in the same way as on the income statement. Consider cash and securities. In 1995, this account represented $6,263,000/$114,805,000 = 0.0546 = 5.46% of sales. This percentage of sales amount is shown in Column 2. The 1996 forecast is created by multiplying the percentage of sales by the 1996 revenue forecast, so 0.0546($126,268,000) = $6,889,000, which is shown in Column 3 of Table 13.4.

2. Accounts such as notes payable and long-term lease obligations are carried over into 1996 at their 1995 values. One or more of these accounts will probably have to be changed later in the analysis.

3. Next, add the forecasted 1996 depreciation expense from the income statement to the 1995 accumulated depreciation account on the balance sheet to get the 1996 forecast for accumulated depreciation: $4,543,000 + $25,160,000 = $29,703,000.

4. Then, add the net income for 1996, which is all retained within the firm, to the 1995 balance sheet fund balance amount to obtain the projected fund balance for 1996: $9,316,000 + $107,364,000 = $116,680,000.

5. Finally, fill in the missing values in Column 3 by merely adding or subtracting as necessary.

The projected 1996 asset accounts sum to $164,379,000. This is less than a 10 percent increase, because accumulated depreciation, which is a contra asset account, increased by about 18 percent. Thus, to support a revenue increase of 10 percent, Bayside must increase its assets from $151,278,000 to $164,379,000. The projected liability and fund accounts sum to $161,630,000. Again, this is less than a 10 percent increase because (1) several accounts were held at their 1995 levels, and (2) the fund balance increased by less than 10 percent.

At this point, the balance sheet does not balance: assets total $164,379,000, but only $161,630,000 of liabilities and fund capital is projected. Thus we have a shortfall, or *external funding requirement (EFR)*, of $2,749,000, which will have to be raised by bank borrowings and/or by selling securities, or by changing operating variables—such as charges—to generate more revenue and hence more retained earnings.

Financing the external funding requirement

Assuming no change in operating variables, Bayside could use short-term notes payable, long-term debt, increased solicitations, or a combination of these sources to make up the $2,749,000 shortfall. Ordinarily, Bayside would base this choice on its target capital structure, the relative costs of different types of securities, maturity matching considerations, its ability to increase contributions above the forecasted level, and so on.

If Bayside's managers decided to raise the external funds needed using a mix of 25 percent notes payable and 75 percent long-term debt, then the $2,749,000 external funding requirement would be met as follows:

Notes payable: 0.25($2,749,000) = $ 687,000
Long-term debt: 0.75($2,749,000) = 2,062,000

Total external funding $2,749,000

However, the use of external funds will change the first approximation income statement for 1996 as set forth in Column 3 of Table 13.3. The issuance of new debt will increase the hospital's 1996 interest expense. Bayside's managers are forecasting that new short-term debt will cost 12 percent, and that new long-term debt, which will be tax-exempt, will cost 7 percent.

If Bayside financed in 1996 as outlined above, and if the external financing occurred on January 1, 1996, then its income statement interest expenses would increase by the following amount:

Short-term interest: 0.12($687,000) = $ 82,440
Long-term interest: 0.07($2,062,000) =   144,340

Total additional interest $226,780 ≈ $227,000

This added interest expense will increase the 1996 interest expense forecast to $1,542,000 + $227,000 = $1,769,000.

The projected 1996 income statement and balance sheet, including financing feedback effects, are shown in Column 4 (second pass) of

Tables 13.3 and 13.4. We see that although $2,749,000 were added to Bayside's liabilities, the hospital is still $164,379,000 − $164,152,000 = $227,000 short in meeting its financing requirements, because the additional interest expense associated with external financing reduced the projected net income by $9,316,000 − $9,089,000 = $227,000, and hence reduced the fund balance by $116,680 − $116,453 = $227,000. Bayside's managers could repeat the preceding process with an additional $227,000 of external (notes payable and long-term debt) financing and create a third-pass income statement and balance sheet. The projected fund balance would be further reduced by additional interest requirements, but the balance sheet would be closer to being in balance. Successive iterations would continue to reduce the discrepancy. If the budget process were computerized, as would be true for most firms, an exact solution could be reached very rapidly. (We discuss this point later in the chapter.) Otherwise, firms would go through two or three iterations and then stop. At this point, the projected statements would generally be very close to being in balance, and they would certainly be close enough for practical purposes, given the uncertainty inherent in the projections themselves.

We completed the forecasting iterations using a spreadsheet model. The final-pass forecasted financial statements could then be used (1) to create the pro forma statement of cash flows and (2) to check Bayside's critical financial ratios. This is done in Table 13.5. Here we see that Bayside's base case forecast projects the hospital to have positive operating cash flow, but that it must still raise almost $3 million in external debt financing to meet its capital investment requirements. Furthermore, there is a slight deterioration in the hospital's profitability, and its use of debt financing increases slightly, although its liquidity remains unchanged.

The base case pro forma financial statements, along with the corresponding financial and operating analyses that we discussed in Chapter 12, are then reviewed by Bayside's executive committee for consistency with the hospital's financial objectives. Generally, they will make changes in the initial assumptions that will result in a new set of pro forma financial statements, which are then analyzed and reviewed, and so on, until the forecast is finalized.

The forecasting process undertaken by Ann Arbor Health Systems, a for-profit hospital, is very similar to that used by Bayside. The only real difference is that a for-profit firm has to deal with the fact that it uses stock rather than fund financing. This fact presents three complications. (1) The firm may pay dividends, so net income must be reduced by

Table 13.5   Bayside Memorial Hospital: 1996 Pro Forma
Statement of Cash Flows and Selected Ratios
(thousands of dollars)

Statement of Cash Flows:

Cash Flow from Operations

Income from operations	$ 6,398
Depreciation expense	4,543
Change in accounts receivable	(2,184)
Change in inventories	(318)
Change in accounts payable	471
Change in accruals	565
Net cash flow from operations	$ 9,475

Cash Flow from Investing Activities

Investment in plant and equipment	($14,516)

Cash Flow from Financing Activities

Additional long-term debt	$ 2,247
Additional notes payable	749
Net cash flow from financing	$ 2,996

Nonoperating Cash Flow

Contributions and grants	$ 2,253
Investment income	418
Nonoperating gain (loss)	$ 2,671
Net increase (decrease) in cash	$ 626

Beginning cash and securities	$ 6,263
Ending cash and securities	$ 6,889

Selected Ratios:

	1995	1996
Current ratio	2.3	2.3
Profit (total) margin	7.5%	7.2%
Total asset turnover	0.8	0.8
Debt ratio	29.0%	29.2%
Return on assets (ROA)	5.7%	5.5%
Return on equity (ROE)	8.0%	7.8%

the forecasted dividend payment to find the amount of capital that is retained within the firm, and hence which flows to the balance sheet. (2) The firm has the option of issuing common stock to meet its external financing needs. (3) The financing feedback effect must be expanded to include dividend payments if new common stock is issued.

Finally, note that forecasted financial statements must be checked for internal consistency. That is, accumulated depreciation on the balance sheet must be consistent with the depreciation expense shown on the income statement, and the fund balance (or retained earnings account) on the balance sheet must be consistent with the retentions shown on the income statement. There is a dependency between some income statement items and some balance sheet accounts, and the pro forma statements must recognize these dependencies.

Self-Test Questions:

Briefly describe the mechanics of percentage of sales forecasting.

Why is the external financing requirement so important to the planning process?

Do you think that most health care firms use the percentage of sales method to develop pro forma financial statements, or do they use some other methodology?

Factors That Influence the External Financing Requirement

The five factors that have the greatest influence on a firm's external financing requirement are (1) its projected revenue growth; (2) its initial fixed asset utilization rate, or excess capacity situation; (3) its capital intensity; (4) its profit margin; and (5) its dividend policy. In this section, we discuss each of these factors in some detail.

Revenue growth rate

The faster Bayside's revenues are forecasted to grow, the greater its need for external financing will be. At growth rates less than 8.2 percent, Bayside will need no external financing; indeed, all required funds can be obtained by spontaneous increases in current liability accounts plus retained earnings, and the hospital will even generate surplus capital. However, if Bayside's projected sales growth rate is greater than 8.2 percent, then it must seek outside financing, and the greater the projected growth rate, the greater will be its external financing requirement. The reasoning here is as follows:

1. Increases in revenues normally require increases in assets. If sales are not projected to grow, no new assets will be needed.

2. Any projected asset increases require financing of some type. Some of the required financing will come from spontaneously generated liabilities. Also, assuming a positive profit margin (and for investor-owned firms, a payout ratio of less than 100 percent), the firm will generate some retained earnings.

3. If the revenue growth rate is low enough, spontaneously generated funds plus retained earnings will be sufficient to support the asset growth. However, if the growth rate exceeds a certain level, then external funds will be needed. If management foresees difficulties in raising this capital—perhaps because it has no more debt capacity—then the feasibility of the firm's expansion plans may have to be reconsidered.

Capacity utilization

In determining Bayside's external financing requirement for 1996, we assumed that the hospital's fixed assets were being fully utilized. Thus, any significant increase in revenues would require an increase in fixed assets. What would be the effect if Bayside had been operating its fixed assets at less than full capacity? Assume that Bayside's managers consider 90 percent occupancy to be full capacity. Since the hospital had 75.9 percent occupancy in 1995, it was actually operating at $75.9/90 = 84\%$ of capacity. Under this condition, fixed assets could remain constant until sales reach that level at which fixed assets were being fully utilized, defined as *capacity sales,* which is calculated as follows:

$$\text{Utilization rate (\% of capacity)} = \frac{\text{Actual sales}}{\text{Capacity sales}},$$

so

$$\text{Capacity sales} = \frac{\text{Actual sales}}{\text{Utilization rate}}.$$

Since Bayside had been operating in 1995 at 84 percent of capacity, then its capacity sales *without any new fixed assets* would be $140,006,000:

$$\text{Capacity sales} = \frac{\$114,805,000}{0.82} = \$140,006,000.$$

In reality, Bayside could have increased total operating revenue all the way to $140,006,000 with no increase in fixed assets, so to reach its projected revenues of $126,286,000 in 1996, it would require no new fixed assets. Thus, its external financing requirement would decrease by $14,516,000 (the projected increase in gross plant and equipment), and hence Bayside would generate surplus capital in 1996.

In general, operating at less than full capacity can be incorporated into the pro forma balance sheet as follows:

1. Calculate the gross plant and equipment percentage of sales multiplier on the basis of capacity sales rather then on actual sales. To illustrate, assume that Bayside had been operating at 95 percent of capacity in 1995. Then, its capacity sales would be $114,805,000/0.95 = $120,847,000, and its gross fixed assets percentage of sales multiplier would be $145,158,000/$120,847,000 = 120.12% versus the 126.44 percent multiplier used in Table 13.4.

2. Use the new percentage of sales multiplier to forecast Bayside's 1996 level of gross plant and equipment. The new 1996 level would be $126,286,000(1.2012) = $151,695,000, rather than the $159,674,000 originally projected. Thus, operating at only 95 percent of capacity in 1995 reduces 1996 projected gross plant and equipment by $159,674,000 − $151,695,000 = $7,979,000. This decrease in projected assets, in turn, reduces the external financing requirement by a like amount. Obviously, operating at less than full capacity has a significant impact on the need for external funds.

Capital intensity

The amount of assets required per dollar of sales (total assets/sales) is often called the *capital intensity ratio*, which is the reciprocal of the total asset turnover ratio. Capital intensity has a major effect on capital requirements to support any level of sales growth. If the capital intensity ratio is low, such as for home health care firms, then sales can grow rapidly without much outside capital. However, if the firm is capital-intensive, such as a hospital, then even a small growth in output will require a great deal of outside capital if the firm is operating at full capacity.

Profitability

Profitability is also an important determinant of external financing requirements: the higher the profit margin, the lower the external financing requirement, other factors held constant. Bayside's profit (total) margin in 1995 was 7.5 percent, while its operating margin was 5.1 percent. Now suppose its profit margin increased to 10 percent through higher reimbursements and better expense control. This would increase net income, and hence retained earnings, which in turn would decrease the requirement for external funds.

Dividend policy

For investor-owned firms, dividend policy also affects external capital requirements. When Ann Arbor Health Systems projects its 1996 financial statements, if it foresees difficulties in raising capital, it might want to consider a reduction in its dividend payout ratio. However, before making this decision, management should consider the possible effects of a dividend cut on stock price.[6]

Self-Test Question:

How do the following factors affect the external financing requirement?

1. Sales growth rate
2. Capacity utilization
3. Capital intensity
4. Profitability
5. For investor-owned firms, dividend policy.

Sustainable Growth

We have often mentioned that investor-owned companies other than start-up firms generally try to avoid issuing new common stock for two reasons: (1) high issuance costs must be incurred to sell common stock, but no such costs are incurred on retained earnings; and (2) information asymmetries lead investors to view stock issues as bad news, and stock prices decline when a new stock issue is announced. These two factors combine to make equity raised by selling stock much more costly than equity obtained by retaining earnings. In a not-for-profit situation, the firm is unable to issue new common stock. Therefore, regardless of ownership, managers are often confronted with this question: How fast can the firm grow (or how many new services can be offered) using only retention and debt financing; that is, what is the firm's *sustainable growth rate?* If we make some assumptions, a relatively simple model can be used to answer that question.[7]

We begin by defining these key terms:

M = projected profit (total) margin, or net income divided by total sales.

b = target retention rate = $1 -$ Target payout ratio.

D/E = target debt-to-equity ratio.

A/S = ratio of total assets to sales, the reciprocal of the total asset turnover ratio.

If the firm is operating at full capacity, and if it is currently at its target capital structure, then the sustainable growth rate, g^*, can be found using this equation:

$$g^* = \frac{M(b)(1 + D/E)}{A/S - M(b)(1 + D/E)}. \tag{13.1}$$

To illustrate the use of Equation 13.1, consider the situation facing Bayside Memorial Hospital. From the data in Tables 13.3 and 13.4 presented earlier in the chapter, Bayside's 1995 profit (total) margin = Excess of revenues over expenses/Total operating revenue = \$8,572/\$114,805 = 7.47%; since Bayside is a not-for-profit hospital, its retention rate = 1.00; its book value debt-to-equity ratio = Total debt/Total funds = (\$13,332 + \$30,582)/\$107,364 = 0.41; and its assets-to-sales ratio = Total assets/Total operating revenue = \$151,278/\$114,805 = 1.32. If we assume (1) that these values will hold for 1996; (2) that Bayside's current book value structure is also its target market value target; (3) that depreciation cash flows are being used to replace worn-out assets; and (4) that financing feedback effects are small, and hence can be ignored, then the firm's sustainable growth rate is 8.7 percent:

$$g^* = \frac{M(b)(1 + D/E)}{A/S - M(b)(1 + D/E)} = \frac{7.47\%(1.00)(1 + 0.41)}{1.32 - 0.0747(1.00)(1 + 0.41)}$$

$$= \frac{10.53\%}{1.32 - 0.11} = \frac{10.53\%}{1.21} = 8.7\%.$$

Thus, according to the sustainable growth model, Bayside's revenues can grow as much as 8.7 percent in 1996 without requiring the firm to increase its use of financial leverage. Using a spreadsheet forecasting model, and our initial Table 13.3 and Table 13.4 assumptions, we find that Bayside can grow at 9.8 percent in 1996 without increasing its debt ratio, so Equation 13.2 must be viewed as a rough approximation.

An actual sales growth rate that differs from the sustainable rate has important implications for the firm, and managers must actively develop growth targets and financial objectives that are mutually consistent. If the sales growth rate is less than the sustainable rate, then the firm will generate more than enough capital to meet its capital investment needs, and its financial plans must call for an increase in cash and marketable securities, a reduction in the amount of debt outstanding, a merger program, stock repurchases or a dividend increase (for investor-owned firms), or some combination of these actions. Conversely, if the sales growth rate is greater then g^*, then financial leverage must be increased, or for investor-owned firms, new equity must be sold or the payout ratio reduced. If these are not viable options, then the growth rate itself must be scaled back.

In Bayside's actual case, with its excess capacity and a forecasted sales growth rate of only 10 percent, it did not require any external financing for 1996. However, Bayside's managers are well aware of its sustainable growth rate, and of the implications of expanding beyond that rate.

Self-Test Question:

Why is it important for hospital managers to know their firms' sustainable growth rate?

Problems with the Percentage of Sales Approach

For the percentage of sales method to produce accurate forecasts, each spontaneous asset and liability item must increase in the same proportion as sales. In graph form, this assumption suggests the existence of the type of relationship indicated in Figure 13.2(a), where we graph inventory versus sales for a fictional firm. Here the plotted relationship is linear and passes through the origin. Thus, if the company grows and sales double, from $200 million to $400 million, inventories will also double, from $100 million to $200 million.

The assumption of constant ratios is appropriate at times, but there are times when it is incorrect. Four such conditions are described in the following sections.

Revenue growth is due to pricing rather than volume changes

Earlier, we emphasized that revenue growth can be due to changes in either unit volume or pricing (reimbursement). If revenue growth is due solely to reimbursement changes, then there will be no impact on income statement items such as labor expenses or on balance sheet

Figure 13.2   Four Possible Ratio Relationships (millions of dollars)

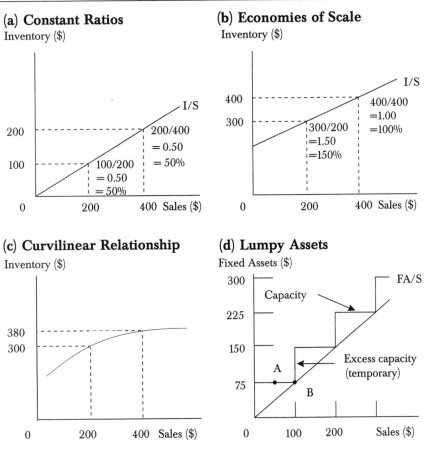

Source: E. F. Brigham and L. C. Gapenski. 1994. *Financial Management: Theory and Practice,* 7th ed. Fort Worth, TX: The Dryden Press.

items such as inventories, payables, and fixed asset requirements. Since the percentage of sales method ties most items and accounts directly to dollar sales, it can give very misleading forecasts when reimbursement changes rather than volume changes are driving the revenue forecast.

Economies of scale

There are economies of scale in the use of many kinds of assets, and when they occur, the ratios are likely to change over time as the size of the firm increases. Often, for example, firms need to maintain base stocks of different inventory items, even if sales levels are quite low. Then, as sales expand, inventories tend to grow less rapidly than sales, so the ratio of inventory to sales declines. This situation is depicted in Figure 13.2(b). Here we see that the inventory-to-sales ratio is 1.50, or 150 percent, when sales are $200 million, but the ratio declines to 1.00 when sales climb to $400 million.

Panel (b) still shows a linear relationship between inventories and sales, but even this is not necessarily the case. Indeed, as we will see in Chapter 15, if a firm employs the EOQ model to establish inventory levels, then inventory will rise with the square root of sales. This type of situation is illustrated in Figure 13.2(c).

Lumpy assets

In many industries, technological considerations dictate that if a firm is to be competitive, it must add fixed assets in large, discrete units. For example, in the hospital industry, it is usually not economically feasible to add, say, ten beds, so when hospitals expand capacity, they typically do so in large increments. This type of situation is depicted in Panel (d) of Figure 13.2. Here, we assume that the plant with the minimum feasible size has a cost of $75 million, and that such a plant can produce enough output to attain a sales level of $100 million per year. If the firm is to be competitive, it simply must have at least $75 million of fixed assets.

This situation has a major effect on the fixed assets/sales (FA/S) ratio at different sales levels, and consequently on financial requirements. At Point A in Panel (d), which represents a sales level of $50 million, the fixed assets are $75 million, so the ratio FA/S = $75/$50 = 1.5. However, sales can expand by $50 million, out to $100 million, with no required increase in fixed assets. At that point, represented by Point B, the ratio FA/S = $75/$100 = 0.75. If the firm is operating at full capacity, even a small increase in sales would require the firm to double its plant capacity, so a small projected sales increase would bring with it very large financial requirements.

Several other points should be noted about Panel (d) of Figure 13.2. First, if the firm is operating at a sales level of $100 million or less, then any expansion that calls for a sales increase above $100 million would require a *doubling* of fixed assets. Much smaller percentage increases would be involved if the firm were large enough to be operating a number of facilities. Second, firms generally go to multiple shifts and take other actions to minimize the need for new fixed asset capacity as they approach Point B. However, these efforts can go only so far, and eventually a fixed asset expansion is required. Finally, firms can sometimes make arrangements to purchase excess capacity output from other firms in their industry, or to sell excess capacity to other firms.

Cyclical/Seasonal changes

All of the asset projections in a forecast should be based on target, or optimal, relationships between sales and assets. Actual sales, however, often differ from projected sales, and the actual asset/sales ratio for a given period might be quite different from the optimal ratio. To illustrate, the firm depicted in Panel (b) of Figure 13.2 might, when its sales are at $200 million and its inventories at $300 million, predict a sales expansion to $400 million, and then increase its inventories to $400 million in anticipation of the sales expansion. But suppose a seasonal or cyclical downturn holds sales to only $300 million. In this case, actual inventories would be $400 million versus only about $350 million needed to support sales of $300 million. In this situation, if the firm is forecasting its financial requirements, it must recognize that sales can be expanded by $100 million with no increase in inventories, but that any sales expansion beyond $100 million would require additional financing to build inventories. In other words, the percentage of sales multipliers must be based on the optimal relationships to sales, which are not necessarily the relationships indicated on the latest financial statements.

If any of the problems noted here are encountered in practice— and generally many of them are—then the simple percentage of sales method of forecasting financial statements should not be used. Rather, other techniques must be used to forecast asset and liability levels and the resulting external financing requirements. Some of these methods are discussed in the next section.

Self-Test Questions:

Describe several conditions under which the percentage of sales method can give questionable results.

Do these conditions happen often in "real world" forecasting?

Real World Forecasting

We have emphasized that the percentage of sales method is generally not used in actual forecasting situations. The overall approach of fore-casting first the firm's income statement, then its balance sheet, then its external funding requirement, and so on, is used; but techniques other than percentage of sales are used to forecast the specific income statement items and balance sheet accounts. In this section, we discuss the four forecasting techniques that are used in practice: (1) simple linear regression, (2) curvilinear regression, (3) multiple regression, and (4) specific item forecasting.

Simple linear regression

Simple linear regression is often used to estimate asset requirements. To illustrate, Bayside's inventories and total operating revenue over the last five years are given in the lower section of Figure 13.3, and the regression plot is shown in the upper section. The estimated regression equation, as found using a spreadsheet, is as follows (in thousands of dollars):

$$\text{Inventories} = \$1,336 + 0.0158(\text{Sales}).$$

The plotted points are quite close to the regression line. In fact, the correlation coefficient between inventories and sales is 0.97, indicating that there is a very strong linear relationship between these two variables. Why might this be the case for Bayside? According to the EOQ model, which we will discuss in Chapter 15, inventories should increase with the square root of sales, which would cause the regression to be nonlinear—the true regression line would rise at a decreasing rate. However, Bayside has greatly expanded its service line over the last decade, and the base stocks associated with these new services have caused inventories to rise. Also, inflation has had a similar impact on both sales and inventory levels. These three influences—economies of scale in existing products, base stocks for new products, and inflationary effects—are offsetting, resulting in the observed linear relationship between inventories and sales.

We can use the estimated relationship between inventories and sales to forecast the 1996 inventory level. Since 1996 sales are projected at \$126,286,000, 1996 inventories should be \$3,331,000:

$$\text{Inventories} = \$1,336 + 0.0158(\$126,286)$$
$$= \$1,336 + \$1,995 = \$3,331.$$

This is \$3,495,000 − \$3,331,000 = \$164,000 less than our earlier forecast based on the percentage of sales method. The difference occurs because the percentage of sales method assumes that the ratio of inventories to sales remains constant, but the ratio actually declines because the inventories regression line in Figure 13.3 does not pass through the origin.

Figure 13.3   Bayside Memorial Hospital: Linear Regression on
Inventories (thousands of dollars)

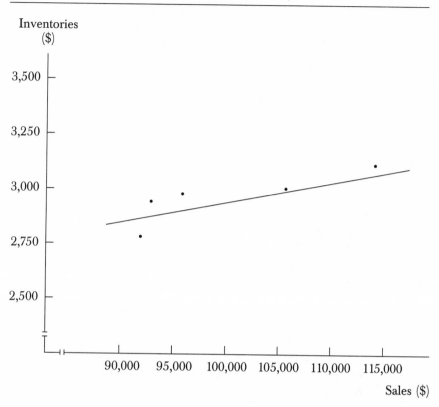

Year	Sales	Inventories
1991	$ 91,477	$2,752
1992	92,568	2,838
1993	97,351	2,896
1994	106,757	2,981
1995	114,805	3,177

We could run linear regressions on all the items on the income
statement and all the accounts on the balance sheet that need to be

forecasted to determine those that might be forecasted using this technique. Those items and accounts that produce a high correlation (those for which there is a strong linear relationship) may then be forecasted in this way. Then, we could use these relationships in Tables 13.3 and 13.4 in lieu of the percentage of sales multipliers, and thus create new financial statements based on linear regressions rather than percentage of sales.

Curvilinear regression

Simple linear regression, as discussed previously, is based on the assumption that a straight-line relationship exists between a particular account and sales. Although linear relationships between financial statement variables and sales frequently do exist, this is not a universal rule. For example, if the EOQ relationship had dominated the inventory-sales relationship, the plot of inventory versus sales would be a concave curve such as the one depicted in Panel (c) of Figure 13.2 rather than a line. If we forecasted the inventory level needed to support sales using a linear relationship, our forecast would be too high.

Firms have in their databases historical data on their own company by divisions, by product lines, and by individual products. They also have or can easily obtain certain types of data for other firms in their industry. These data can be analyzed using computer programs based on advanced statistical techniques (1) to help determine whether a relationship is curvilinear or linear and (2) to estimate the curvilinear relationship should one exist. Once the best-fit relationship has been estimated, it can be used to project future levels of items such as inventories, given the sales forecast.[8]

Multiple regression

If the relationship between a variable, such as inventories, and sales is such that the individual points are widely scattered about the regression line (and hence the correlation coefficient is low), but a curvilinear relationship does not appear to exist, then there is a good chance that other factors in addition to sales affect the level of that variable. For example, inventory levels might be a function of both sales level and number of different services offered (or products sold). In this case, we would obtain the best forecast for inventory level by using multiple regression techniques, where inventories would be regressed against both sales and the number of services offered. Then the projected inventories would be based on forecasts of number of services in addition to total sales. Most computer installations now have complete regression software packages, making it easy to apply multiple and curvilinear regression techniques. One can even do multiple regression analysis with spreadsheet programs.

Specific item forecasting

A final technique, and the one that is often most useful in practice, is to develop a specific model for each income statement item and balance sheet account that must be forecasted. For example, salaries could be projected using payroll records; inventories could be forecasted by the EOQ model; receivables could be forecasted by using the payments pattern approach; gross fixed assets could be forecasted on the basis of the firm's capital budget; and depreciation could be forecast on the basis of the firm's aggregate depreciation schedule.[9] Of course, projected volume (but not reimbursement) is the driving force behind each of these specific item forecasts.

Specific item forecasting is especially useful when input costs and output prices are affected by different forces, and hence are expected to grow at different rates. In today's health care environment, this is probably the rule rather than the exception.

Comparison of forecasting methods

The percentage of sales method assumes that different financial statement items vary directly (proportionally) with sales. It is the easiest method, but often its forecasts are of questionable accuracy. Simple linear regression differs from the percentage of sales method in that regression does not assume constant ratios. This technique can improve on the forecasts for many financial statement items. Note too that curvilinear and multiple regression techniques can provide especially accurate forecasts when relationships either (1) are not linear or (2) depend on other variables in addition to sales. Finally, specific item forecasting that utilizes various decision models can be used.

As we move down the list of forecasting methods, accuracy may or may not increase, but costs are sure to increase. The need to employ more complicated, and consequently more costly, methods varies from situation to situation. As in all applications, the costs of using more refined techniques must be balanced against the benefits obtained. Unfortunately, there is no assurance that the use of more sophisticated forecasting methods will lead to better forecasts. Furthermore, the use of more complicated forecasting methods often hides the assumptions inherent in the forecast.

Self-Test Questions:

Identify several techniques that can be used instead of percentage of sales forecasting.

Which of these techniques do you think would be the most accurate? The most costly?

Computerized Financial Planning Models

Although the types of financial forecasting described thus far in the chapter can be done with a hand calculator, even the smallest health care firms now have at least a personal computer and can employ some type of computerized financial planning model. Such models can be programmed to show the effects of different volume and reimbursement rates, different relationships between sales and operating assets, and even different assumptions about sales prices and input costs (labor, materials, and so forth). Plans are then made regarding how projected external financing requirements are to be met—through short-term bank loans, by selling long-term bonds, or, in the case of investor-owned firms, by selling new common stock. Pro forma balance sheets, income statements, and statements of cash flows are generated under the different financing plans, and key risk and return ratios, such as the current ratio, debt/assets ratio, times-interest-earned ratio, return on assets, and return on equity, are calculated.

Depending on how these projections look, management may need to modify the base case, or initial, forecast. For example, management might conclude that the projected volume growth rate must be cut because external funding requirements exceed the firm's ability to raise money. Or management could decide to raise more funds internally, if possible. Alternatively, the company might investigate production processes or services that require fewer fixed assets, or it might consider the possibility of contracting out some services rather than offering them in house.

Scenario analysis

The most important benefit of a computerized forecasting model is that it permits financial managers to see the effects of changing both basic assumptions and specific financial policies. The pro forma financial statements could be rerun over and over, each time creating a new scenario that changes one or more of the basic operating assumptions inherent in the model. For example, what if there is a significant reduction in Medicare payments? What if we lose a large managed care contract to a competitor? What if we experience a nurses' strike during the coming year? What if a competitor opens a new outpatient surgery center? Changes in basic assumptions about Medicare reimbursement, labor costs, or competitors' actions have a significant effect on volume, reimbursement, cost relationships, profit margins, and so on. A computerized forecasting model permits managers to quickly develop forecasts to match numerous different assumptional scenarios, although the forecasts are only as good as the managers' ability to predict the impact of each scenario on key forecasting parameters.

We could also rerun the model with changes in financial variables, such as changing the external financing mix or interest rate forecasts. It is important, however, to note (1) that managers still must interpret the results of all of the forecasts and (2) that the analysis could encompass virtually hundreds of combinations of operating assumptions and financial policies, and thus hundreds of different sets of pro forma financial statements could easily be created.

One way to reduce the number of possible scenarios is to perform a sensitivity analysis to determine the effect of each assumption—those assumptions that have little effect on the key financial integrity and profitability ratios need not be changed from their base case levels. Another approach to reducing the number of scenarios is to perform a Monte Carlo simulation analysis. For example, instead of specifying volume, reimbursement levels, labor costs, and so on, at discrete levels, probability distributions could be specified. Then, the key results would be presented as distributions rather than as point estimates.[10]

Self-Test Question:

Why are computerized planning models playing an increasingly important role in corporate management?

A Useful Forecasting Tool: Percentage Changes

Percentage change analysis was discussed in Chapter 12 as one of the tools commonly used in financial statement analysis. This technique is also useful in evaluating the validity of forecasted financial statements.

To illustrate, consider Table 13.6, which shows the annual percentage change in each balance sheet account from its 1995 value. It is very easy for Bayside's managers to scan down Column 2 of Table 13.6 to get a feel for the percentage change forecasted for each account. Since the percentage of sales method was used to forecast the Column 3 projections, and since sales were forecasted to increase by 10 percent, most of the balance sheet accounts show an increase of 10 percent. However, if other techniques had been used to forecast the 1996 accounts, then there would be much more variability in the percentage changes. Managers can review the percentage changes inherent in the baseline forecast and then use their judgment to make changes to any accounts that appear to be inconsistent with the assumptions of the forecast.

Note that percentage changes can even be used to create the baseline forecast. Here, some inherent change in volume is forecasted, say, an increase of 10 percent. Then each item on the income statement and balance sheet account would be forecasted to increase by more or less than 10 percent depending on how the volume growth forecast, inflation, and other factors are predicted to affect each item and account. Of course, the consistency among income statement and balance sheet accounts regarding retentions and depreciation must still be preserved.

Self-Test Question:

Why is percentage change analysis a useful tool in evaluating financial statement forecasts?

Financial Controls

Financial forecasting and planning is vital to corporate success, but planning is for nought unless the firm has a control system that both (1) ensures implementation of the planned policies and (2) provides an information feedback loop that permits rapid adjustments if the assumed market conditions change. In a financial control system, the key question is not "How is the firm doing in 1996 as compared with 1995?" Rather, it is "How is the firm doing in 1996 as compared with our forecasts, and if actual results differ from the budget, what can we do to get back on track?"

The basic tools of financial control are *budgets* and *pro forma financial statements*. These documents set forth expected performance, and hence they express management's targets. These targets are then compared with actual corporate performance—on a daily, weekly, or

Table 13.6   Bayside Memorial Hospital: Historical and Projected Balance Sheets (thousands of dollars)

	1995 (1)	Percentage Change (2)	1996 Projection (3)
Cash and securities	$ 6,263	10.0%	$ 6,889
Accounts receivable	21,840	10.0	24,024
Inventories	3,177	10.0	3,495
Total current assets	$ 31,280	10.0%	$ 34,408
Gross plant and equipment	$145,158	10.0%	$159,674
Accumulated depreciation	25,160	18.1	29,703
Net plant and equipment	$119,998	8.3%	$129,971
Total assets	$151,278	8.7%	$164,379
Accounts payable	$ 4,707	10.0%	$ 5,178
Accrued expenses	5,650	10.0	6,215
Notes payable	825	83.3	1,512
Current portion of long-term debt	2,150	0.0	2,150
Total current liabilities	$ 13,332	12.9%	$ 15,055
Long-term debt	$ 28,750	7.2%	$ 30,812
Capital lease obligations	1,832	0.0	1,832
Total long-term liabilities	$ 30,582	6.8%	$ 32,654
Fund balance	$107,364	8.5%	$116,453
Total liabilities and funds	$151,278	8.5%	$164,152

monthly basis—to determine the *variances*, which are defined here as the difference between realized values and target values. Thus, the control system identifies those areas where performance is not meeting target levels. If a firm's actuals are better than its targets, this could signify that its managers are doing a great job, but it could also mean that the targets were set too low and thus should be raised in the future. Conversely, failure to meet the financial targets could mean that market conditions are changing, that some managers are not performing up to par, or that the targets were set initially at unrealistic, unattainable levels. In any event some action should be taken—and perhaps quickly if the situation is deteriorating rapidly. By focusing on variances, managers can "manage by exception," concentrating on those operations most in need of improvement and leaving alone those operations that are running smoothly.

Of course, entire textbooks have been written on financial controls, and much of the subject of financial control overlaps with managerial, or cost, accounting. Here, we want only to emphasize that financial controls are as critical to financial performance as are financial planning and forecasting. We must also add that financial control systems are not costless. Thus, the control system must balance its costs against the savings it is intended to produce.

Self-Test Questions:

What are the purposes of a financial control system?

What are the basic financial control tools and how do they work?

Summary

This chapter described in broad outline how firms forecast their financial statements and estimate their future capital requirements. The key concepts covered are listed next.

- The primary planning documents are *strategic plans, operating plans,* and *financial plans.*

- *Financial forecasting* generally begins with a forecast of the firm's revenues, in terms of both volume and reimbursement, for some future time period.

- *Pro forma,* or *projected, financial statements* are developed to determine the firm's financial requirements.

- The *percentage of sales method* of forecasting financial statements is based on the assumptions (1) that most income statement items and balance sheet accounts vary directly with sales and (2) that the firm's existing levels of spontaneous assets and liabilities are optimum for its sales volume.

- A firm can determine the amount of the *external financing requirement (EFR)* by estimating the amount of assets necessary to support the forecasted level of sales and then subtracting from that amount the forecasted total claims. The firm can then plan to raise the EFR through bank borrowing, by issuing securities, or both.

- Additional external capital means additional interest and/or dividends, which lowers the amount of forecasted retained earnings. Thus, raising external funds creates a *financing feedback* effect that must be incorporated in the forecasting process.

- Four factors have the greatest impact on the external financing requirement. (1) The higher a firm's *sales growth rate*, the greater will be its need for external financing. (2) The greater the *capital intensity*, the greater the EFR. (3) The higher the *profit margin*, the lower the EFR. (4) Finally, the larger a firm's *dividend payout*, the greater its need for external funds.

- A formula can be used to estimate a firm's *sustainable growth rate*, which is the growth rate that can be sustained without issuing new common stock.

- The percentage of sales method is often inadequate to deal with real world situations such as *volume and reimbursement changes, economies of scale, excess capacity,* or *lumpy assets.*

- *Linear regression, curvilinear regression, multiple regression,* and *specific item forecasting techniques* can be used to forecast asset requirements when the percentage of sales method is not appropriate.

- Even the smallest firms now use *computerized financial planning models* to forecast both their financial statements and their external financing needs.

- *Financial controls* should be an integral part of a firm's planning system.

The type of forecasting described in this chapter is important for several reasons. First, if the projected operating results are unsatisfactory, management can go "back to the drawing board," reformulate its plans, and develop more reasonable targets for the coming year. Second, it is possible that the funds required to meet the forecast simply cannot be obtained; if so, it is obviously better to know this in advance and to scale back the projected level of operations than suddenly to run out of cash and have operations grind to a halt. Third, even if the required funds can be raised, it is desirable to plan for their acquisition well in advance.

Notes

1. In a log-linear regression, sales amounts are converted to natural logarithms and regressed against time. The slope coefficient of the regression line,

which is 0.0597 = 5.97% in this case, is the *continuous* growth rate over the five-year period. The continuous growth rate is converted to a *compound annual* growth rate as follows:

$$e^{0.0597} - 1 \approx 6.2\%.$$

2. This assumption does not imply that Bayside's 1995 occupancy rate was 100 percent. A hospital is operating at full capacity when its average occupancy is somewhere around 80 to 90 percent. A few times during the year, a hospital may operate at 100 percent capacity, but most hospital managers prefer to maintain a reserve capacity to meet emergency situations.

3. It might be more logical to relate nursing services expenses to net patient services revenue (thereby excluding other operating revenue), while such items as administrative services might be more logically tied to total operating revenue. For simplicity, we are expressing all items as a percentage of total operating revenue. Since the proportion of other operating revenue to total operating revenue is only 5.4 percent, any errors will be small.

4. We generated the forecast with a spreadsheet model, so the amounts that we show in Column 2 will be different from those obtained by a calculator if the percentage of sales multiplier is rounded.

5. Some assets, such as marketable securities, are not tied directly to operations, so do not vary directly with sales. In fact, marketable securities, if they were held, could be run down to zero, thus reducing external funding requirements. We assume that Bayside's securities holdings are minimal, and hence that cash and securities will increase proportionally with sales.

6. Dividend policy is not discussed in this book. However, most managers believe that dividend cuts have a severe negative impact on stock price, and this belief is generally supported by empirical testing. For a full discussion of dividend policy, see E. F. Brigham and L. C. Gapenski, *Intermediate Financial Management* (Ft. Worth, TX: Dryden Press, 1996), chap. 13.

7. For a more complete discussion of sustainable growth, see R. C. Higgins, "How Much Growth Can a Firm Afford?" *Financial Management* (Fall 1977): 7–16.

8. Often, a plot of the data will suggest a nonlinear relationship. The data— inventories in this case—can then be converted to logarithms if it appears that the regression points slope down, or raised to a power if the slope of the points seems to be increasing. We often use the graphics capabilities of spreadsheets to identify nonlinear relationships.

9. We will discuss the payments pattern approach to receivables management in Chapter 16.

10. This is a good time to mention the basic axiom of computer modeling: GIGO, which meas "garbage in, garbage out." Stated another way, the output of a financial model is no better than the assumptions and other inputs used to construct it. So when you build models, proceed with caution. Note, though, that one advantage of computer modeling is that it does bring the key assumptions out into the open, where their realism can be examined. One strong advocate of models made this statement: "Critics of our models

generally attack our assumptions, but they forget that in their own forecasts, they simply assume the answer."

Selected Additional References

Anderson, D. 1985. "Impact of Strategic Financial Planning in the Health Care Industry." *Topics in Health Care Financing* (Summer): 1–6.

Armstrong, J. S. 1990. *Long Range Forecasting.* New York: Wiley.

Cook, D. 1990. "Strategic Plan Creates a Blueprint for Budgeting." *Healthcare Financial Management* (May): 21–27.

Dixon, L. H., and S. K. Bossert. 1993. "The Commercial Bank as Investment Advisor for Hospital Investable Assets." *Topics in Health Care Financing* (Summer): 58–68.

Fallon, R. P. 1991. "Not-For-Profit ≠ No Profit: Profitability Planning in Not-For-Profit Organizations." *Health Care Management Review* (Summer): 47–61.

Folger, J. C. 1989. "Integration of Strategic, Financial Plans Vital to Success." *Healthcare Financial Management* (January): 22–32.

Glenesk, A. E. 1990. "Six Myths That Can Cloud Strategic Vision." *Healthcare Financial Management* (May): 38–43.

Green, L. A. 1993. "Cash Management: Acceleration and Information Strategies." *Topics in Health Care Financing* (Summer): 44–57.

Kelly, V. K. 1993. "Banks As a Source of Capital." *Topics in Health Care Financing* (Summer): 21–34.

Makridakis, S., and S. C. Wheelwright. 1983. *Forecasting Methods for Management.* New York: Wiley.

Nyp, R. G., and I. Angermeier. 1990. "Financial Plan Charts a Hospital's Course for Success." *Healthcare Financial Management* (May): 30–36.

Scarborough, S. P. 1993. "Establishing Banking Relationships." *Topics in Health Care Financing* (Summer): 69–79.

Schmitz, V., G. M. Masters, and W. Dilts. 1989. "Better Forecasting Ensures Profitability, Quality of Care." *Healthcare Financial Management* (January): 60–66.

Thomas, L. M., and R. R. Johnson. 1988. "Financial Modeling: Creating a Plan for the Future." *Healthcare Financial Management* (February): 70–78.

Case 13

St. Margaret's Hospital (B): Financial Forecasting

St. Margaret's Hospital is a 210-bed, not-for-profit, acute care hospital with a long-standing reputation for quality service to the community. For a more thorough description of the hospital, along with its 1996 financial statements, see Case 12 (St. Margaret's Hospital [A]).

As the newly hired assistant administrator, you have completed the financial and operating analysis (Case 12) assigned by Sister Mary Frances, the hospital's administrator. In fact, your presentation to the board of trustees went so well that Sister Mary Frances asked you to present the hospital's preliminary five-year financial plan at the next board meeting. To aid in the planning process, she provided the following information:

(1) Given your knowledge of the historical situation for St. Margaret's and the health care and hospital industries, and the situation faced by hospitals today, use your own best judgment to create the hospital's financial plan. Make any assumptions you believe to be necessary to create the financial plan, including assumptions about inpatient and outpatient volume growth, reimbursement patterns, hospital staffing patterns, cost inflation, and so on. Be sure to completely document your assumptions in the report. The quality of your forecast will be judged as much (or more) on the validity of your assumptions as on the mechanics of the forecasting process. (You have very limited specific information about St. Margaret's, so use your general knowledge about trends in the hospital industry and your own local market to make the forecasts.)

(2) The emphasis should be on the forecast for next year (1997), but you should also create rough pro forma income statements and balance sheets for the coming five years, including key financial indicators.

(3) The five primary methods for forecasting income statement items and balance sheet accounts are (a) percentage of sales, (b) simple linear regression, (c) curvilinear regression, (d) multiple regression, and (e) specific item forecasting. You will probably need to use several of these methods in your forecast. Although you may use any forecasting software available, don't forget that spreadsheets have a regression capability.

(4) Use the financial analysis from Case 12 to help with the forecast. Those areas where hospital performance has been poor should be improved, and your forecasts should reflect such anticipated improvements where applicable.

(5) Do not get so involved in the mechanics of the forecasting process that you forget to apply common sense to your forecasts. Think about what has happened in the past and what is likely to happen in the future in regard to utilization, prices, costs, and asset requirements. If the forecast doesn't make sense, modify it until it does. For example, a blind application of statistical forecasting techniques might lead to a forecast containing five years of net operating losses. Regardless of statistical "fit," such a forecast makes no sense because any hospital, if it expects to survive, will have to take actions to adjust either utilization or costs to ensure positive operating results. Thus, the "blindly" forecasted values do not represent what is likely to happen in the future, even though they might be a perfect reflection of historical trends.

In closing, Sister Mary Frances gave you the following guidance: "Here's my view of a good financial plan. First, the plan should consist of the pro forma financial statements along with a table that summarizes the internal and external financing requirements. Second, key financial ratios should be calculated, and the hospital's future financial condition should be assessed, with special emphasis on changes from the hospital's current condition. Third, make sure that your pro forma financial statements are consistent with one another. The last assistant administrator couldn't figure out that some balance sheet accounts—namely fund capital and accumulated depreciation—are tied to income statement items, so he didn't last very long. Finally, be sure to make all your assumptions clear, and be prepared to answer questions from the board concerning the impact of changes in your assumptions on the financial plan."

Part VII

Working Capital Management

14

Cash Management and Short-Term Financing

In Chapters 6 through 13, we generally focused on long-term, strategic decisions. However, another important element of health care financial management involves short-term assets and financing, which is the topic of the next two chapters of the text. This chapter contains an overview of short-term financial management, a discussion of cash management, which includes the management of cash substitutes (marketable securities), and a discussion of short-term financing.

An Overview of Short-Term Financial Management

Although short-term financial management involves all current assets and most current liabilities, one of its most important goals is to ensure that the firm maintains its *liquidity*. As used here, liquidity means the ability to meet cash obligations as they become due. A firm that is liquid can by definition support its operational goals, since it has the funds that are needed to pay salaries, taxes, interest, supplies invoices, and so on. Conversely, a firm that is illiquid cannot easily generate the cash needed to make these payments, and thus its operations suffer. In some situations, illiquidity may be due to seasonal or cyclical factors, and hence only be temporary, but in other cases it may be the first symptom of severe problems that could ultimately lead to bankruptcy.

Basic definitions

Short-term financial management uses some unique terminology which must be understood by all health care managers.

1. *Working capital,* sometimes called *gross working capital,* simply refers to current assets.

2. *Net working capital* is defined as current assets minus current liabilities.

3. The *current ratio,* which we discussed in Chapter 12, is defined as current assets divided by current liabilities. The current ratio is intended to measure a firm's liquidity, but a high current ratio does not necessarily ensure that a firm will have the cash required to meet its needs. If cash is not on hand, and inventories are not sold or receivables are not collected in a timely manner, then the apparent safety reflected in a high current ratio could be illusory.

4. The *quick ratio,* also discussed in Chapter 12, is defined as current assets less inventories, all divided by current liabilities. The quick ratio removes inventories from current assets because they are typically the least liquid of current assets, and hence it is designed to be a more stringent measure of liquidity than the current ratio. However, like the current ratio, the quick ratio could give a false signal regarding a firm's liquidity position.

5. *Days liquidity on hand* is another liquidity measure. It is defined as liquid assets (cash, marketable securities, and receivables) divided by projected daily cash operating expenses, and it measures the number of days that the firm can operate solely on the basis of its present liquid assets. Daily cash operating expenses are best obtained from the projected cash budget (which we discuss later in the chapter), but a reasonable proxy can be obtained by dividing annual cash operating costs by 360 (or 365). This ratio recognizes, at least partially, that true liquidity stems from cash flows rather than stocks of assets, although it still focuses on the stock of liquid assets rather than on the inflow of cash.

6. *Days cash on hand,* defined as cash plus marketable securities, divided by daily cash operating expenses, is similar to the days liquidity on hand ratio, but it is even more restrictive in its interpretation of liquidity. The days cash on hand ratio recognizes that cash and marketable securities are the only absolutely liquid assets.

7. By far the best and most comprehensive picture of a firm's liquidity position is obtained by examining its *cash budget.* This forecast of cash inflows and outflows focuses on what really counts, the firm's ability to generate cash inflows as needed to meet required outflows. We will

discuss cash budgeting in detail in a later section.

8. *Liquidity management* involves the planned acquisition and use of liquid resources over time to meet cash obligations as they become due. Liquidity management is more encompassing than current asset management, as liquidity management includes planned sales of fixed assets, issuance of long-term securities, and all other long-term activities that affect the firm's liquidity.

A simple illustration

Table 14.1 contains the December 31, 1995, and May 31, 1996, balance sheets of Sun Coast Clinics, Inc., a for-profit operator of four ambulatory care clinics in the Fort Lauderdale area. Note that, according to the definitions given, Sun Coast's December 31 working capital is $200,000, and its net working capital is $200,000 − $150,000 = $50,000. Also, Sun Coast's year-end current ratio is 1.33, and its quick ratio is 1.23. Finally, if the firm's daily cash operating expenses are $10,000, then its end-of-year days liquidity on hand ratio is 18.5, and its days cash on hand is 3.0.

Sun Coast's total current liabilities of $150,000 include the current portion of long-term debt, which is $20,000. This account is unaffected by short-term financing decisions, since it is a function of past long-term financing decisions. Thus, even though accountants define long-term debt coming due in the next accounting period as a current liability, it is not a short-term management variable. However, this cash flow certainly must be considered by Sun Coast's managers when assessing the firm's liquidity position.

The requirement for external working capital financing

The provision of ambulatory care services in Fort Lauderdale is a seasonal business. The peak season for Sun Coast is December through May, when the population of the area soars due to tourism, and even more important to Sun Coast, the arrival of the "snow birds" (retired individuals who typically live in the North during the summer and fall months, but move to their residences in Florida for the winter). In December of each year, Sun Coast has just finished its slow season and is preparing for its busy season. Thus, the firm's accounts receivables are relatively low, but its cash and marketable securities and inventories are relatively high. By the end of May, Sun Coast has completed its busy season, so its accounts receivable are relatively high, but its cash and

Table 14.1   Sun Coast Clinics, Inc.: December and May Balance
Sheets (thousands of dollars)

	December 1995	May 1996
Cash and marketable securities	$ 30	$ 20
Accounts receivable	155	210
Inventories	15	10
Total current assets	$200	$240
Net fixed assets	500	500
Total assets	$700	$740
Accounts payable	$ 30	$ 40
Accrued wages	5	10
Accrued taxes	10	15
Notes payable	85	105
Current portion of long-term debt	20	20
Total current liabilities	$150	$190
Long-term debt	150	140
Common equity	400	410
Total liabilities and equity	$700	$740

marketable securities and inventories are relatively low in preparation
for the slow summer season. On the current liabilities side, Sun Coast's
accounts payable and accruals are relatively high in May, just after the
busy season.

Now consider what happens to Sun Coast's current assets and
current liabilities over the period. Current assets increase from $200,000
to $240,000, so the firm must raise $40,000: a net increase on the
left side of the balance sheet must be financed by an increase on the
right-hand side. However, the higher volume of both purchases and
labor expenditures associated with increased services causes accounts
payable and accruals to increase *spontaneously*, on net, by $20,000—from
$30,000 + $5,000 + $10,000 = $45,000 to $40,000 + $10,000 + $15,000
= $65,000. The end result is a $20,000 projected current asset financing
requirement, which Sun Coast obtained from the bank as a short-term
loan. Therefore, on May 31, 1996, Sun Coast showed notes payable of
$105,000, up from $85,000 on December 31, 1995.

These fluctuations for Sun Coast resulted from seasonal factors. Similar fluctuations in current asset requirements, and hence in financing needs, can occur due to business cycles: typically, financing needs contract during recessions, and they expand during good times.

Self-Test Questions:

Briefly define the following terms:

1. Working capital
2. Net working capital
3. Current ratio
4. Quick ratio
5. Days liquidity on hand
6. Days cash on hand
7. Cash budget
8. Liquidity management.

Describe how both seasonal and cyclical sales fluctuations influence current asset levels and financing requirements.

Working Capital Investment and Financing Policies

Working capital financial policy involves two basic questions: (1) What is the appropriate level for current assets, both in total and by specific accounts? (2) How should current assets be financed?

Working capital investment policies

Figure 14.1 shows three alternative policies regarding the total amount of working capital carried. Essentially, *working capital investment policies* differ in that different amounts of current assets are carried to support a given level of sales. The line with the steepest slope represents a *high investment policy*, where relatively large amounts of cash, marketable securities, and inventories are carried for a given sales level, and where sales are stimulated by the use of a credit policy that provides liberal financing to customers and a corresponding high level of receivables. Conversely, with the *low investment policy*, the holdings of cash, securities, inventories, and receivables are minimized at each sales level. The *moderate investment policy* falls between the two extremes.

Under conditions of certainty—when volume, operating costs, collection times, and so on, are known for sure—all firms would hold only

Figure 14.1   Alternative Working Capital Investment Policies
(thousands of dollars)

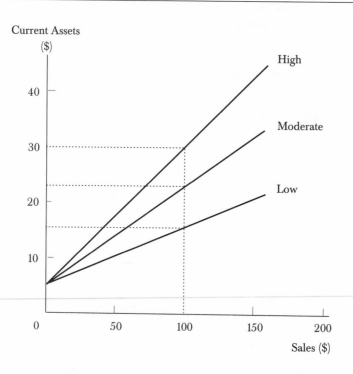

Policy	Current Assets to Support Sales of $100
High	$30
Moderate	23
Low	16

Note: The Sales/Current Assets relationship is shown here as being linear, but the relationship is often curvilinear.

Source: E. F. Brigham and L. C. Gapenski. 1994. *Financial Management: Theory and Practice*, 7th ed. Fort Worth, TX: The Dryden Press.

minimal levels of current assets, and hence follow a low working capital investment policy. Any larger amounts would increase the need for external funding, and hence increase costs, without a corresponding increase in profits. Any smaller holdings would involve late payments to labor and suppliers, production and service inefficiencies because of inventory shortages, and lost sales due to an overly restrictive credit policy.

However, the picture changes when uncertainty is introduced. Now, the firm requires some minimum amount of cash and inventories to meet expected needs, plus additional amounts, or *safety stocks,* which enable it to deal with realizations that differ from expectations. Similarly, accounts receivable levels are determined by credit terms (payer mix and collections policy), and the tougher the credit terms, the lower the receivables for any given level of sales. With a low working capital investment policy, the firm would hold minimal levels of safety stocks for cash and inventories, and it would have a tight credit policy. A low working capital investment policy generally provides the highest expected return on investment, but it entails the greatest risk, while the converse is true under a high working capital investment policy. The moderate policy falls in between the two extremes in terms of expected risk and return.

As we will see in the next chapter, companies can often reduce current assets without adversely affecting sales or operating costs through the use of just-in-time inventory procedures and the like. It should also be noted that the profit penalty for holding current assets is very much dependent upon how they are financed. Therefore, corporate policy with regard to the level of current assets is never set in isolation: it is always established in conjunction with the firm's working capital financing policy, which we consider next.

Working capital financing policies

Most businesses experience seasonal fluctuations, as illustrated earlier with Sun Coast Clinics. Similarly, most businesses must build up current assets when the economy is strong, but they then sell off inventories and have reductions in receivables when the economy slacks off. Still, current assets never drop to zero, and this realization has led to the concept of permanent versus temporary assets. Although firms in the health care industry face cyclical and seasonal variations in volume, these variations are often not as large as those found in most other industries. Nevertheless, an understanding of permanent and temporary assets is vital to understanding working capital financing policies.

Consider Sun Coast Clinics. Table 14.1 suggests that, at this stage in its life, the firm's total assets fluctuate between $700,000 and $740,000. Thus, Sun Coast has $700,000 in *permanent assets,* composed of $500,000 of fixed assets and $200,000 in *permanent current assets,* plus *seasonal,* or *temporary, current assets* which fluctuate from zero to a maximum of $40,000. The manner in which the permanent and temporary current assets are financed defines the firm's *working capital financing policy.*

One policy, *maturity matching* or a *moderate financing policy*, calls for the firm to match asset and liability maturities as shown in Panel (a) of Figure 14.2. This strategy minimizes the risk that the firm will be unable to pay off its maturing obligations. To illustrate, suppose Sun Coast borrows on a one-year basis and uses the funds obtained to build and equip a new clinic. Cash flows from the clinic (profits plus depreciation) would almost never be sufficient to pay off the loan at the end of only one year, so the loan must be renewed. If for some reason the lender refuses to renew the loan, then Sun Coast would have problems. Had the clinic been financed with long-term debt, however, the required loan payments would have been better matched with cash flows from profits and depreciation, and the problem of loan renewal would not have arisen.

At the limit, a firm could attempt to match exactly the maturity structure of its assets and liabilities. Inventory expected to be sold in 30 days could be financed with a 30-day bank loan; a machine expected to last for five years could be financed by a five-year loan; a 20-year building could be financed by a 20-year mortgage bond; and so forth. Actually, three factors make this exact maturity matching strategy both unpractical and wrong: (1) there is uncertainty about the lives of assets, (2) some common equity (or fund capital) must be used, and this capital has no maturity, and (3) to develop a meaningful working capital financing policy it is necessary to consider whether an asset is permanent or temporary.

The proper framework for defining working capital financing policies requires us to use the concept of permanent and temporary assets. Thus, assets are not classified by their accounting definitions of current and long-term, but rather as either permanent or temporary. In this framework, maturity matching calls for the permanent portion of cash, receivables, and inventories (permanent assets) to be financed with *permanent capital* (long-term debt and equity or fund capital) even though accountants classify these assets as current assets, which implies that to match maturities they should be financed with short-term liabilities. The key here is that each dollar of cash, each individual receivable, and each dollar of inventory may well be short-term in that these items will be quickly turned over or converted to cash. However, as each individual item is converted, it will be replaced by a like item if it is permanent

Figure 14.2 Alternative Working Capital Financing Policies

(a) Moderate Approach (Maturity Matching)

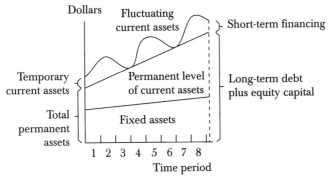

(b) Relatively Aggressive Approach

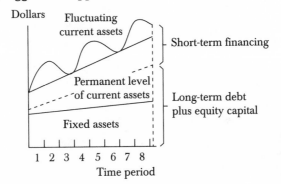

(c) Conservative Approach

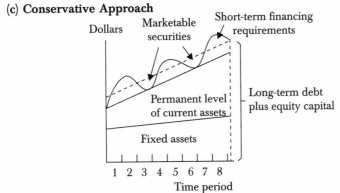

Source: E. F. Brigham and L. C. Gapenski. 1994. *Financial Management: Theory and Practice,* 7th ed. Fort Worth, TX: The Dryden Press.

in nature, and hence such short-term assets are actually carried permanently over the long term.

Panel (b) of Figure 14.2 illustrates an *aggressive financing policy.* Here, the firm finances all of its fixed assets with long-term capital but part of its permanent current assets with short-term, nonspontaneous credit. A look back at Table 14.1 will show that Sun Coast actually follows this strategy. Assuming that the $20,000 current portion of long-term debt will be refinanced with new long-term debt, Sun Coast has $500,000 in net fixed assets and $570,000 of long-term capital, leaving only $70,000 of long-term capital to finance $200,000 in permanent current assets. Additionally, Sun Coast has a minimum of $45,000 of "costless" spontaneous short-term credit consisting of accounts payable and accruals. Thus, Sun Coast uses $85,000 of short-term notes payable to help finance its permanent level of current assets.

Returning to Figure 14.2, note that we used the term "relatively" in the title for Panel (b), because there can be different *degrees* of aggressiveness. For example, the dashed line in Panel (b) could have been drawn *below* the line designating fixed assets, indicating that all of the permanent current assets and part of the fixed assets were financed with short-term credit; this would be a highly aggressive, extremely unconservative position, and the firm would be very much subject to dangers from rising interest rates as well as to loan renewal problems. However, short-term debt is often cheaper than long-term debt, and some firms are willing to sacrifice safety for the chance of higher profits.

As shown in Panel (c) of Figure 14.2, the dashed line could also be drawn above the line designating permanent current assets, indicating that permanent capital is being used to finance all permanent asset requirements and also to meet some or all of the temporary demands. In the situation depicted in our graph, the firm uses a small amount of short-term, nonspontaneous credit to meet its peak requirements, but it also meets a part of its seasonal needs by "storing liquidity" in the form of marketable securities during the off-season. The humps above the dashed line represent short-term financing; the troughs below the dashed line represent short-term security holdings. Panel (c) represents a very safe, *conservative working capital financing policy.*

As with working capital investment policy, the choice among alternative working capital financing policies involves a risk/return trade-off. The aggressive policy has the highest expected return, but also the highest risk, while the conservative policy has the lowest expected return and lowest risk. The maturity matching policy falls between the extremes. Unfortunately, there is no underlying finance theory that managers can use to pick the "correct" financing policy. In general, firms that have low business risk can afford to take on more financial risk. Thus, such firms tend to have more debt in their target capital structures and are more likely to use an aggressive working capital financing policy. Conversely, firms with high business risk usually take a conservative view regarding added financial risk.

Self-Test Questions:

What two key issues does working capital policy involve?

What is involved in the working capital investment decision?

What is involved in the working capital financing decision?

What is meant by the term "permanent assets"? By the term "permanent current assets"?

Cash Management

Cash is often called a "nonearning asset." It is needed to pay for labor and materials, to buy fixed assets, to pay taxes, to service debt, and so on. However, cash itself (and also commercial checking accounts) earns no interest. Thus, the goal of cash management is to minimize the amount of cash the firm must hold to conduct its normal business activities, yet, at the same time, have sufficient cash (1) to take trade discounts, (2) to maintain its credit rating, and (3) to meet unexpected cash needs. We begin our discussion of cash management with the cash budget.

The cash budget

A firm estimates its liquidity (cash) needs as part of its general budgeting, or forecasting, process. First, it forecasts both fixed asset and inventory requirements, along with the times when payments must be made. This information is combined with projections about the delay in collecting accounts receivable, wage payment dates, interest payment dates, and so on. All of this information is summarized in the *cash budget,* which shows the firm's projected cash inflows and outflows over some specified period. Generally, firms use a monthly cash budget forecasted over the next year, plus a more detailed daily or weekly cash budget for the coming month. The monthly cash budget is used for liquidity planning purposes and the daily or weekly budget for actual cash control.

We shall illustrate the process with a monthly cash budget covering the last six months of 1996 for Madison Drug Company, a producer of nonprescription drugs. Madison's drugs are sold year-round, but the bulk of the company's sales occurs from July through November, with a peak in September, when retailers are stocking up for the flu and cold season. All sales are made on terms that allow a 2 percent cash discount for payments made within 10 days, and if the discount is not taken, the full amount is due in 40 days. (Such terms are called "credit terms," which we will discuss in detail later in the chapter.) However, like most other companies, Madison finds that some of its customers delay payment up to 90 days. Experience shows that on 20 percent of the sales, payment is made during the month in which the sale is made; on 70 percent of the sales, payment is made during the first month after the month of the sale; and on 10 percent of the sales, payment is made during the second month after the month of the sale. Virtually all payments received in the month of sale are discount sales.

Rather than produce at a uniform rate throughout the year, Madison manufactures drugs shortly before they are required for delivery to reduce losses due to limited shelf life inventory obsolescence. The costs of chemicals, bottles, and other materials that go into the final products, on average, amount to 70 percent of sales prices. Such materials are bought the month before the company expects to sell the finished product. Its own purchase terms permit Madison to delay payment on purchases for one month. Accordingly, if July sales are forecasted at $10 million, then materials purchases during June will amount to $7 million, and this amount will actually be paid in July.

Such other cash expenditures as wages and rent are also built into the cash budget, and Madison must make tax payments of $2 million on September 15 and on December 15, while payment for a plant renovation must be made in October. Assuming that the company's target cash balance is $2.5 million, and that it has $3 million on hand on July 1, what are Madison's monthly cash requirements for the period from July through December?

The monthly cash requirements are worked out in Table 14.2. The top of the table provides a worksheet for calculating both collections on sales and payments on purchases. Line 1 gives the gross sales forecast for the period from May through December. (May and June sales are necessary to determine collections for July and August.) Next, on Lines 2a through 2c, cash collections are given. Line 2a shows that 20 percent of the sales during any given month are collected during that month. Customers who pay in the month of sale, however, typically take the discount, so the cash collected in the month of sale is reduced by 2 percent. For example, collections during July for the $10 million of sales

Table 14.2 Madison Drug Company: July through December Cash Budget (thousands of dollars)

	May	Jun	Jul	Aug	Sep	Oct	Nov	Dec
Collections and Purchases Worksheet								
1. Gross sales	$5,000	$5,000	$10,000	$15,000	$20,000	$10,000	$10,000	$5,000
2. Collections								
a. During month of sale			1,960	2,940	3,920	1,960	1,960	980
b. First month after sale			3,500	7,000	10,500	14,000	7,000	7,000
c. Second month after sale			500	500	1,000	1,500	2,000	1,000
3. Total collections			$ 5,960	$10,440	$15,420	$17,460	$10,960	$ 8,980
4. Purchases		$7,000	$10,500	$14,000	$ 7,000	$ 7,000	$ 3,500	
5. Payments for purchases			$ 7,000	$10,500	$14,000	$ 7,000	$ 7,000	$ 3,500
Cash Gain or Loss								
6. Total collections			$ 5,960	$10,440	$15,420	$17,460	$10,960	$ 8,980
7. Purchases			$ 7,000	$10,500	$14,000	$ 7,000	$ 7,000	$ 3,500
8. Wages and salaries			750	1,000	1,250	750	750	500
9. Rent			250	250	250	250	250	250
10. Other expenses			100	150	200	100	100	50
11. Taxes					2,000			2,000
12. Payment for capital assets						5,000		
13. Total payments			$ 8,100	$11,900	$17,700	$13,100	$ 8,100	$ 6,300
14. Net cash gain (loss)			($ 2,140)	($ 1,460)	($ 2,280)	$ 4,360	$ 2,860	$ 2,680
Cash Surplus (Loan Requirement)								
15. Cash at beginning with no borrowing			$ 3,000	$ 860	($ 600)	($ 2,880)	$ 1,480	$ 4,340
16. Cumulative cash			$ 860	($ 600)	($ 2,880)	$ 1,480	$ 4,340	$ 7,020
17. Target cash balance			2,500	2,500	2,500	2,500	2,500	2,500
18. Cumulative surplus cash (loan balance)			($ 1,640)	($ 3,100)	($ 5,380)	($ 1,020)	$ 1,840	$ 4,520

in that month will be 20 percent times sales less the 2 percent discount = 0.2($10,000,000)0.98 = $1,960,000. Line 2b shows the collections on the previous month's sales; 70 percent of the $5,000,000 June sales, or $3,500,000, will be collected in July. Line 2c gives collections from sales two months earlier, or 10 percent of sales in that month; for example, the July collections for May sales are 0.10($5,000,000) = $500,000. Total collections in July represent 20 percent of July sales (minus the discount) plus 70 percent of June sales plus 10 percent of May sales, or $5,960,000 in total. This amount is shown on Line 3.

Next, payments for purchases of materials are shown. July sales are forecasted at $10 million, so Madison will purchase 0.70($10) = $7 million of materials in June (Line 4) and pay for these purchases in July (Line 5). Similarly, Madison will purchase 0.70($15) = $10.5 million of materials in July to produce the drugs necessary to meet August's forecasted sales of $15 million.

With the top section of Table 14.2 completed, the center section can be constructed. Cash from collections is shown on Line 6. Lines 7 through 12 list payments made during each month, and these payments are summed on Line 13. The difference between cash receipts and cash payments (Line 6 minus Line 13) is the net cash gain or loss during the month; for July there is a net cash loss of $2,140,000, as shown on Line 14.

In the bottom section of the table, we first determine Madison's cash balance at the start of each month, assuming no borrowing is done; this is shown on Line 15. We assume that Madison will have $3 million on hand on July 1. The beginning cash balance (Line 15) is then added to the net cash gain or loss during the month (Line 14) to obtain the cumulative cash that would be on hand if no financing were done (Line 16); at the end of July, Madison forecasts a cumulative cash balance of $860,000 in the absence of borrowing.

The target cash balance, $2.5 million, is then subtracted from the cumulative cash balance to determine the firm's borrowing requirements, shown in parentheses, or its surplus cash. Because Madison expects to have cumulative cash, as shown on Line 16, of only $860,000 in July, it will have to borrow $1,640,000 to bring the cash account up to the target balance of $2,500,000. Assuming that this amount is indeed borrowed, loans outstanding will total $1,640,000 at the end of July. (We assume that Madison did not have any loans outstanding on July 1 because its beginning cash balance exceeded the target balance.)

The cash surplus or required loan balance is given on Line 18; a positive value indicates a cash surplus, whereas a negative value indicates a loan requirement. Note that the surplus cash or loan requirement shown on Line 18 is a *cumulative amount*. Thus, Madison must borrow $1,640,000 in July; it has a cash shortfall during August of $1,460,000 as reported on Line 14, so its total loan requirement at the end of August is $1,640,000 + $1,460,000 = $3,100,000, as reported on Line 18. Madison's arrangement with its bank permits it to increase its outstanding loans on a daily basis, up to a prearranged maximum, just as you could increase the amount you owe on a credit card. Madison will use any surplus funds it generates to pay off its loans, and because the loan can be paid down at any time, on a daily basis, the firm will never have both a cash surplus and an outstanding loan balance.

This same procedure is used in the following months. Sales will peak in September, accompanied by increased payments for materials purchases, wages, and other items. Receipts from sales will also go up, but the firm will still be left with a $2,280,000 net cash outflow during the month. The total loan requirement at the end of September will hit a peak of $5,380,000. This amount equals the $3,100,000 needed at the end of August plus the $2,280,000 cash deficit for September.

Sales, purchases, and payments for past purchases will fall sharply in October, but collections will be the highest of any month because they will reflect the high September sales. As a result, Madison will enjoy a healthy $4,360,000 net cash gain during October. This net gain can be used to pay off borrowings, so loans outstanding will decline by $4,360,000, to $1,020,000.

Madison will have another cash surplus in November, which will permit it to pay off all its loans. In fact, the company is expected to have $1,840,000 in surplus cash by the month's end, and another cash surplus in December will swell the excess cash to $4,520,000. With such a large amount of unneeded funds, Madison's treasurer will certainly want to invest in interest-bearing securities, or to put the funds to use in some other way.

Before concluding our discussion of the cash budget, we should make some additional points:

• Madison's cash budget does not reflect any bad debt losses. If such losses are expected, they can be incorporated easily into the cash budget by altering the collections percentages so that they add to less than 100 percent.

• Madison's cash budget does not reflect interest on loans or income from the investment of surplus cash. This refinement could easily be added.

- If cash inflows and outflows are not uniform during the month, a monthly cash budget could seriously understate the firm's peak financing requirements. The data in Table 14.2 show the situation expected on the last day of each month, but on any given day during the month it could be quite different. For example, if all payments had to be made on the fifth of each month, but collections came in uniformly throughout the month, the firm would need to borrow much larger amounts than those shown in Table 14.2. In this case, we would have to prepare a cash budget on a daily basis.

- Since depreciation is a noncash charge, it does not appear on the cash budget other than through its effect on taxes paid.

- Since the cash budget represents a forecast, all the values in the table are *expected* values. If actual sales, materials purchases, and so on, are different from the forecasted levels, then the projected cash deficits and surpluses will also be incorrect. Thus, Madison might end up needing to borrow larger amounts than are indicated on Line 18, so it should arrange a line of credit in excess of that amount.

- Spreadsheet programs are particularly well suited for constructing and analyzing cash budgets, especially with respect to the sensitivity of cash flows to changes in sales levels, collection periods, and the like. We could change any assumption, say the projected monthly sales or the time customers take to pay, and the cash budget would automatically and instantly be recalculated. This would show us exactly how the firm's borrowing requirements would change if other factors changed. Also, with a spreadsheet model, it is easy to add features like interest paid on loans, interest earned on marketable securities, and so on.

- Finally, we should note that the target cash balance probably will be adjusted over time, rising and falling with seasonal patterns and with long-term changes in the scale of the firm's operations. Thus, Madison will probably plan to maintain larger cash balances during August and September than at other times, and as the company grows, so will its required cash balance. Also, Madison's managers might even be able to set the firm's target cash balance at zero: this could be done if the firm carried a portfolio of marketable securities which could be sold to replenish the cash account, or if it had an arrangement with its bank that permitted it to borrow the funds it needed on a daily basis. In that event, the cash budget would simply stop with Line 14, and the amounts on that line would represent the projected loans outstanding or surplus cash. Note, though, that most firms would find it difficult to operate with a zero-balance bank account, just as you would, and the costs of such an operation would in most instances offset the opportunity cost associated with maintaining a positive cash balance. Therefore, most firms do set a positive target cash balance.

Using Monte Carlo simulation to set the target cash balance

In discussing Madison's cash budget, we assumed a target cash balance of $2,500,000. There are several models that can be used to set a firm's target cash balance, including trial and error. In this section, we use the Madison Drug Company cash budget presented in Table 14.2 to illustrate the use of *Monte Carlo simulation* to set the target bash balance.

Sales and collections are the driving forces in the cash budget. In the Table 14.2 cash budget, we used expected values for sales, and these values were used to derive most of the other cash flow forecasts. Now we repeat the cash budget, but with the assumption that sales are subject to a probability distribution about the expected value. Specifically, we assume that the distribution of sales for each month is normal, with a coefficient of variation (CV) of 0.10 and a standard deviation which varies with the sales level. In effect, we assume that the relative variability of sales is constant from month to month. Thus, in May, when expected sales are $5 million, the standard deviation of sales is $500,000:

$$CV = 0.10 = \frac{\sigma_{Sales}}{\text{Expected sales}} = \frac{\sigma_{Sales}}{\$5,000,000}$$

$$\sigma_{Sales} = 0.10(\$5,000,000) = \$500,000.$$

Similarly, the standard deviation of sales in the peak month of September is found to be $2 million, and so forth.

Of course, collections are based on actual sales rather than on expected sales, so the collections pattern will reflect realized sales. If we assume that the sales realized in any month will not change Madison's expectations for future sales, then purchases in any month will be based on 70 percent of next month's expected sales, but with upward or downward adjustments to reflect excess inventories on hand due to the current month's sales being less than expected or inventory shortages that result from above-normal sales. Other payments, such as wages, rent, and so on, were assumed to be fixed for the analysis, although uncertainty could be built into them, too.

Based on these assumptions, we ran a Monte Carlo simulation of Madison's cash budget. The simulation analysis focuses on Line 14 of Table 14.2, the net cash gain (loss) during the month. Table 14.3

summarizes the results and compares the range of likely cash gains or losses with the point estimates taken from Line 14 of Table 14.2.

Now suppose Madison's managers want to be 90 percent confident that the firm will not run out of cash during July. They would set the beginning-of-month balance at $2,897,000 (rather than $2,500,000), because there is a 90 percent probability that the July cash flow will be no worse than a $2,897,000 net outflow. Thus, with a beginning cash balance of $2,897,000, there would be only a 10 percent probability that the firm would run out of cash during July. This type of analysis could be extended for the other months, and it could be used in lieu of the fixed $2.5 million as the target beginning-of-month cash balance.

Note that in our simulation we assumed that sales are independent from month to month. Alternatively, we could have assumed some type of dependence such that a lower-than-expected sales level in July would signal a trend toward lower sales in the following months. This type of dependency would increase the firm's uncertainty with regard to cash flows in any given month and, consequently, increase the required cash balance needed to provide any prescribed level of confidence regarding running out of cash.

Firms actually set their target cash balances as the larger of (1) their transactions balances plus precautionary (safety stock) balances or (2) their required compensating balances as determined by their agreements with banks. (Compensating balances are discussed in detail in a later section.) Transactions balances and precautionary balances depend upon the firm's volume of business, the degree of uncertainty inherent in its forecasts of cash inflows and outflows, and its ability to borrow on short notice to meet cash shortfalls. Consider again the cash budget shown for Madison Drug Company in Table 14.2, in which the

Table 14.3   Madison Drug Company: Cash Budget Monte Carlo Simulation (thousands of dollars)

Month	Net Cash Flow from Table 14.2	Probability of Achieving at Least the Indicated Amount				
		90%	*70%*	*50%*	*30%*	*10%*
July	($2,140)	($2,897)	($2,454)	($2,161)	($1,832)	($1,354)
August	(1,460)	(2,810)	(2,043)	(1,512)	(855)	(130)
September	(2,280)	(4,088)	(2,989)	(2,302)	(1,587)	(489)
October	4,360	2,407	3,606	4,394	5,097	6,268
November	2,860	1,737	2,324	2,868	3,328	4,002
December	2,680	1,753	2,259	2,661	3,077	3,651

target cash balance is shown on Line 17. Other factors held constant, the target cash balance would increase if Madison expanded, whereas it would decrease if Madison contracted. Similarly, Madison could afford to operate with a smaller target balance if it could forecast better and thus be more certain that inflows would come in as scheduled and that no unanticipated outflows, such as might result from uninsured fire losses, lawsuits, and the like, would occur.

Statistics are not available on whether transactions balances or compensating balances actually control most firms' target cash balances. Compensating balance requirements sometimes dominate, especially during periods of high interest rates and tight money, but, for most firms at most times, transactions balances determine the target.

Cash management techniques

Cash management has changed significantly over the last 20 years as a result of two factors. First, until recently, interest rates had been relatively high, pushing up the opportunity cost of holding cash and forcing managers to search for more efficient ways of managing the firm's cash. Second, new technologies, particularly computerized electronic fund transfer mechanisms, have provided a means to optimize cash transactions on a real-time basis.

Cash management techniques fall generally into four categories: (1) synchronizing cash flow, (2) using float, (3) accelerating collections, and (4) controlling disbursements. We discuss the most commonly used techniques for accomplishing these tasks in the following sections.[1]

Cash flow synchronization

If you as an individual were to receive income once a year, you would probably put it in the bank, draw down your account weekly, and have an average balance during the year equal to about half your annual income. If you received income monthly instead of once a year, you would operate similarly, but your average balance would be much smaller. If you could arrange to receive income daily and to pay rent, tuition, and other charges on a daily basis, and if you were quite confident of your forecasted inflows and outflows, then you could hold a very small average cash balance.

Exactly the same situation applies to businesses: by improving their forecasts and by arranging things so that their cash receipts coincide with required cash outflows, firms can reduce their transactions balances to a minimum. Recognizing this point, many companies bill customers on a regular "billing cycle" throughout the month that matches their own outflows. This improves the *synchronization of cash flows,* which in turn enables a firm to reduce its cash balances, decrease its bank loans, lower interest expenses, and boost profits.

Using float

Float is defined as the difference between the balance shown in a firm's (or individual's) checkbook and the balance on the bank's records. Suppose a firm writes, on the average, checks in the amount of $5,000 each day, and it takes six days for these checks to clear and to be deducted from the firm's bank account. This will cause the firm's own checkbook to show a balance $30,000 smaller than the balance on the bank's records; this difference is called *disbursement float.*

Now suppose the firm also receives checks in the amount of $5,000 daily, but it loses four days while they are being deposited and cleared. This will result in $20,000 of *collections float.* In total, the firm's *net float*— the difference between the $30,000 positive disbursement float and the $20,000 negative collections float—will be $10,000.

If the firm's own collection and clearing process is more efficient than that of the recipients of its checks—which is generally true of larger, more efficient firms—then the firm could actually show a *negative* balance on its own books but have a *positive* balance on the records of its bank. Some firms indicate that they *never* have positive book cash balances. One medical equipment manufacturer stated that while its checking account, according to its bank's records, shows an average cash balance of about $200,000, its *book* balance is *minus* $200,000; it has $400,000 of net float. Obviously the firm must be able to forecast its disbursements and collections accurately in order to make such heavy use of float.

Basically, a firm's net float is a function of its ability to speed up collections on checks received and to slow down collections on checks written. Efficient firms go to great lengths to speed up the processing of incoming checks, thus putting the funds to work faster, and they try to stretch their own payments out as long as possible, without engaging in unethical or illegal practices.

Acceleration of receipts

Managers have searched for ways to collect receivables faster since credit transactions began. Although cash collection is the responsibility of a firm's managers, the speed with which checks are cleared is dependent on the banking system. Several techniques are now used both to speed collections and to get funds where they are needed, but the two most popular are lockbox services and concentration banking. For health care providers, electronic claims processing is a way of speeding collections, but we will defer this discussion until the next chapter.

Lockboxes are one of the oldest cash management tools. The concept was first used on a large scale by RCA (now part of General Electric), but now virtually all banks that offer cash management services also offer lockbox services. In a lockbox system, incoming checks are sent to post office boxes rather than to corporate headquarters. For example, Health SouthWest, a regional HMO headquartered in Oklahoma City, has its Texas customers send their payments to a box in Dallas, its New Mexico customers send their checks to Albuquerque, and so on, rather than having all checks sent to Oklahoma City. Several times a day a local bank will collect the contents of each lockbox and deposit the checks into the company's local account. The bank would then provide the firm with daily records of the receipts collected, usually via an electronic data transmission system in a format that permits on-line updating of the firm's receivables accounts.

A lockbox system reduces the time required for a firm to receive incoming checks, to deposit them, and to get them cleared through the banking system so that the funds are available for use. This time reduction occurs because mail time and check collection time are both reduced if the lockbox is located in the geographic area where the customer is located. Lockbox services can often increase the availability of funds by one to four days over the "regular" system for firms with customers over a large geographical area.

Lockbox systems, although efficient in speeding up collections, result in the firm's cash being spread around among many banks. The primary purpose of *concentration banking* is to mobilize funds from decentralized receiving locations, whether they be lockboxes or decentralized company locations, into one or more central cash pools. In a typical concentration system, the firm's collection banks record deposits received each day. Then, based on disbursement needs, the funds are transferred from these collection points to a concentration bank. Concentration accounts allow firms to take maximum advantage of economies of scale in cash management and investment. Health SouthWest uses an Oklahoma City bank as its concentration bank. The HMO's cash manager then uses this pool for short-term investing or reallocation among the HMO's other banks.

One of the keys to concentration banking is the ability to quickly transfer funds from collecting banks to concentration banks. The advent of electronic transfer mechanisms makes such transfers easy. *Automated clearinghouses* are communications networks that provide a means of sending data from one financial institution to another. Instead of using paper checks, computer files are created, and all entries for a particular bank are placed on a single file which is sent to that bank. Some banks send and receive their data on tapes, while others have direct computer links to the clearinghouse. In addition to automated clearinghouses, the *Federal Reserve wire system* can be used for cash concentration or for other cash transfers. This system is used to move large sums that occur on a sporadic basis, such as would occur if Humana borrowed $10 million in the commercial paper market.

Disbursement control

Accelerated collections represent one side of cash management, and controlling funds outflows is the flip side of the coin. Of course, efficient cash management can only result if both inflows and outflows are effectively managed.

No single action controls disbursements more effectively than *payables centralization.* This permits the firm's managers to evaluate the payments coming due for the entire firm and to schedule cash transfers to meet these needs on a company-wide basis. Centralized disbursement also permits more efficient monitoring of payables and float balances. Of course, there are also disadvantages to a centralized disbursement system: regional offices may not be able to make prompt payment for services rendered, which can create ill will with suppliers.

Zero-balance accounts (ZBAs) are special disbursement accounts having a zero-dollar balance on which checks are written. Typically, a firm establishes several ZBAs in the concentration bank and funds them from a master account. As checks are presented to a ZBA for payment, funds are automatically transferred from the master account. If the master account goes negative, it is replenished by borrowing from the bank against a line of credit, by borrowing in the commercial paper market, or by selling some securities from the firm's marketable securities portfolio. Zero-balance accounts simplify the control of disbursements and cash balances, and hence reduce the amount of idle (non-interest-bearing) cash.

Whereas zero-balance accounts are typically established at concentration banks, *controlled disbursement accounts* can be set up at any bank. In fact, controlled disbursement accounts were initially used only in relatively remote banks, so this technique was originally called *remote disbursement.* The basic technique is simple: controlled disbursement accounts are not funded until the day's checks are presented against the account. The key to controlled disbursement is the ability of the bank having the account to report the total daily amount of checks received for clearance by 11 a.m., New York time. This early notification gives a firm's managers sufficient time (1) to wire funds to the controlled disbursement account to cover the checks presented for payment and (2) to invest excess cash at midday, when money market trading is at a peak.

Matching the costs and benefits of cash management

Although a number of techniques have been discussed to reduce cash balance requirements, implementing these procedures is not a costless operation. How far should a firm go in making its cash operations more efficient? As a general rule, the firm should incur these expenses only so long as the marginal returns exceed the marginal costs.

For example, suppose that by establishing a lockbox system, a firm can reduce its investment in cash by $1 million without increasing the risk of running short of cash. Further, suppose the firm borrows at a cost of 12 percent. The lockbox system will release $1 million, which can be used to reduce bank loans and thus save $120,000 per year. If the costs of setting up and operating the lockbox system are less than $120,000, the move is a good one, but if the costs exceed $120,000, the improvement in efficiency is not worth the cost.

The value of careful cash management depends upon the costs of funds invested in cash, which in turn depends upon the current rate of interest. For example, in the early 1980s, with interest rates at relatively high levels, firms were devoting a great deal of care to cash management. Today, with interest rates much lower, the value of cash management is reduced. It is clear that larger firms, with larger cash balances, can better afford to hire the personnel necessary to maintain tight control over their cash positions. Cash management is one element of business operations in which economies of scale are present. Banks have also placed considerable emphasis on developing and marketing cash management services. Because of scale economies, banks can generally provide these services to smaller companies at lower costs than companies can achieve by operating in-house cash management systems.

Self-Test Questions:

Briefly describe the construction and use of a cash budget.

How can Monte Carlo simulation be used to set the target cash balance?

What is float? How do firms use float to increase cash management efficiency?

What are some methods firms can use to accelerate receipts? To control disbursements?

Marketable Securities Management

Realistically, cash and marketable securities management cannot be separated—management of one implies management of the other. In the previous section of the chapter, we focused on cash management. Now we turn to marketable securities management.

Rationale for holding marketable securities

Many firms hold large portfolios of temporary investments called *marketable securities.* There are two underlying reasons for these holdings: (1) they serve as a substitute for cash balances and (2) they are used as a temporary investment.

Marketable securities as a substitute for cash

Some firms hold portfolios of marketable securities in lieu of larger cash balances, liquidating part of the portfolio to increase the cash account when cash outflows exceed inflows. In most cases, the securities are held primarily for precautionary purposes: most firms prefer to rely on bank credit to make temporary transactions or to meet speculative needs, but they may still hold some liquid assets to guard against a possible shortage of bank credit.

Marketable securities as a temporary investment

Temporary investments in marketable securities generally occur in one of the following two situations:

1. *To finance seasonal or cyclical operations.* If the firm has a conservative financing policy as we defined it in Panel (c) of Figure 14.2, then its long-term capital will exceed its permanent assets, and marketable securities will be held when inventories and receivables are low. On the other hand, with a highly aggressive policy, the firm will never carry any securities, and it will borrow heavily to meet peak needs. With a moderate policy, in which maturities are matched, permanent assets will be matched with long-term financing, most seasonal increases in inventories and

receivables will be met by short-term loans, and the firm will also carry marketable securities at certain times.

2. *To meet known financial requirements.* Marketable securities are frequently built up immediately preceding quarterly corporate tax payment dates. Further, if a major plant construction program is planned for the near future, if an acquisition is planned, or if a bond issue is about to mature, a firm may build up its marketable securities portfolio to provide the required funds.

Not-for-profit hospitals often have particularly large marketable securities holdings compared with similar-sized businesses in other industries. As a whole, not-for-profit hospitals sit atop financial assets of some $200 billion, including cash, stocks, bonds, and pension funds. One hospital system alone, Methodist Hospital System in Houston, has accumulated almost $800 million in financial assets. There are four reasons why not-for-profit hospitals typically carry large marketable securities portfolios:

1. Not-for-profit hospitals often set aside funds for future asset replacement rather than acquire the funds at time of replacement.

2. Many hospitals self-insure at least part of their professional liability exposure, and hence establish an investment pool to meet actuarial needs.

3. Many hospitals have defined benefit pension plans, which require a firm-sponsored pension fund.

4. Not-for-profit hospitals receive endowment gifts that must be managed over time.

In addition to these reasons, many managers are predicting rough times ahead for hospitals, so a large cash holding is a prudent hedge against a potentially harsh future.

Criteria for selecting marketable securities

A wide variety of securities and investment strategies are available to firms that hold marketable securities. In this section, we first consider the risk characteristics of different securities, and then we discuss how financial managers select the specific instruments held in their marketable securities portfolios.

Default (credit) risk

The risk that a borrower will be unable to make interest or principal payments is known as *default,* or *credit, risk.* If the borrower is the U.S.

Treasury, default risk is essentially zero, so Treasury securities are risk free with regard to default risk. Corporate securities, and bonds issued by state and local governments, are subject to some degree of default risk.

Event risk

The probability that some event that suddenly increases a firm's default risk, such as a recapitalization or a leveraged buyout (LBO), will occur, and hence lower the value of its outstanding bonds, is called *event risk*. Bonds issued by industrial and service companies generally have more event risk than bonds issued by regulated companies such as banks or electric utilities. Also, long-term securities have more event risk than short-term securities, because longer maturities mean more time for an event to happen. Treasury securities do not carry any event risk, barring national disaster.

Price risk

Bond prices vary with changes in interest rates. Further, the prices of long-term bonds are much more sensitive to shifts in interest rates than are the prices of short-term securities—long-term bonds have much more *price risk*. Therefore, even Treasury securities are not free of all risk; they are subject to risk due to interest rate fluctuations. If Bayside's treasurer purchased at par $1 million of 25-year U.S. government bonds paying 9 percent interest, and if interest rates rose to 14.5 percent, then the market value of the bonds would fall from $1 million to approximately $638,000—a loss of almost 40 percent. (This actually happened from 1980 to 1982.) Had 90-day Treasury bills been held, the capital loss resulting from the change in interest rates would have been negligible.

Purchasing power risk

Another type of risk is *purchasing power risk*, or the risk that inflation will reduce the purchasing power of a given sum of money. This risk is important both to firms and to individual investors during times of inflation, and it is generally regarded as being lower on assets whose returns can be expected to rise during inflation than on assets whose returns are fixed. Thus, real estate and common stocks are often thought of as being better "hedges against inflation" than are bonds and other long-term, fixed-income securities.

Liquidity (marketability) risk

An asset that can be sold on short notice for close to its "fair value" is defined as being highly *liquid*. If Bayside purchased $1 million of infrequently traded bonds issued by a relatively obscure company, it would probably have to accept a price reduction to sell the bonds on short notice. On the other hand, if Bayside bought $1 million worth of U.S. Treasury bonds, or bonds issued by AT&T, General Motors, or Exxon, it would be able to dispose of them almost instantaneously at close to the current market price. These latter bonds are said to have very little *liquidity risk*.

Returns on securities

As we know from earlier chapters, the higher a security's risk, the higher its expected and required rates of return. Thus, managers, like other investors, must make a trade-off between risk and return when choosing investments for their marketable securities portfolios. Since marketable securities are generally held for a specific known need, or else for use in emergencies, the firm might be financially embarrassed should the portfolio decline in value. Accordingly, the marketable securities portfolio is generally confined to safe, highly liquid, short-term securities issued by either the U.S. government or the very strongest corporations. However, the cash managers of larger firms with substantial marketable security holdings often use sophisticated hedging strategies that permit them to be more aggressive in constructing their portfolios.

Types of marketable securities

Larger corporations, with large amounts of surplus cash, often directly own Treasury bills, commercial paper, negotiable certificates of deposit, and even Euromarket securities (dollar denominated loans held outside the United States). In addition, large taxable firms often hold preferred stock because of its 70 percent dividend exclusion from federal income taxes. Smaller firms, on the other hand, are more likely to invest with a bank or with a money market or preferred stock mutual fund, because the small firm's volume of investment simply does not warrant its hiring specialists to manage a marketable securities portfolio. Firms can use a mutual fund and then literally write checks on the fund to meet cash needs as they arise. Interest rates on mutual funds are somewhat lower than rates on direct investments of equivalent risk because of management fees, but for smaller companies net returns may well be higher on mutual funds.

Self-Test Questions:

Why do firms hold marketable securities portfolios?

What are some securities commonly held as marketable securities? Why are these the securities of choice?

Short-Term Financing

In the previous section, we discussed short-term investment of excess cash. Now, we turn our attention to short-term financing. The three possible working capital financing policies described earlier in the chapter were distinguished by the relative amounts of short-term debt used under each policy. The aggressive policy called for the greatest use of short-term debt, while the conservative policy called for the least. Maturity matching fell in between.

Advantages and disadvantages of short-term credit

Although using short-term credit is generally riskier than using long-term credit, short-term credit does have some significant advantages. The pros and cons of short-term financing are considered in this section.

Speed

A short-term loan can be obtained much faster than long-term credit. Lenders will insist on a more thorough financial examination before extending long-term credit, and the loan agreement will have to be spelled out in considerable detail because a lot can happen during the life of a 10- or 20-year loan. Therefore, if funds are needed in a hurry, the firm should look to the short-term markets.

Flexibility

If its needs for funds are seasonal or cyclical, a firm may not want to commit itself to long-term debt for three reasons: (1) Flotation costs are generally high when raising long-term debt but trivial for short-term credit. (2) Although long-term debt can be repaid early, provided the loan agreement includes a prepayment provision, prepayment penalties can be expensive. Accordingly, if a firm thinks its need for funds may diminish in the near future, it should choose short-term debt for the flexibility it provides. (3) Long-term loan agreements always contain restrictive covenants that constrain the firm's future actions. Short-term credit agreements are generally much less onerous in this regard.

Cost

The yield curve is normally upward sloping, indicating that interest rates are generally lower on short-term than on long-term debt. Thus, under normal conditions, interest costs at the time the funds are obtained will be lower if the firm borrows on a short-term rather than a long-term basis.

Risk

Even though short-term debt is often less expensive than long-term debt, short-term credit subjects the firm to more risk than does long-term financing. This occurs for two reasons. (1) If a firm borrows on a long-term basis, its interest costs will be relatively stable over time, but if it uses short-term credit, its interest expense will fluctuate widely, at times possibly going quite high. For example, the short-term rate banks charge large corporations (the prime rate) more than tripled over a two-year period in the 1980s, rising from 6.25 to 21 percent. Many firms that had borrowed heavily on a short-term basis simply could not meet their rising interest costs, and as a result bankruptcies hit record levels during that period. (2) If a firm borrows heavily on a short-term basis, it may find itself unable to repay this debt, and it may be in such a weak financial position that the lender will not extend the loan; this too could force the firm into bankruptcy.

Sources of short-term financing

Statements about the flexibility, cost, and riskiness of short-term versus long-term debt depend, to a large extent, on the type of short-term credit that is actually used. There are numerous sources of short-term funds, and in the following sections we described four major types: (1) accruals, (2) accounts payable (trade credit), (3) bank loans, and (4) commercial paper.

Accruals

Firms generally pay employees on a weekly, biweekly, or monthly basis, so the balance sheet will typically show some accrued wages. Similarly, the firm's own estimated income taxes (if applicable), the social security and income taxes withheld from employee payrolls, and the sales taxes collected are generally paid on a weekly, monthly, or quarterly basis, so the balance sheet will typically show some accrued taxes along with accrued wages.

Accruals increase automatically, or spontaneously, as a firm's operations expand. Further, this type of debt is "free" in the sense that no explicit interest is paid on funds raised through accruals. However, a firm cannot ordinarily control its accruals: The timing of wage payments is set by economic forces and industry custom, while tax payment dates are established by law. Thus, firms use all the accruals they can, but they have little control over the levels of these accounts.

Accounts payable (trade credit)

Firms generally make purchases from other firms on credit, recording the debt as an *account payable*. Accounts payable, or *trade credit*, is the largest single category of short-term debt for many firms. Because small companies often do not qualify for financing from other sources, they rely especially heavily on trade credit.[2]

Trade credit is a spontaneous source of financing in the sense that it arises from ordinary business transactions. For example, suppose a hospital purchases an average of $2,000 a day of supplies on terms of net 30, meaning that it must pay for goods 30 days after the invoice date. On average, the hospital will owe 30 times $2,000, or $60,000, to its suppliers, assuming that the hospital's managers act rationally and do not pay before the credit is due. If the hospital's sales, and consequently its purchases, were to double, then its accounts payable would also double, to $120,000. Simply by growing, the hospital would have spontaneously generated an additional $60,000 of financing. Similarly, if the terms under which it bought were extended from 30 to 40 days, the hospital's accounts payable would expand form $60,000 to $80,000. Thus, lengthening the credit period, as well as expanding sales and purchases, generates additional financing.

Firms that sell on credit have a *credit policy* that includes certain *terms of credit*. For example, Midwestern Metals Company sells on terms of 2/10, net 30, meaning that a 2 percent discount is given if payment is made within 10 days of the invoice date, with the full invoice amount being due and payable within 30 days if the discount is not taken. Suppose Chicago Surgical Instruments, Inc. buys an average of $12 million of high quality stainless steel from Midwestern each year, less a 2 percent discount, for net purchases of $11,760,000/360 = $32,666.67 per day. For simplicity, suppose Midwestern is Chicago Surgical's only supplier. If Chicago Surgical takes the discount, paying at the end of the tenth day, its payables will average (10)($32,666.67) = $326,667; Chicago Surgical will, on average, be receiving $326,667 of credit from its only supplier, Midwestern Metallurgical Company.

Now suppose Chicago Surgical decides not to take the discount; what will happen? First, Chicago Surgical will begin paying invoices after 30 days, so its accounts payable will increase to 30($32,666.67) = $980,000.[3] Midwestern will now be supplying Chicago Surgical with $980,000 − $326,667 = $653,000 of additional credit. Chicago Surgical could use this additional credit to pay off bank loans, to expand inventories, to increase fixed assets, to build up its cash account, or even to increase its own accounts receivable.

Chicago Surgical's new credit from Midwestern has a cost: Chicago Surgical is forgoing a 2 percent discount on its $12 million of purchases, so its costs will rise by $240,000 per year. Dividing this $240,000 cost by the amount of additional credit, we find the implicit cost of the added trade credit as follows:

$$\text{Approximate percentage cost} = \frac{\$240,000}{\$653,333} = 36.7\%.$$

Assuming that Chicago Surgical can borrow from its bank (or from other sources) at an interest rate less than 36.7 percent, it should not expand its payables by forgoing discounts.

The following equation can be used to calculate the approximate percentage cost, on an annual basis, of not taking discounts:

$$\text{Approximate percentage cost} = \frac{\text{Discount percent}}{100 - \text{Discount percent}} \times$$

$$\frac{360}{\text{Days credit received} - \text{Discount period}}. \qquad (14.1)$$

The numerator of the first term, Discount percent, is the cost per dollar of credit, while the denominator in this term, 100 − Discount percent, represents the funds made available by not taking the discount. Thus, the first term is the periodic cost of the trade credit—Chicago Surgical must spend $2 to gain $98 of credit. The second term shows how many times each year this cost is incurred. To illustrate the equation, the approximate cost of not taking a discount when the terms are 2/10, net 30, is computed as follows:

$$\text{Approximate percentage cost} = \frac{2}{98} \times \frac{360}{20} = 0.0204(18)$$

$$= 0.367 = 36.7\%.$$

In effective annual interest terms, the rate is even higher. The discount amounts to interest, and with terms of 2/10, net 30, the firm gains use of the funds for 30 − 10 = 20 days, so there are 360/20 = 18 "interest periods" per year. Remember that the first term in Equation 14.1, Discount percent/(100 − Discount percent) = 2/98 = 0.0204, is the periodic interest rate. This rate is paid 18 times each year, so the effective annual rate cost of trade credit is 43.8 percent:

$$\text{Effective annual rate} = (1.0204)^{18} - 1.0$$
$$= 1.438 - 1.0 = 0.438 = 43.8\%.$$

Thus, the 36.7 percent approximate cost calculated with Equation 14.1 understates the true cost of trade credit.

Notice, however, that the cost of trade credit can be reduced by paying late. Thus, if Chicago Surgical could get away with paying in 60 days rather than in the specified 30, the effective credit period would become 60 − 10 = 50 days, and the approximate cost would drop from 36.7 percent to (2/98)(360/50) = 14.7%. The effective annual rate would drop from 43.8 percent to 15.7 percent. In recessionary periods, firms may be able to get away with late payments, but they will also suffer a variety of problems associated with "stretching" accounts payable and being branded a "slow payer" account.

The cost of the additional trade credit that results from not taking discounts can be worked out for other purchase terms. Some illustrative costs are shown below:

	Cost of Additional Credit if the Cash Discount Is Not Taken	
Credit Terms	Approximate Cost	Effective Annual Cost
1/10, net 20	36%	44%
1/10, net 30	18	20
2/10, net 20	73	107
3/15, net 45	37	44

As these figures show, the cost of not taking discounts can be substantial.

A firm's policy with regard to taking or not taking discounts can have a significant effect on its financial statements. To illustrate, assume that Chicago Surgical is just beginning its operations. On the first day, it makes net purchases of $32,666.67. This amount is recorded on its balance sheet under accounts payable.[4] The second day it buys another $32,666.67. The first day's purchases are not yet paid for, so at the end of the second day, accounts payable total $65,333.34. Accounts payable increase by another $32,666.67 on the third day, for a total of $98,000, and after 10 days, accounts payable are up to $326,667.

If Chicago Surgical takes discounts, then on the 11th day it will have to pay for the $32,666.67 of purchases made on the first day, which will reduce accounts payable. However, it will buy another $32,666.67, which will increase payables. Thus, after the 10th day of operations, Chicago Surgical's balance sheet will level off, showing a balance of $326,667 in accounts payable, assuming that the company pays on the 10th day to take the discount.

Now suppose the firm decides not to take the discount. In this case, on the 11th day it will add another $32,666.67 to payables, but it will not pay for the purchases made on the 1st day. Thus, the balance sheet figure for accounts payable will rise to 11($32,666.67) = $359,333.37. This build-up will continue through the 30th day, at which point payables will total 30($32,666.67) = $980,000. On the 31st day, Chicago Surgical will buy another $32,667 of goods, which will increase accounts payable, but it will also pay for the purchases made the 1st day, which will reduce payables. Thus, the balance sheet item accounts payable will stabilize at $980,000 after 30 days, assuming Chicago Surgical does not take discounts.

The top part of Table 14.4 shows Chicago Surgical's balance sheet after it reaches a steady state, under the two trade credit policies. Total assets are unchanged by this policy decision, and we also assume that the accruals and common equity accounts are unchanged. The differences show up in accounts payable and notes payable; when Chicago Surgical elects to take discounts and thus gives up some of the trade credit it otherwise could have obtained, it will have to raise $653,333 from other sources. It could have sold more common stock, or it could have used long-term bonds, but it chose to use bank credit, which has a 10 percent cost and is reflected in the notes payable account.

The bottom part of Table 14.4 shows Chicago Surgical's income statement under the two policies. If the company does not take discounts, then its interest expense will be zero, but it will have a $240,000 expense for discounts lost. On the other hand, if it does take discounts, it will incur an interest expense of $65,333, but it will avoid the cost of discounts lost. Since discounts lost exceed the interest expense, the take-discounts policy results in a higher cash flow to the firm.

On the basis of the preceding discussion, trade credit can be divided into two components: (1) *free trade credit*, which involves credit received during the discount period and which for Chicago Surgical amounts to 10 days' net purchases, of $326,667, and (2) *costly trade credit*, which involves credit in excess of the free credit, and whose cost is an implicit one based on the foregone discounts. Chicago Surgical could obtain $653,333, or 20 days' net purchases, of nonfree trade credit at a cost of

Table 14.4   Chicago Surgical Instruments: Financial Statements
with Different Trade Credit Policies

	Take Discounts	Do Not Take Discounts
Balance Sheets		
Cash and marketable securities	$ 500,000	$ 500,000
Accounts receivable	1,000,000	1,000,000
Inventories	2,000,000	2,000,000
Net fixed assets	2,980,000	2,980,000
Total assets	$ 6,480,000	$ 6,480,000
Accounts payable	$ 326,667	$ 980,000
Accruals	500,000	500,000
Notes payable	653,333	0
Common equity	5,000,000	5,000,000
Total liabilities and equity	$ 6,480,000	$ 6,480,000
Income Statements		
Sales	$15,000,000	$15,000,000
Less:		
Purchases	11,760,000	11,760,000
Labor	2,000,000	2,000,000
Interest	65,333	0
Discounts lost	0	240,000
Net income before taxes	$ 1,174,667	$ 1,000,000
Taxes (40%)	469,867	400,000
Net income	$ 704,800	$ 600,000

approximately 37 percent. Firms should always take the free component, but they should use the costly component only after analyzing the cost of this capital to make sure that it is less than the cost of funds which could be obtained from other sources. As we pointed out earlier, under the terms of trade found in most industries, the costly component will involve a relatively high percentage cost, so stronger firms will avoid using it.

Bank loans

Commercial banks, whose loans generally appear on firms' balance sheets under the notes payable account, are another important source of short-term financing.[5] The banks' influence is actually greater than it appears from the dollar amounts they lend, because banks provide *nonspontaneous* funds. As a firm's financing needs increase, it requests its bank to provide the additional funds. If the request is denied, the firm may be forced to abandon attractive growth opportunities.

Although banks do make longer-term loans, the bulk of their lending is on a short-term basis—about two-thirds of all bank loans mature in a year or less. Bank loans to businesses are frequently written as 90-day notes, so the loan must be repaid or renewed at the end of 90 days. Of course, if a borrower's financial position has deteriorated, the bank may well refuse to renew the loan. This can mean serious trouble for the borrower.

When a bank loan is approved, the agreement is executed by signing a *promissory note*. The note specifies (1) the amount borrowed; (2) the percentage interest rate; (3) the repayment schedule, which can involve either a lump sum or a series of installments; (4) any collateral that might have to be put up as security for the loan; and (5) any other terms and conditions to which the bank and the borrower may have agreed. When the note is signed, the bank credits the borrower's checking account with the amount of the loan, while on the borrower's balance sheet, both cash and notes payable increase.

Banks sometimes require regular borrowers to maintain an average demand deposit (checking account) balance equal to from 10 percent to 20 percent of the face amount of the loan. This is called a *compensating balance,* and such balances raise the effective interest rate on the loans. For example, suppose Pine Garden, a nursing home, needs a $80,000 bank loan to pay off maturing obligations. If the loan requires a 20 percent compensating balance, then the nursing home must borrow $100,000 to obtain a usable $80,000. If the stated interest rate is 8 percent, the effective cost is actually 10 percent: 0.08($100,000) = $8,000 interest divided by $80,000 of usable funds equals 10 percent.

A *line of credit,* sometimes called a *revolving credit agreement* or just *revolver,* is a formal understanding between the bank and the borrower indicating the maximum credit the bank will extend to the borrower. For example, on December 31 a bank loan officer might indicate to Pine Garden's manager that the bank regards the nursing home as being "good" for up to $80,000 during the forthcoming year. If on January

10, Pine Garden's manager signs a promissory note for $15,000 for 90 days, this would be called "taking down" $15,000 of the total line of credit. This amount would be credited to the nursing home's checking account at the bank, and before repayment of the $15,000, Pine Garden could borrow additional amounts up to a total of $80,000 outstanding at any one time. Lines of credit are generally for one year or less, and borrowers typically have to pay an up front commitment fee of about 0.5 to 1 percent of the total amount of the line.

Revolvers can involve large sums over longer periods. To illustrate, in 1995, Colorado Health Systems negotiated a revolving credit agreement for $100 million with a group of banks. The banks were formally committed for four years to lend the firm up to $100 million if the funds were needed. Colorado Health Systems, in turn, paid an annual commitment fee of one-quarter of 1 percent on the unused credit to compensate the banks for making the commitment. Thus, if Colorado Health Systems did not take down any of the $100 million commitment during a year, it would still be required to pay a $250,000 annual fee, normally in monthly installments of $20,833.33. If it borrowed $50 million on the first day of the agreement, the unused portion of the line of credit would fall to $50 million, and the annual fee would fall to $125,000. Of course, interest would also have to be paid on the money Colorado Health Systems actually borrowed. As a general rule, the rate of interest on credit lines is pegged to the prime rate, so the cost of the loan varies over time as interest rates change.[6] Colorado Health Systems' rate was set at prime plus 0.5 percentage points.

Individuals whose only contact with their bank is through the use of its checking services generally choose a bank for the convenience of its location and the competitive cost of its services. However, a business that borrows from banks must look at other criteria, and a potential borrower seeking banking relations should recognize that important differences exist among banks. Some of these differences are listed here.

1. *Willingness to assume risks.* Banks have different basic policies toward risk. Some banks are inclined to follow relatively conservative lending practices, while others engage in what are called "creative banking practices." These policies reflect partly the personalities of officers of the bank and partly the characteristics of the bank's deposit liabilities. Thus, a bank with fluctuating deposit liabilities in a static community will tend to be a conservative lender, while a bank with constantly growing deposits may follow more aggressive credit policies. A large bank with

broad diversification over geographic regions or across industries can obtain the benefits of loan portfolio diversification. Thus, marginal credit risks that might be unacceptable to a small bank or to a specialized unit bank can be pooled by a branch banking system to reduce the overall risk of a group of marginal accounts.

2. *Advice and counsel.* Some bank loan officers are active in providing counsel and in stimulating development loans to firms in their formative years. Certain banks have specialized departments that make loans to firms expected to grow and thus to become more important customers. The personnel of these departments can provide valuable counseling to customers: the bankers' experience with other firms in growth situations may enable them to spot, and then to warn their customers about, developing problems.

3. *Loyalty to customers.* Banks differ in the extent to which they will support the activities of the borrower in bad times. This characteristic is referred to as the degree of *loyalty* of the bank. Some banks may put great pressure on a business to liquidate its loan when the firm's outlook becomes clouded, whereas others will stand by the firm and work diligently to help it get back on its feet.

4. *Specialization.* Banks differ greatly in their degrees of loan specialization. Larger banks have separate departments that specialize in different kinds of loans—for example, real estate loans, farm loans, and commercial loans. Within these broad categories, there may be a specialization by line of business, such as steel, machinery, cattle, or health care. The strengths of banks are also likely to reflect the nature of the business and the economic environment in which they operate.

5. *Maximum loan size.* The size of a bank can be an important factor. Since the maximum loan a bank can make to any one customer is limited to 15 percent of the bank's capital account (common equity plus retained earnings), it is generally not appropriate for large firms to develop borrowing relationship with small banks.

6. *Other services.* As we discussed earlier, banks also provide cash management services, assist with electronic funds transfers, help firms obtain foreign exchange, and the like, and such services should be taken into account when selecting a bank. Also, if the firm is a small business whose manager owns most of its stock, the

bank's willingness and ability to provide trust and estate services should also be considered.

Commercial paper

Commercial paper is a type of unsecured promissory note issued by large, strong firms, and it is sold primarily to other business firms, to insurance companies, to pension funds, to money market mutual funds, and to banks. Although the amount of commercial paper outstanding is smaller than bank loans outstanding, this form of financing has grown rapidly in recent years.

Maturities of commercial paper generally vary from one to nine months, with an average of about five months.[7] The rate on commercial paper fluctuates with supply and demand conditions—it is determined in the market place, varying daily as conditions change. Recently, commercial paper rates have generally ranged from 1½ to 2½ percentage points below the stated prime rate, and about ½ of a percentage point above the T-bill rate. Also, since compensating balances are not required for commercial paper, the *effective* cost differential may be wider.[8]

The use of commercial paper is restricted to a comparatively small number of concerns that are exceptionally good credit risks. Dealers prefer to handle the paper of firms whose net worth is $100 million or more and whose annual borrowing exceeds $10 million. One potential problem with commercial paper is that a debtor who is in temporary financial difficulty may receive little help, because commercial paper dealings are generally less personal then are bank relationships. Thus, banks are generally more able and willing to help a good customer weather a temporary storm than is a commercial paper dealer. On the other hand, using commercial paper permits a corporation to tap a wide range of credit sources, including financial institutions outside its own area and industrial corporations across the country, and this can reduce interest costs.

Secured loans

Thus far, we have not addressed the question of whether or not loans are secured. Commercial paper loans are rarely secured by specific collateral, but all the other types of loans can be if this is deemed necessary or desirable. Given a choice, it is ordinarily better to borrow on an unsecured basis, since the bookkeeping costs of secured loans are often high. However, weak firms may find (1) that they can borrow only if they put up some type of security to protect the lender, or (2) that by using some security they can borrow at a much lower rate.

Several different kinds of collateral can be employed, including marketable securities, land or buildings, equipment, inventory, and accounts receivable. Marketable securities make excellent collateral, but few firms hold portfolios of stocks and bonds. Similarly, both real property (land and buildings) and equipment are good forms of collateral, but, because of maturity matching, they are generally used as security for long-term loans rather than for short-term loans. Therefore, most secured short-term business borrowing involves the use of accounts receivable or inventories, or both as collateral. Note, however, that owners of small businesses are often required to pledge personal assets as collateral for bank loans.

Accounts receivable financing involves either the pledging of receivables or the selling of receivables (factoring). The *pledging of accounts receivable* is characterized by the fact that the lender not only has a claim against the receivables but also has recourse to the borrower: If the person or the firm that bought the goods does not pay, the selling firm must take the loss. Therefore, the risk of default on the accounts receivable pledged remains with the borrowing firm. Also, the buyer of the goods is not ordinarily notified about the pledging of the receivables, and the financial institution that lends on the security of accounts receivable is generally either a commercial bank or one of the large industrial finance companies such as General Electric Capital Corporation.

Factoring, or *selling accounts receivable,* involves the purchase of accounts receivable by the lender, generally without recourse to the borrowing firm. In a typical transaction, the buyer pays the seller about 90 percent to 95 percent of the face value of the receivables. When receivables are factored, the original buyer of the goods or services is often notified of the transfer and is asked to make payment directly to the company that bought the receivables. Since the factoring firm assumes the risk of default on bad accounts, it must do a credit check. Accordingly, factors can provide not only money but also a credit department for the borrower. Incidentally, the same bank and other financial institutions that make loans against pledged receivables also serve as factors. Thus, depending on the circumstances and the wishes of the borrower, a financial institution will provide either form of receivables financing.

Because health care providers tend to carry relatively large amounts of receivables, such firms are prime candidates for receivables financing.[9] To illustrate the potential size of the receivables financing market, hospitals alone have accounts receivable that total nearly $15 billion. The selling of these receivables, especially by hospitals that are experiencing liquidity problems, represents one way to reduce working capital and stimulate cash flow.

To illustrate receivables financing for hospitals, consider the program recently instituted between Chase Manhattan Bank and Presbyterian Hospital, New York City's largest hospital. This program provides $15 million in advance funding of receivables over a three-year period. Presbyterian sells its accounts receivable to Chase for cash. Chase, in turn, obtains the cash it needs by selling commercial paper. The payers of the receivables technically make payments directly to Chase, although Chase actually pays Presbyterian a fee to service the receivables accounts. Chase charges an up-front fee for the program, and then charges an interest rate of about one percent to one-and-a-half percent above the prime rate on the amount advanced.

Interestingly, the expanding volume of health care receivables financing has created a new class of receivables-backed securities. For example, Prudential Securities recently placed $40 million in medium-term, taxable, AAA-rated notes issued by NPF III, a company created solely to buy receivables from cash-strapped providers. The notes are backed by the Medicare, Medicaid, and commercial insurance receivables of 21 hospitals nationwide. Under the plan, the hospitals sell their receivables to NPF III each week, and hence get cash in less than 10 days versus the 70 or so days commonly required to collect from third party payers.

Although receivables financing is a way to reduce working capital, and hence working capital financing costs, critics contend that such programs are too expensive. Furthermore, they do not solve underlying cash management problems. Because of these factors, most receivables financing programs are used by providers that have serious liquidity problems, although programs are being developed that can provide benefits even to well-run companies that are not facing a liquidity crunch. Although the illustrations here have focused on the use of receivables financing by hospitals, such financing is also used by medical group practices and other health care providers.

Receivables financing dominates health care providers' use of secured financing, but health care equipment manufacturers and pharmaceutical firms are more likely to obtain credit secured by business inventories. If a firm is a relatively good credit risk, the mere existence of the inventory may be sufficient to obtain an unsecured loan. However, if the firm is a relatively poor risk, the lending institution may insist upon security, which can take the form of a blanket lien against all inventory or either trust receipts or warehouse receipts against specific inventory items. The *inventory blanket lien* gives the lending institution a lien against all the borrower's inventories. However, the borrower is free to sell inventories, so the value of the collateral can be reduced below the level that existed when the loan was granted. Because of the inherent weakness of the blanket lien, another procedure for inventory financing was developed—the *security instrument* (also called a *trust receipt*), which is an instrument acknowledging that the goods are held in trust for the lender. When trust receipts are used, the borrowing firm, upon receiving funds from the lender, signs and delivers a trust receipt for the goods. The goods can be stored in a public warehouse or held on the premises of the borrower. The trust receipt acknowledges that the goods are held in trust for the lender and that any proceeds from the sale of trust goods must be transmitted to the lender at the end of each day. Automobile dealer financing is one of the best examples of trust receipt financing.

Self-Test Questions:

What are accruals, and what is their role in short-term financing?

What is the difference between free and costly trade credit?

How might a hospital that expects to have a cash shortage sometime during the coming year make sure that needed funds will be available?

What are some types of current assets that might be pledged as security for short-term loans?

Summary

This chapter examined cash management and short-term financing. The key concepts covered are listed next.

- The essence of short-term financial planning is assuring that the firm's *liquidity* is adequate to meet cash obligations as they become due.

- Under a *high working capital investment policy,* a firm holds relatively large amounts of each type of current asset. A *low working capital investment policy* entails holding minimal amounts of these items.

- *Permanent assets* are those assets that the firm holds even during slack times, whereas *temporary assets* are the additional assets, usually current assets, that are needed during seasonal or cyclical peaks. The method used to finance permanent and temporary assets defines the firm's *working capital financing policy.*

- A *moderate* approach to working capital financing involves matching, to the extent possible, the maturities of assets and liabilities, so that temporary current assets are financed with temporary financing and permanent assets are financed with permanent financing. Under an *aggressive* approach, some permanent current assets and perhaps even some fixed assets are financed with short-term debt. A *conservative* approach would be to use long-term capital to finance all permanent assets and some of the temporary current assets.

- The *primary goal of cash management* is to reduce the amount of cash held to the minimum necessary to conduct business. Some cash is necessary so the firm (1) can take trade discounts, (2) can maintain its credit rating, and (3) can meet unexpected cash needs.

- A *cash budget* is a schedule showing projected cash inflows and outflows over some period. The cash budget is used to predict cash surpluses and shortages, and thus it is the primary short-term financial management planning tool.

- *Monte Carlo simulation* provides a probability distribution of net cash flows which can be used to set a target balance which holds the probability of a shortfall to an acceptable level.

- *Cash management techniques* generally fall into four categories: (1) *synchronizing cash flows*, (2) *using float*, (3) *accelerating collections*, and (4) *controlling disbursements*.

- *Lockboxes* are used to accelerate collections. Then, a *concentration banking system* consolidates the collections into a centralized pool that can be managed more efficiently than a large number of individual accounts.

- Three techniques for controlling disbursements are (1) *payables centralization*, (2) *zero-balance accounts*, and (3) *controlled disbursement accounts*.

- The implementation of a sophisticated cash management system is costly, and all cash management actions must be evaluated to ensure that the *benefits exceed the costs*.

- Firms can reduce their cash balances by holding *marketable securities*. Marketable securities serve both as a substitute for cash and as a temporary investment for funds that will be needed in the near future. Safety is the primary consideration when selecting marketable securities.

- The advantages of short-term credit are (1) the *speed* with which short-term loans can be arranged, (2) increased *flexibility*, and (3) the fact that short-term *interest rates* are generally *lower* than long-term rates. The principal disadvantage of short-term credit is the *extra risk* that borrowers must bear because (1) lenders can demand payment on short notice, and (2) the cost of the loan will increase if interest rates rise.

- *Accruals,* which are continually recurring short-term liabilities, represent free spontaneous credit.

- *Accounts payable,* or *trade credit,* arises spontaneously as a result of purchases on credit. Firms should use all the *free trade credit* they can obtain, but they should use *costly trade credit* only if it is less expensive than other forms of short-term debt.

- *Bank loans* are an important source of short-term credit. When a bank loan is approved, a *promissory note* is signed.

- Banks sometimes require borrowers to maintain *compensating balances,* which are deposit requirements set at between 10 percent and 20 percent of the loan amount. Compensating balances raise the effective rate of interest on bank loans.

- *Lines of credit,* or *revolving credit agreements,* are formal understandings between the bank and the borrower indicating the maximum amount of credit the bank will extend to the borrower.

- *Commercial paper* is unsecured short-term debt issued by businesses. Although the cost of commercial paper is lower than the cost of bank loans, commercial paper's maturity is effectively limited to 270 days, and it can be used only by large firms with exceptionally strong credit ratings.

- Sometimes a borrower will find that it is necessary to borrow on a *secured basis,* in which case the borrower pledges assets such as real estate, securities, equipment, inventories, or accounts receivable as collateral for the loan.

Notes

1. Our discussion of cash management is necessarily brief. For a much more detailed discussion of cash management within the health care industry, see A. G. Seidner and W. O. Cleverly, *Cash and Investment Management for the Health Care Industry* (Rockville, MD.: Aspen, 1990).
2. In a credit sale, the seller records the transaction as a receivable; the buyer, as a payable. We will examine accounts receivable as an asset investment in

Chapter 15. Our focus in this chapter is on accounts payable, a liability item. We might also note that if a firm's accounts payable exceed its receivables, it is said to be *receiving net trade credit*, whereas if its receivables exceed its payables, it is *extending net trade credit*. Smaller firms frequently receive net credit; larger firms generally extend it.

3. A question arises here: Should accounts payable reflect gross purchases or purchases net of discounts? Although generally accepted accounting principles permit either treatment on the grounds that the difference is not material, most accountants prefer to record payables net of discounts, and then to report the higher payments that result from not taking discounts as an additional expense, called "discounts lost." From a finance perspective, the true cost of a purchase is the price available to cash customers—any charge above that is a financing cost—so accounts payable should reflect the net, or "true," price.

4. Inventories also increase by \$32,666.67, but we are not now concerned with inventories. Again note that both inventories and receivables are generally recorded net of discounts regardless of whether discounts are taken.

5. Although commercial banks remain the primary source of short-term loans, other sources are available. For example, in 1995 GE Capital Corporation had over \$2 billion in commercial loans outstanding. Firms such as GE Capital, which was initially established to finance consumers' purchases of General Electric's durable goods, often find business loans to be more profitable than consumer loans.

6. The prime rate is the interest rate charged to a bank's very best customers. Each bank sets its own prime rate, but, because of competition, most banks' prime rates are identical. Furthermore, most banks follow the lead of the large New York City banks.

7. The maximum maturity without SEC registration is 270 days. Also, commercial paper can only be sold to "sophisticated" investors; otherwise, SEC registration would be required even for maturities of 270 days or less.

8. However, this factor is offset to some extent by the fact that firms issuing commercial paper are required by commercial paper dealers to have unused revolving credit agreements to back up their outstanding commercial paper, and fees must be paid on these lines. In other words, to sell \$1 million of commercial paper, a firm must have revolving credit available to pay off the paper when it matures, and commitment fees on this unused credit line (about 0.5 percent) increase the effective cost of the paper. Note also that commercial paper and T-bill rates are quoted on a discount basis, whereas the prime rate is on an annual yield basis.

9. For more information on the use of receivables financing by health care providers, see T. J. Kincaid, "Selling Accounts Receivable to Fund Working Capital," *Healthcare Financial Management* (May 1993): 27–32.

Selected Additional References

Anderson, A. M. 1993. "Enhancing Hospital Cash Reserves Management." *Healthcare Financial Management* (July): 91–95.

Coyne, J. S. 1987. "Corporate Cash Management in Health Care: Can We do Better?" *Healthcare Financial Management* (September): 76–79.

Dixon, L. H., and S. K. Bossert. 1993. "The Commercial Bank as Investment Advisor for Hospital Investable Assets." *Topics in Health Care Financing* (Summer): 58–68.

Edwards, D. E., W. C. Hamilton, and R. Hauser. 1991. "Financial Reserve: Hospitals Leery of Credit Lines, Factoring Receivables." *Healthcare Financial Management* (October): 82–88.

Ferconio, S., and M. R. Lane. 1991. "Financing Maneuvers: Two Opportunities to Boost a Hospital's Working Capital." *Healthcare Financial Management* (October): 74–80.

Green, L. A. 1993. "Cash Management: Acceleration and Information Strategies." *Topics in Health Care Financing* (Summer): 44–57.

Hauser, R. C., D. E. Edwards, and J. T. Edwards. 1991. "Cash Budgeting: An Underutilized Resource Management Tool in Not-for-Profit Health Care Entities." *Hospital & Health Services Administration* (Fall): 439–446.

Kelly, V. K. 1993. "Banks As a Source of Capital." *Topics in Health Care Financing* (Summer): 21–34.

Masonson, L. N. 1992. "Banks Aggressively Marketing Cash Management Services." *Healthcare Financial Management* (December): 59–60.

McFadden, D. R. 1989. "How to Gain Maximum Returns through Cash Management." *Healthcare Financial Management* (October): 44–53.

Reiss, J. B., and S. J. Di Cioccio. 1991. "Where There's a Will: How to Finance Medicare Receivables—Legally." *Healthcare Financial Management* (October): 90–96.

Seidner, A. G. 1987. "Reviewing the Basics of Investment Management." *Healthcare Financial Management* (October): 68–72.

Smith, D., and L. C. McPherson. 1988. "Improving Hospital Investments Using a Disciplined Approach." *Healthcare Financial Management* (July): 32–41.

Case 14

Medical Research Supply Company: Cash Budgeting

Medical Research Supply Company is a very small California company that manufactures highly specialized cultures used in the biotechnology industry. Richard Ratacek, the firm's treasurer, was recently summoned to the office of Sonia Mason, the firm's president and chief executive officer. When he got to Mason's office, Ratacek found her shuffling through a set of spreadsheet models. She told him that she had just received a phone call from the head of commercial lending at BankWest, the firm's bank. Because of a forecasted reduction in bank deposits, and hence funds available to make commercial loans, BankWest has asked each of its loan customers for an estimate of its borrowing requirements for the first half of 1997.

Mason had a previously scheduled meeting at BankWest the following Monday to discuss cash management services, so she asked Ratacek to come up with an estimate of the firm's line of credit requirements to submit at that time. Mason was going away on a hiking expedition, a trip that had already been delayed several times, and she would not be back until just before her meeting at the bank.

Mason therefore asked Ratacek to prepare a cash budget while she was away. No one had taken the time to prepare a cash budget recently, although a spreadsheet model that had been constructed a few years ago was available for use. From information previously developed, Ratacek knew that no loans would be needed from BankWest before January, so he decided to restrict his budget to the period from January through June 1997. As a first step, he obtained the sales forecast contained in Table 1 from the firm's marketing manager. In 1995 and early 1996, sales ran about $100,000 a month without much seasonal variation. However, special needs by Endocino Laboratories, one of the firm's best customers, has resulted in the highly variable sales forecast shown in Table 1.

The company's credit policy is 2/10, net 30, and hence a 2 percent discount is allowed if payment is made within 10 days of the sale. Otherwise, payment in full is due 30 days after the date of sale. On the basis of a previous study conducted by the firm's marketing manager, Ratacek estimates that, on average, 15 percent of the firm's customers take the discount, 65 percent pay within 30 days, and 20 percent pay late, with the late payments averaging about 60 days after the invoice date. For monthly budgeting purposes, discount sales are assumed to be collected in the month of the sale, net sales in the month following the sale month, and late sales two months after the month of sale.

Medical Research Supply Company begins production of goods two months before the anticipated sale date. Variable production costs are made up entirely of raw materials and labor, which total 60 percent of forecasted sales—20 percent for materials and 40 percent for labor. All materials are purchased just before production begins, or two months before the sale of the final product. On average, Medical Research pays 50 percent of the materials cost in the month it receives the materials, and the remaining 50 percent the next month, or one month prior to the sale. Labor expenses follow a similar pattern, but only 30 percent is paid two months prior to the sale, while 70 percent is paid one month before the sale.

The firm pays fixed general and administrative expenses of approximately $30,000 a month, while lease obligations amount to $12,000

Table 1   Medical Research Supply Company

Year	Month	Sales
1996	November	$100,000
	December	160,000
1997	January	200,000
	February	240,000
	March	280,000
	April	380,000
	May	260,000
	June	200,000
	July	100,000
	August	80,000

Note: Sales listed are gross amounts, that is, before discounts.

per month. Both expenditures are expected to continue at the same level throughout the forecast period. The firm estimates miscellaneous expenses to be $10,000 monthly, and fixed assets are currently being depreciated by $16,000 per month. Medical Research has a $400,000 long-term bank loan outstanding with BankWest that has a 10 percent annual rate, with interest paid semiannually on January 15 and July 15. Also, the company is planning to replace an old machine in June with a new one costing $200,000. The old machine has both a zero book and a zero market value. Federal and state income taxes are expected to be $30,000 quarterly, and payments must be made on the 15th of December, March, June, and September. Medical Research must maintain a minimum cash balance of $120,000 at BankWest due to compensating balance requirements on its long-term loan. This amount, but no more, is expected to be on hand on January 1, 1997.

If a daily cash budget is required, some additional assumptions about sales and payment patterns are required:

1. Because of the fragile nature of the production process and the resulting products, Medical Research Supply Company normally operates seven days a week.

2. Sales are made at a more or less constant rate throughout the month, so the daily sales forecast will be 1/(Number of days in the month) multiplied by the sales forecast for that month.

3. Daily sales follow the 15 percent, 65 percent, 20 percent collection breakdown.

4. Discount purchasers take full advantage of the 10-day discount period before paying, and "on time" purchasers wait the full 30 days to pay. Late sales are collected 60 days after the sale date.

5. The lease payment is made on the first of the month.

6. Fifty percent of both labor costs and general and administrative expenses are paid on the 1st of the month and 50 percent are paid on the 15th of the month.

7. Materials are delivered on the 1st of the month and paid for on the 5th of the month.

8. Miscellaneous expenses are incurred and paid evenly throughout each month.

9. Required interest payments are made on the 15th.

10. The compensating balance of $120,000 must be in the bank on each day.

In addition to the cash budget itself, Mason asked Ratacek to consider several additional issues:

1. Will the company need to request a line of credit for the period and, if so, how big should the line be?

2. Perhaps a monthly budget may not reveal the full extent of the borrowing requirements actually encountered in the future. To see if her concern is valid, Mason suggested that Ratacek construct a daily cash budget for the month having the highest net cash loss.

3. The existing cash budget model does not include any lines for interest paid on line of credit borrowings or interest earned on cash surpluses. Mason suggested that the monthly cash budget be modified to include these items. Currently, the interest rate on a BankWest line of credit is 7 percent compounded monthly and BankWest pays 5 percent compounded monthly on temporary investments of excess cash.

4. Although the target cash balance has been based on BankWest's compensating balance requirement, the loan will be paid off in July 1997. Mason asked how the firm might go about setting its target cash balance when no compensating balance is required.

5. Mason is well aware of the fact that the cash budget is a forecast, so most of the cash flows shown are expected values rather than amounts known with certainty. If actual sales, and hence collections, were different from the forecasted levels, then the forecasted surpluses and deficits would be incorrect. Mason is very interested in knowing how various changes in key assumptions would affect the funds surplus or deficit. For example, if sales fell below the forecasted level, or if collections were stretched out, what effect would that have?

6. Finally, Mason believes that the surge in sales over the forecast period is bound to result is some cash surpluses, and she wants to know what the company should do with them.

Assume that your administrative residency rotation has just placed you in the treasurer's office. (Talk about bad timing.) Richard Ratacek has asked you to do the work on the cash budget, and to be prepared to discuss your analysis with him at the next treasurer's staff meeting.

15

Receivables and Inventory Management

The typical firm has about 20 percent of its assets in receivables and another 20 percent in inventories, although health care providers normally have a smaller investment in inventories and a larger investment in receivables. Regardless of the exact percentages, a firm's effectiveness in managing these two accounts is obviously important to its profitability and risk. In this chapter, we focus on receivables management, including credit policy, and inventory management.

Receivables Management

In general, firms would rather sell for cash than on credit, but competitive pressures force most firms to offer credit. The problem is even more acute in the health services industry, where the third party payment system forces firms to extend credit to most patients. In a credit sale, goods are shipped or services are provided, inventories are reduced, and an account receivable is created. Eventually, the customer or third party payer will pay the account, at which time the firm will receive cash and its receivables will decline. Carrying receivables has both direct and indirect costs, but it also has an important benefit for many firms—granting credit will increase sales. One could certainly open, say, an ambulatory clinic for cash customers only, but sales would be much lower as compared with a clinic that accepts assignment from all insurance companies and managed care plans. The optimal credit policy from a financial perspective is the one that maximizes the firm's net cash flows over time, giving consideration to the risks involved.

Technically, receivables management begins with the decision of whether or not to grant credit, but for most firms, industry standards and practices dictate a firm's credit policy. In this section, we discuss the manner in which a firm's receivables build up, and we also present several alternative means of monitoring receivables. A monitoring system is important, because without it, receivables will build up to excessive levels, cash flows will decline, and bad debts will offset profits on sales. Corrective action is often needed, and the only way to know whether the situation is getting out of hand is to set up and then follow a good receivables control system.

The accumulation of receivables

The total amount of accounts receivable outstanding at any given time is determined by two factors: (1) the volume of credit sales and (2) the average length of time between sales and collections. For example, suppose Home Infusion, Inc., a home health care firm, begins operations on January 1 and, starting the first day, provides services to patients billed at $1,000 each day. For simplicity, assume that all patients have the same insurance, that it takes Home Infusion 10 days to submit patients' bills, and it takes the insurer another 10 days to make the payments, for a total of 20 days from delivery of service to receipt of payment. Also for simplicity, assume Home Infusion must pay its $800 of salaries and other expenses at the end of each day.

At the end of the first day, Home Infusion's accounts receivable will be $1,000; they will rise to $2,000 by the end of the second day; and by January 20, they will have risen to 20($1,000) = $20,000. On January 21, another $1,000 will be added to receivables, but, assuming that the insurer pays the full amount on the 20th day, payments for services provided on January 1 will reduce receivables by $1,000, so total accounts receivable will remain constant at $20,000. In general, once Home Infusion's operations have stabilized, this situation will exist:

$$\text{Accounts receivable} = \text{Credit sales per day} \times \text{Length of collection period}$$
$$= \quad \$1,000 \quad \times \quad 20 \text{ days}$$
$$= \quad \$20,000$$

If either credit sales or the collection period changes, such changes will be reflected in accounts receivable.

Notice that Home Infusion's $20,000 investment in receivables must be financed. To illustrate, suppose that when the firm began services on January 1, Home Infusion's shareholders had put up $800 as common stock and used this money to pay wages and other expenses on the first day. The services costing $800 will be sold for $1,000; thus, Home Infusion's gross profit on the $800 investment is $200 or 25 percent. In this situation, Home Infusion's starting balance sheet would be as follows:

Cash	$800	Common equity	$800
Total assets	$800	Total claims	$800

Note that the firm would need other assets such as fixed assets and inventory. Also, overhead costs and taxes would have to be deducted, so retained earnings would be less than the figures shown here. We abstract from these details so that we may focus on receivables. At the end of the day, Home Infusion's balance sheet would look like this:

Cash	$ 0	Common equity	$ 800
Accounts receivable	1,000	Retained earnings	200
Total assets	$1,000	Total claims	$1,000

In order to remain in business, Home Infusion must replenish its cash, because $800 in salaries and other expenses must be paid on the second day. Assuming that Home Infusion borrows that $800 from the bank, the balance sheet at the start of the second day will be as follows:

Cash	$ 800	Notes payable	$ 800
Accounts receivable	1,000	Common equity	800
		Retained earnings	200
Total assets	$1,800	Total claims	$1,800

At the end of the second day, the cash will have been converted into receivables, and the firm will have to borrow another $800 to meet expenses on the third day.

This process will continue, provided the bank is willing to lend the necessary funds, until the beginning of the 21st day, when the balance sheet reads as follows:

Cash	$ 800	Notes payable	$16,000
Accounts receivable	20,000	Common equity	800
		Retained earnings	4,000
Total assets	$20,800	Total claims	$20,800

From this point on, $1,000 of receivables will be collected every day, and $800 of these funds can be used to meet expenses, so the receivables and payables accounts will stabilize at the above values.

This example should make it clear (1) that accounts receivable depend jointly on the level of credit sales and the collection period, (2) that any increase in receivables must be financed in some manner, but (3) that the entire amount of receivables does not have to be financed because the profit portion ($200 of each $1,000 of sales) does not represent a cash expense associated with creating the receivables. In our example, we assumed bank financing, but, as we noted in Chapter 14, there are many alternative ways to finance current assets.

Monitoring the receivables position

If a sale is made for cash, the profit is definitely earned, but if the sale is on credit, the profit is not actually earned until the account is collected. Of course, if the account is never collected, the profit is never earned. Firms have been known to encourage "sales" to very weak customers in order to report high profits. This could boost the firm's stock price, at least until credit losses begin to lower earnings, at which time the stock price will fall. Analysis along the lines suggested in the following sections will detect any such questionable practice, as well as any unconscious deterioration in the quality of accounts receivable. Such early detection can help health care managers take corrective action before the situation gets out of hand.

Average collection period (ACP)

Suppose Adolph Weiss & Sons, a manufacturer of surgical instruments, manufactures and sells 200,000 instruments a year at an average sales price of $198 each. Furthermore, assume that all sales are on credit, with terms of 2/10, net 30. Finally, assume that 70 percent of the firm's customers take discounts and pay on Day 10, while the other 30 percent pay on Day 30.

Weiss's *average collection period (ACP)*, often called *days sales outstanding (DSO)* or *days in receivables*, is 16 days.

$$\text{ACP} = 0.7(10 \text{ days}) + 0.3(30 \text{ days}) = 16 \text{ days.}$$

Weiss's *average daily sales (ADS)*, assuming a 360-day year, is $110,000:

$$\text{ADS} = \frac{\text{Annual sales}}{360} = \frac{(\text{Units sold})(\text{Sales price})}{360}$$
$$= \frac{200,000(\$198)}{360} = \frac{\$39,600,000}{360} = \$110,000.$$

If the company had made cash as well as credit sales, we would have concentrated on credit sales only and calculated average daily *credit* sales.

Weiss's accounts receivable, assuming a constant, uniform rate of sales all during the year, will at any point in time be $1,760,000.[1]

$$\text{Receivables} = (\text{ADS})(\text{ACP}) = (\$110,000)(16) = \$1,760,000.$$

The ACP is a measure of the average length of time it takes Weiss's customers to pay off their credit purchases, and the ACP is often compared with an industry average ACP. For example, if all surgical instrument manufacturers sell on the same credit terms, and if the industry average ACP is 25 days versus Weiss's 16-day ACP, then Weiss either has a higher percentage of discount customers or else its credit department is exceptionally good at ensuring prompt payment.

The ACP can also be compared with the firm's own credit terms. For example, suppose Weiss's ACP had been running at a level of 35 days versus its 2/10, net 30 credit terms. With a 35-day ACP, some customers would obviously be taking more than 30 days to pay their bills. In fact, if some customers were paying within 10 days to take advantage of the discount, the others would, on average, have to be taking much longer than 35 days. One way to check this possibility is to use an aging schedule, described next.

Aging schedules

An *aging schedule* breaks down a firm's receivables by age of account. Table 15.1 contains the December 31, 1995, aging schedules of two surgical instrument manufacturers, Weiss and Cutright. Both firms offer the same credit terms, 2/10, net 30, and both show the same total receivables. However, Weiss's aging schedule indicates that all of its customers pay on time—70 percent pay on Day 10, while 30 percent pay on Day 30. Cutright's schedule, which is more typical, shows that many of its customers are not abiding by its credit terms—some 27 percent of its receivables are more than 30 days past due, even though Cutright's credit terms call for full payment by Day 30.

Aging schedules cannot be constructed from the type of summary data that are reported in a firm's financial statements; they must be developed from the firm's accounts receivable ledger. However, well-run firms have computerized their accounts receivable records, so it is easy to determine the age of each invoice, to sort electronically by age categories, and thus to generate an aging schedule. Although changes in aging schedules over time do provide more information than does the overall ACP taken alone, and although aging schedules are valuable for monitoring individual accounts, there is a better way to monitor the aggregate performance of the credit department, as we demonstrate in the next section.

The payments pattern approach

The primary point in analyzing the aggregate accounts receivable situation is to see if payers are slowing down their payments. If so, the firm will have to increase its receivables financing, which will increase its cost of carrying receivables. Furthermore, the payment slowdown may signal an increase in bad debt losses down the road. The ACP and aging schedule are useful in monitoring credit operations, but both are affected by increases and decreases in a firm's level of sales. Thus, changes in sales levels, including normal seasonal or cyclical changes, can change a firm's ACP and aging schedule even though its customers' payment behavior has not changed at all. For this reason, a procedure called the *payments pattern approach* has been developed to measure any changes that might be occurring in customers' payment behavior.

Table 15.1   Aging Schedules for Two Firms

Age of Account (Days)	Weiss Value of Account	Weiss Percentage of Total Value	Cutright Value of Account	Cutright Percentage of Total Value
0–10	$1,232,000	70%	$ 825,000	47%
11–30	528,000	30	460,000	26
31–45	0	0	265,000	15
46–60	0	0	179,000	10
Over 60	0	0	31,000	2
Total	$1,760,000	100%	$1,760,000	100%

To illustrate the payments pattern approach, consider the credit sales of Hanover Pharmaceutical Company, a small drug manufacturer which commenced operations in January 1995. Table 15.2 contains Hanover's credit sales and receivables data for 1995. Column 2 shows that Hanover's credit sales are seasonal, with the lowest sales in the fall and winter months and the highest sales during the summer.

Now assume that 10 percent of Hanover's customers pay in the same month that the sale is made, that 30 percent pay in the first month following the sale, that 40 percent pay in the second month, and that the remaining 20 percent pay in the third month. Furthermore, assume that Hanover's customers have the same payment behavior throughout the year; that is, they always take the same length of time to pay. On the basis of this payment pattern, Column 3 of Table 15.2 contains Hanover's receivables balance at the end of each month. For example, during January, Hanover has $60,000 in sales. Ten percent of the customers paid during the month of sale, so the receivables balance at the end of January was $60,000 − 0.1($60,000) = (1.0 − 0.1)($60,000) = 0.9($60,000) = $54,000. By the end of February, 10% + 30% = 40% of the customers had paid for January's sales, and 10 percent had paid for February's sales.

Table 15.2   Hanover Pharmaceutical Company: Receivables Data (thousand of dollars)

Month (1)	Credit Sales (2)	Receivables (3)	Quarterly ADS* (4)	Quarterly ACP† (5)	Year to Date ADS* (6)	Year to Date ACP† (7)
January	$ 60	$ 54				
February	60	90				
March	60	102	$2.00	51	$2.00	51
April	60	102				
May	90	129				
June	120	174	3.00	58	2.50	70
July	120	198				
August	90	177				
September	60	132	3.00	44	2.67	49
October	60	108				
November	60	102				
December	60	102	.00	51	2.50	41

* Average daily sales.

† Average collection period (in days).

Thus, the receivables balance at the end of February was 0.6($60,000) + 0.9($60,000) = $90,000. By the end of March, 80 percent of January's sales had been paid, 40 percent of February's had been paid, and 10 percent of March's had been paid, so the receivables balance was 0.2($60,000) + 0.6($60,000) + 0.9($60,000) = $102,000; and so on.

Columns 4 and 5 give Hanover's average daily sales (ADS) and average collection period (ACP) respectively, as these measures would be calculated from quarterly statements. For example, in the April–June quarter, ADS = ($60,000 + $90,000 + $120,000)/90 = $3,000, and the end-of-quarter (June 30) ACP = $174,000/$3,000 = 58 days. Columns 6 and 7 also show ADS and ACP, but here they are calculated on the basis of accumulated sales throughout the year. For example, at the end of June, ADS = $450,000/180 = $2,500 and ACP = $174,000/$2,500 = 70 days. (For the entire year, sales are $900,000, ADS = $2,500, and ACP at year-end = 41 days. These last two figures are shown in the lower right corner of the table.)

The data in Table 15.2 illustrate two major points. First, when the level of sales changes, the ACP changes, which suggests that customers are paying faster or slower, even though we know that customers' payment patterns are actually not changing at all. The rising monthly sales trend causes the calculated ACP to rise, whereas falling sales (as in the third quarter) cause the calculated ACP to fall, even though nothing is changing with regard to when customers pay. Second, we see that the ACP depends on an averaging procedure, but regardless of whether quarterly, semiannual, or annual data are used, the ACP is still unstable even though payment patterns are *not* changing. Therefore, it is difficult to use the ACP as a monitoring device if the firm's sales exhibit seasonal or cyclical patterns.

Seasonal or cyclical variations also make it difficult to interpret aging schedules. Table 15.3 contains Hanover's aging schedules at the end of each quarter of 1995. At the end of June, Table 15.2 shows that Hanover's receivables balance was $174,000. Eighty percent of April's $60,000 of sales had been collected, 40 percent of May's $90,000 of sales had been collected, and 10 percent of June's $120,000 of sales had been collected. Thus, the end-of-June receivables balance consisted of 0.2($60,000) = $12,000 of April sales, 0.6($90,000) = $54,000 of May sales, and 0.9($120,000) = $108,000 of June sales. Note again that Hanover's customers had not changed their payment patterns. However, rising sales during the second quarter created the impression of faster payments when judged by an aging schedule, and falling sales after July created the opposite appearance. Thus, neither the ACP nor the aging schedule provides managers with an accurate picture of customers' payment patterns if sales fluctuate during the year or are trending up or down.

With this background, we can now examine the *uncollected balances schedule,* which is shown in Table 15.4. At the end of each quarter, the dollar amount of receivables remaining from each of the three month's sales is divided by that month's sales to obtain three receivables-to-sales ratios. For example, at the end of the first quarter, $12,000 of the $60,000 January sales, or 20 percent, are still outstanding; 60 percent of February sales are still out; and 90 percent of March sales are uncollected. Exactly the same situation is revealed at the end of each of the next three quarters. Thus, Table 15.4 shows that the payments pattern of Hanover's customers has remained constant.

Recall that at the beginning of the example we assumed the existence of a constant payments pattern. In a normal situation, the payments pattern would probably vary somewhat over time. Such variations would be shown in the last column of the uncollected balances schedule. For example, suppose customers began, in the second quarter, to pay their accounts slower. That might cause the second quarter uncollected balances schedule to look like this (in thousands of dollars):

Quarter and Month	Sales	Remaining Receivables	Receivables/ Sales Ratio
Quarter 2			
April	$ 60	$ 16	27%
May	90	70	78
June	120	110	92
		$196	197%

We see that the receivables-to-sales ratios are now higher than in the corresponding months of the first quarter. This causes the total

Table 15.3 Hanover Pharmaceutical Company: Aging Schedules (thousands of dollars)

Age of Account (Days)	Value and Percentage of Value at the End of Each Quarter							
	March 31		June 30		September 30		December 31	
0–30	$ 54	53%	$108	47%	$ 54	41%	$ 54	53%
31–60	36	35	54	31	54	41	36	35
61–90	12	12	12	7	24	18	12	12
Total	$102	100%	$174	85%	$132	100%	$102	100%

Table 15.4   Hanover Pharmaceutical Company: Uncollected
Balances Schedule (thousands of dollars)

Quarter and Month	Sales	Remaining Receivables	Receivables/ Sales Ratio
Quarter 1			
January	$ 60	$ 12	20%
February	60	36	60
March	60	54	90
		$102	170%
Quarter 2			
April	$ 60	$ 12	20%
May	90	54	60
June	120	108	90
		$174	170%
Quarter 3			
July	$120	$ 24	20%
August	90	54	60
September	60	54	90
		$132	170%
Quarter 4			
October	$ 60	$ 12	20%
November	60	36	60
December	60	54	90
		$102	170%

uncollected balances percentage to rise from 170 percent to 197 percent, which in turn should alert Hanover's managers that customers are paying slower than they did earlier in the year.

The uncollected balances schedule permits a firm to monitor its receivables better, and it can also be used to forecast future receivables balances. When Hanover's pro forma 1996 quarterly balance sheets are constructed, management can use the receivables-to-sales ratios, coupled with the 1996 sales estimates, to project each quarter's receivables balance using the historical payments pattern from 1995. For example, Hanover's projected end-of-June 1996 receivables balance might be forecasted as follows:

Projected Quarter 2	Projected Sales	Receivables/ Sales Ratio	Projected Receivables
April	$ 70,000	20%	$ 14,000
May	100,000	60	60,000
June	140,000	90	126,000
	Total projected receivables =		$200,000

The payments pattern approach permits managers to remove the effects of seasonal sales variation or cyclical sales variation, or both, and to construct an accurate measure of customers' payments patterns. Thus, it provides financial managers with better aggregate information than such crude measures as the average collection period or aging schedule.

Use of computers in receivables management

Except possibly in the inventory and cash management areas, nowhere in the typical firm have computers had more of an impact than in accounts receivable management. A well-run business will use a computer system to record sales, to send out bills, to keep track of when payments are made, to alert managers when an account becomes past due, and to ensure that actions are taken to collect past due accounts (for example, to prepare form letters requesting payment). Additionally, the payment history of each customer can be summarized and used to help establish credit limits for customers and classes of customers, and the data on each account can be aggregated and used for the firm's accounts receivable monitoring system. Finally, historical data can be stored in the firm's data base and used to develop inputs for pro forma financial statements and for studies related to credit policy changes.

The unique problems faced by health care providers

Although the general principles discussed up to this point are applicable to all businesses, health care providers face some unique problems in managing their receivables accounts.

The most obvious problem is the complexities in billing created by the third party payer system. For example, rather than having a single billing system which applies to all customers, providers have to deal with the rules and regulations of many different governmental and private insurers using different payment methodologies. Thus, providers have to maintain large staffs of specialists who operate under the firm's *patient accounts manager.* To illustrate the problem, consider Table 15.5, which contains the receivables mix for the hospital industry. Of course, there are multiple payers within many of the categories listed in the table, so the actual number of different payers can easily run into the hundreds, or even thousands.

Table 15.6 provides information on how long it takes hospitals to collect receivables. Because of the large number of payers and the complexities involved with billing and follow-up actions, which lead to high error rates, it is clear that hospitals have a great deal of difficulty in collecting bills in a timely manner. On average, it takes 64.1 days to collect a receivable. However, this figure has tended downward in recent years as hospital managers have become increasingly aware of the costs associated with carrying receivables and as automated systems have made the collections process more efficient. In spite of the positive trend, 24.9 percent of receivables still were over 90 days old. In addition, 5.2 percent of patient bills were never paid at all, with 3.4 percent being charged off as bad debt losses and 1.8 percent going to charity care.

The complexities involved in billing scores of different payers cannot be overstated. St. Joseph Health System in Orange County, California, deals with more than 2,000 different payers in the system's eight hospitals. Each one of the payers requires a slightly different version of the UB-92, a paper billing form that can be translated into electronic format. Some of the differences are very minor, such as whether the patient's name is filled in last-name-first or first-name-first, but even such trivial differences means added expense and potential problems. The

Table 15.5   Hospital Industry's Receivables Mix

Payer	Percentage of Total Accounts Receivable
Medicare	30.2%
Commercial insureers	19.5
Medicaid	14.0
Self-pay	13.4
HMO/PPO	9.7
Blue Cross	8.1
CHAMPUS	5.1
	100.0%

Source: Zimmerman Associates. 1993. *Hospital Accounts Receivable Analysis (HARA)* (Third quarter).

Table 15.6   Hospital Industry's Collection Performance

Aggregrate Aging Schedule:

Age of Account (Days)	Percentage of Total Accounts Receivable
0–30	42.5%
31–60	21.4
61–90	11.2
91–120	7.8
Over 120	17.1
	100.0%

Average Collection Period:
(Days in Patient Accounts Receivable)

Percentile Values	Average Collection Period (Days)
10th	42.7days
25th	54.1
Median	64.1
75th	74.8
90th	88.0

Sources: Zimmerman Associates. 1993. *Hospital Accounts Receivable Analysis (HARA)* (Third quarter). Center for Healthcare Industry Performance Studies. 1994. *Almanac of Hospital Financial and Operating Indicators.*

lack of true uniformity in billing format is estimated to cost the hospital industry alone billions of dollars each year.

One development of note in provider collections is the movement toward electronic claims processing. In 1991, new standards were promulgated for the *electronic data interchange (EDI)* of health care claims, which over time will facilitate widespread adoption of electronic claims processing and payment systems. In such a system, claims information is electronically transmitted over telephone lines in a standard format so that it can be processed by receiving firms without human intervention. Because the health services reimbursement system is paper intensive, mountains of paper claims are currently produced, which leads to high error rates and numerous delays. Although some Medicare intermediaries, as well as other third party payers, are currently passing information to providers on magnetic tape, these systems tend to be payer unique and require providers to have relatively sophisticated computer systems.

To illustrate an EDI system, the University of Virginia Medical Center sends electronic claims to Health Communications Services, a wholly owned subsidiary of Blue Cross/Blue Shield of Virginia, which, in turn, transmits the claims received to a variety of payers in five states. About 55 percent of all of the hospital's claims are processed through the EDI system, which has a series of automated checks that immediately reject improper claim submissions. The advantages to the hospital include (1) much greater efficiency in claims origination and tracking, which has led to a significant decrease in the number of personnel allocated to claims processing, and (2) quicker collections, which have meant lower receivables carrying costs. Although EDI systems put pressure on payers to pay faster, and hence lose some of the payment float advantages that they currently enjoy, processing by payers is also reduced significantly, so net cost savings are available to both providers and payers.[2]

In perhaps the most ambitious attempt to date to reduce billing and collections costs, Medicare is planning to have a new streamlined automated processing system online by 2000. The system will have a single electronic claims processing and payment system that providers will use to submit bills directly to HCFA, bypassing the current set of 80 carriers and intermediaries that use 11 different claims processing systems. In addition, Medicare will electronically forward claims to secondary payers, which eliminates the need for providers to file multiple claims on the same patient encounter. Clearly, increased uniformity, consolidation, and automation in billing and collection has the potential for significantly increasing the efficiency, and hence lowering the costs, of our health care system.

Self-Test Questions:

Explain how a firm's receivables balance is built up over time.

Briefly discuss several means by which a firm can monitor its receivables position.

What are some of the unique problems faced by health care providers in managing receivables, and what trends are occurring in billing and collections?

Credit Policy

The success or failure of a business depends primarily on the demand for its products or services—as a rule, the higher its sales, the larger its profits and the better its financial condition. Sales, in turn, depend on a number of factors, some exogenous, but others under the control of the firm. The major controllable variables that affect demand are sales prices, product quality, advertising, and the firm's *credit policy*. Credit policy, in turn, consists of four variables:

1. The *credit period*, which is the length of time buyers are given to pay for their purchases

2. The *credit standards*, which refer to the minimum financial strength of acceptable credit customers, and the amount of credit available to different customers

3. The firm's *collection policy*, which is measured by its toughness or laxity in following up on slow-paying accounts

4. Any *discounts* given either for bulk purchases, such as contracts with managed care plans, or for early payment, including the discount amount and period.

The credit manager has the responsibility for administering the firm's credit policy. However, because of the pervasive importance of credit, the credit policy itself is normally established by the executive committee, which usually consists of the firm's president and vice presidents in charge of finance, marketing, and operations.

Setting the credit period and standards

A firm's regular credit terms, which include the *credit period*, might call for sales on a 2/10, net 30 basis to all "acceptable" customers. Its *credit standards* would be applied to determine which customers qualify for the regular credit terms, and the amount of credit available to each customer. The focal point when considering credit standards is the likelihood that a given customer will pay slowly, or end up as a bad debt loss. This requires a measurement of *credit quality*, which is defined in terms of the probability of default. The probability estimate for a given customer is, for the most part, a subjective judgment, but credit evaluation is a well-established practice, and a good credit manager can make reasonably accurate judgments regarding the probability of default by different classes of customers.

Credit-scoring systems

Although most credit decisions are subjective, many firms now use a sophisticated statistical method called *multiple discriminant analysis (MDA)* to assess credit quality. MDA is similar to multiple regression analysis. The dependent variable is, in essence, the probability of default, and the independent variables are factors associated with financial strength and the ability to pay off the debt if credit is granted. For example, if a firm such as Walgreen Drug Stores evaluated consumers' credit quality, then the independent variables in the credit scoring system would be such factors as these: (1) Does the credit applicant own his or her own home? (2) How long has the applicant worked at his or her current job? (3) What is the applicant's outstanding debt in relation to his or her annual income? (4) Does the potential customer have a history of paying his or her debts on time?

One major advantage of an MDA credit-scoring system is that a customer's credit quality is expressed in a single numerical value, rather than as a subjective assessment of various factors. This is a tremendous advantage for a large firm that must evaluate many customers in many different locations using many different credit analysts, for without an automated procedure the firm would have a hard time applying equal standards to all credit applicants. To illustrate credit scoring, suppose Hanover Pharmaceuticals has historical information on 500 of its customers, all of whom are retail drug stores. Of these 500, assume that 400 have always paid on time, but the other 100 either paid late or, in some cases, went bankrupt and did not pay at all. Furthermore, the firm has historical data on each customer's quick ratio, times-interest-earned ratio, debt ratio, years in existence, and so on. Multiple discriminant analysis relates the experienced record (or historical probability) of late payment or nonpayment with various measures of a firm's financial condition, and MDA assigns weights for the critical factors. In effect, MDA produces an equation that looks much like a regression equation, and when data on a customer are plugged into the equation, then a credit score for that customer is produced.

Assume that Hanover's multiple discriminant analysis indicates that the critical factors affecting prompt payment are its customers' times-interest-earned ratio (TIE), quick ratio, debt/assets ratio, and number of years in business. Here is the discriminant function:

$$\text{Score} = 3.5(TIE) + 10.0(\text{Quick ratio})$$
$$- 25.0(\text{Debt-to-assets ratio}) + 1.3(\text{Years in business}).$$

Furthermore, assume that a score less than 40 indicates a poor credit risk, 40 to 50 indicates an average credit risk, and a score above 50 signifies a good credit risk. Now, suppose a store with the following conditions applies for credit:

$$\text{TIE} = 4.2$$
$$\text{Quick ratio} = 3.1$$
$$\text{Debt-to-assets ratio} = 0.30$$
$$\text{Years in business} = 10$$

This store's credit score would be $3.5(4.2) + 10(3.1) - 25.0(0.30) + 1.3(10) = 51.2$. Therefore, it would be considered a good credit risk, and consequently Hanover would offer it favorable credit terms.

Sources of credit information

Two major sources of credit information are available. The first is a set of *credit associations,* which are local groups that meet frequently and correspond with one another to exchange information on credit customers. These local groups have also banded together to create Credit Interchange, a system developed by the National Association of Credit Management for assembling and distributing information about debtors' past performance. The interchange reports show the paying records of different debtors, the industries from which they are buying, and the geographic areas in which they are making purchases.

The second source of external information is the work of the *credit-reporting agencies,* which collect credit information and sell it for a fee. The best known of these agencies are Dun & Bradstreet (D&B) and TRW, Incorporated. D&B, TRW, and other agencies provide factual data that can be used in credit analysis, and they also provide ratings similar to those available on corporate bonds.

Managing a credit department requires fast, accurate, up-to-date information, and to help get such information, the National Association of Credit Management (a group with 43,000 member firms) persuaded TRW to develop a telecommunication network for the collection, storage, retrieval, and distribution of consumer credit information. The TRW system contains credit reports that are available within seconds to its thousands of subscribers. Dun & Bradstreet has a similar electronic system that covers businesses, plus another service that provides more detailed reports through the U.S. mail.

A typical business credit report would include the following pieces of information:

1. A summary balance sheet and income statement
2. A number of key ratios, with trend information

3. Information obtained from the firm's suppliers telling whether it has been paying promptly or slowly, and whether it has recently failed to make any payments

4. A verbal description of the firm's operations

5. A verbal description of the backgrounds of the firm's owners, including any previous bankruptcies, lawsuits, divorce settlement problems, and the like

6. A summary rating, ranging from A for the best credit risks down to F for those that are deemed likely to default.

Although a great deal of credit information is available, it must still be processed in a judgmental manner. Computerized information systems can assist in making better credit decisions, but, in the final analysis, most credit decisions are really exercises in informed judgment. Even credit scoring systems require judgment in deciding where to draw the lines, given the set of derived scores.

Setting the collection policy

Collection policy refers to the procedure the firm follows to collect past-due accounts. For example, a letter may be sent to customers when a bill is ten days past due; a more severe letter, followed by a telephone call, may be used if payment is not received within 30 days; and the account may be turned over to a collection agency after 90 days.

The collection process can be expensive in terms of both out-of-pocket expenditures and lost good will, but at least some firmness is needed to prevent an undue lengthening of the collection period and to minimize outright losses. Again, a balance must be struck between the costs and benefits of different collection policies.

Changes in collection policy influence sales, the collection period, the bad debt loss percentage, and the percentage of customers who take discounts. The effects of a change in collection policy, along with changes in the other credit policy variables, will be analyzed later in the chapter.

It should be noted that collection policy is probably the most important credit policy variable for health care providers. In effect, providers are prohibited from setting credit standards, because they must treat all patients needing care (at least sufficiently to stabilize the condition). Since providers must accept all patients, the importance of collection policy is enhanced. The key here is, first, to identify which patients can be collected from immediately, and how much, and whether or not credit cards should be accepted for payment. Then the patients must be segregated into categories on the basis of probability of payment: say, (1) most likely to pay full amount, (2) likely to pay partial amount, and (3) unlikely to pay. This allows the patient accounts manager to best use the provider's collection resources. Most effort should be directed toward the "most likely to pay" patients, while the least effort should be applied to the "unlikely to pay" patients. A rational approach to collection policy should result in the greatest amount of collections for the lowest cost.

Cash discounts

The last element in the credit policy decision, the use of *cash discounts* for early payment, is analyzed by balancing the costs and benefits of different cash discounts. For example, a firm might decide to change its credit terms from "net 30," which means that customers must pay within 30 days, to "2/10, net 30," which means that it will allow a 2 percent discount if payment is received within 10 days, while the full invoice price must otherwise be paid within 30 days. This change should produce two benefits: (1) it should attract new customers who consider discounts to be a price reduction, and (2) the discounts should cause a reduction in the average collection period, since some established customers will pay more promptly in order to take advantage of the discount. Offsetting these benefits is the dollar cost of the discounts taken.[3] The optimal discount is established at the point where the marginal costs and benefits are exactly offsetting. The methodology for analyzing changes in the discount is developed in the next section.

Analyzing proposed changes in credit policy

If the firm's credit policy is *eased* by such actions as lengthening the credit period, relaxing credit standards, following a less tough collection policy, or offering cash discounts, then sales should increase: *easing the credit policy stimulates sales.* Of course, if credit policy is eased and sales rise, then costs will also rise because more labor, materials, and so on will be required to produce the additional goods or services. Additionally, receivables outstanding will also increase, which will increase carrying costs, and bad debt or discount expenses, or both, may also rise. Thus, the key question when deciding on a proposed credit policy change is this: Will sales revenues rise more than costs, including credit-related costs, causing cash flow to increase, or will the increase in sales revenues be more than offset by the higher costs?

Table 15.7 illustrates the general idea behind credit policy analysis. Column 1 shows the projected 1996 income statement for Medical Equipment Supply Corporation (MESC) under the assumption that the firm's current credit policy is maintained throughout the year. Column 2 shows the expected effects of easing the credit policy by extending the credit period, offering larger discounts, relaxing credit standards, and easing collection efforts. Specifically, MESC is analyzing the effects of changing its credit terms from 1/10, net 30, to 2/10, net 40, relaxing its credit standards, and putting less pressure on slow-paying customers. Column 3 shows the projected income statement incorporating the expected effects of an easing in credit policy. The generally looser policy is expected to increase sales and lower collection costs, but discounts and several other types of costs would rise. The overall, bottom-line effect is a $7 million increase in projected net income. In the following paragraphs, we explain how the numbers in the table were calculated.

MESC's annual sales are $400 million. Under its current credit policy, 50 percent of those customers who pay do so on Day 10 and take the discount, 40 percent pay on Day 30, and 10 percent pay late, on Day 40. Thus, MESC's average collection period is $0.50(10) + 0.40(30) + 0.10(40) = 21$ days, and discounts total $0.01(\$400,000,000)0.50 = \$2,000,000$.

Table 15.7 Medical Equipment Supply Corporation: Credit Policy Change Analysis (millions of dollars)

	Projected 1996 Net Income Under Current Credit Policy	*Effect of Policy Change*	*Projected 1996 Net Income Under New Credit Policy*
Gross sales	$400	+$130	$530
Less discounts	2	+ 4	6
Net sales	$398	+$126	$524
Variable costs	280	+ 91	371
Profit before credit costs and taxes	$118	+$ 35	$153
Credit related costs:			
Cost of carrying receivables	3	+ 2	5
Analysis and collection costs	5	− 3	2
Bad debt losses	10	+ 22	32
Profit before taxes	$100	+$ 14	$114
Taxes (50%)	50	+ 7	57
Net income	$ 50	+$ 7	$ 57

The cost of carrying receivables is equal to the average receivables balance times the variable cost percentage times the cost of money used to carry receivables. The firm's variable cost ratio is 70 percent, and its pre-tax cost of capital to finance receivables is 20 percent. Thus, its cost of carrying receivables is $3 million:

Cost of carrying receivables

$= \text{ACP}(\text{Sales per day})(\text{Variable cost ratio})(\text{Cost of funds})$

$= 21(\$400,000,000/360)(0.70)0.20$

$= \$3,266,667 \approx \$3 \text{ million.}$

Only variable costs enter this calculation because this is the only cost element in receivables that must be financed. We are seeking the cost of carrying receivables, and variable costs represent the firm's investment in the cost of goods sold.

Even though MESC spends $5 million annually to analyze accounts and to collect from late payers, 2.5 percent of sales will never be collected. Bad debt losses therefore amount to $0.025(\$400,000,000) =$ $10,000,000.

MESC's new credit policy would be 2/10, net 40 versus the old policy of 1/10, net 30, so the new policy calls for a larger discount and a longer payment period, as well as a relaxed collection effort and lower credit standards. The company believes that these changes will lead to a $130 million increase in sales, to $530 million per year. Under the new terms, management believes that 60 percent of the customers who pay will take the 2 percent discount, so discounts will increase to $0.02(\$530,000,000)0.60 = \$6,360,000 \approx \$6$ million. Half of the nondiscount customers will pay on Day 40, and the remainder on Day 50, so the new ACP is estimated to be 24 days:

$0.60(10) + 0.20(40) + 0.20(50) = 24 \text{ days.}$

Also, the cost of carrying receivables will increase to $5 million:[4]

$24(\$530,000,000/360)(0.70)(0.20) = \$4,946,667 \approx \$5 \text{ million.}$

The company plans to reduce its annual credit analysis and collection expenditures to $2 million. The reduced credit standards and the relaxed collection effort are expected to raise bad debt losses to about 6 percent of sales, or to $0.06(\$530,000,000) = \$31,800,000 \approx \$32,000,000$, which is an increase of $22 million from the current level.

The combined effect of all the changes in credit policy is a projected $7 million annual increase in net income. There would, of course, be corresponding changes on the projected balance sheet—the higher sales would necessitate somewhat larger cash balances, inventories, and, depending on the capacity situation, perhaps more fixed assets. Since these asset increases, like the increase in receivables, would have to be financed, certain liabilities or equity, or both, would have to be increased. The Table 15.7 analysis does not include such costs, so if they are significant, they would have to be added to the analysis.

The $7 million expected increase in net income is, of course, an estimate, and the actual effects of the proposed credit policy change could be quite different than anticipated. In the first place, there is uncertainty—perhaps quite a lot—about the projected $130 million increase in sales. Conceivably, if MESC's competitors matched its credit policy changes, sales would not rise at all. Similar uncertainties must be attached to the number of customers who would take discounts, to production costs at higher or lower sales levels, to the costs of carrying additional receivables, and to bad debt losses. In the final analysis, the decision will be based on judgment, especially concerning the risks involved, but the type of quantitative analysis set forth above is essential to the process.

Self-Test Questions:

What are the four credit policy variables?

What is a credit-scoring system?

Describe how a proposed change in credit policy could be evaluated.

Inventory Management

Inventories are an essential part of virtually all business operations. As is the case with accounts receivable, inventory levels depend heavily upon sales. However, whereas receivables build up *after* sales have been made, inventories must be acquired *ahead* of sales. This is a critical difference, and the necessity of forecasting sales before establishing target inventory levels makes inventory management a difficult task. Also, since errors in the establishment of inventory levels quickly lead either to lost sales or to excessive carrying costs, inventory management is as important as it is difficult. In the health services industry, inventory management is even more critical, because an inventory stock-out could lead to catastrophic consequences for patients.

To illustrate inventory concepts, consider the situation facing American Vaccine Company. American must order large amounts of biological materials in May, and it must take delivery by July to be sure of having enough materials to make the vaccines necessary to meet the heavy August–September demand caused by school registration. There are several alternative vaccines that can be required by school districts, so the firm must order its materials on the basis of its best guess on what vaccines will be ordered by its customers. American will lose potential sales if its stocks are too small, but it will be forced to lower prices on its vaccines, or even write off some stock entirely, if its stocks are too high or the wrong types.

The effects of inventory changes on the balance sheet are important. For simplicity, assume that American has a $10 million base stock of vaccines, financed by common stock. Its balance sheet is as follows (in thousands of dollars):

Inventories (base stock)	$10,000	Common stock	$10,000
Total assets	$10,000	Total claims	$10,000

Now it anticipates that it will sell $5 million of vaccines in August and September. Dollar sales will actually be greater than $5 million, since American makes about $200,000 in profits for every $1 million of inventory sold. American finances its seasonal inventory with bank loans, so its pre-fall balance sheet would look like this (in thousands of dollars):

Inventories (seasonal)	$ 5,000	Notes payable to bank	$ 5,000
Inventories (base stock)	10,000	Common stock	10,000
Total assets	$15,000	Total claims	$15,000

If everything works out as planned, sales will be made, inventories will be converted to cash, the bank loan will be retired, and the company will earn a profit. The balance sheet, after a successful vaccine season, might look like this (in thousands of dollars):

Cash	$ 1,000	Notes payable to bank	$ 0
Inventory (seasonal)	0	Common stock	10,000
Inventory (base stock)	10,000	Retained earnings	1,000
Total assets	$11,000	Total claims	$11,000

The company is now in a highly liquid position and will be ready when the next school registration season comes around.

But suppose the season had not gone well, and American had only sold $1 million of its vaccine inventory. In October, its balance sheet would look like this (in thousands of dollars):

Cash	$ 200	Notes payable to bank	$ 4,000
Inventory (seasonal)	4,000	Common stock	10,000
Inventory (base stock)	10,000	Retained earnings	200
Total assets	$14,200	Total claims	$14,200

Now suppose the bank insists on repayment of the $4 million outstanding on the loan, and it wants cash, not vaccine serum. But if the vaccines did not sell well in the busy pre-school season, how easy will it be to sell them now? Assume that American is forced to mark the vaccines down to half their cost to sell them to raise cash to repay the bank loan. The result will be as follows (in thousands of dollars):

Cash	$ 2,200	Notes payable to bank	$ 4,000
Inventory (base stock)	10,000	Common stock	10,000
		Retained earnings	(1,800)
Total assets	$12,200	Total claims	$12,200

At this point, American is in serious trouble. It does not have the cash to pay off the loan, and the firm's shareholders have lost $1.8 million of their original $10 million equity investment. If the bank will not extend the loan, and if other sources of cash are not available, American will have to mark down its base stock prices in an effort to stimulate sales, and if this does not work, American could be forced into bankruptcy. Clearly, poor inventory decisions can spell trouble.

Proper inventory management requires close coordination among the sales, purchasing, production, and finance departments. The marketing department is generally the first to spot changes in demand. These changes must be worked into the company's purchasing and operating schedules, and the financial manager must arrange any financing that will be needed to support the inventory buildup. Improper communication among departments, poor sales forecasts, or both, can lead to disaster.

Inventory management focuses on three basic questions: (1) How many units should be ordered (or produced) at a given time? (2) At what point should inventory be ordered (or produced)? (3) What inventory items warrant special attention? The remainder of the chapter is devoted to providing answers to these questions.

Inventory costs

The goal of inventory management is to provide at the lowest total cost the inventories required to sustain operations. The first step in inventory management is to identify all the costs involved in purchasing and maintaining inventories. Table 15.8 gives a listing of the typical costs that are associated with inventories. In the table, we have broken down costs into three categories: those associated with carrying inventories, those associated with ordering and receiving inventories, and those associated with running short of inventories. Of course, the costs reported here are just rough averages. Inventory costs vary widely across firms depending on the nature and size of the inventories held.

Although they may well be the most important element, we shall at this point disregard the third category of costs—the costs of running short. These costs are dealt with by adding safety stocks, as we will discuss later. Similarly, we shall discuss quantity discounts in a later section. The

Table 15.8 Typical Costs Associated with Inventories

	Approximate Annual Cost as a Percentage of Inventory Value
Carrying Costs	
Cost of capital tied up in inventories	12.0%
Storage and handling costs	0.5
Insurance	0.5
Inventory taxes	1.0
Depreciation and obsolescence	<u>12.0</u>
	<u>26.0%</u>
Ordering, Shipping, and Receiving Costs	
Cost of placing orders, including set-up costs	Varies
Shipping and handling costs	2.5%
Costs of Running Short	
Loss of sales	Varies
Loss of customer goodwill	Varies
Disruption of production (service) schedules	Varies
Litigation losses	Varies

costs that remain for consideration at this stage, then, are carrying costs and ordering, shipping, and receiving costs.

Carrying costs

Carrying costs generally rise in direct proportion to the average amount of inventory carried. Inventories carried, in turn, depend on the frequency with which orders are placed. To illustrate, if a firm uses S units per year, and if it places equal-sized orders N times per year, then S/N units will be purchased with each order. If the inventory is used evenly over the year, and if no safety stocks are carried, then the average inventory, A, will be:

$$A = \frac{\text{Units per order}}{2} = \frac{S/N}{2}. \tag{15.1}$$

For example, if S = 120,000 units in a year, and N = 4, then the firm will order 30,000 units at a time, and its average inventory will be 15,000 units.

$$A = \frac{S/N}{2} = \frac{120,000/4}{2} = \frac{30,000}{2} = 15,000 \text{ units.}$$

Just after a shipment arrives, the inventory will be 30,000 units; just before the next shipment arrives, it will be zero; and on average, 15,000 units will be carried.

Now assume the firm purchases its inventory at a price P = \$2 per unit. The average inventory value is, thus, $(P)(A) = \$2(15,000) = \$30,000$. If the firm has a cost of capital used to carry inventory of 10 percent, it will incur \$3,000 in financing charges to carry the inventory for one year. Furthermore, assume that each year the firm incurs \$2,000 of storage costs (space, utilities, security, taxes, and so forth), that its inventory insurance costs are \$500, and that it must mark down inventories by \$1,000 because of depreciation and obsolescence. The firm's total costs of carrying the \$30,000 average inventory is thus \$3,000 + \$2,000 + \$500 + \$1,000 = \$6,500, so the annual percentage cost of carrying the inventory is \$6,500/\$30,000 = 0.217 = 21.7%.

Defining the annual percentage carrying cost as C, we can, in general, find the annual total carrying cost, TCC, as the percentage carrying cost, C, times the price per unit, P, times the average number of units, A:

$$TCC = \text{Total carrying cost} = (C)(P)(A). \tag{15.2}$$

In our example,

$$TCC = (0.217)(\$2)(15,000) \approx \$6,500.$$

Ordering costs

Although we assume that carrying costs are entirely variable and rise in direct proportion to the average size of inventories, we assume that all ordering costs are fixed. For example, the costs of placing and receiving an order—interoffice memos, long-distance telephone calls, costs to the supplier of setting up a production run (if necessary), and taking delivery—are essentially fixed regardless of the size of an order, so this part of inventory costs is simply the fixed cost of placing and receiving orders times the number of orders placed per year.[5] We define the fixed costs associated with ordering inventories as F, and if we place N orders per year, the total ordering cost is given by Equation 15.3:

$$\text{Total ordering cost} = TOC = (F)(N). \tag{15.3}$$

Here TOC = total ordering cost, F = fixed costs per order, and N = number of orders placed per year.

Equation 15.1 may be rewritten as $N = S/2A$, and then substituted into Equation 15.3:

$$\text{Total ordering cost} = TOC = F\left(\frac{S}{2A}\right). \tag{15.4}$$

To illustrate the use of Equation 15.4, if $F = \$100$, $S = 120,000$ units, and $A = 15,000$ units, then TOC, the total annual ordering cost, is \$400:

$$TOC = \$100\left(\frac{120,000}{30,000}\right) = \$100(4) = \$400.$$

Total inventory costs

Total carrying cost, TCC, as defined in Equation 15.2, and total ordering cost, TOC, as defined in Equation 15.4, may be combined to find total inventory costs, TIC, as follows:

$$\text{Total inventory costs} = TIC = TCC + TOC$$
$$= (C)(P)(A) + F\left(\frac{S}{2A}\right). \tag{15.5}$$

Recognizing that the average inventory carried is $A = Q/2$, or one-half the size of each order quantity, Q, we may rewrite Equation 15.5 as follows:

$$TIC = TCC + TOC$$
$$= (C)(P)\left(\frac{Q}{2}\right) + (F)\left(\frac{S}{Q}\right). \tag{15.6}$$

Here we see that total carrying cost equals average inventory in units, $Q/2$, multiplied by unit price, P, times the percentage annual carrying cost, C. Total ordering cost equals the number of orders placed per year, S/Q, multiplied by the fixed cost of placing and receiving an order, F. We will use Equation 15.6 in the next section to develop the optimal inventory ordering quantity.

The economic ordering quantity (EOQ) model

Inventories are obviously necessary, but it is equally obvious that a firm's profitability will suffer if it has too much or too little inventory. How can we determine the optimal inventory level? In general, inventory levels are set on the basis of experience, which, after all, is the best teacher. However, managers can gain a feel for those factors that affect inventory levels by examining the *economic ordering quantity (EOQ) model*, which is described in this section.

Derivation of the EOQ model

Figure 15.1 illustrates the basic premise on which the EOQ model is built: namely, that some costs rise with larger inventories while other costs decline, and there is an optimal order size (and associated average inventory) that minimizes the total costs associated with inventories. First, as noted earlier, the average investment in inventories depends on how frequently orders are placed and the size of each order— if we order every day, average inventories will be much smaller than if we order once a year. Furthermore, as Figure 15.1 shows, a firm's carrying costs rise with larger orders: larger orders mean larger average inventories, so warehousing costs, capital costs associated with carrying inventory, insurance, and obsolescence costs will all increase. However, ordering costs decline with larger orders and inventories: the cost of placing orders, suppliers' production setup costs, and order handling costs will all decline if we order infrequently and consequently hold larger quantities.

If the carrying and ordering cost curves in Figure 15.1 are added, the sum represents total inventory costs, *TIC*. The point where *TIC* is minimized defines the *economic ordering quantity (EOQ)*, and this, in turn, determines the optimal average inventory level.

Figure 15.1   The EOQ Concept

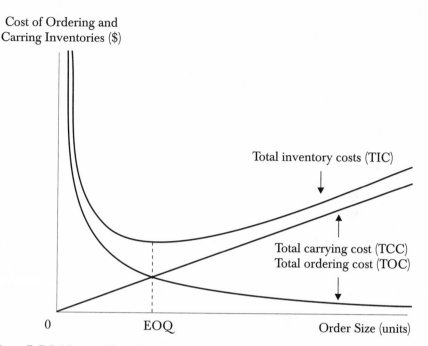

Source: E. F. Brigham and L. C. Gapenski. 1994. *Financial Management: Theory and Practice,* 7th ed. Fort Worth, TX: The Dryden Press.

The *EOQ* is found by differentiating Equation 15.6 with respect to ordering quantity, Q, and setting the derivative equal to zero:

$$\frac{d(TIC)}{dQ} = \frac{(C)(P)}{2} - \frac{(F)(S)}{Q^2} = 0.$$

Now, solving for Q, we obtain:

$$\frac{(C)(P)}{2} = \frac{(F)(S)}{Q^2} \tag{15.7}$$

$$Q^2 = \frac{2(F)(S)}{(C)(P)}$$

$$EOQ = \sqrt{\frac{2(F)(S)}{(C)(P)}}.$$

Here

> EOQ = economic ordering quantity, or the optimum quantity to be ordered each time an order is placed.
>
> F = fixed costs of placing and receiving an order.
>
> S = annual sales in units.
>
> C = annual carrying costs expressed as percentage of average inventory value.
>
> P = purchase price the firm must pay per unit of inventory.

Equation 15.7 is the EOQ model. The assumptions of the model, which will be relaxed shortly, include the following: (1) sales can be forecasted perfectly, (2) sales are evenly distributed throughout the year, and (3) orders are received when expected.

EOQ model illustration

To illustrate the EOQ model, consider the following data, supplied by Bayside Memorial Hospital. One of the items used by several of Bayside's laboratories is a biological hazard bag used to dispose of biological wastes. For this item:

> S = annual usage = 11,250 bags per year.
>
> C = percentage carrying cost = 25 percent of inventory value.
>
> P = purchase price per bag = \$1.00 per bag.
>
> F = fixed cost per order = \$100.

Substituting these data into Equation 15.7, we obtain an EOQ of 3,000 bags:

$$EOQ = \sqrt{\frac{2(F)(S)}{(C)(P)}} = \sqrt{\frac{2(\$100)\,11{,}250}{0.25(\$1.00)}} = \sqrt{9{,}000{,}000} = 3{,}000.$$

With an EOQ of 3,000 bags and annual usage of 11,250 bags, Bayside will place 11,250/3,000 = 3.75 orders per year. Notice that average inventory holdings depend directly on the EOQ: this relationship is illustrated graphically in Figure 15.2, where we see that average inventory = $EOQ/2$. Immediately after an order is received, 3,000 bags are in stock. The sales rate, or usage rate in this case, is 216 bags per week (11,250/52 weeks), so inventories are drawn down by this amount each week. Thus, the actual number of units held in inventory will vary from 3,000 bags just after an order is received to zero just before a new order arrives. With a 3,000 beginning balance, a zero ending balance, and a uniform usage rate, inventories will average one-half the EOQ, or 1,500 bags, during the year. At a cost of $1.00 per bag, the average investment in inventories will be 1,500($1.00) = $1,500. If inventories are financed by bank loans, the loan balance will vary from a high of $3,000 to a low of $0, but the average amount outstanding over the course of a year will be $1,500.

Notice that the EOQ, and hence average inventory holdings, rises with the square root of usage. Therefore, a given increase in sales will result in a less-than-proportional increase in inventories, so the inventory/sales ratio will tend to decline as a firm grows. For example, Bayside's EOQ is 3,000 bags at an annual sales level of 11,250, and the average inventory is 1,500 bags, or $1,500. However, if usage of biological hazard bags were to increase by 100 percent, to 22,500 bags per year, the EOQ would rise only to 4,243 units, or by about 41 percent, and the average inventory would rise by this same percentage. This suggests that there are economies of scale in holding inventories.[6]

Figure 15.2   Bayside Memorial Hospital: Inventory Position
                        without Safety Stock

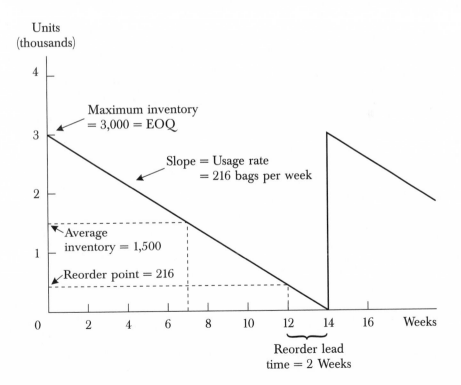

Finally, look at Bayside's total inventory costs for the year, assuming that the EOQ is ordered each time. Using Equation 15.6, we find total inventory costs are $750:

$$TIC \quad = \qquad TCC \qquad + \qquad TOC$$

$$= \qquad (C)(P)\left(\frac{Q}{2}\right) \quad + \quad (F)\left(\frac{S}{Q}\right)$$

$$= 0.25(\$1.00)\left(\frac{3{,}000}{2}\right) + \$100\left(\frac{11{,}250}{3{,}000}\right)$$

$$= \qquad \$375 \qquad + \qquad \$375 \qquad = \$750.$$

Note these two points: (1) The $750 total inventory cost represents the total of carrying costs and ordering costs, but this amount does *not* include the 11,250($1.00) = $11,250 annual purchasing cost of the inventory itself. (2) As we see both in Figure 15.1 and in the numbers just preceding, at the *EOQ*, total carrying cost (*TCC*) equals total ordering cost (*TOC*). This property is not unique to our Bayside illustration; it always holds.

Setting the reorder point

If a two-week lead time is required for order processing and shipping, what is Bayside's *reorder point*? If we use a 52-week year, Bayside uses $11{,}250/52 \approx 216$ bags per week. Thus, if a two-week lag occurs between placing an order and receiving goods, Bayside must place the order when there are 2(216) = 432 bags on hand. During the two-week processing and shipping period, Bayside will use 432 bags, so the inventory balance will hit zero just as the order of new bags arrives.

If Bayside knew for certain that both the usage rate and the order lead time would never vary, it could operate exactly as shown in Figure 15.2. However, usage does change, and processing delays or shipping delays, or both, are frequently encountered. To guard against these events, the hospital must carry additional inventories, or safety stocks, as discussed in the next section.

The concept of safety stocks

Safety stocks protect Bayside against increased usage rates and delivery delays. First, note that the slope of the usage line measures the expected use rate. Bayside *expects* to use 216 bags per week, but let us assume that the maximum likely usage rate is twice this amount, or 432 bags each week. Furthermore, assume that Bayside sets the safety stock at 432 bags, so it initially orders 3,432 bags, the EOQ of 3,000 plus the 432-unit safety stock. Subsequently, it reorders the EOQ whenever the inventory level falls to 864 bags, the safety stock of 432 bags plus the 432 bags expected to be used while awaiting delivery of the order.

Notice that the hospital could, over the two-week delivery period, use 432 bags a week, or double its normal expected sales. The condition that makes this higher maximum sales rate possible is the safety stock of 432 bags. The safety stock is also useful to guard against delays in receiving orders. The expected delivery time is two weeks, but with a 432-bag safety stock, the hospital could maintain usage at the expected rate of 216 bags per week for an additional two weeks if processing or shipping delays held up an order.

However, carrying a safety stock has a cost. The average inventory is now $EOQ/2$ plus the safety stock, or $3,000/2 + 432 = 1,500 + 432 = 1,932$ bags, and the average inventory value is now $1,932(\$1.00) = \$1,932$. This increase in average inventory causes an increase in annual inventory carrying costs equal to (Safety stock)$(P)(C) = 432(\$1.00)(0.25) = \$108$. Although this may seem like a small amount, when applied to thousands of items, the cost of carrying safety stocks can be substantial.

The optimal safety stock for any item varies from situation to situation, but, in general, it *increases* (1) with the uncertainty of usage forecasts, (2) with the costs (in terms of lost sales or good will, or production or service inefficiencies, or, most important for health care providers, negative health outcomes) that result from inventory shortages, and (3) with the probability that delays will occur in receiving shipments. The optimal safety stock *decreases* as the cost of carrying this additional inventory increases.

Quantity discounts

Now suppose the biological hazard bag manufacturer offered Bayside a *quantity discount* of 2 percent on large orders. If the quantity discount applied to orders of 2,000 or more, then Bayside would continue to place the EOQ order of 3,000 bags and take the quantity discount. However, if the quantity discount required orders of 5,000 or more, then Bayside's managers would have to compare the savings in purchase price that would result if its ordering quantity were increased to 5,000 units with the increase in total inventory costs caused by the departure from the hospital's 3,000-unit EOQ.

First, consider the total costs associated with Bayside's EOQ of 3,000 units. We found earlier that total inventory costs are $750:

$$TIC = \qquad TCC \qquad + \qquad TOC$$

$$= \qquad (C)(P)\left(\frac{Q}{2}\right) \quad + \quad (F)\left(\frac{S}{Q}\right)$$

$$= 0.25(\$1.00)\left(\frac{3,000}{2}\right) + \$100\left(\frac{11,250}{3,000}\right)$$

$$= \qquad \$375 \qquad + \qquad \$375 \qquad = \$750.$$

Now, what would total inventory costs be if Bayside ordered 5,000 units instead of 3,000? The answer is $837.50:

$$TIC = 0.25(\$0.98)\left(\frac{5,000}{2}\right) + \$100\left(\frac{11,250}{5,000}\right)$$

$$= \qquad \$612.50 \qquad + \qquad \$225 \qquad = \$837.50.$$

Notice that when the discount is taken, the price, P, is reduced by the amount of the discount; the new price per unit would be 0.98($1.00) = $0.98. Also, note that when the ordering quantity is increased, carrying costs increase because the firm is carrying a larger average inventory, but ordering costs decrease since the hospital is placing fewer orders per year. If we were to calculate total inventory costs at an ordering quantity of 2,000, we would find that carrying costs would be less than $375, and ordering costs would be more than $375, but total inventory costs would be more than $750 since they are at a minimum when 3,000 units are ordered.

We see, then, that inventory costs would increase by $837.50 − $750 = $87.50 if Bayside were to increase its order size to 5,000 bags. *However, this cost increase must be compared with Bayside's savings if it takes the discount.* Taking the discount would save 0.02($1.00) = $0.02 per bag. Over the year, Bayside orders 11,250 bags, so the annual savings is $0.02(11,250) = $225. Here is a summary:

Reduction in purchase price	= 0.02($1.00)(11,250)	= $225.00
Less: Increase in total inventory costs	= $837.50 − $750	= 87.50
Net savings from taking discounts		$137.50

Obviously, Bayside should order 5,000 units at a time and take advantage of the quantity discount.

Inflation

Moderate inflation—say 3 percent per year—can largely be ignored for purposes of inventory management, but higher rates of inflation must be explicitly considered. If the rate of inflation in the types of goods the firm stocks tend to be relatively constant, it can be dealt with quite easily—simply deduct the expected annual rate of inflation from the carrying cost percentage, C, in Equation 15.7, and use this modified version of the EOQ model to establish the working stock. The reason for making this deduction is that inflation causes the value of inventories to rise, thus offsetting somewhat the effects of depreciation and other carrying costs factors. Since C will now be smaller, the calculated EOQ, and the average inventory, will increase. However, the higher the rate of inflation, the higher are interest rates and hence carrying costs, so C will increase, which in turn lowers the EOQ and average inventories.

On balance, there is no evidence that inflation either raises or lowers the optimal inventories of firms in the aggregate. Inflation should still be explicitly considered, however, because it will raise the individual firm's optimal holdings if the rate of inflation for its own inventories is above average (and hence is greater than the effects of inflation on interest rates), and vice versa if the rate of inflation on inventories is below average.

Seasonal demand

For some firms, it is unrealistic to assume that the demand for an inventory item is uniform throughout the year. What happens when there is seasonal demand, as would be the case for an ambulatory care clinic in a resort area such as Vail? Here the standard annual EOQ model is obviously not appropriate. However, it does provide a point of departure for setting inventory parameters, which are then modified to fit the particular seasonal pattern. The procedure here is to divide the year into seasons in which annualized sales are relatively constant, say summer, spring and fall, and winter. Then, the EOQ model can be applied separately to each period. During the transitions between seasons, inventories would be either run down or else built up with special seasonal orders.

EOQ range

Thus far, we have interpreted the EOQ, and the resulting inventory variables, as single point estimates. It can be easily demonstrated that small deviations from the EOQ do not appreciably affect total inventory costs, and, consequently, that the optimal ordering quantity should be viewed more as a range than as a single value.[7]

To illustrate this point, we can examine the sensitivity of total inventory costs to ordering quantity for Bayside's biological hazard bags.

Table 15.9 contains the results of our sensitivity analysis. We conclude that the ordering quantity could range from 2,000 to 4,000 units without affecting total inventory costs by more than 8.3 percent. Thus, we see that managers can adjust the ordering quantity within a fairly wide range without fear of significantly increasing total inventory costs.

Inventory control systems

In addition to setting inventory levels, inventory management also involves establishing *inventory control systems*. Inventory control systems run the gamut from very simple to extremely complex, depending on the size of the firm and the nature of its inventories. For example, one simple control procedure is the *redline method*: inventory items are stored in a bin, a red line is drawn around the inside of the bin at the level of the order point, and the inventory clerk places an order when the red line shows. The *two-bin method* has inventory items stocked in two bins. When the working bin is empty, an order is placed and inventory is drawn from the second bin. These procedures work well for small components in a manufacturing process, or for many laboratory items.

Computerized systems

Larger companies employ *computerized inventory control systems*. The computer starts with an inventory count in memory. As withdrawals are made, they are recorded in the computer, and the inventory balance is revised. When the order point is reached, the computer automatically places an order, and when the order is received, the recorded balance is increased.

Table 15.9   Bayside Memorial Hospital: EOQ Sensitivity Analysis

Ordering Quantity	Total Inventory Costs	Percentage Deviation from Optimum
1,000 units	$1,250.00	+66.7%
1,500	937.50	+25.0
2,000	812.50	+8.3
2,500	762.50	+1.7
3,000	750.00	0.0
3,500	758.93	+1.2
4,000	781.25	+4.2
4,500	812.50	+8.3
5,000	850.00	+13.3

Retailers such as Wal-Mart have carried this system quite far: each item has a magnetic bar code, and, as an item is checked out, the code is read, a signal is sent to the computer, and the inventory balance is adjusted at the same time the price is fed into the cash register tape. When the balance drops to the reorder point, an order is placed directly from the store's computers to those of its suppliers.

A good inventory control system is dynamic. A large company may stock thousands of different items. The sales (or usage) of these various items can rise or fall quite separately from rising or falling overall corporate sales. As the usage rate for an individual item begins to rise or fall, the inventory manager must adjust its balance to avoid running short or ending up with obsolete items. If the change in the usage rate appears to be permanent, then the EOQ should be recomputed, the safety stock level should be reconsidered, and the computer model used in the control process should be reprogrammed.

Just-in-time systems

A relatively new approach to inventory control called *just-in-time (JIT)* is gaining popularity in all industries, including health care. To illustrate the use of just-in-time systems in the health care industry, consider St. Luke's Episcopal Hospital in Houston, which consumes large quantities of medical supplies each year. A few years ago, the hospital maintained a 25,000 square foot warehouse to hold its medical supplies. But, as cost pressures mounted, the hospital closed its warehouse and sold the inventory to Baxter International, a major hospital supplier. Now, Baxter is a full-time partner of St. Luke's in ordering and delivering Baxter's hospital supplies, as well as the products of 400 other companies.

The inventory streamlining process began with daily deliveries to the hospital's loading dock, but soon expanded to a JIT system called *stockless inventory*. Now, Baxter fills orders in exact, sometimes small, quantities and delivers them directly to departments, including the operating rooms and nursing floors, inside St. Luke's. St. Luke's managers estimate that the stockless system has saved the hospital about $1.5 million a year since it was instituted, including $350,000 from staff reductions and $650,000 from inventory reductions. Additionally, the hospital has converted space that was previously used as storerooms to patient care and other cash-generating uses. The distributors that offer stockless inventory systems typically add 3 to 5 percent service fees, but many hospitals still can realize a large savings on total inventory costs.

Of course, the stockless inventory concept has its own set of problems. The major concern is that a stockout will cause a serious problem.

"We walk very carefully and slowly, because we can't afford a glitch," said a Baxter spokesperson. "The first morning that an operating room doesn't open, we've got a problem." Also, some hospital managers are concerned that such systems create too much dependence on a single supplier, and eventually the cost savings will disappear as prices are increased.

As stockless inventory systems become more prevalent in hospitals, more and more hospitals are decreasing their in-house inventory management (or *materials management*, as it is often called in the hospital industry) in favor of outside contractors who assume both inventory management and supplier roles. In effect, hospitals are beginning to "outsource" inventory management, as discussed next.

Outsourcing

Another important development related to inventories is *outsourcing*, which is the practice of purchasing goods and services rather than doing them in-house. Thus, if Baxter International arranged to purchase certain medical supply items from suppliers rather than making them in-house, it would be increasing its use of outsourcing. Outsourcing is often combined with just-in-time systems to reduce inventory levels. However, perhaps the major reason for outsourcing in many industries has nothing to do with inventory policy: heavily unionized companies can often buy goods and services from nonunionized suppliers at a lower cost than it would take to do the same thing in-house because of wage-rate and benefit differentials.

As noted earlier, some hospitals are beginning to use outsourcing for inventory management. For example, some hospitals are experimenting with an inventory management program known as *point-of-service distribution*, which is one generation ahead of stockless systems. Under point-of-service programs, the supplier delivers supplies, intravenous solutions, medical forms, and so on, to the supply rooms that it runs on the hospital's nursing floors. The supplier owns the products in the supply rooms until used by the hospital, at which time the hospital pays for the items. This system has been used by supplier Owens & Minor to deliver supplies to 200 inventory locations at UCLA Medical Center. By introducing more sophisticated inventory management techniques, inventory turnover at UCLA Medical Center has been raised from 8.5 times in 1989 to 11.5 times in 1993. In addition to reducing inventories, outside inventory managers are good at ferreting out waste. For example, an inventory management company recently found that one hospital was spending $600 for products used in open heart surgery while another was spending only $420. Since there was no real difference in surgery procedures or outcomes, the higher-cost hospital was able to change its procedures and pocket the difference.

In an even more advanced form of inventory management, some hospitals are just beginning to negotiate with suppliers to furnish materials on the basis of how much medical care is delivered, rather than the type and number of products used. In such agreements, providers pay suppliers a set fee for each "unit of patient service" provided, say, $125 for each case-mix–adjusted patient day. Under this type of system, a hospital ties its supplies expenditures to its revenues, which, at least for now, are for the most part tied to the number of units of patient service. The end of the evolution of inventory management techniques for health care providers is expected to be some form of capitated payment, whereby providers will pay suppliers a previously agreed-upon fee regardless of actual future patient usage, and hence regardless of materials actually consumed.

Self-Test Questions:

Why is good inventory management important to a firm's success?

What is the EOQ model, and what does it tell us about inventory management?

Describe some recent trends in inventory management by health care providers.

Summary

- When a firm sells goods to a customer on credit, an *account receivable* is created.

- Firms can use an *aging schedule* and the *average collection period (ACP)* to help keep track of their receivables position and to help avoid the buildup of possible bad debts.

- The *payments pattern approach* is the best way to monitor receivables. The primary tool in this approach is the *uncollected balances schedule*.

- A firm's *credit policy* consists of four elements: (1) credit period, (2) discounts given for early payment, (3) credit standards, and (4) collection policy. The first two, when combined, are called the firm's *credit terms*.

- Two major sources of external credit information are available: *credit associations*, which are local groups that meet frequently and correspond with one another to exchange information on credit customers, and *credit reporting agencies*, which collect credit information and sell it for a fee.

- The *basic objective* of credit sales is to increase profitable sales by extending credit to worthy customers and therefore adding value to the firm.

- If a firm *eases its credit policy*, its sales should increase. Actions that ease the credit policy include lengthening the credit period, relaxing credit standards and collection policy, and offering cash discounts. Each of these actions, however, increases costs. A firm should ease its credit policy only if the costs of doing so will be more than offset by higher sales revenues.

- *Inventory management* involves determining how much inventory to hold, when to place orders, and how many units to order at a time. Because the cost of holding inventory is high, inventory management is important.

- *Inventory costs* can be divided into three types: carrying costs, ordering costs, and stock-out costs. In general, carrying costs increase as the level of inventory rises, but ordering costs and stock-out costs decline with larger inventory holdings.

- The *economic ordering quantity (EOQ) model* is a formula for determining the order quantity that will minimize total inventory costs. It provides many insights, but its real world use is limited.

- The *reorder point* is the inventory level at which new items must be ordered.

- *Safety stocks* are held to avoid shortages if (1) demand becomes greater than expected or (2) shipping delays are encountered.

- Firms use inventory control systems, such as the *red-line method* and the *two-bin method*, as well as *computerized inventory control systems*, to help them keep track of actual inventory levels and to insure that inventory levels are adjusted as sales change. *Just-in-time (JIT)* systems are also used to hold down inventory costs and, simultaneously, to improve operations.

Notes

1. Note that the ACP can be calculated, given a firm's accounts receivable balance and its average daily credit sales (ADS), as follows:

$$\text{ACP} = \frac{\text{Receivables}}{ADS} = \frac{\$1,760,000}{\$110,000} = 16 \text{ days.}$$

2. For a more complete description of EDI systems, see J. J. Moynihan, M. K. Bednar, and K. C. Norman, "Standards Opening a Door to Electronic Payments." *Healthcare Financial Management* (March 1991): 21–31.

3. Note that some firms offer discounts only to customers who pay cash on the spot, because the cost of giving such discounts is offset by the reduction in receivables accounting costs.

4. Since the credit policy change will result in a longer ACP, the firm will have to wait longer to receive its profit on the goods it sells. Therefore, the firm will incur an opportunity cost due to not having the cash from these profits available for investment. The dollar amount of this opportunity cost is equal to the old sales per day times the change in ACP times the contribution margin (1 − Variable cost ratio) times the firm's cost of carrying receivables, or

$$\begin{aligned} \text{Opportunity cost} &= (\text{Old sales}/360)(\Delta DSO)(1 - V)k \\ &= (\$400/360)(3)0.20 \\ &= \$0.2 = \$200,000. \end{aligned}$$

For simplicity, we have ignored this opportunity cost in our analysis. For a more complete discussion of credit policy change analysis, see E. F. Bringham and L. C. Gapenski, *Intermediate Financial Management.* (Fort Worth, TX: Dryden Press, 1996).

5. Note that in reality both carrying and ordering costs can have variable and fixed cost elements, at least over certain ranges of inventory. For example, security and utilities charges are probably fixed in the short run over a wide range of inventory levels. Similarly, labor costs in receiving inventory could be tied to the quantity received, and hence could be variable. To simplify matters, we treat all carrying costs as variable and all ordering costs as fixed. However, if these assumptions do not fit the situation at hand, the cost definitions can be changed. For example, one could add another term for shipping costs if there are economies of scale in shipping, such that the cost of shipping one unit is smaller if shipments are larger. However, in most situations, shipping costs are not sensitive to order size, so total shipping costs are simply the shipping cost per unit times the number of units ordered during the year. Under this condition, shipping costs are not influenced by inventory policy, so they may be disregarded for purposes of determining the optimal inventory level and the optimal order size.

6. Note, however, that these scale economies relate to each particular item, and not to the entire firm. For example, a large distributor of hospital supplies might have a higher inventory/sales ratio than a much smaller distributor if the small firm has only a few high-sales-volume items while the large firm distributes a great many low-volume items.

7. This is somewhat analogous to the optimal capital structure in that small

changes in capital structure around the optimum do not have much effect on the firm's weighted average cost of capital.

Selected Additional References

Anderson, H. J. 1989. "Patient Accounts Managers Share Views on Receivables." *Healthcare Financial Management* (December): 42–46.

Berling, R. J., Jr., and J. T. Geppi. 1989. "Hospitals Can Cut Materials Costs by Managing Supply Pipeline." *Healthcare Financial Management* (April): 19–26.

Bruch, N. M., and L. L. Lewis. 1994. "Using Control Charts to Help Manage Accounts Receivable." *Healthcare Financial Management* (July): 44–48.

Clarkin, J. F. (ed.). 1990. "Managing Accounts Receivable." *Topics in Health Care Financing* (Fall issue).

Dias, K., and D. Stockamp. 1992. "Nursing Process Approach Improves Receivables Management." *Healthcare Financial Management* (September): 55–64.

Folk, M. D., and P. R. Roest. 1995. "Converting Accounts Receivable into Cash." *Healthcare Financial Management* (September): 74–78.

Frohlich, R. M., Jr. 1994. "Effective Reassignment of Accounts Can Decrease Bad Debt." *Healthcare Financial Management* (July): 37–42.

Funsten, R. S. (ed.). 1993. "Accounts Receivable Management." *Topics in Health Care Financing* (Fall issue).

Groenevelt, C. J. 1990. "Applying Japanese Management Tips to Patient Accounts." *Healthcare Financial Management* (April): 46–55.

Kincaid, T. J. 1993. "Selling Accounts Receivable to Fund Working Capital." *Healthcare Financial Management* (May): 27–32.

Kowalski, J. C. 1991. "Materials Management Crucial to Overall Efficiency." *Healthcare Financial Management* (January): 40–44.

———. 1991. "Inventory to Go: Can Stockless Deliver Efficiency." *Healthcare Financial Management* (November): 21–34.

Ladewig, T. L., and B. A. Hecht. 1993. "Achieving Excellence in the Management of Accounts Receivable." *Healthcare Financial Management* (September): 25–32.

Marshall, S. 1993. "Cost Justifying the Electronic Billing Decision." *Healthcare Financial Management* (June): 68–72.

Moynihan, J. J. 1993. "Improving the Claims Process with EDI." *Healthcare Financial Management* (January): 48–52.

Melson, L. M., and M. K. Schultz. 1989. "Overcoming Barriers to Operating Room Inventory Control." *Healthcare Financial Management* (April): 28–34.

Newton, R. L. 1993. "Measuring Accounts Receivable Performance: A Comprehensive Method." *Healthcare Financial Management* (May): 33–36.

Prince, T. R., and R. Ramanan. 1992. "Collection Performance: An Empirical Analysis of Not-for-Profit Community Hospitals." *Hospital & Health Services Administration* (Summer): 181–196.

Robinson, E. F. 1989. "Automated Collection Systems Improve Cash Flow." *Healthcare Financial Management* (December): 31–40.

Sen, S., and J. P. Lawler. 1995. " Securitizing Receivables Offers Low-Cost Financing Option." *Healthcare Financial Management* (May): 32–37.

Slater, R. M., R. Corti, and J. Privitera. 1991. "Giving Receivables an 'Outside' Chance." *Healthcare Financial Management* (October): 56–66.

Souders, R. V. 1990. "Electronic Claims Can be a Remedy for Cash Flow Troubles." *Healthcare Financial Management* (June): 62–68.

Spiegel, M. 1989. "Selling Accounts Receivable Can Improve Cash Flow." *Healthcare Financial Management* (September): 40–46.

Swarzman, G. F. 1994. "Does Your Patient Accounting System Pass the Systems Test?" *Healthcare Financial Management* (July): 27–34.

Zimmerman, D. 1993. *Cash is King* (Franklin, WI: Eagle Press).

Case 15A

Puget Sound Pharmaceuticals, Inc.: Receivables Management

Mark Spence received his M.S. in pharmacology ten years ago from the University of Washington. While there, he became very interested in the business side of drug distribution, and stayed on for an extra 18 months to earn his M.B.A. After graduation, he went to work for a major drug manufacturer, where he assisted in the development of a new allergy drug. Although the drug passed all FDA trials and was certified for general use, the company in the next year developed a similar drug that was cheaper to produce and equally effective in treating most allergy symptoms. Thus, Mark's employer decided not to proceed with production of the earlier drug. However, it was willing to license production and distribution rights to another company. Mark thought that this might be a golden opportunity, so he quit his job with the firm and founded his own company, Puget Sound Pharmaceuticals. The sole purpose of the new company is to obtain the license for, produce, and distribute the new drug, which Mark dubbed SneezeRelief.

Mark is currently working on the business plan that he will present at a venture capital conference to be held in Seattle. The main purpose of the conference is to match entrepreneurs with venture capitalists who are interested in providing capital to fledgling firms. Mark has spent a lot of time thinking about how his proposed firm's receivables should be managed; he is concerned about this issue because he is aware of several small drug manufacturers that have gotten into serious financial difficulty due to poor receivables management.

The proposed firm initially would sell exclusively to drug wholesalers in Washington that specialized in nonprescription drugs. If demand proved solid, the firm would expand its sales area. Sales are expected to be highly seasonal: allergy drug sales are slow during the

694

cooler winter months, but they pick up dramatically in the spring, when plant pollen levels reach a peak. Business falls off again in the summer, but it picks up in the fall when the ragweed season begins. Mark's sales forecasts for the first six months of operations are given in Table 1.

Mark does not plan to give discounts for early payment—discounts are not widely used in the industry. Approximately 30 percent of the customers (by dollar value) are expected to pay in the month of sale, 50 percent are expected to pay in the month following the sale, and the remaining 20 percent are expected to pay two months after the sale. Mark does not foresee any problems with bad debt losses—he plans to screen his customers very carefully, and he thinks this will eliminate such losses. On average, Mark believes that 40 percent of receivables will contribute to profits, so 60 percent of receivables represent variable costs. Furthermore, banks are currently charging about 12 percent annually to finance receivables.

In spite of his optimism regarding bad debt losses, Mark is concerned about the company's potential level of receivables, and he wants to have a monitoring system in place that will allow him to spot quickly any adverse trends if they develop. Mark's total sales forecast for the company's first full year of operations is 285,000 bottles at a sales price of $5 per package of 12 tablets. As a first approximation, Mark assumes that 30 percent of the firm's customers will pay 10 days after the sale, 50 percent will pay on the 30th day, and 20 percent will pay on the 60th day.

Mark would like you, an outside consultant, to develop the following data for the venture capital conference:

1. The firm's projected average collection period (ACP)
2. The firm's projected average daily sales (use a 360-day year)
3. The firm's projected average receivables level
4. The end-of-year balance sheet figures for accounts receivable

Table 1   Puget Sound Pharmaceuticals: Sales Forecasts

Month	Sales
January	$ 50,000
February	125,000
March	200,000
April	300,000
May	225,000
June	150,000

and notes payable assuming that notes payable are used to finance the investment in receivables

5. The projected annual dollar cost of carrying the receivables

6. The receivables level at the end of March and the end of June; note that the receivables level forecasts, and all forecasts required by items 7 through 10, which follow, should be based on these assumptions: (a) the monthly sales forecasts given in Table 1 are realized, and (b) the firm's customers pay exactly as predicted

7. The firm's forecasted average daily sales for the first three months of operations and for the entire half year

8. The implied average collection period (ACP) at the end of March and at the end of June

9. Aging schedules as of the end of March and the end of June

10. Uncollected balances schedules as of the end of March and the end of June.

Mark anticipates that the venture capitalists will ask some questions concerning both the interpretation of the receivables data that is developed and the sensitivity of the results to the basic assumptions. Thus, be prepared to discuss thoroughly the results of your analysis.

Case 15B

Narragansett Regional Medical Center: Inventory Management

Narragansett Regional Medical Center is a 350-bed, not-for-profit, acute care hospital that carries more than 10,000 different items in inventory. These items vary widely in price, order lead times, and stockout costs. (Stockout costs are all the costs, from higher costs of service due to scheduling delays to lost profits to the risk of negative outcomes and potential lawsuits, that result from running out of stock of a particular item.) Narragansett uses the ABC method of inventory classification, along with a variety of inventory control methods, to manage its different inventory items. The ABC inventory classification system works in this way. Narragansett maintains data on the average annual usage and cost of each item. Based on these data, plus the multiplier values given in Table 1, Narragansett's managers assign a numerical *inventory importance value* to each item using the following formula:

$$\begin{matrix} \text{Inventory} \\ \text{importance} \\ \text{value} \end{matrix} = \begin{bmatrix} \text{Average} \\ \text{annual} \\ \text{usage} \end{bmatrix} \times \begin{bmatrix} \text{Cost} \\ \text{per} \\ \text{unit} \end{bmatrix} \times \begin{bmatrix} \text{Lead} \\ \text{time} \\ \text{multiplier} + \begin{matrix} \text{Stockout} \\ \text{multiplier} \end{matrix} \end{bmatrix}.$$

For example, a customized probe used in cardiac catheterization costs Narragansett $250, and the hospital uses 1,000 units per year. The probes require an order lead time of ten days, and they are in the average consequence class. Thus, the inventory importance value of the probes is $1,250,000:

$$\text{Inventory importance value} = (1,000)(\$250)(2 + 3)$$
$$= \$1,250,000.$$

Table 1   Narragansett's Hospital: Inventory Multiplier Values

Order Lead Time Multipliers:	
Lead Time Class	*Lead Time Multiplier*
0–2 days	0
3–7 days	1
8–30 days	2
1–3 months	4
4–6 months	8
7–12 months	12
Stockout Consequence Multipliers:	
Consequence Class	*Stockout Multiplier*
Unimportant	1
Average	3
Critical	5

No particular significance can be attached to the value $1,250,000—it is just a number that is used to compare the relative importance of this item with other inventory items.

Each of the hospital's inventory items is analyzed similarly; the inventory importance values for the various items are arrayed from highest to lowest, each item's percentage of the total importance value is calculated, and then the *cumulative* percentage values are plotted as shown in Figure 1. Finally, the items are separated into three classes, labeled A, B, and C. Note that only 10 percent of the inventory items— those in the A class—account for 50 percent of the total importance value, while 60 percent of the number of items fall into Class C, but these items constitute only 18 percent of the total importance value.

To better utilize the limited resources available for inventory management, Narragansett's managers focus most of their attention on the A category items. For items in this class, the hospital's managers review usage rates, stock positions, and delivery times on a monthly basis, and adjust the control and ordering system as necessary. Class B items are reviewed every quarter, while Class C items are reviewed only annually.

Even though this process has served Narragansett well, Roger Moran, the hospital's newly hired chief financial officer (CFO), thinks the hospital is carrying excess inventories. He notes that Narragansett has never come close to having a stockout, even when the hospital has been running at near 100 percent occupancy. Moran believes that a

Figure 1   ABC Inventory Classification Chart

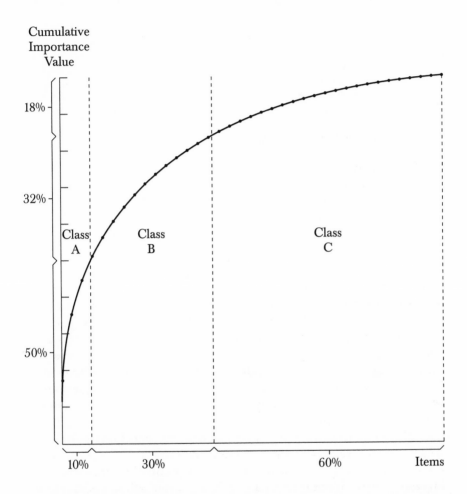

thorough review should be undertaken of all Class A items, and that it might be possible to increase inventory turnover 25 percent by trimming current stocks. To convince the hospital's president and CEO, Moran plans to perform an inventory analysis, focusing initially on a single item, the cardiac catheterization probe. Table 2 contains inventory cost and delivery data on this item.

    Narragansett currently uses a single source for the probe, Atwood Medical Supplies, known at the hospital as Supplier A. Supplier A requires an $800 setup fee on each order, in addition to the basic cost per

Table 2   Cost and Usage Data: Cardiac Catheterization Probe

Expected annual usage	1,000 units
Cost per unit	$250
Inventory carrying costs:	
Depreciation	1%
Storage and handling	8
Interest expense	10
Property taxes	2
Insurance	2
Total carrying costs	23%
Inventory ordering costs:	
Supplier A	$1,000
Supplier B	$ 500
Delivery lead times:	
Supplier A	10 days
Supplier B	20 days

unit, and it delivers in ten days. Although the probe is basically a standard item, Narragansett, as a local leader in cardiac care, customizes the probe slightly to conform to the wishes of its cardiology staff. Narragansett is considering another supplier, Bateman Health Products (Supplier B), which charges only a $300 setup fee, but which takes 20 days to deliver. It costs Narragansett another $200 to process each order, regardless of which supplier is used. Thus, the total order cost is $1,000 for Supplier A and $500 for Supplier B.

Moran wants to use EOQ concepts to examine the probe inventory situation and to select the supplier. His primary areas of concern are the number of orders placed each year, reorder points (in units), and total inventory costs. In addition to an analysis without safety stocks, Moran is also concerned about the impact of safety stocks on the decision. Narragansett currently carries a safety stock of 75 probes to protect itself against stockouts due to delivery delays or an increase in the usage rate, or both. However, if it decides to switch to Supplier B, Narragansett would need to increase the safety stock to 150 units to reflect Supplier B's longer lead time. Of particular interest is the impact of safety stocks on inventory costs, and the safety margins that such stocks would provide against higher-than-expected usage and shipping delays.

Also, Moran has heard the rumor that Supplier A, the current supplier, is about to offer a 2 percent discount on the $250 per unit purchase price on orders of 250 or more units. He wants to know what impact this would have, if it comes about, on the optimal order amount and the supplier decision.

Finally, Moran knows that it is unlikely that the probes would be ordered exactly as prescribed by the EOQ model, so he would like to know the impact of ordering variations on total inventory costs. In closing, Moran expressed some doubt about the value of the EOQ model in making "real world" inventory decisions. "If I'm right in my concerns," he asked, "what other inventory control methods are available to us?"

Part VIII

Other Topics

16

Lease Financing

Firms generally own fixed assets, but it is the use of buildings and equipment that is important to businesses, not their ownership. One way to obtain the use of assets is to raise debt or equity capital, and then to use this capital to buy the assets. An alternative way to obtain the use of assets is to lease them. Prior to the 1950s, leasing was generally associated with real estate—land and buildings. Today, however, it is possible to lease almost any kind of capital asset, and leasing is used extensively in the health care industry. In fact, it is estimated that about 40 percent of all medical equipment used in the industry is now leased rather than purchased.[1]

Operating versus Financial Leases

Historically, leases have been informally classified as either operating leases or financial leases. In later sections, we will discuss more formal classifications used by accountants and by the Internal Revenue Service (IRS).

Operating leases

Operating leases, sometimes called *service leases,* generally provide for both *financing* and *maintenance.* IBM was one of the pioneers of operating lease contracts, and computers and office copying machines, together with automobiles, trucks, and some medical diagnostic equipment, are the primary types of equipment involved in operating leases. Note that the user of a leased asset is called the *lessee,* while the owner of the equipment, usually the manufacturer or a leasing company, is called the *lessor.* (The term "lessee" is pronounced "less-ee," not "lease-ee," and "lessor" is pronounced "less-or.") Ordinarily, operating leases require the lessor to maintain and service the leased equipment, and the cost of the maintenance is built into the lease payments.

Another important characteristic of operating leases is the fact that they are *not fully amortized*. In other words, the payments required under the lease contract are not sufficient for the lessor to recover the full cost of the equipment. However, the lease contract is written for a period considerably less than the expected economic life of the leased asset, and the lessor expects to recover all costs eventually either by lease renewal payments, by releasing the equipment to other lessees, or by sale of the equipment.

A final feature of operating leases is that they frequently contain a *cancellation clause* which gives the lessee the right to cancel the lease and to return the equipment before the expiration of the basic lease agreement. This is an important consideration to the lessee, for it means that the equipment can be returned if it is rendered obsolete by technological developments or if it is no longer needed because of a decline in the lessee's business.

Financial leases

Financial leases, which are called *capital leases* by accountants, are differentiated from operating leases in that (1) they typically do not provide for maintenance service, (2) they typically are not cancelable, (3) they are generally for a period that approximates the economic life of the asset, and (4) they are hence fully amortized (that is, the lessor receives rental payments equal to the full cost of the leased asset plus a return on the funds employed). In a typical financial lease, the user firm (lessee) selects the specific item it requires, and then it negotiates the price and delivery terms with the manufacturer. The lessee then arranges to have a leasing company (lessor) buy the equipment from the manufacturer, and the lessee simultaneously executes a lease agreement with the lessor. The terms of the lease call for full amortization of the lessor's investment, plus a rate of return on the unamortized balance that is close to the percentage rate the lessee would have paid on a secured term loan. For example, if a radiology group practice would have to pay 10 percent for a term loan to buy an x-ray machine, then a rate of about 10 percent would be built into the lease contract by the lessor.

A *sale and leaseback* is a special type of financial lease that can be arranged by a user that currently owns some asset. Here, the user sells the asset to another party and simultaneously executes an agreement to lease the property back for a stated period under specific terms. In a sale and leaseback, the lessee receives an immediate cash payment in exchange for a future series of lease payments that must be made to rent the use of the asset sold.

The parallel to borrowing is obvious in a financial lease. Under a secured loan arrangement, the lender would normally receive a series of equal payments just sufficient to amortize the loan and to provide a specified rate of return on the outstanding loan balance. Under a financial lease, the lease payments are set up exactly the same way: the payments are just sufficient to return the full purchase price to the lessor, plus a stated return on the lessor's investment.

In general, a financial lease cannot be canceled unless the lessor is completely paid off. Also, the lessee generally pays the property taxes and insurance on the leased property. Since the lessor receives a return *after,* or *net of,* these payments, this type of lease is often called a "net, net" lease.

Although the distinction between operating and financial leases has historical significance, today many lessors offer leases under a wide variety of terms. Therefore, in practice, leases often do not fit exactly into the operating lease or financial lease category but, rather, combine some features of each. To illustrate, cancellation clauses are normally associated with operating leases, but some of today's financial leases also contain cancellation clauses. However, in financial leases these clauses generally include prepayment provisions whereby the lessee must make penalty payments sufficient to enable the lessor to recover some portion of the unamortized cost of the leased property.

Self-Test Questions:

What is the difference between an operating lease and a financial lease?

What is a sale and leaseback?

Tax and Third Party Payer Effects

For both investor-owned and not-for-profit health care firms, tax and third party payer effects can play an important role in the lease-versus-buy decision.

Tax effects

For investor-owned firms, the full amount of lease payments is a tax-deductible expense for the lessee *provided that the Internal Revenue Service agrees that a particular contract is a genuine lease and not simply a loan that is called a lease.* This makes it important that a lease contract be written in a form acceptable to the IRS. A lease that complies with all of the IRS requirements is called a *guideline,* or *tax-oriented, lease.* In a guideline lease, ownership tax benefits accrue to the lessor, but the lessee's lease payments are fully tax deductible. A lease that does not meet the tax guidelines is called a *non-tax-oriented lease.* For this type of lease, the lessee can only deduct the implied interest portion of each lease payment. However, the lessee is effectively the owner of the leased equipment; thus, the lessee can take the tax depreciation.

The main provisions of the tax guidelines are as follows:

1. The lease term (including any extensions or renewals at a fixed rental rate) must not exceed 80 percent of the estimated useful life of the equipment at the commencement of the lease transaction. Thus, at the end of the lease, the equipment must have an estimated remaining life equal to at least 20 percent of its original life. Furthermore, the remaining useful life must not be less than one year. This requirement limits the maximum term of a lease to 80 percent of the asset's useful life. Note that an asset's useful life is normally much longer than its Modified Accelerated Cost Recovery Sytem (MACRS) depreciation class life.

2. The equipment's estimated value (in constant dollars without adjustment for inflation) at the expiration of the lease must equal at least 20 percent of its value at the start of the lease. Note that the estimated value of the asset at the end of the lease is called the *residual value.* This requirement also has the effect of limiting the maximum lease term.

3. Neither the lessee nor any related party can have the right to purchase the property from the lessor at a fixed price predetermined at the lease's inception. However, the lessee can be given a fair market value purchase option.

4. Neither the lessee nor any related party can pay or guarantee payment of any part of the price of the leased equipment. Simply put, the lessee cannot make any investment in the equipment, other than through the lease payments.

5. The leased equipment must not be "limited use" property, defined as equipment that can only be used by the lessee or a related party at the end of the lease.

The reason for the IRS's concern about lease terms is that, without restrictions, a company could set up a "lease" transaction calling for very rapid lease payments, which would be tax deductions. The effect would be to depreciate the equipment over a much shorter period than the IRS allows in its depreciation guidelines. For example, suppose that HealthSource, Inc., an investor-owned company that owns clinical laboratories in New Hampshire, Maine, Massachusetts, and Vermont, planned to acquire a $2 million computer which has a three-year MACRS class life. The annual depreciation allowances would be $660,000 in Year 1, $900,000 in Year 2, $300,000 in Year 3, and $140,000 in Year 4. If the firm were in the 40 percent federal-plus-state tax bracket, the depreciation would provide a tax savings of 0.40($660,000) = $264,000 in Year 1, $360,000 in Year 2, $120,000 in Year 3, and $56,000 in Year 4, for a total savings of $800,000. At a 6 percent discount rate, the present value of these tax savings would be $757,441.

Now suppose HealthSource could acquire the computer through a one-year lease arrangement with Bank of New England for a payment of $2 million, with a one dollar purchase option. If the $2,000,000 payment were treated as a lease payment, it would be fully deductible, so it would provide a tax saving of 0.40($2,000,000) = $800,000 versus a present value of only $757,441 for the depreciation shelters associated with ownership. Thus, the lease payment and the depreciation would both provide the same total amount of tax savings (40 percent of $2 million, or $800,000), but the savings would come in faster, and hence have a higher present value, with the one-year lease. Therefore, if just any type of contract could be called a lease and given tax treatment as a lease, then the timing of the tax shelters could be speeded up compared with ownership depreciation tax shelters. This speedup would benefit companies, but it would be costly to the government, and hence to individual taxpayers. For this reason, the IRS has established the rules described above for defining a lease for tax purposes.

Even though leasing can be used only within limits to speed up the effective depreciation schedule, there are still times when very substantial tax benefits can be derived from a leasing arrangement. For example, if an investor-owned hospital has a very large construction program that has generated so much accelerated depreciation that it has no current tax liabilities, then depreciation shelters are not very useful. In this case, a leasing company set up by a very profitable company like General Electric can buy the equipment, receive the depreciation shelters, and then share these benefits with the hospital by charging lower lease payments.[2] This issue will be discussed in detail later in the chapter, but the point to be made now is that if firms are to obtain tax benefits from leasing, the lease contract must be written in a manner that will qualify it as a true lease under IRS guidelines. Any questions about the tax status of a lease contract must be resolved by the lessee's lawyers prior to signing the contract.

Not-for-profit firms also benefit from tax laws, but in a different way. Since not-for-profit firms do not obtain tax benefits from depreciation, the ownership of assets has no tax value. However, lessors, which are taxable businesses, do benefit from ownership. In effect, when assets are owned by not-for-profit firms, the depreciation tax benefit is lost, while when assets are leased, the tax benefit is realized, but by the lessor rather than the lessee. This realized benefit, in turn, can be shared with the lessee in the form of lower rental payments. Note, however, that the cost of tax-exempt debt to not-for-profit firms can be lower than the after-tax cost of debt to taxable firms, so leasing is not automatically less costly to not-for-profit firms than borrowing in the tax-exempt markets and buying.

Third party payer effects

As we have discussed in other chapters, some third party payers reimburse providers, usually hospitals, for capital costs separately from operating costs. Such capital payments, which include reimbursement for interest expense, depreciation, and lease payments, are called *capital pass-through payments.* Just as tax effects can influence the lease versus buy decision, so can capital pass-through payments.

If a provider owns an asset, then any capital pass-through payments made will include reimbursement for the asset's depreciation, as well as for any interest expense associated with financing the asset, regardless of whether the provider is investor-owned or not-for-profit. If that same asset is leased, then the lessee will not be reimbursed for depreciation and interest expense because those costs are being borne by the lessor. Instead, the lessee will be reimbursed for the lease payments. Since capital pass-through payments are becoming rare, we will not include them in our examples. Recognize, however, that capital pass-through payments, if applicable, must be considered in any lease-versus-buy analysis.[3]

Self-Test Questions:

What is the difference between a tax-oriented lease and a non-tax-oriented lease?

What are some provisions that would make a lease non-tax-oriented?

Why should the IRS care about lease provisions?

What are capital pass-through payments, and should they be considered in a lease-versus-buy decision?

Financial Statement Effects

Under certain conditions, neither the leased asset nor the liabilities under the lease contract appear on the lessee's balance sheet. For this reason, leasing is often called *off-balance sheet* financing. This point is illustrated in Table 16.1 by the balance sheets of two hypothetical firms, B and L. Initially, the balance sheets of both firms are identical, and they both have debt ratios of 50 percent. Next, each firm decides to acquire a fixed asset costing $100. Firm B borrows $100 and buys the asset, so both an asset and a liability go on its balance sheet, and its debt ratio rises from 50 percent to 75 percent. Firm L leases the equipment. The lease may call for fixed charges as high or even higher than the loan, and the obligations assumed under the lease may have equal or even more potential to force the firm into bankruptcy, but the firm's debt ratio remains at only 50 percent.

To correct this problem, accountants require firms that enter into financial leases to restate their balance sheets to report the leased asset as a fixed asset and the present value of the future lease payments as a liability. This process is called *capitalizing* the lease, and hence such a lease is called a *capital lease.* The net effect of capitalizing the lease is to cause Firms B and L to have similar balance sheets, both of which will, in essence, resemble the one shown for Firm B.[4]

The logic here is as follows. If a firm signs a capital lease contract, its obligation to make lease payments is just as binding as if it had signed a loan agreement: the failure to make lease payments has the potential to bankrupt a firm just as the failure to make principal and interest payments on a loan can result in bankruptcy. Therefore, under most circumstances, a capital lease has the same impact on a firm's financial condition as does a loan. This being the case, if a firm signs a capital lease agreement, this has the effect of raising its effective debt ratio. Therefore, if the firm had previously established a target capital structure, and if there is no reason to think that the optimal capital structure has changed, then using lease financing requires additional equity support exactly like debt financing.

Table 16.1   Effects of Leasing on Balance Sheets

Before Asset Increase:

Firms B and L

Current assets	$ 50	Debt	$ 50
Fixed assets	50	Equity	50
Total assets	$100		$100
Debt/assets ratio			50%

After Asset Increase:

Firm B, Which Borrows and Buys

Current assets	$ 50	Debt	$150
Fixed assets	150	Equity	50
Total assets	$200		$200
Debt/assets ratio			75%

Firm L, Which Leases

Current assets	$ 50	Debt	$ 50
Fixed assets	50	Equity	50
Total assets	$100		$100
Debt/assets ratio			50%

Note, however, that there are some legal differences between loans and leases, mostly involving the rights of lessors versus lenders when a company in financial distress reorganizes or liquidates. In most financial distress situations, lessors fare better than lenders, so lessors may be more willing to deal with firms in poor financial condition than are lenders. At a minimum, lessors may be willing to accept lower rates of return than lenders when dealing with financially distressed firms since risks are lower.

If disclosure of the lease in our Table 16.1 example were not made, then Firm L's investors could be deceived into thinking that its financial position is stronger than it really is. Thus, even before firms were required to place financial leases on the balance sheet, they were required to disclose the existence of long-term leases in footnotes to their financial statements. At that time, whether or not investors recognized fully the impact of leases was debated—whether, in effect, they would see that Firms B and L were in essentially the same financial position. Some people argued that leases were not fully recognized, even by sophisticated investors. The question of whether investors were truly deceived was debated but never resolved. Those who believe strongly in efficient markets thought that investors were not deceived and that footnotes were sufficient, while those who questioned market efficiency thought that all leases should be capitalized. Current accounting requirements represent a compromise between these two positions, though one that is tilted heavily toward those who favor capitalization.

A lease is classified as a capital lease, and thus is capitalized and shown directly on the balance sheet, if one or more of the following conditions exist:

- Under the terms of the lease, ownership of the property is effectively transferred from the lessor to the lessee.

- The lessee can purchase the property at less than its true market value when the lease expires.

- The lease runs for a period equal to or greater than 75 percent of the asset's life. Thus, if an asset has a ten-year life and the lease is written for eight years, the lease must be capitalized.

- The present value of the lease payments is equal to or greater than 90 percent of the initial value of the asset. The discount rate used to calculate the present value of the lease payments must be the lower of (1) the rate used by the lessor to establish the lease payments (this rate is discussed later in the chapter) or (2) the rate of interest that the lessee would have to pay for new debt with a maturity equal to that of the lease. Also note that any maintenance payments embedded in the lease payment must be stripped out prior to checking this condition.

These rules, together with strong footnote disclosure rules for operating leases, are sufficient to ensure that no one will be fooled by lease financing. In effect, a financial lease for a particular asset has the same economic consequences for the firm as does a loan in which the asset is pledged as collateral. Thus, leases are regarded as debt for capital structure purposes, and they have roughly the same effects as debt on the financial condition of the firm.

In closing, note that the rules that accountants follow in making the decision of whether or not to capitalize a lease are not identical to the rules that the IRS follows to decide whether or not the lease is a guideline lease. In most cases, however, leases that meet IRS guidelines are operating leases that will not be capitalized, while leases that do not meet IRS guidelines are financial leases that will be capitalized. Remember, however, that even operating (noncapitalized) leases must be disclosed in the footnotes to the firm's financial statements.

Self-Test Questions:

Why is lease financing sometimes called "off-balance sheet financing"?
How are leases treated by accountants?

Evaluation by the Lessee

Leases are evaluated by both the lessee and the lessor. The lessee must determine whether leasing an asset is less costly than obtaining equivalent alternative financing and buying the asset, and the lessor must decide what the lease payments must be to produce a rate of return consistent with the riskiness of the investment. This section focuses on the analysis by the lessee.

In the typical case, the events leading to a lease arrangement follow the sequence described next. We should note that a degree of uncertainty exists regarding the theoretically correct way to evaluate lease-versus-purchase decisions, and some very complex decision models have been developed to aid in the analysis. However, the simple analysis given here, coupled with judgment, is sufficient to avoid situations where a lessee enters into a lease agreement that is clearly not in its best interests.

1. The firm decides to acquire a particular building or piece of equipment; this decision is based on the standard capital budgeting procedures discussed in Chapters 10 and 11. The decision to acquire the asset is not at issue in the typical lease analysis—this decision was made previously as part of the capital budgeting process. In lease analysis, we are concerned simply with whether to obtain the use of the asset by lease or by purchase.

2. Once the firm has decided to acquire the asset, the next question is how to finance its acquisition. A well-run business does not have excess cash lying around and, even if it does, there are opportunity costs associated with its use.

3. Funds to purchase the asset could be obtained by borrowing, by retaining earnings, or, if the firm is investor owned, by selling new equity. If the firm is not-for-profit, perhaps the funds could be raised by soliciting contributions for the project. Or, some combination of these sources could be used. Alternatively, the asset could be leased. Because of the capitalization/disclosure provisions for leases, leasing is assumed to have the same impact on a firm's financial condition as debt financing (borrowing).

As indicated earlier, a lease is comparable to a loan in the sense that the firm is required to make a specified series of payments, and that failure to meet these payments could result in bankruptcy. Thus, the most appropriate comparison when making lease decisions is the cost of lease financing versus the cost of debt financing, *regardless of how the asset actually would be financed if it were not leased.* The asset may be purchased with available cash if not leased or financed by a new equity sale or a cash contribution, but since leasing is a substitute for debt financing, the appropriate comparison would still be to debt financing.

To illustrate the basic elements of lease analysis, consider this simplified example. Nashville Radiology Group (NRG) requires the use of an asset for two years that costs $100, and the Group must choose between leasing and buying the asset. (The actual cost is $100,000, but let's keep the numbers simple.) If the asset is purchased, the bank would lend NRG the $100 at a rate of 10 percent on a two-year, simple interest loan. Thus, the firm would have to pay the bank $10 in interest at the end of each year, plus return the $100 in principal at the end of Year 2. For simplicity, assume that NRG could depreciate the asset over two years for tax purposes by the straight line method if it were purchased, resulting in tax depreciation of $50 in each year. Also for simplicity, assume that the asset's value at the end of two years (its residual value) is estimated to be $0.

Alternatively, the Group could lease the asset under a guideline lease for two years for a payment of $55 at the end of each year. Finally, assume that none of NRG's revenues come from third party payers making separate capital payments, so there are no capital pass-through cash flows to consider, and NRG's tax rate is 40 percent. The analysis for the lease-versus-buy decision consists of (1) estimating the cash flows associated with borrowing and buying the asset, that is, the flows associated with debt financing, (2) estimating the cash flows associated with leasing the asset, and (3) comparing the two financing methods to determine which has the lower cost. Here are the borrow-and-buy flows:

Cash Flows if NRG Buys	*Year 0*	*Year 1*	*Year 2*
Equipment cost	($100)		
Loan amount	100		
Interest expense		($10)	($ 10)
Tax savings from interest		4	4
Principal repayment			(100)
Tax savings from depreciation		20	20
Net cash flow	$ 0	$14	($ 86)

The net cash flow is zero in Year 0, positive in Year 1, and negative in Year 2. Since the operating cash flows (the revenues and operating costs) will be the same regardless of whether the asset is leased or purchased, they can be ignored. Cash flows that are not affected by the decision at hand are *nonincremental* to the decision.

Here are the cash flows associated with the lease:

Cash Flows if NRG Leases	*Year 0*	*Year 1*	*Year 2*
Lease payment		($55)	($55)
Tax savings from payment	___	22	22
Net cash flow	$0	($33)	($33)

Note that the two sets of cash flows reflect the tax savings associated with interest expense, depreciation, and lease payments, as appropriate. If the lease had not met IRS guidelines, then ownership would effectively reside with the lessee, and NRG would depreciate the asset for tax purposes whether it was "leased" or purchased. Furthermore, only the implied interest portion of the lease payment would be tax deductible. Thus, the analysis for a nonguideline lease would consist of simply comparing the after-tax financing flows on the loan with the after-tax lease payment stream.

To compare the cost streams of buying and leasing, we must put them on a present value basis. As we explain later, the correct discount rate is the after-tax cost of debt, which for NRG is $10\% (1 - T) = 10\% (1 - 0.4) = 6.0\%$. Applying this rate, we find the present value cost of buying to be $63.33, and the present value cost of leasing to be $60.50. Since leasing has the lower present value of costs, it is the less costly financing alternative and the Group should lease the asset.

This simplified example shows the general approach used in lease analysis, and it also illustrates a concept that can simplify the cash flow estimation process. Look back at the loan-related cash flows if NRG buys the asset. The after-tax loan-related flows are −$6 in Year 1 and −$106 in Year 2. When these flows are discounted to Year 0 at the 6.0 percent after-tax cost rate, their present value is −$100, the negative of the loan amount shown in Year 0. This equality results because we first used the cost of debt to estimate the future financing flows, and we then used this same rate to discount the flows back to Year 0, all on an after-tax basis. In effect, the loan amount positive cash flow and the loan cost negative cash flows cancel one another out. Here is the cash flow stream associated with buying the asset after the Year 0 loan amount and the related Year 1 and Year 2 flows have been removed:

Cash Flows if NRG Buys	Year 0	Year 1	Year 2
Cost of asset	($100)		
Tax savings from payments	_____	$20	$20
Net cash flow	($100)	$20	$20

The present value cost of buying here is, of course, $63.33, the same number we found earlier. This result will always occur regardless of the specific terms of the debt financing: as long as the discount rate is the after-tax cost of debt, the cash flows associated with the loan can be ignored.

To examine a more realistic example of lease analysis, consider the following lease-versus-buy decision facing the Nashville Radiology Group:

1. NRG plans to acquire a new computer system which will automate the Group's clinical records as well as its accounting, billing, and collection process. The computer has an economic life of eight years and costs $200,000, delivered and installed. However, NRG plans to lease the equipment for only four years, because it believes that computer technology is changing rapidly, and it wants the opportunity to reevaluate the situation at that time.

2. NRG can borrow the required $200,000 from its bank at a before-tax cost of 10 percent.

3. The computer's estimated scrap value is $5,000 after eight years of use, but its estimated residual value when the lease expires after four years of use is $20,000. Thus, if NRG buys the equipment, it would expect to receive $20,000 before taxes when the equipment is sold in four years.

4. NRG can lease the equipment for four years at a rental charge of $57,000, payable at the beginning of each year, but the lessor will own the equipment upon the expiration of the lease. (The lease payment schedule is established by the potential lessor, as described in the next major section, and NRG can accept it, reject it, or negotiate.)

5. The lease contract stipulates that the lessor will maintain the computer at no additional charge to NRG. However, if the Group borrows

and buys the computer, it will have to bear the cost of maintenance, which would be performed by the equipment manufacturer at a fixed contract rate of $2,500 per year, payable at the beginning of each year.

6. The computer falls in the MACRS five-year class life, the Group's marginal tax rate is 40 percent, and the lease qualifies as a guideline lease under a special IRS ruling.

7. None of NRG's payers reimburse the Group for capital expenses by making capital pass-through payments.

Dollar cost analysis

Table 16.2 shows the steps involved in a complete dollar cost analysis. Again, our approach here is to compare the cost of owning (borrowing and buying) the computer to the cost of leasing the computer. All else the same, the lower cost alternative is preferable. Part I of the table is devoted to the costs of borrowing and buying. Here, Line 1 gives the equipment's cost and Line 2 shows the maintenance expense; both are cash costs, or outflows. Note that whenever an analyst is setting up cash flows on a time line, the first decision that must be made is what time interval will be used, that is, months, quarters, years, or some other period. As a starting point, we generally assume that all cash flows occur at the end of each year. If, at some point later in the analysis, we conclude that another interval is better, we change. Longer intervals, such as years, simplify the analysis, but introduce some inaccuracies because all cash flows do not actually occur at year end. For example, tax benefits occur quarterly, because businesses pay taxes on a quarterly basis. On the other hand, shorter intervals, such as months, complicate the model and often imply a degree of forecasting accuracy that just does not exist.

Line 3 gives the maintenance tax savings: since maintenance expense is tax deductible, NRG saves 0.40 ($2,500) = $1,000 in taxes by virtue of paying the maintenance fee. Line 4 contains the depreciation tax savings, which is the depreciation expense times the tax rate. For example, the MACRS allowance for the first year is 20 percent, so the depreciation expense is 0.20($200,000) = $40,000 and the depreciation tax savings is 0.40 ($40,000) = $16,000.

Lines 5 and 6 contain the residual value cash flows. The residual value is estimated to be $20,000, but the tax book value after four years of depreciation is $34,000, so the Group is losing $14,000 for tax purposes, which results in a 0.40 ($14,000) = $5,600 tax savings, which is shown as

Table 16.2 Lessee's Dollar Cost Analysis

	Year 0	Year 1	Year 2	Year 3	Year 4
I. Cost of Owning (Borrowing and Buying)					
1. Net purchase price	($200,000)				
2. Maintenance cost	(2,500)	($ 2,500)	($ 2,500)	($ 2,500)	
3. Maintenance tax savings	1,000	1,000	1,000	1,000	
4. Depreciation tax savings		16,000	25,600	15,200	$ 9,600
5. Residual value					20,000
6. Residual value tax					5,600
7. Net cash flow	($201,500)	$14,500	$24,100	$13,700	$35,200
8. PV cost of owning =	($126,987)				
II. Cost of Leasing					
9. Lease payment	($ 57,000)	($57,000)	($57,000)	($57,000)	
10. Tax savings	22,800	22,800	22,800	22,800	
11. Net cash flow	($ 34,200)	($34,200)	($34,200)	($34,200)	$ 0
12. PV cost of leasing =	($125,617)				

III. Cost Comparison

13. Net advantage to leasing (NAL) = PV cost of leasing − PV cost of owning

$$= -\$125,617 - (-\$126,987) = \underline{\$1,370}.$$

Notes:

a. The MACRS depreciation allowances are 0.20, 0.32, 0.19, and 0.12 in Years 1 through 4, respectively.

b. In practice, a lease analysis such as this would be done using a spreadsheet program.

an inflow. Line 7, which sums the component cash flows, contains the net cash flows associated with borrowing and buying.

Part II of Table 16.2 contains an analysis of the cost of leasing. The lease payments, shown on Line 9 are $57,000 per year; this rate, which includes maintenance, was established by the prospective lessor and offered to NRG. If the Group accepts the lease, the full amount will be a deductible expense, so the tax savings, shown on Line 10, is 0.40(Lease payment) = 0.40($57,000) = $22,800. The net cash flows associated with leasing are shown on Line 11.

The final step is to compare the net cost of owning with the net cost of leasing. However, we must first put the annual cash flows associated with owning and leasing on a common basis. This requires converting them to present values, which brings up the question of the proper rate at which to discount the net cash flows. We know that the riskier the cash flows, the higher will be the discount rate used to find the present value. This same principle was observed in our discussion of security valuation and capital budgeting, and it applies to all discounted cash flow analyses, including lease analysis. Just how risky are the cash flows under consideration here? Most of them are relatively certain, at least when compared with the types of cash flow estimates associated with stock investments or with NRG's operating cash flows. For example, the loan payment schedule is set by contract, as is the lease payment schedule. The depreciation expenses are also established by law and not subject to change, and the annual maintenance fee is fixed by contract as well. The tax savings are somewhat uncertain, but they will be as projected so long as NRG's marginal tax rate remains at 40 percent. The residual value is the least certain of the cash flows, but even here, NRG's management is fairly confident because the estimated residual value distribution is relatively tight.

Since the cash flows under the lease and under the borrow-and-purchase alternatives are both relatively certain, they should be discounted at a relatively low rate. Most analysts recommend that the company's cost of debt financing be used, and this rate seems reasonable in our example. However, NRG's cost of debt, 10 percent, must be adjusted to reflect the tax deductibility of interest payments since this benefit of borrowing and buying is not accounted for in the cash flows. Thus, NRG's effective cost of debt becomes (Before-tax cost)$(1 - $ Tax rate$) = 10\%(0.6) = 6.0\%$. Accordingly, the cash flows in Lines 7 and 11 are discounted at a 6.0 percent rate. The resulting present values are $126,987 for the cost of owning and $125,617 for the cost of leasing, as shown on Lines 8 and 12. Leasing is the lower cost financing alternative, so NRG should lease, rather than buy, the computer.

The cost comparison can be formalized by defining the *net advantage to leasing (NAL)* as follows:

$$NAL = \text{PV cost of leasing} - \text{PV cost of owning}$$
$$= -\$125,617 - (-\$126,987) = \$1,370.$$

Since leasing is advantageous—the *NAL* is positive—NRG should lease the equipment. The *NAL* tells us that the value of NRG is increased by $1,370 if the Group leases, rather than buys, the computer.[5]

Percentage cost analysis

NRG's lease-versus-buy decision can also be analyzed by looking at the effective cost rate on the lease, and comparing it to the effective cost rate on the loan. Here we know the after-tax cost of debt, 6.0 percent, so we must find the after-tax cost rate implied in the lease contract and compare it with the cost of the loan. Signing a lease is similar to signing a loan contract: the firm has the use of equipment, but it must make a series of payments under either type of contract. We know the rate built into the loan; it is 6.0 percent. If the after-tax cost rate in the lease is less than 6.0 percent, then there is an advantage to leasing.

Table 16.3 sets forth the cash flows needed to determine the percentage cost of the lease. Here is an explanation of the table:

1. The first step is to calculate the lease-versus-own cash flows. To do this, we merely subtract the owning cash flows, Line 7 from Table 16.2, from the leasing cash flows, Line 11 from Table 16.2. The differences are the cash flows that NRG obtains if it leases rather than buys the computer.

2. Note that Table 16.3 consolidates the analysis shown in Table 16.2 into a single set of cash flows. At this point, we can discount the consolidated cash flows shown on Line 3 by 6.0 percent to obtain the NAL, $1,370. In Table 16.2, we discounted the owning and leasing cash flows separately, and then subtracted their present values to obtain the NAL. In Table 16.3, we subtracted the cash flows first to obtain a single set of flows, and then found their present value. The end result is the same.

3. The consolidated cash flows provide a good insight into the economics of leasing. If NRG leases the computer, it avoids the Year 0 cash outlay required to buy the equipment, but it is then obligated to a series of cash outflows in Years 1 through 4.

4. By inputting the leasing versus owning cash flows listed in Table 16.3 into the cash flow registers of a calculator and solving for IRR, or by using a spreadsheet's @IRR function, we can find the cost rate inherent in the cash flow stream: it is 5.6 percent. This is the equivalent after-tax cost rate implied in the lease contract. Since this cost rate is less than the 6.0 percent after-tax cost of a regular loan, leasing is cheaper than borrowing and buying. Thus, the percentage cost analysis confirms the NAL analysis.

Table 16.3 Lessee's Percentage Cost Analysis

	Year 0	Year 1	Year 2	Year 3	Year 4
1. Leasing cash flow	($ 34,200)	($34,200)	($34,200)	($34,200)	$ 0
2. Less: Owning cash flow	(201,500)	(14,500)	(24,100)	(13,700)	(35,200)
3. Leasing versus owning CF	$167,300	($48,700)	($58,300)	($47,900)	($35,200)

NAL = $1,370.
IRR =   5.6%.

Some additional points about the lessee's analysis

So far, we have discussed the main features of a lessee's analysis. However, before we move on to the lessor, note the following points:

1. The dollar cost and percentage cost approaches will always lead to the same decision. Thus, one method is as good as the other from a decision standpoint.

2. If the net residual value cash flow (residual value and tax effect) is considered to be much riskier than the other cash flows in the analysis, it is possible to account for this risk by applying a higher discount rate to this flow, which results in a lower present value. Since the net residual value flow is an inflow in the cost of owning analysis, a lower present value leads to a higher present value cost of owning. Thus, increasing residual value risk decreases the attractiveness of owning an asset.

   To illustrate, assume that NRG's managers believe that the computer's residual value is much riskier than the other flows in Table 16.2. Furthermore, they believe that 10.0 percent, rather than 6.0 percent, is the appropriate discount rate to apply to the residual value flows. When the Table 16.2 analysis is modified to reflect this risk, the present value cost of owning increases to $129,780, while the NAL increases to $4,163. The riskier the residual value, all else the same, the more favorable leasing becomes, because residual value risk is borne by the lessor.

3. Remember that net present value (NPV) is the dollar present value of a project assuming that it is financed using debt and equity financing. In lease analysis, the NAL is the additional dollar present value of a project attributable to leasing, as opposed to conventional financing. Thus, as an approximation of the value of a leased asset to the firm, the project's *NPV* can be increased by the amount of *NAL*:

$$\text{Adjusted } NPV = NPV + NAL.$$

The value added through leasing, in some cases, can turn unprofitable (negative NPV) projects into profitable (positive adjusted NPV) projects.

Self-Test Questions:

Explain how the cash flows are structured in conducting a dollar-based (NAL) analysis.

What discount rate should be used when lessees perform lease analyses?

What is the economic interpretation of the net advantage to leasing?

What is the economic interpretation of a lease's IRR?

Evaluation by the Lessor

Thus far we have considered leasing only from the lessee's viewpoint. It is also useful to analyze the transaction as the lessor sees it: Is the lease a good investment for the party that *writes* the lease (i.e., the party that must put up the money to buy the asset)? The lessor will generally be a specialized leasing company, a bank or bank affiliate, or a manufacturer such as General Electric Medical Systems that uses leasing as a sales tool.

Any potential lessor needs to know the rate of return on the capital invested in the lease, and this information is also useful to the prospective lessee: lease terms on large leases are generally negotiated, so the lessor and the lessee should know one another's position. The lessor's analysis involves (1) determining the net cash outlay, which is usually the invoice price of the leased equipment less any lease payments made in advance; (2) determining the periodic cash inflows, which consist of the lease payments minus both income taxes and any maintenance expense the lessor must bear; (3) estimating the after-tax residual value of the property when the lease expires; and (4) determining whether the rate of return on the lease is adequate for the risk of the investment.

To illustrate the lessor's analysis, we assume the same facts as for the NRG lease, as well as this situation: (1) The potential lessor is Medicomp, Inc., a commercial leasing company that specializes in leasing computers to health care providers. Medicomp's marginal federal-plus-state tax rate is 40 percent. (2) To provide maintenance to NRG, Medicomp must contract with the computer manufacturer under the same terms available to NRG, that is, $2,500 at the beginning of each year. (3) Medicomp views computer lease arrangements as relatively low-risk investments. There is, however, some small chance of default on the lease, so Medicomp typically assumes that a lease investment is about as risky as buying AA-rated corporate bonds. Since four-year AA-rated bonds are yielding about 9 percent, Medicomp could earn an after-tax yield of $(9.0\%)(1 - T) = (9.0\%)(0.6) = 5.4\%$ on such investments. This is the after-tax return that Medicomp can obtain on alternative investments of similar risk.

The lease analysis from the lessor's standpoint is developed in Table 16.4. Here we see that the cash flows to the lessor are similar to those for the lessee shown in Table 16.2. Line 1 contains the purchase price of the computer, $200,000. Line 2 contains the maintenance costs, while Line 3 lists the tax savings attributable to these costs. Line 4 contains the depreciation tax savings, or tax shields, that accrue to the owner of the computer. On Line 5, we show the annual lease rental payment as an inflow, while the taxes that must be paid on the rental payments are shown in Line 6. Lines 7 and 8 contain the residual value and resulting taxes (tax savings in this case). Finally, the cash flows are summed in Line 9.

The net present value (NPV) of the lease to Medicomp can be easily found by discounting the Line 9 cash flows at the firm's after-tax opportunity cost of capital, 5.4 percent, and then summing the resultant present values. For Medicomp, the NPV of the lease investment is $815, which means that the firm is somewhat better off, on a present value basis, if it writes the lease rather than invests in comparable-risk AA-rated bonds. Conversely, if the NPV of the lease were negative, Medicomp would be better off investing in the bonds. Since we saw earlier that the lease is also advantageous to NRG, the transaction is beneficial to both parties.

We can also calculate Medicomp's expected percentage rate of return on the lease by finding the IRR of the net cash flows shown on Line 9 of Table 16.4. Simply use the IRR function on a financial calculator, or a spreadsheet's @IRR function. The answer is 5.6 percent. Thus, the lease provides a 5.6 after-tax return to Medicomp, which exceeds the 5.4 percent after-tax return available on alternative investments of similar

Table 16.4   Lessor's Analysis

	Year 0	Year 1	Year 2	Year 3	Year 4
1. Net purchase price	($200,000)				
2. Maintenance cost	(2,500)	($ 2,500)	($ 2,500)	($ 2,500)	
3. Maintenance tax savings	1,000	1,000	1,000	1,000	
4. Depreciation tax savings		16,000	25,600	15,200	$ 9,600
5. Lease payment	57,000	57,000	57,000	57,000	
6. Tax on lease payment	(22,800)	(22,800)	(22,800)	(22,800)	
7. Residual value					20,000
8. Tax on residual value					5,600
9. Net cash flow	($167,300)	$48,700	$58,300	$47,900	$35,200

NPV = $815.
IRR = 5.6%.

risk, AA-rated four-year bonds. So, using either the dollar rate of return (NPV) method or the percentage rate of return (IRR) method, the lease appears to be a satisfactory investment for Medicomp.

Note, however, that the lease investment is actually slightly more risky than the alternative bond investment because the residual value cash flow is less certain than a principal repayment. Thus, Medicomp would probably require a rate of return somewhat above the 5.4 percent promised on the bond investment, and the higher the risk of the residual value, the higher the required return. Also, note that the lessor's NPV analysis could be extended by using a higher discount rate on the residual value cash flows than used on the other flows. This would lower the NPV, and hence make the lease investment look less attractive vis-a-vis the bond investment.

Lease analysis symmetry

Stop for a moment and compare the cash flows in Tables 16.2 and 16.4. Upon examination, we find that the cash flows to the lessee and lessor are symmetrical. They differ in sign, but the values are the same. This symmetry occurs because there are only two parties to a lease transaction, and our example assumed that the parties would pay the same amount for the computer, and that they also paid taxes at the same rate, forecasted the same residual value, and so on. Thus, what is a cash inflow to one party becomes a cash outflow to the other. Taken one step further, if the cost of debt to the lessee equaled the opportunity cost to the lessor, then the NAL to the lessee would be equal, but opposite in sign, to the lessor's NPV. When there is symmetry between the lessor and the lessee (same tax rates, costs, and so on), leasing is a *zero-sum game*.[6] If the lease is attractive to the lessee, the lease is unattractive to the lessor, and vice versa. However, conditions are often such that leasing can provide net benefits to both parties. This situation arises because of asymmetries, generally in taxes, estimated residual values, or the ability to bear residual value risk. We will explore this issue in detail in a later section.

Setting the lease payment

In the preceding sections we evaluated the lease assuming that the lease payments had already been specified. However, as a general rule, in large leases the parties will sit down and work out the terms of the lease, including the size of the lease payments. In situations where the lease terms are not negotiable, which is often the case for small leases, the lessor must still go through the same type of analysis, setting terms which provide a target rate of return, and then offering these terms to the potential lessee on a take it or leave it basis.

Competition among leasing companies forces lessors to build market-related returns into their lease payment schedules. To illustrate all of this, suppose Medicomp, after examining other alternative investment opportunities, decides that the 5.4 percent return on the NRG lease is too low, and that the lease should provide an after-tax return of 6.0 percent. What lease payment schedule would provide this return?

To answer this question, note again that Table 16.4 contains the lessor's cash flow analysis. If the basic analysis is computerized, it is very easy to change the lease payment until the lease's NPV = $0 at a 6.0 percent discount rate or, equivalently, its IRR = 6.0 percent. We did this with our spreadsheet lease evaluation model, and found that the lessor must set the lease payment at $57,622 to obtain an expected after-tax rate of return of 6.0 percent. However, if this lease payment is not acceptable to NRG, then it may not be possible to strike a deal.

Leveraged lease analysis

When leasing began, only two parties were involved in a lease transaction—the lessor, which put up the front money, and the lessee, which used the asset. In recent years, however, a new type of lease, the *leveraged lease*, has come into widespread use. Under a leveraged lease, the lessor arranges to borrow all or part of the required funds, generally giving the lender a first mortgage on the plant or a lien on the equipment being leased. The lessor still receives the tax benefits associated with depreciation. However, the lessor now has a riskier position because of the use of debt financing. Leveraged leases are an important part of the financial scene today. Incidentally, whether or not a lease is leveraged is not important to the lessee; from the lessee's standpoint, the method of analyzing a proposed lease is unaffected by whether or not the lessor borrows part of the required capital.

The analysis in Table 16.4 can be easily modified if the lessor borrows all or part of the required $200,000, making the transaction a leveraged lease. First, we would add a set of lines to Table 16.4 to show the financing cash flows. The interest component would represent another tax deduction, while the loan repayment would constitute an additional cash outlay. The "initial cost" would be reduced by the amount of the loan. With these changes made, a new NPV and IRR could be calculated and used to evaluate whether or not the lease represents a good investment.

To illustrate, assume that Medicomp can borrow $100,000 of the $200,000 purchase price at a rate of 9 percent on a 4-year simple interest loan. Table 16.5 contains the lessor's leveraged lease analysis. Line 1 contains the unleveraged lease cash flows from Table 16.4, while the leveraging cash flows are shown on Lines 2 through 5. The net cash flows to Medicomp are shown on Line 6. The NPV of the leveraged lease is $815, which is the same as for the unleveraged lease.[7] Note, though, that the lessor has a net investment of only $67,300 on the leveraged lease compared to a net investment of $167,300 on the unleveraged lease. Therefore, the lessor could invest in a total of $167,300/$67,300 = 2.5 similar leveraged leases for the same $167,300 investment required to finance a single unleveraged lease, producing a total net present value of 2.5($815) = $2,038.

The effect of leverage on the lessor's return is also reflected in the leveraged lease's IRR. The IRR of the leveraged lease is 9.1 percent, which is substantially higher than the 5.6 percent after-tax return on the unleveraged lease.

Typically, leveraged leases provide lessors with higher expected rates of return (IRRs) and higher NPVs per dollar of invested capital than unleveraged leases. However, such leases are also riskier for the same reason that any leveraged investment is riskier. Since leveraged leases

Table 16.5   Leveraged Lease Analysis

	Year 0	Year 1	Year 2	Year 3	Year 4
1. Unleveraged cash flow	($167,300)	$48,700	$58,300	$47,900	$ 35,200
2. Loan amount	100,000				
3. Interest		(9,000)	(9,000)	(9,000)	(9,000)
4. Interest tax savings		3,600	3,600	3,600	3,600
5. Principal repayment					(100,000)
6. Net cash flow	($ 67,300)	$43,300	$52,900	$42,500	($ 70,200)

NPV = $815.
IRR =   9.1%.

are a relatively new development, no standard methodology has been developed for analyzing them in a risk/return framework. However, sophisticated lessors are now developing simulations similar to those described in Chapter 11. Then, given the apparent riskiness of the lease investment, the lessor can decide whether the returns built into the contract are sufficient to compensate for the risks involved.

Self-Test Questions:

What discount rate is used in a lessor's NPV analysis?

What is the economic interpretation of the lessor's NPV? Of the lessor's IRR?

What is meant by the term "lease analysis symmetry"? What impact does this symmetry have on the economic viability of leasing?

What is a leveraged lease? What is the usual impact of lease leveraging on the lessor's expected rate of return and risk?

Motivations for Leasing

We noted earlier that leasing is a zero-sum game unless there are differentials between the lessee and the lessor. In this section, we discuss some of the differentials that motivate lease agreements.

Tax differentials

Many leases are driven by tax differentials. Historically, the typical tax asymmetry arose between highly taxed lessors and lessees with sufficient tax shields (primarily depreciation) to drive their tax rates very low, even to zero. Here, the asset's depreciation tax benefits could be taken by the lessor and then this value shared with the lessee. However, many other possible tax motivations exist, including tax differentials between not-for-profit providers and investor-owned lessors as well as the alternative minimum tax, discussed next.

Taxable corporations are permitted to use accelerated depreciation and other tax shelters to reduce their actual taxes paid, but then to use straight line depreciation for stockholder reporting, and hence to report higher profits to shareholders than to the IRS. In the early 1980s, many very profitable companies reported high earnings yet paid little or no federal income taxes. The *alternative minimum tax (AMT)*, which is figured at 20 percent of profits *reported to shareholders*, is designed to force profitable companies to pay at least some taxes.

Many companies are exposed to heavy tax liabilities under the AMT, so they are looking for ways to reduce reported income. Leasing can be beneficial here: companies can use a relatively short period for the lease and consequently have a high annual payment, resulting in lower reported profits and a lower AMT liability. Note that the lease payments do not have to qualify as a deductible expense for regular tax purposes—all that is needed is that they reduce reported income as shown on a firm's income statement.

Lessors have designed spreadsheet models to deal with AMT considerations, and they are generating a substantial amount of leasing business as a direct result of the alternative minimum tax. Thus, one of the important motivations for leasing is tax differentials.

Ability to bear obsolescence (residual value) risk

Leasing is an attractive financing alternative for many high-tech items that are subject to rapid and unpredictable technological obsolescence. For example, assume that a small, rural hospital wants to acquire a magnetic resonance imaging (MRI) device. If it buys the MRI equipment, it is exposed to the risk of technological obsolescence. In a relatively short time, some new technology might be developed that makes the current system almost worthless, and this large economic depreciation could create a severe financial burden on the hospital. Since it does not use much equipment of this nature, the hospital would bear a great deal of risk if it buys the MRI device. Conversely, a lessor that specializes in state-of-the-art medical equipment might be exposed to significantly less risk. By purchasing and then leasing many different high-tech items, the lessor benefits from diversification—over time some items will lose more value then the lessor expected, but these losses will be offset by other items that retain more value than expected. Also, since leasing companies are especially familiar with the markets for used medical equipment, they can both estimate residual values better and negotiate better prices when the asset is resold than can a hospital. Since the lessor is better able to bear residual value risk than the hospital, the lessor could charge a premium for bearing this risk that is less than the premium inherent in ownership.

Some lessors also offer programs that guarantee that the leased asset is modified as necessary to keep it abreast of technological advancements. For an increased rental fee, lessors will provide upgrades to keep the leased equipment current regardless of the cost. To the extent that lessors are better able to forecast such upgrades, negotiate better terms from manufacturers, and, by greater diversification, control the risks involved with such upgrades, it may be cheaper for lessees to ensure state-of-the art equipment by leasing than by buying.

Ability to bear volume risk

A type of lease that is gaining popularity among health care providers is the *per procedure lease*. In this type of lease, instead of a fixed annual or monthly payment, the lessor charges the lessee a fixed amount for each procedure performed. For example, the lessor may charge the hospital $300 for every scan performed using a leased MRI device. Or it may charge $400 per scan for the first 100 scans in each month and $200 for each scan above 100. Since the hospital's reimbursement for MRI scans typically depends on usage, and since the per procedure lease changes the hospital's costs for the MRI from a fixed payment to a variable payment, the hospital's risk is reduced.

Conversely, the payment stream to the lessor is converted from a fixed stream to an uncertain stream, so the lessor's risk increases. This type of arrangement can be beneficial to both parties if the lessor is better able to bear the usage risk than the lessee. As before, if the lessor has written a large number of per procedure leases, then some of the leases will be more profitable than expected and some will be less profitable than expected, but if the lessor's expectations are unbiased, the aggregate return on all of the leases will be quite close to that expected.

Ability to bear project life risk

Leasing can also be attractive when a firm is uncertain about how long an asset will be needed. Again, consider the hospital industry. Hospitals sometimes offer services that are dependent on a single staff member—for example, a physician who does liver transplants. To support the physician's practice, the hospital might have to invest millions of dollars in equipment that can be used only for this particular procedure. The hospital will charge for the use of the equipment, and if things go as expected, the investment will be profitable. However, if the physician dies or leaves the hospital staff, and if no other qualified physician can be recruited to fill the void, then the project is dead and the equipment becomes useless to the hospital. In this situation, the annual usage may be quite predictable, but the need for the asset could suddenly cease. A lease with a cancellation clause would permit the hospital to simply return the equipment to the lessor. The lessor would charge something for the cancellation clause, because such clauses increase the riskiness of the lease to the lessor. The increased lease cost would lower the expected profitability of the project, but it would provide the hospital with an option to abandon the equipment, and such an option could have a value that exceeds the incremental cost of the cancellation clause. The leasing company would be willing to write this option because it is in a better position to remarket the equipment, either by writing another lease or by selling it outright.

Maintenance services

Some companies find leasing attractive because the lessor is able to provide maintenance services on favorable terms. For example, MEDTRANS, Inc., a for-profit ambulance and medical transfer service that operates in Pennsylvania, recently leased 25 ambulances and transfer vans. The lease agreement, with a large leasing company that specializes in purchasing, maintaining, and then reselling automobiles and trucks, permitted the replacement of an aging fleet that MED-TRANS had built up over seven years. "We are pretty good at providing emergency services and moving sick people from one facility to another, but we aren't very good at maintaining an automotive fleet," said MEDTRANS's CEO.

Lower information search costs

Leasing may be financially attractive for smaller firms that have limited access to debt markets. For example, a small, recently formed physician group practice may need to finance one or more diagnostic devices, such as an EKG machine. The group has no credit history, so it would be relatively difficult, and hence costly, for a bank to assess the group's credit risk. Some banks might think the loan is not even worth the effort, while others might be willing to make the loan, but the high cost of credit assessment will be built into the loan rate. On the other hand, Medical Equipment Leasing Company has a division which specializes in leasing to group practices. Their analysts have assigned credit ratings to hundreds of group practices, and it would be relatively easy for them to make the credit judgment. Thus, a specialized leasing company might be more willing to provide the financing, and charge lower rates because of lower credit analysis costs, than conventional lenders.

Lower risk in bankruptcy

Finally, leasing may be less expensive than buying to firms that are poor credit risks. As discussed earlier, in the event of financial distress leading to reorganization or liquidation, lessors generally have more secure claims than do lenders. Thus, lessors may be willing to write leases to firms with poor financial characteristics that are less costly than loans offered by lenders, if such loans are even available.

There are other reasons that might motivate firms to lease an asset rather than buy it. Often these reasons are difficult to quantify, so they cannot be easily incorporated into a numerical analysis. Nevertheless, a sound lease analysis must begin with a quantitative analysis, and then qualitative factors can be considered before making the final lease-or-buy decision.

Self-Test Questions:

What are some economic factors that motivate leasing? That is, what asymmetries might exist that make leasing beneficial to both lessors and lessees?

Would it ever make sense to lease an asset that has a negative NAL when evaluated by a conventional lease analysis? Explain.

Other Issues in Lease Analysis

Leasing terminology, the basic methods of analysis used by lessees and lessors, and some rationales for leasing were presented in the previous sections. However, some other issues associated with leasing also warrant discussion.

Estimated residual value

It is important to note that the lessor owns the property upon expiration of a lease; thus, the lessor has claim to the asset's residual value. Superficially, it would appear that if residual values are expected to be large, owning would have an advantage over leasing. However, this apparent advantage is usually eliminated by market forces. If expected residual values are large—as they may be under inflation for certain types of equipment and also if real estate is involved—competition between leasing companies will force lease rates down to the point where potential residual values are fully recognized in the lease payment. Thus, the existence of large residual values is not likely to result in materially higher costs for leasing.

Increased credit availability

There are those who argue that leasing has an advantage for firms that are seeking the maximum degree of financial leverage. First, it is sometimes argued that firms can obtain more money, and for longer terms, under a lease arrangement than under a loan secured by a specific piece of equipment. Second, since some leases do not appear on the balance sheet, lease financing has been said to give the firm a stronger appearance in a *superficial* credit analysis, and thus permits the firm to use more (or cheaper) debt financing than would be possible if it did not lease.

There may be some truth to these claims for smaller firms or for firms facing financial distress. However, since firms are required to capitalize financial leases and to report them on their balance sheets, and to disclose operating leases in the footnotes to the financial statements, this point is of questionable validity for any financially sound firm large enough to have audited financial statements.

Computer models

Lease analysis is particularly well-suited for computer analysis. Both the lessee and lessor can create computer models for their analyses. Setting the analysis up on a computer is especially useful when negotiations are under way. When investment banking houses such as Merrill Lynch are working out a leasing deal between a group of investors and a company, the analysis is always computerized.

Self-Test Questions:

Does leasing lead to increased credit availability?

Do larger residual values favor owning over leasing? Explain.

Summary

In this chapter, we discussed the leasing decision from the standpoints of both the lessee and lessor. The key concepts covered are listed below.

- Lease agreements are often categorized as (1) *operating leases* or (2) *financial,* or *capital, leases.*

- The IRS has specific guidelines that apply to lease arrangements. A lease that meets these guidelines is called a *guideline,* or *tax-oriented, lease* because the IRS permits the lessee to deduct the lease payments. A lease that does not meet IRS guidelines is called a *non-tax-oriented lease.* In these leases, ownership effectively resides with the lessee rather than the lessor.

- *FASB Statement 13* spells out the conditions under which a lease must be *capitalized* (shown directly on the balance sheet), as opposed to being shown only in the notes to the financial statements. Generally, leases that run for a period equal to or greater than 75 percent of the asset's life must be capitalized.

- The lessee's analysis consists basically of a comparison of the costs and benefits associated with leasing the asset and the costs and benefits associated with owning the asset. There are two analytical techniques that can be used: (1) the *dollar cost (NAL) method* and (2) the *percentage cost (IRR) method.*

- One of the key issues in the lessee's analysis is the appropriate discount rate. Since the cash flows in a lease analysis are known with relative certainty, the appropriate discount rate is the *lessee's after-tax cost of debt.* A higher discount rate may be used on the *residual value* if it is substantially riskier than the other flows.

- In a *lessor's analysis,* the return on a lease investment is compared with the return available on alternative investments of similar risk.

- In a *leveraged lease,* the lessor borrows part of the funds required to buy the asset. Generally, the asset is pledged as collateral for the loan.

- Leasing is motivated by differentials between lessees and lessors. Some of the more common reasons for leasing are (1) *tax rate differentials*, (2) *alternative minimum taxes*, (3) *residual risk bearing*, and (4) *lack of access* to conventional debt markets.

Notes

1. For more information about the motivating forces and extent of leasing in the hospital industry, see L. C. Gapenski and B. Langland-Orban, "Leasing Capital Assets and Durable Goods: Opinions and Practices in Florida Hospitals," *Health Care Management Review* (Summer 1991): 73–81.
2. In fact, General Electric has a subsidiary, GE Capital Corporation, which is one of the largest lessors in the world. The subsidiary was originally set up to finance consumers' purchases of GE's durable goods such as refrigerators and wash machines, but it has become a major player in the commercial loan and leasing markets.
3. See Note 5.
4. Financial Accounting Standards Board (FASB) Statement 13, "Accounting for Leases," spells out in detail both the conditions under which the lease must be capitalized and the procedures for capitalizing it. FASB is empowered by the American Institute of Certified Public Accountants to promulgate rules that form the basis of generally accepted accounting principles, which in turn guide the preparation of all financial statements.
5. If any of NRG's third party payers made capital pass-through payments, the analysis would be modified in two ways. First, capital pass-through payments on interest would lower NRG's effective cost of debt, so the discount rate (after-tax cost of debt) would be multiplied by $(1 - P)$, where P is the proportion of total interest offset by such payments. Second, the dollar amount of capital pass-through payments for depreciation attributable to the project, along with their tax consequences, would be included in the Table 16.2 analysis.
6. The zero-sum game feature of leasing can be useful in debugging lease analysis models. Whenever we build a new spreadsheet model that contains both lessee's and lessor's analyses, we test it by trying symmetrical input values for the lessee and lessor. If the lessee's NAL and lessor's NPV are not equal but opposite in sign, there is something wrong with the model!
7. In this situation, leveraging had no impact on the lessor's per-lease NPV. This is because the cost of the loan to the lessor (5.4 percent after taxes) equals the discount rate, and thus the leveraging cash flows are netted out on a present value basis.

Selected Additional References

Beggan, J. F., and L. K. McNulty. 1991. "Restrictions on Depreciation Where Tax-Exempt Entities are Involved." *Topics in Health Care Financing* (Fall): 62–69.

Berg, I. J., and A. N. Frankel. 1988. "Equipment Leasing: How, When, and If." *Health Progress* (15 November): 22–26.

Conbeer, G. P. 1990. "Leasing Can Add Flexibility to High-Tech Asset Management." *Healthcare Financial Management* (July): 26–34.

Dine, D. D. 1988. "Equipment Leasing Firms Offer Deals to Hospitals." *Modern Healthcare* (18 November): 50–51.

Grant, L., and D. O'Donnell. 1990. "Watch for Pitfalls When Analyzing Lease Options." *Healthcare Financial Management* (July): 36–43.

"Leasing: Three Experts Discuss the Advantages of Equipment Leasing." *HealthWeek* November 1989, 51–53.

Meyers, S. C., D. A. Dill, and A. J. Bautista. 1976. "Valuation of Financial Lease Contracts." *Journal of Finance* (June): 799–819.

Rosenthal, R. A. 1992. "Creative Leasing Strategies for Medical Office Buildings." *Healthcare Financial Management* (December): 30–34.

Case 16

Chicago Medical Center: Leasing Decisions

Chicago Medical Center is a 600-bed not-for-profit referral hospital associated with a large private university. The hospital is well known for its extensive medical research program, and to support the program it acquires millions of dollars of state-of-the-art equipment each year.

In the last several years, the hospital has been working diligently to perfect noninvasive brain surgery techniques. One of the most promising procedures involves stereotactic radiosurgery using a linear accelerator. This procedure allows the surgeon to effectively remove certain lesions in the brain without surgery. Stereotactic radiosurgery is especially useful in the treatment of arteriovenous malformations, but it can also be used to treat certain types of benign tumors and even some small malignant lesions. The main benefit to the patient is the significant reduction in the risk associated with surgery, because radiosurgery eliminates dangerous surgical procedures for patients with deeper lesions where the morbidity or mortality rate is substantial. Furthermore, patients who are considered too risky for surgery can be treated using stereotactic radiosurgery.

The procedure calls for a team approach including a neurosurgeon, radiation physicist, radiologist, and radiation therapist. The neurosurgeon selects the patients appropriate for the procedure and performs the stereotactic process required to localize the target area. The radiation physicist works with a computer program to compute the appropriate dosimetry, while the radiologist performs a CT scan, MRI scan, angiogram, or a combination of the three to help the neurosurgeon localize the lesion.

The dosimetry calculations are especially complex. Since differing thicknesses of skull and brain will attenuate the beam in varying amounts, the amount of radiation applied is highly dependent on where the lesion is located and the size and shape of the patient's skull. The actual application of the radiation generally takes only between 20 and 30 minutes, and the patient can be released from the hospital after only a short period of observation.

Chicago Medical Center plans to upgrade some of the equipment required for this procedure. The equipment has an invoice price of $1,275,000, including delivery and installation charges, and it falls into the modified accelerated cost recovery system (MACRS) five-year class, with current allowances of 0.20, 0.32, 0.19, 0.12, 0.11, and 0.06 in Years 1–6, respectively. The manufacturer of the equipment will provide a maintenance contract for $25,000 per year, payable at the beginning of each year, if the hospital decides to buy the equipment. If purchased, the equipment would be financed by a four-year simple interest bank note which would carry an interest rate of 10 percent.

Regardless of whether the equipment is purchased or leased, the hospital's managers do not think that it will be used for more than four years, at which time the hospital plans to open a new radiation therapy facility. Land on which to construct a larger facility has already been acquired, and the building should be ready for occupancy at that time. The new facility is designed to enable Chicago Medical Center to use several new radiosurgery procedures. Thus, the current equipment is viewed as a "bridge" to serve only until the new facility is ready four years from now. The expected physical life of the equipment is ten years, but medical equipment of this nature is subject to unpredictable technological obsolescence.

After considerable debate among the hospital's managers, they concluded that there is a 25 percent probability that the residual value will be $0, a 50 percent probability that it will be $200,000, and a 25 percent probability that it will be $600,000, which makes the residual value quite risky. However, the managers are not sure which residual value estimate should be used in the base case analysis; the most likely value of $200,000, or the expected value of $250,000. If the residual value is judged to have high risk, the hospital's normal procedure is to apply a 3 percentage point risk adjustment to the base discount rate used on the other lease analysis flows to obtain the appropriate rate for the residual value flows.

Great Lakes Capital (GLC), Inc., the leasing subsidiary of Great Lakes National Bank, has presented an initial offer to lease the equipment to the hospital for annual payments of $340,000, with the first payment due upon delivery and installation, and additional payments due at the beginning of each succeeding year of the four-year lease term. This price includes a service contract under which the equipment would be maintained in good working order. GLC would buy the equipment from the manufacturer under the same terms that were offered to the hospital, and GLC would have to enter into a maintenance contract with the manufacturer for $25,000 per year.

Unlike the hospital, GLC forecasts a $300,000 residual value. Their estimate is based on the following facts: (1) There is no competing equipment on the horizon that would make the equipment obsolete. (2) The equipment has a physical life estimated to be two and one-half times longer than the four-year lease term. (3) GLC is more skilled in selling used equipment than is Chicago Medical Center. GLC's federal-plus-state tax rate is 40 percent, and if the lease is not written, GLC could invest the funds in a four-year term loan of similar risk yielding 8.0 percent before taxes.

Pam Ridgeway, the hospital's CFO, has the final say on all of Chicago Medical Center's lease-versus-purchase decisions, but the actual analysis of the relevant data will be conducted by the hospital's capital funds manager, Tom Halvorson. In the past, Ridgeway and Halvorson tended to pretty much agree on analytical methodologies, but in discussing this lease analysis, they ended up in a heated discussion about the appropriate discount rate to use in calculating the present values of the cash flows.

Ridgeway argues that the cash flows associated with performing stereotactic radiosurgery are very uncertain. She is convinced that insurers are not going to be nearly as generous in the future as they have been in the past in funding such procedures, so the revenue stream is highly speculative. Furthermore, the negative influence of managed care plans on reimbursement rates will be accelerating in the future. Accordingly, she thinks that a high discount rate should be used in the analysis. Halvorson, on the other hand, believes that leasing is a substitute for other "financing," which means a blend of debt and fund capital. Consequently, he believes that the lease analysis cash flows should be discounted at the hospital's weighted average cost of capital. In addition to the discount rate dispute, there is also some disagreement about how the lease will be handled on the hospital's financial statements, so that has to be resolved.

Both Ridgeway and Halvorson believe that lessees should not blindly accept the first offer made by potential lessors, but rather that they conduct a complete analysis from the viewpoint of both parties, and then, using this knowledge, negotiate the best deal possible. Thus, it is important to know the range of lease payments that is acceptable to both parties.

There is a possibility that the hospital will move to its new radiation facility earlier than anticipated, and hence prior to the expiration of the lease. Furthermore, if the neurosurgeon who is the primary user of this procedure leaves the staff, there is some question about whether he could be replaced, and this could render the equipment useless. Thus, Ridgeway is considering asking GLC to include a cancellation clause in the lease contract. Under such a clause, the hospital would be able to return the equipment to GLC at any time during the lease term after giving a minimum two weeks notice. Before negotiations begin, the hospital must assess the impact of such a clause on the riskiness of the lease to both parties, and any consequences that it might have on the terms of the lease.

In addition to a cancellation clause, Ridgeway is aware that many lessors are now writing per-procedure leases, whereby the lease payment is based on the number of procedures performed rather than a fixed amount. She wonders whether the hospital might be better off negotiating for this type of lease, and what the consequences would be for both the lessee and lessor.

There is some chance that the hospital would be able to finance the equipment with tax-exempt debt issued by the Cook County Health Facilities Authority. If so, the cost of this tax-exempt (municipal) debt would be only 7 percent. To complicate matters even more, the hospital currently has over $2,000,000 in excess funds invested in marketable securities earning 4 percent that could be used to purchase the equipment.

Finally, Ridgeway's brother-in-law, who works at GLC, found out that GLC will probably obtain a $500,000, 9 percent, simple interest loan from its parent bank, which it will use to leverage the lease. Such leveraging could affect the hospital's ability to negotiate lower lease payments, so it is important that Chicago Medical Center understand its impact, both from the perspective of the lessee and the lessor.

17

Mergers and Acquisitions

$\mathbf{M}$ost of the growth in health care businesses occurs through internal expansion, which takes place when a firm's existing operations grow through normal capital budgeting activities. However, the most dramatic examples of growth result from mergers and acquisitions, the focus of this chapter. For legal and accounting purposes, there are distinctions between a merger and an acquisition, but those distinctions do not affect the fundamental business and financial considerations involved. Thus, we will not distinguish between the two, but instead we will refer to all combinations in which a single business unit is formed from two or more existing units as a *merger*. We will begin our discussion of mergers with some general background information. Later, we will focus on mergers in the health care industry, including a discussion of the factors that must be considered when investor-owned and not-for-profit firms merge.

Level of Merger Activity

To better understand mergers, it is useful to review the level of merger activity in the United States, including activity in the health care industry.

Merger waves

Five major *merger waves* have occurred in the United States. The first was in the late 1800s, when consolidations took place within the oil, steel, tobacco, and other basic industries. The second occurred in the 1920s, when the buoyant stock market helped promoters consolidate firms in a number of industries, including utilities, communications, and automobiles. The third was in the 1960s, when conglomerate mergers (mergers among unrelated firms) were the rage.

The fourth wave of mergers was the "merger mania" of the 1980s. This wave was fueled by many factors, including (1) the relatively depressed condition of the stock market at the beginning of the decade (in early 1982, the Dow Jones Industrial Index was below its 1968 level); (2) the unprecedented level of inflation that existed during the 1970s and early 1980s, which increased the replacement value of firms' assets; (3) a political climate that fostered a more tolerant attitude toward mergers; (4) the general belief among major natural resource companies that it was cheaper to "buy reserves on Wall Street" than to explore and find them in the field; (5) the development of an active junk bond market, which helped acquirers obtain the capital needed to do the deals; and (6) the decline of the dollar, which made U.S. firms relatively cheap for foreign firms to acquire, combined with huge U.S. trade deficits, which gave foreign firms large pools of funds to invest in the United States.

The final merger wave began in 1992, and in 1996 it is still going strong. The current wave is significantly different from the wave of the 1980s. Most 1980s mergers were primarily financial transactions in which buyers were seeking to acquire companies that were selling at less than their true value due to poor management. In the 1990s, however, most mergers are strategic in nature—companies are merging to enable the consolidated enterprise to better position itself to compete in the future. Indeed, many of the recent mergers have involved companies in the defense, media, computer, and health care industries, all of which are undergoing rapid structural change and intense competition.

Another major difference between mergers in the 1990s and those in the 1980s is the way in which they are financed and the form of payment to the acquired firms' stockholders. In the 1980s wave, cash was the preferred method of payment, because a cash tender offer that was large enough could convince even the most reluctant shareholders to approve the deal, and this put great pressure on the managements of firms being acquired. Moreover, the cash for the deal was generally obtained by borrowing, often with junk bonds, which gave the combined firm a heavy debt burden that left it vulnerable to economic downturns. In the current wave, the preferred method of payment has been the stock swap, because (1) there are fewer lenders willing to supply debt for mergers, and (2) in strategic mergers, it is easier to convince shareholders and managers of target companies that the merger should take place, so stock swaps are easier to sell. Also, in a stock swap, managers of target companies are much more motivated to work for the common good of the combined company if a merger does take place. Even the cash mergers have tended to be different: in the 1980s, companies typically borrowed the cash needed; but in the 1990s, corporate cash flows have often been high enough to fund acquisitions internally, especially smaller ones.

Merger activity in the health care industry

Prior to the current wave, mergers in the health care industry were not as frequent nor as large as mergers in some other industries. First, the health care industry, at least in its current form, is relatively new, not having really developed until after World War II. Second, the motivations that fueled the wave of the 1980s only partially applied to health care, so the industry was not one of the major participants in that wave (although there were some spectacular mergers between for-profit hospital chains). As seen in Table 17.1, however, merger activity in the health care industry is now off and running, and preliminary data for 1995 indicate another record year.

To illustrate some recent health care mergers, consider the following deals that were either announced or completed in 1995/96:

1. Aetna agreed to buy U.S. Healthcare for $8.9 billion in cash and stock. The deal, which would link the insurance giant with an aggressive HMO operator, would create the nation's largest managed care company.

2. Columbia/HCA Healthcare acquired Healthtrust for $5.6 billion. The deal added 116 hospitals to Columbia/HCA, giving the combined firm over 300 hospitals.

Table 17.1   Merger Activity in the Health Care Industry (millions of dollars)

Year	Number of Deals	Aggregate Value
1988	93	$14,593
1989	172	36,787
1990	215	10,438
1991	263	5,459
1992	404	8,091
1993	394	24,945
1994	406	44,808

Source: Fortune, 1995. (15 February).

3. National Medical Enterprises acquired American Medical International for $3.3 billion. The combined company, which is now the second largest hospital chain in the United States, has been renamed Tenet Healthcare.

4. American Healthcare Systems and Premier Health Alliance, two major hospital alliances, announced plans to merge. The combined alliance will serve over 1,400 hospitals, or about one-fourth of all community hospitals. It is expected that the alliance will buy about $8 billion annually in goods and services for its member hospitals.

5. Eli Lilly & Co. announced plans to acquire PCS Health Systems, a unit of McKesson Corporation, for $4 billion. PCS is a management company that oversees the drug benefits programs of major employers and health plans. The deal would give Lilly, a major drug manufacturer, entree to a growing business with potentially valuable information on prescription patterns. The acquisition would also give Lilly a captive distribution channel, although the Federal Trade Commission has indicated that anticompetitive behavior would cause the merger to be reviewed.

6. Abbey Healthcare Group and Homedco Group merged to form Apria Healthcare Group, a powerhouse in home health care. The $1.1 billion merger created a company that is the largest provider of home respiratory care and the second largest provider of home infusion services.

As can be seen from this list and Table 17.1, health care mergers are currently taking place at a dizzying pace.

The deal frenzy in the health care industry is occurring because providers are convinced that size is the key to success in the evolving health care market. This view is based on the trend toward managed care, in which buyers are grouping together as never before. HMOs are growing rapidly, worker groups are expanding and contracting as single entities, and insurers are combining to form increasingly formidable alliances. In response, providers are seeking greater size and scope of services to spread overhead, shift risk and, most importantly, to offer the full range of services required by large payers. Current thinking mandates that providers must offer more types of services over larger geographic areas at lower prices to gain market share, and hence ensure survival in changing market conditions. Furthermore, mergers fuel mergers because providers are afraid to sit on the sidelines while others are merging around them. Although the health care megamergers are occurring on the for-profit side, all providers are subject to the same industry trends, so there has also been considerable merger activity among not-for-profit providers, including mergers between investor-owned and not-for-profit firms.

Self-Test Questions:

What are the five major merger waves that have occurred in the United States?

What are the differences between the waves of the 1980s and the 1990s?

What is the factor fueling the current merger wave in the health care industry?

The Good, the Bad, and the Ugly: Motives for Mergers

In the previous section, we presented some factors that fueled merger waves in the past. In this section, we take a more detailed look at some of the motives behind business mergers, along with some views regarding the validity of these motives.

Synergy

From an economic perspective, the best motivation for mergers is to increase the value of the combined enterprise. If Companies A and B merge to form Company C, and if C's value exceeds that of A and B taken separately, then *synergy* is said to exist. When synergy drives a merger, value is created, and hence society benefits. Furthermore, such a merger can be beneficial to both A's and B's stockholders if the companies are investor owned.

Synergistic effects can arise from four sources: (1) *operating economies*, which result from economies of scale in management, marketing, contracting, operations, or distribution, including mergers that better position a firm strategically; (2) *financial economies*, including lower transactions costs, access to additional capital markets, and better coverage by security analysts; (3) *differential efficiency*, which implies that the management of one firm is inefficient, and that the firm's assets will be used more productively after the merger; and (4) *increased market power* due to reduced competition. Operating and financial economies are socially desirable, as are mergers that increase managerial efficiency. To some extent, increased market power can also be beneficial to society, such as the contracting savings that result when major purchasers buy health care services. However, too much market power can result in monopoly or monopsony power, which can be harmful to society, and hence is both undesirable and illegal.

Excess cash

Mergers are an easy, perhaps too easy, way for firms to get rid of excess cash. If a firm has a shortage of internal investment opportunities compared with its cash flow, it could (1) increase its dividend or repurchase stock if investor owned, (2) invest in marketable securities, or (3) purchase another firm. Marketable securities often provide a good temporary parking place for money, but generally the rate of return on such securities is less than the return on real asset investments.

Although there is nothing inherently wrong with using excess cash to buy other companies, the acquisition must create value to be economically worthwhile. Just making a company larger may benefit managers, but it does not necessarily benefit stockholders or society at large. If the return on a potential acquisition is not as high as the opportunity cost of the capital used, then the capital should be used for other purposes. If the firm is investor owned, the capital should be returned to the firm's investors, while if the firm is not-for-profit, it should be used to retire debt or invested temporarily until better uses can be found.

Purchase of assets at below replacement cost

Sometimes a firm will be touted as a possible acquisition candidate because the cost of replacing its assets is considerably higher than its market value. For example, suppose that a small, rural hospital can be acquired for $5 million, while the cost to construct a similar hospital from the ground up is $10 million. There might be a strong temptation to say that the hospital is a good "buy" because it can be bought for less than its replacement value.

However, the true value of any business should be based on its earning power, which sets the economic value of its assets. The real question, then, is not whether the hospital can be acquired for less than its replacement cost, but rather whether it can be acquired for less than its *economic value*, which is a function of the cash flows that the hospital is expected to produce in the future. If the rural hospital's earning power gives it a value of $7 million, then it is a good buy at $5 million, but this conclusion is based on economic, not replacement, value.

Diversification

Managers often claim that diversification into other lines of business is a reason for mergers. They contend that diversification helps to stabilize the firm's earnings stream, and thus benefits its owners. Stabilization of earnings is certainly beneficial to managers, employees, suppliers, customers, and other stakeholders, but its value is less certain from the standpoint of stockholders. If a stockholder is worried about the variability of a firm's earnings, he or she could diversify more easily than could the firm. Why should Firms A and B merge to stabilize earnings when a stockholder in Firm A could sell half of his or her stock in A and use the proceeds to purchase stock in Firm B? Stockholders can create diversification more easily than can the firm.

Also, if a stockholder is concerned about the relative performance of different industry segments, he or she can solve the problem more easily through portfolio diversification than can managers through mergers. For example, assume that a stockholder who holds primarily hospital stocks is concerned that the increased purchasing power of managed care plans will erode hospital profits, and hence value, over time. It is easier for the stockholder to purchase HMO stocks than it is for hospitals to diversify into managed care.

Of course, there are some situations where mergers for diversification do make sense from a stockholder's perspective. For example, if you were the owner-manager of a closely held firm, it might be nearly impossible for you to sell part of your stock to diversify, because this would dilute your ownership and perhaps also generate a large capital gains tax liability. In this case, a diversification merger might well be the best way to achieve personal diversification. Also, as mentioned earlier, diversification mergers that better position firms to deal with future events are worthwhile, because such mergers can create operating synergies.

Even though diversification, without synergy, does not benefit shareholders directly, it clearly benefits a firm's other stakeholders. Thus, diversification-motivated mergers can be beneficial to not-for-profit firms. Furthermore, stockholders can obtain indirect benefits from diversification, because making the firm less risky to managers, creditors, suppliers, customers, and the like, could have positive implications for shareholders' wealth.

Personal incentives

Economists like to think that business decisions are based only on economic considerations. However, there can be no question that some business decisions are based more on managers' personal motivations than on economic analyses. Many people, business leaders included, like power, and more power is attached to running a larger corporation than a smaller one. Obviously, no executive would ever admit that his or her ego was the primary reason behind a merger, but knowledgeable observers are convinced that egos do play a prominent role in many mergers. It has also been observed that executive salaries, prestige, and perquisites are highly correlated with company size—the bigger the company, the higher these executive benefits. This too could play a role in the aggressive acquisition programs of some corporations.

Managers' personal incentives as a basis for mergers constitute another example of the agency problem. Of course, there is nothing wrong with executives feeling good about increasing the size of their firms, or with their getting a better compensation package as a result of growth through mergers—provided the mergers make economic sense.

Self-Test Questions:

Define synergy. Is synergy a valid rationale for mergers? Describe several situations that might produce synergistic gains within the health care industry.

Suppose your firm could purchase another firm for only half of its replacement value. Would this be sufficient justification for the acquisition?

Discuss the merits of diversification as a rationale for mergers.

Can managers' personal incentives motivate mergers? Explain.

Types of Mergers

Economists have traditionally classified mergers into four groups: (1) horizontal, (2) vertical, (3) congeneric, and (4) conglomerate. A *horizontal merger* occurs when one firm combines with another in its line of business—for example, when one hospital acquires another, or one home health care firm merges with a second. The merger of Columbia/HCA Healthcare and Healthtrust was a horizontal merger, because both firms were in the hospital industry.

A *vertical merger* occurs when a company merges with a supplier. An example of a vertical merger is a drug manufacturer's acquisition of a pharmaceutical distribution company, such as Eli Lilly's acquisition of PCS Health Systems. Congeneric means "allied in nature or action";

hence, a *congeneric merger* involves related enterprises, but not producers of the same product (horizontal) or firms in a producer-supplier relationship (vertical). For example, in 1995, Madison Regional Medical Center, a not-for-profit hospital in Atlanta, acquired ProperCare, Inc., a local home health care agency. A *conglomerate merger* occurs when unrelated enterprises combine. Since all health care firms, at a minimum, are in related lines of business, mergers between such firms could not be classified as conglomerate.

Operating economies (and also anticompetitive effects) are at least partially dependent on the type of merger involved. Vertical and horizontal mergers generally provide the greatest synergistic operating benefits, but they are also the ones most likely to be attacked by federal or state authorities as anticompetitive. In any event, it is useful to think of these economic classifications when analyzing the feasibility of a prospective merger.

Self-Test Questions:

What are the four economic classifications of mergers?

Briefly describe the characteristics of each classification.

Hostile versus Friendly Takeovers

In the vast majority of merger situations, one firm (the *acquirer*) simply decides to another company (the *target*), negotiates a price with the target firm's management, and then acquires the company. Occasionally, the acquired firm will initiate the action, but it is much more common for a firm to seek acquisitions than to seek to be acquired.

Once an acquiring company has identified a possible target, it must (1) establish a suitable price, or range of prices; and (2) tentatively set the terms of payment—will it offer cash, its own common stock, bonds, or a mix of securities? Next, the acquiring firm's managers must decide how to approach the target company's managers. If the acquiring firm has reason to believe that the target's management will support the merger, then it will simply propose a merger and try to work out suitable terms. If an agreement is reached, then the two management groups will issue statements indicating that they approve the merger and, if the firms are investor owned, recommend that stockholders agree to the merger. Generally, the stockholders of acquiring firms must merely vote to approve the merger, but the stockholders of target firms are asked to tender (or send in) their shares to a designated financial institution, along with a signed power of attorney that transfers ownership of the shares to the acquiring firm. The target firm's stockholders then receive the specified payment, be it common stock of the acquiring company (in which case the target company's stockholders become stockholders of the acquiring company), cash, bonds, or some mix of cash and securities. This type of merger is called a *friendly merger,* or a *friendly tender offer.*

The 1993 acquisition of HCA (Hospital Corporation of America) by Columbia Healthcare typifies a friendly merger. First, the boards of directors of the two firms announced that HCA had agreed to be acquired by Columbia in a stock-swap transaction. (HCA stockholders received 1.05 shares of Columbia stock for each share held.) The merger was approved by shareholders of both companies and by the Justice Department, and then the acquisition was completed. Richard Scott, Columbia's CEO, said that the merger would provide Columbia with broader opportunities to achieve economies of scale and increased market share in selected markets, which would enable it to negotiate better contracts with managed care companies. In addition, operating economies would be achieved in markets where Columbia and HCA hospitals provided duplicative services.

Another example of a friendly merger is the previously mentioned combination of Abbey Healthcare Group and Homedco Group to form Apria Healthcare Group. In the deal, each holder of Homedco stock received two shares of the new firm per share held, while each Abbey holder received 1.4 shares of the new company for each share held. Because the two companies competed in some of the same markets, about 100 of the combined 450 offices were expected to be closed, resulting in a pre-tax savings of between $30 and $40 million dollars. Analysts praised the merger as a smart combination that would add Abbey's strength in home infusion to Homedco's strength in home respiration, resulting in one company that could offer a single package contract to an increasingly cost-conscious managed care industry.

Often, however, the target company's management resists the merger. Perhaps the managers feel that the price offered for the stock is too low, or perhaps they simply want to retain their autonomy. In either case, the acquiring firm's offer is said to be hostile rather than friendly, and the acquiring firm must make a direct appeal to the target firm's stockholders. In a *hostile merger,* the acquiring company will again make a tender offer, and again it will ask the stockholders of the target firm to tender their shares in exchange for the offered price. This time, though, the target firm's managers will urge stockholders not to tender their shares, generally stating that the price offered (cash, bonds, or stocks in the acquiring firm) is too low.

The recent battle between Regal Care Group, an Illinois-based long-term care company, and Clover Holdings illustrates a failed hostile merger attempt. It began in the summer of 1993, when Regal's stock was trading at under $10 a share. At the time, many analysts had declared that Regal was a likely takeover candidate because of its sluggish stock performance but good earnings and spotless image in an industry that has many questionable players. Then, Clover Holdings, the investment vehicle of the George Wray family, purchased five percent of Regal's stock, proposed a friendly takeover, was rebuffed, and made a $15-per-share hostile tender offer. Regal responded to the unwanted offer (1) by selling a chunk of its stock to a newly established employee stock ownership plan (ESOP), (2) by selling another chunk to a friendly investor (a *white squire*), and (3) by buying back 30 percent of its outstanding shares at $17 a share. To finance all of this, Regal added $40 million in bank debt. Additionally, Regal restructured its operations by cutting its work force by 15 percent. Clover responded to these actions (1) by initiating a proxy fight to elect new directors on Regal's board and (2) by filing a lawsuit challenging the legitimacy of Regal's defensive maneuvers.

After nine months of heated exchanges between the companies, an accord was reached in March 1994. Regal agreed to pay Clover $5 million in compensation for expenses incurred in the battle, plus repurchase all of Regal's shares held by Clover at $15 per share. For its part, Clover promised not to seek control of Regal for ten years. Finally, Clover agreed to drop all litigation, as well as its proxy fight. Although defeated, Clover ended up making about $10 million before taxes, considering both the cash settlement and the profit on the Regal shares that it owned. Charles Wray, Clover's president, said that the decision to settle was sealed by an Illinois court decision that upheld Regal's defenses. "It isn't that we went away quietly; we tried as hard as we could," he said. Regal ended up with more debt, although it still has a strong balance sheet, and a $12.50-per-share stock price. Regal's president and CEO, Michael Roberts, said "The fundamental changes and initiatives put in place during this period made us stronger, despite the pressure."

Although many hostile takeover bids fail, many others succeed. It is very difficult to defend against a hostile takeover attempt if the bidder has a large amount of resources that it is willing to spend on the battle. In such situations, the acquiring firm can offer enough cash to shareholders to overcome even the most adamant managerial resistance.

Self-Test Questions:

What is the difference between a hostile and a friendly merger?

Describe the mechanics of a typical friendly takeover and of a typical hostile takeover.

Merger Regulation

Merger regulation falls into two broad categories: (1) regulation concerning the procedures acquiring companies must follow in making hostile bids and (2) antitrust regulation to ensure that mergers do not lead to monopoly power.

Bid procedure regulation

Prior to the mid-1960s, friendly acquisitions generally took place through simple exchange-of-stock mergers, and the proxy fight was the primary weapon used in a hostile control battle. However, in the mid-1960s, corporate raiders began to operate differently. First, they noted that it took a long time to mount a proxy fight: they had to first request a list of the target company's stockholders, then be refused, and finally get a court order forcing management to turn over the list. During that time, management could think through and then implement a strategy to fend off the raider. As a result, the instigator lost most proxy fights.

Then raiders began saying to themselves, "If we could take an action that would bring the decision to a head quickly, before management could take countermeasures, that would greatly increase the probability of a successful takeover." That led raiders to turn from proxy fights to tender offers, which have a much shorter response time. For example, the stockholders of a company whose stock was selling for $20 might be offered $25 per share and be given two weeks to accept. The raider, meanwhile, would have accumulated a substantial block of the shares in open market purchases, and additional shares might have been purchased by institutional friends of the raider who promised to tender their shares in exchange for the tip that a raid was to occur, even though such actions are illegal.

Faced with a well-planned raid, managements were generally overwhelmed. The stock might actually still be undervalued at the offered price, at least in the opinion of management of the target firm, but such management simply might not have time to get this message across to stockholders, or to find a friendly competing bidder (called a *white knight*), or to take any other action. This situation was thought to be unfair and, as a result, Congress passed the Williams Act in 1968. This law had two main objectives: (1) to regulate the way in which acquiring firms can structure takeover offers and (2) to force acquiring firms to disclose more information about their offers. Basically, Congress wanted to put target managements in a better position to defend against hostile offers. Additionally, Congress believed that shareholders needed easy access to information about tender offers—including information on any securities that might be offered in lieu of cash—in order to make a rational decision.

The Williams Act placed the following three major restrictions on the activities of acquiring firms. (1) Acquirers must disclose their current holdings and future intentions within ten days of amassing at least 5 percent of a company's stock, and they must disclose the source of the funds to be used in the acquisition. (2) The target firm's shareholders must be allowed at least 20-days to tender their shares; that is, the offer must be "open" for at least 20 days. (3) If the acquiring firm increases the offer price during the 20-day open period, all shareholders who tendered prior to the improved offer must receive the higher price. In total, these restrictions were intended to reduce the ability of the acquiring firm to surprise management and to stampede target shareholders into accepting the offer. Prior to the Williams Act, offers were generally made on a first-come, first-served basis, and they were often accompanied by an implicit threat to lower the bid price after 50 percent of the shares were in hand. The legislation also gave target managements more time to mount a defense, and it gave rival bidders and white knights a chance to enter the fray and thus help a target's stockholders obtain a better price.

Many states have also passed laws designed to protect firms in their states from hostile takeovers. At first, these laws focused on disclosure requirements, but by the late 1970s, several states had enacted takeover statutes so restrictive that they virtually precluded hostile takeovers. The constitutionality of state laws regulating takeover bids was challenged and, at first, the state laws were struck down. For example, the U.S. Supreme Court ruled that an Illinois anti-takeover law put undue burden on interstate commerce. The opinion also stated that the market for securities is a national market, and even though the issuing firm might be incorporated in Illinois, the State of Illinois could not regulate interstate securities transactions.

In spite of such decisions, states kept trying to protect their state-headquartered companies and, in 1987, the U.S. Supreme Court upheld an Indiana law that radically changed the rules of the takeover game.

Specifically, the Indiana law first defined "control shares" as enough shares to give an investor 20 percent of the vote, and it went on to state that when an investor buys control shares, those shares can be voted only after approval by a majority of "disinterested shareholders," defined as those who are neither officers nor inside directors of the company, nor associates of the raider. Thus, a hostile acquirer that owned 20 percent of a target company's shares could not force a takeover by gaining only 31 percent more but, rather, would have to get 51 percent of the remaining 80 percent, or 41 percent more. The law also gives the buyer of control shares the right to insist that a shareholders' meeting be called within 50 days to decide whether the shares may be voted. The Indiana law dealt a major blow to raiders, mainly because it slowed down the action. Delaware (the state in which most large companies are incorporated) later passed a similar bill, and so did New York and a number of other states.

The new state laws also have some features that protect target stockholders from their own managers. Included are limits on the use of *golden parachutes*, which are lucrative compensation plans given to managers who lose their jobs as a result of takeovers, and the elimination of some types of *poison pills*, which are actions that managers of beleaguered firms can take to "kill off their own companies" to make them less attractive as targets. Since these types of state laws do not regulate tender offers per se but, rather, govern the practices of firms in the state, they have thus far withstood all legal challenges.

Antitrust regulation

Antitrust laws are intended to ensure that no organization attains enough market power to act as a monopoly. Such laws are based on the assumption that vigorous competition is the most effective way to ensure that consumers receive the best possible goods and services at the lowest cost. There are two primary laws that govern antitrust litigation: the Sherman Act and the Clayton Act. The *Sherman Act*, which dates to 1890, prohibits contracts, conspiracies, and combinations that restrain trade. The *Clayton Act*, passed in 1914, prohibits all mergers, acquisitions, and joint ventures that may substantially lessen competition or allow creation of a monopoly.

The two agencies that are charged with enforcing antitrust laws are the *Federal Trade Commission (FTC)* and the *Justice Department (JD)*. The FTC and JD classify potential antitrust violations into two categories: per se and rule of reason. *Per se* violations are those so unlikely to produce redeeming consumer benefits that they are immediately presumed to be illegal. Examples would be two hospitals agreeing to fix prices for certain procedures or agreeing to allocate specific markets. Actions that are not considered per se violations are evaluated using *rule of reason* analysis. Under rule of reason analysis, the FTC or JD must first determine whether a merger (or other combination) will enable a firm to exercise market power in an anticompetitive manner. If so, the agency must then analyze whether the activity produces economic efficiencies that outweigh the anticompetitive effects. If the benefits outweigh the anticompetitive consequences, then the merger is allowed to take place. Mergers within the health care industry generally fall into the rule of reason category, so a great deal of leeway exists in implementing the antitrust laws.

Regulators are informed of pending mergers by premerger notification laws, which require companies involved in mergers to file certain information with federal and state agencies. Such agencies, including the FTC and JD, have 30 days time to request additional information, approve the application, or file suit to prevent the merger.

Clearly, the manner in which antitrust laws are enforced have a significant impact on merger activity, and hence on the future structure of the health care system. Before the 1990s, when fee-for-service insurance prevailed, physicians competed with one another for patients and hospitals competed for inpatient business. Today, however, the health services industry is being transformed by the growth of managed care, selective contracting, and vertical integration, in which an organization provides both insurance and medical services. This transformation means that the FTC and JD have their hands full figuring out how and when to apply antitrust laws. For example, two hospitals may merge to increase their bargaining power with insurers. If insurers now have fewer hospitals with which to negotiate, they cannot drive nearly as hard a bargain as before, so the merger may be anticompetitive. But, by merging, the hospitals may be able to reduce duplicative services and achieve other operating efficiencies that could lead to lower prices, which would be good for the insurers, and ultimately for consumers. The question then, becomes: Which merger policy—vigorous or lax enforcement—should the FTC and JD follow to ensure good health policy?

The answer is not easy to find. For example, consider the case of Ukiah Valley Medical Center, a 94-bed not-for-profit hospital company located some 120 miles north of San Francisco. The company was created by the recent merger of two rural hospitals: one with 51 beds and one with 43 beds. However, the merger was initially challenged by the

FTC, which charged that it violated antitrust laws because it injured consumers by reducing competition among acute care providers. The company resisted the FTC challenge, spending $2 million over a five-year period to save the merger. Finally, in 1994, the commission voted 5–0 to drop the lawsuit, ruling that evidence of anticompetitive effects was weak. Furthermore, the ruling stated that the creation of a larger, more efficient system would provide better medical care than could either of the two hospitals when operated separately. "Obviously, we feel great," said Ukiah's president. "However, the decision is about five years and 2 million dollars late."

The health care industry, led by the American Hospital Association, has been lobbying for antitrust relief, arguing that antitrust laws and enforcement policies have thwarted beneficial collaborative arrangements among hospitals and other providers. However, as shown in Table 17.2, the FTC and JD have requested additional information on only 7 percent of the proposed hospital mergers between 1981 and 1993, and have stopped less than 4 percent from being consummated.

With encouragement from the Clinton administration, in late 1994 the FTC and JD issued a joint policy statement containing "safety zone" guidelines. The statement describes circumstances under which mergers

Table 17.2   Antitrust Actions Against Hospital Mergers

Year	Number of Applications	Number of Requests for Information	Number of Mergers Halted
1981	15	1	0
1982	9	1	1
1983	20	1	1
1984	29	1	0
1985	32	1	1
1986	27	0	0
1987	30	4	2
1988	43	1	1
1989	35	1	1
1990	36	8	1
1991	31	2	2
1992	42	3	1
1993	48	4	4
Total	397	28	15

Source: Modern Healthcare, 1994. (12 September).

between hospitals, physician/network joint ventures, and other health care combinations will not be challenged. For example, a hospital merger will not be challenged if one or both of the hospitals has fewer than 100 beds, fewer than 40 patients per day, and is more than five years old. Also, a physician network will not be contested if the network has no more than 20 percent of the physicians in a specialty in a particular geographical market. Although the guidelines have no effect on court decisions, and hence are no guarantee of legality, most industry representatives agree that the guidelines are needed and are helpful in establishing ground rules for future merger activity.

States are also involved in the antitrust field, both supporting and challenging proposed mergers. For example, four states requested information concerning the impact of the Columbia/HCA–Healthtrust merger on individual markets, and state actions have caused hospital chains involved in large mergers to agree to sell off hospitals in particular markets to avoid antitrust actions. However, for the most part, states have been supportive of mergers in the health care industry. Over 20 states have used the *state action immunity doctrine* to pass laws that grant immunity from federal antitrust laws. However, the doctrine requires states to actively regulate anticompetitive conduct, and there is always the possibility that the FTC or JD might challenge activities permitted by state immunity doctrine legislation because of lax supervision.

The consolidation of the health care industry has produced different views on how aggressively antitrust laws should be enforced. Physicians and hospitals tend to support lenient enforcement, arguing that they can achieve efficiencies only through mergers, acquisitions, and joint ventures. In particular, there is concern over the fact that an insurer or HMO can sign up, say, 70 percent of the physicians in a community, while antitrust laws prohibit even 40 or 50 percent of the physicians in a market from joining together to form their own network. According to an American Medical Association spokesman, "It doesn't make any sense to prevent doctors from getting together. They won't fix prices; they will be subject to market discipline from buyers." Insurers and HMOs, however, tend to argue for strict enforcement of antitrust laws on the grounds that competition will produce maximum efficiency and innovation in the health care system.

Self-Test Questions:

Is there a need to regulate mergers? Explain.

Do the states play a role in merger regulation, or is it all done at the federal level?

How do bidding regulation and antitrust regulation differ?

What two federal agencies enforce antitrust laws?

Do you think that enforcement of antitrust laws should be aggressive or lenient for health care industry mergers? Support your position.

Merger Valuation

In theory, merger analysis is quite simple. The acquiring firm simply performs an analysis to value the target company and then determines whether the target can be bought at that value or, preferably, for less than the assessed value. The target company, on the other hand, should accept the proposal if the price offered exceeds the value of the target firm if it continued to operate independently. Theory aside, however, some difficult issues are involved. In this section, we discuss valuing the target firm, the first step in merger analysis. Then, in later sections, we discuss the remainder of merger analysis: setting the bid price and structuring the bid.

Several methodologies are used to value firms, but we will confine our discussion to the two most commonly used methods in the health care industry: discounted cash flow analysis and market multiple analysis. However, regardless of the valuation methodology, it is crucial to recognize two factors. First, the business being valued typically will not continue to operate as a separate entity, but rather will become part of the acquiring firm's portfolio of assets. Thus, any changes in ownership form or operations occurring as a result of the proposed merger that will affect the value of the business must be considered in the analysis. Second, the goal of merger valuation is to set the value of the target business's equity, or ownership position, because a business is acquired from its owners, not from its creditors. Thus, although we use the phrase "valuing the firm," we are really valuing the firm's equity stake rather than estimating the total value of the firm.

Discounted cash flow analysis

The *discounted cash flow (DCF) approach* to valuing a business involves the application of classical capital budgeting procedures to an entire firm rather than to a single project. To apply this method, two key items are needed: (1) a set of pro forma statements that develop the incremental cash flows expected to result from the merger, and (2) a discount rate, or cost of capital, to apply to these projected cash flows.

The development of accurate postmerger cash flow forecasts is, by far, the most important step in a DCF merger analysis. In a pure *financial merger*, in which no synergies are expected, the incremental postmerger cash flows are simply the expected cash flows of the target firm if it were to continue to operate independently. However, even in this situation, the cash flows for a health care provider may be quite difficult to forecast because the nature of the industry is changing so rapidly. In an *operational merger*, in which the two firms' operations are to be integrated, or if the acquiring firm plans to change the target firm's operations in order to get better results, then forecasting future cash flows is even more complex.

Table 17.3 shows the projected cash flow statements for Doctors' Hospital, an investor-owned hospital that is being evaluated as a possible acquisition by United Health Services Corporation (UHSC), a large integrated health care company. The projected data are for the postmerger period, so all synergistic effects have been included in the cash flow estimates. Doctors' Hospital currently uses 30 percent debt, but if it were acquired, UHSC would increase Doctors' debt ratio to 50 percent. Both UHSC and Doctors' Hospital have 40 percent marginal federal-plus-state tax rates.

Table 17.3   Projected Cash Flow Statements (millions of dollars)

	1997	1998	1999	2000	2001
1. Net revenues	$105.0	$126.0	$151.0	$174.0	$191.0
2. Patient services expenses	80.0	94.0	111.0	127.0	137.0
3. Other expenses	10.0	12.0	13.0	15.0	16.0
4. Depreciation	8.0	8.0	9.0	9.0	10.0
5. Earnings before interest and taxes (EBIT)	$ 7.0	$ 12.0	$ 18.0	$ 23.0	$ 28.0
6. Interest	3.0	4.0	5.0	6.0	6.0
7. Earnings before taxes (EBT)	$ 4.0	$ 8.0	$ 13.0	$ 17.0	$ 22.0
8. Taxes (40 percent)	1.6	3.2	5.2	6.8	8.8
9. Net income	$ 2.4	$ 4.8	$ 7.8	$ 10.2	$ 13.2
10. Plus depreciation	8.0	8.0	9.0	9.0	10.0
11. Cash flow	$ 10.4	$ 12.8	$ 16.8	$ 19.2	$'23.2
12. Less retentions	4.0	4.0	7.0	9.0	12.0
13. Plus terminal value					89.1
14. Net cash flow to UHSC	$ 6.4	$ 8.8	$ 9.8	$ 10.2	$100.3

Line 1 of Table 17.3 contains the forecast for Doctors' net revenues, including patient services revenue, other operating revenue, and nonoperating revenue. Note that all contractual allowances and other adjustments to charges, including collections delays, have been considered, so Line 1 represents actual cash revenues. Note also that any change in Doctors' stand-alone forecasted revenues resulting from synergies have been incorporated into the Line 1 amounts. Lines 2 through 4 contain the expense forecasts, including depreciation. These are the cash costs (except for depreciation) that must be borne to generate the net revenues in Line 1. Again, the expense amounts pertain to the Doctors' Hospital subsidiary assuming that the merger takes place, so savings due to operational efficiencies are included. Line 5, which is merely Line 1 minus Lines 2, 3, and 4, contains the earnings before interest and taxes (EBIT) for each year.

Unlike a typical capital budgeting analysis, merger analyses usually incorporate interest expense, which is shown on Line 6, into the cash flow forecast. This is done for three reasons: (1) acquiring firms often assume the debt of the target firm, so old debt having different coupon rates is often part of the deal; (2) the acquisition is often partially financed by debt; and (3) if the subsidiary is expected to grow in the future, new debt will have to be issued over time to support the expansion. Thus, the debt structure associated with a merger is typically much more complex than the single issue of new debt that is assumed to occur in a normal capital budgeting analysis. The easiest way to properly account for the complexities of merger debt is to explicitly include each year's expected interest expense in the cash flow forecast. In essence, this form of DCF analysis uses the *equity residual,* or *free cash flow, method* to value the target firm, since the net cash flows that are being estimated belong solely to the acquiring firm's shareholders.

Line 7 contains the earnings before taxes (EBT), and Line 8 lists the taxes based on UHSC's 40 percent marginal rate. Note that the tax rate applied in the analysis must reflect the rate that will be applied to the combined enterprise. Line 9 lists each year's net income, but depreciation is added back in Line 10 to obtain each year's cash flow, which is shown on Line 11. Since some of Doctors' assets are expected to wear out or become obsolete, and since UHSC plans to expand the Doctors' Hospital subsidiary should the acquisition occur, some equity funds must be retained and reinvested in the hospital subsidiary. These retentions, which are not available for transfer from the hospital subsidiary to the UHSC parent, are shown on Line 12.

Finally, we have projected only five years of cash flows, but UHSC would likely operate Doctors' Hospital for many years, perhaps 20 or 30 or more. If the cash flows from the hospital are assumed to grow at a constant rate after 2001, the constant growth model can be used to estimate the target firm's *terminal value*. Assuming a constant 5 percent growth rate in net cash flow after 2001, the terminal value is estimated to be $89.1 million:

$$\text{Value of CFs beyond 2001} = \frac{2001 \text{ Cash flow } (1 + \text{Growth rate})}{\text{Required rate of return} - \text{Growth rate}}$$

$$= \frac{(\$23.2 - \$12.0)(1.05)}{0.182 - 0.05} = \$89.1 \text{ million.}$$

This terminal value of Doctors' Hospital, which represents its market value at the end of 2001, is shown on Line 13. Note that the discount rate applied in the terminal value calculation, 18.2 percent, will be estimated shortly.

The net cash flows shown on Line 14 are the flows that would be available to UHSC's stockholders, and these are the basis of the valuation. Of course, the postmerger cash flows attributable to the target firm are extremely difficult to estimate, and in a complete merger valuation, just as in a complete capital budgeting analysis, the component cash flow probability distributions would be specified, and sensitivity, scenario, and Monte Carlo simulation analyses would be conducted. Indeed, in a friendly merger, the acquiring firm would send a team consisting of literally dozens of accountants, financial analysts, engineers, and so forth, to the target firm to go over its books, to estimate required maintenance expenditures, to set values on assets such as real estate, and the like.

The bottom-line net cash flows shown in Line 14 of Table 17.3 belong to UHSC's stockholders, so they should be discounted at a cost of equity rather than at an overall cost of capital. Furthermore, the cost of equity used must reflect the riskiness of the net cash flows in the table, and hence the discount rate is more closely aligned with the cost of equity of Doctors' Hospital, not that of either UHSC or the consolidated postmerger firm.

Although we will not illustrate it here, UHSC would perform a risk analysis on the Table 17.3 net cash flows just as it does on any set of capital budgeting flows. Generally, scenario analysis and Monte Carlo simulation would be used to give UHSC's management some feel for the risks involved with the acquisition. In the illustration, as with many health care mergers, the target company is investor owned but not publicly traded, so it is not possible to obtain a market beta on Doctors' stock. However, we can obtain market betas of the stocks of the major investor-owned hospital chains. Assume that the average market beta of the stock of several hospital chains is 1.28. This value reflects an average 30 percent debt ratio, while Doctors' postmerger debt ratio will be 50 percent, as well as an average 40 percent tax rate, the same as Doctors'.

Hamada's equation, which was first discussed in Chapter 8, can be used to approximate the effects of the leverage change on beta. First, we obtain the unlevered beta of the average hospital's assets, that is, the beta of an average hospital assuming that it is financed entirely with equity:

$$b_{Assets} = \frac{b_{Firm}}{1 + (1 - T)(D/E)} = \frac{1.28}{1 + (1 - 0.40)(0.30/0.70)}$$

$$= \frac{1.28}{1.26} = 1.02.$$

Next, we relever the average hospital's asset beta to reflect the 50 percent debt ratio that would be used in the acquisition:

$$b_{Firm} = b_{Assets}[1 + (1 - T)(D/E)]$$

$$= 1.02[1 + (1 - 0.40)(0.50/0.50)] = 1.02(1.6) = 1.63.$$

Then, we use the Security Market Line to estimate the postmerger cost of equity for the Doctors' Hospital subsidiary. If the risk-free rate is 10 percent and the required rate of return on the market (an average stock with $b = 1.0$) is 15 percent, then the cost of equity of the Doctors' Hospital subsidiary, and hence the discount rate to apply to the Table 17.3 net cash flows, would be about 18.2 percent:

$$\text{Cost of equity} = k_{RF} + (k_M - k_{RF})b$$

$$= 10\% + (15\% = 10\%)1.63 = 18.2\%.$$

Finally, the current value of Doctors' Hospital to UHSC is the present value of the cash flows expected to accrue to UHSC, discounted at 18.2 percent. The present value of the Table 17.3 net cash flows, when discounted at 18.2 percent, is $66.3 million. Thus, if UHSC could acquire Doctors' Hospital for $66.3 million or less, the merger would appear to be acceptable from UHSC's standpoint. Obviously, UHSC would try to buy Doctors' at as low a price as possible, while Doctors' managers would hold out for the highest possible price. The final price is determined by negotiation, with the stronger negotiator capturing most of the incremental value. The larger the synergistic benefits, the more room for bargaining, and the higher the probability that the merger will actually be consummated. We will have more to say about setting the bid price in a later section.

Market multiple analysis

Another method of valuing a business is *market multiple analysis,* which applies a market-determined multiple to some measure of earnings such as net income or earnings per share. Like the DCF valuation method, the basic premise is that the value of any business depends on the earnings that the business produces. The DCF method applies this premise in a precise manner, while market multiple analysis is more ad hoc.

To illustrate the concept, suppose that the net income of Home-Care, Inc., is $700,000. Furthermore, assume that the ratio of stock price to net income per share of a similar home health care firm is found to be 12. That is, its net income per share is $1.50 and its stock is selling for $18, giving it a *market multiple* of 12. To estimate the value of HomeCare, simply multiply its $700,000 net income by the market multiple to obtain the value of $700,000(12) = $8.4 million. Since equity multiples are typically used in such analyses, the resulting value is the equity, or ownership, value of the firm.

The earnings measure that market multiples are most commonly applied to when analyzing health care mergers is *earnings before interest, taxes, depreciation, and amortization (EBITDA).* To apply the EBITDA earnings multiple method to the Doctors' Hospital analysis, note that the hospital's 1997 forecasted EBITDA is $7.0 + $8.0 = $15 million. If an analysis of other investor-owned hospitals produces an average Stock price/EBITDA ratio of 5.0, the value of Doctors' Hospital would be set at $15(5) = $75 million, as compared to $66.3 million using the DCF valuation method.

Clearly, the valuation of a business can only be considered a rough estimate. Although the DCF method has strong theoretical support, one has to be very concerned over the validity of the estimated cash flows and the discount rate applied to those flows. It doesn't take much variation in these estimates to create large differences in estimated value. The market multiple method is more ad hoc, but its proponents argue that earnings estimates for a single year, such as measured by EBITDA, are much more likely to be accurate than a multiple-year cash flow forecast. Furthermore, the market multiple method avoids the problem of having to estimate a discount rate. Of course, the market multiple method has problems of its own. One concern is the comparability between the firm being analyzed and the firm (or firms) that set the market multiple. Another concern is how well does one year of EBITDA, or even an average of several years, capture the value of a firm that will be operated for many years into the future, and whose EBITDA could soar due to merger-related synergies.

Some unique problems in valuing small, privately held firms

It should be obvious that the valuation of potential takeover candidates is a very difficult task, even when the target is a large, publicly traded company. One of the primary difficulties in the process is estimating the right market *capitalization rate*, either the discount rate in the DCF method or the market multiple in the market multiple method. When the target is a small, privately owned company, two additional factors arise that might require modification of a rate based on the analysis of publicly traded firms.

First, ownership of a small firm lacks marketability, which lowers its value relative to the stock of a large firm that is publicly traded on a major exchange or in the over-the-counter market. In effect, a marketability premium should be assessed when valuing small firms, which will raise the discount rate used in the DCF method and lower the multiple used in the market multiple method. Of course, the effect of these adjustments is to lower the value of the target firm. It is very difficult to judge how much lower the value should be because of lack of marketability, but it has been suggested that the value loss is quite large, as high as 50 percent or more.[1]

The second factor that often arises in valuing closely held businesses is that of control. The ability to control a business is very important and, as such, it has value. For example, assume that a business that is valued at $100,000 has three owners, one with 50.2 percent of the stock, and two each with 24.9 percent. The value of the stock owned by the controlling stockholder is worth more than the proportionate amount; that is, worth more than $50,200, perhaps a great deal more. Similarly, the stock of each of the minority stockholders is worth less than $24,900, their proportionate share.

The value of *control interests*, as opposed to *minority interests*, must be taken into account when assessing value, especially when the acquisition will not be for 100 percent of the stock of the target firm. Furthermore, control issues need to be considered when setting the terms of the acquisition offer.

Self-Test Questions:

Briefly describe two methods that are commonly used to value acquisition candidates.

What are some problems that occur when valuing target firms?

What unique considerations arise when valuing small, privately held businesses?

Setting the Bid Price

Assume that UHSC concludes that the value of Doctors' Hospital is $70 million. Furthermore, assume that Doctors' Hospital has 1 million shares of stock outstanding and that it has sold recently in a private sale at $50 a share, so Doctors' total market value is assumed to be $50 million. With an estimated value of $70 million to UHSC, it could offer as much as $70 per share for Doctors' without diluting the value of its own stock.

Figure 17.1 illustrates the situation facing UHSC's managers as they set the bid price. The $70 per share maximum offer price is shown as a point on the horizontal axis, which plots bid price. If UHSC pays less, say, $65 a share, its stockholders will gain $5 per share, or $5 million in total, from the merger. On the other hand, if UHSC pays more than $70 per share, its stockholders will lose value. The line that shows the impact of the per share bid price on UHSC's stockholders is a 45 degree downward sloping line that cuts the X axis at $70. The distance between this diagonal line and the X axis is the amount that UHSC's stockholders will gain (or lose) for each share of Doctors' acquired. The situation facing Doctors' shareholders is depicted by a 45 degree upward sloping line that crosses the X axis at $50. If the hospital is acquired for more than $50 per share, its shareholders will gain value, while they would lose value if the price is less than $50.

Note that there is a bid price range between $50 and $70 where the shareholders of both UHSC and Doctors' benefit from the merger. The range exists because the merger has synergistic benefits that can be divided between the two sets of stockholders. The greater the synergistic benefits, the greater the range of feasible bid prices, and the greater the chance that the merger will be consummated.

The issue of how to divide the synergistic benefit is critically important in any merger analysis. Obviously, both parties will want to gain as much as possible. If Doctors' shareholders knew the maximum price that UHSC is willing to pay, $70, it would hold out for that price. UHSC, on the other hand, will try to acquire the hospital at a price as close

Figure 17.1   Evaluating the Takeover Bid

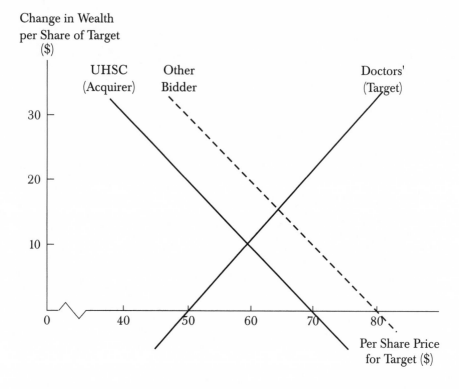

to $50 a share as possible. Where within the $50 to $70 range should UHSC set its initial bid? The answer depends on a number of factors, including whether UHSC will pay with cash or securities, whether the managers of UHSC or Doctors' have the better negotiating skills, and whether another bidder is likely to enter the picture.

The likelihood of a bidding war for Doctors' Hospital plays an important role in setting the initial bid. Suppose first that no other bidder is likely. In this situation, UHSC might make a relatively low take-it-or-leave-it offer, and Doctors' shareholders would probably take it because some gain is better than no gain. On the other hand, assume that Doctors' has a unique situation that makes it attractive to several competing health systems. Now, when UHSC announces its bid, other bidders may enter the fray, and the final price will likely be close to $70 per share. Perhaps another potential acquirer could achieve even greater synergies with Doctors' Hospital than could UHSC, as shown in

Figure 17.1 by the "Other Bidder" dashed line. If so, the bid price could rise above $70, in which case UHSC should drop out of the bidding.

UHSC would, of course, want to keep its maximum bid secret, and it would plan its bidding strategy carefully and consistent with the situation. If UHSC thought that other bidders would emerge, or that Doctors' management would resist a bid to protect their jobs, UHSC might decide to make a high *preemptive*, or *knockout*, *bid* in hopes of scaring off competing bids, eliminating management resistance, or both. On the other hand, if no other bidders were expected, UHSC might make a low-ball bid in hopes of stealing the hospital.

Another factor that influences the initial bid is the employment/control situation. First, consider the situation in which a small, owner-managed firm sells out to a larger concern. The owner-manager may be anxious to retain a high-status position, and he or she may also have developed a camaraderie with the employees and thus be concerned about keeping operating control of the organization after the merger. These points are often stressed during the merger negotiations. When a publicly owned firm not controlled by its managers is merged into another company, the acquired firm's management is also worried about its postmerger position. If the acquiring firm agrees to retain the old management, then management may be willing to support the merger and to recommend its acceptance to the stockholders. If the old management is to be removed, then it will probably resist the merger.

Self-Test Questions:

What impact does the amount of synergistic benefit have on the likelihood of a merger being consummated?

What are some factors that influence the starting and final bid price?

Structuring the Takeover Bid

The acquiring firm's offer to the target's shareholders can be in the form of cash, stock of the acquiring firm, debt of the acquiring firm, or a combination of the three. The structure of the bid is extremely important, since it affects (1) the capital structure of the postmerger firm, (2) the tax treatment of both the acquiring firm and the target's stockholders, (3) the ability of the target firm's stockholders to reap the rewards of future merger-related gains, and (4) the types of federal and state regulations to which the acquiring firm will be subjected. In this section, we focus on how taxes and regulation influence the way in which acquiring firms structure their offers.

The form of payment offered to the target shareholders determines the personal tax treatment of the target's stockholders. Target shareholders do not have to pay taxes on the transaction if they maintain a substantial equity position in the combined firm, defined by the IRS to mean that at least 50 percent of the payment to target shareholders must be in shares (either common or preferred) of the acquiring firm. In such nontaxable offers, target shareholders do not realize any capital gains or losses until the equity securities they receive in the takeover are sold. However, capital gains must be taken and treated as income in the transaction year if an offer consists of over 50 percent of either cash or debt securities, or some combination of the two.

All other things being equal, target stockholders prefer nontaxable offers, especially when they believe that the combined firm will perform well, since they can (1) benefit from the continuing good performance of the combined firm and (2) postpone the realization of capital gains and the payment of taxes. Most target shareholders are thus willing to sell their stock for a lower price in a nontaxable offer than in a taxable offer. As a result, one might expect nontaxable bids to dominate; however, other factors are at work. If a firm pays more than book value for a target firm's assets in a taxable merger, it can write up those assets, depreciate the marked-up value for tax purposes, and thus lower the postmerger firm's taxes vis-à-vis the taxes of the two firms operating separately. However, if the acquiring company writes up the target company's assets for tax purposes, then the target company must pay capital gains taxes in the year the merger occurs. (These taxes can be avoided if the acquiring company elects not to write up acquired assets and depreciates them on their old basis.)

Securities laws also have an effect on the construction of the offer. As we discussed in Chapter 7, the Securities and Exchange Commission (SEC) has oversight over the issuance of new securities, including stock or debt issued in connection with a merger. Therefore, whenever a corporation bids for control of another firm through the exchange of equity or debt, the entire process must take place under the scrutiny of the SEC. The time required for such reviews allows target managements to implement defensive tactics and other firms to make competing offers, and as a result, most hostile tender offers are for cash rather than securities.

Self-Test Questions:

What are some alternative ways of structuring takeover bids?

How do taxes influence the payment structure?

How do securities laws affect the payment structure?

Due Diligence Analysis

One of the most important aspects of a merger is *due diligence analysis.*[2] The primary purposes of a due diligence analysis are (1) to uncover issues that would prevent the acquirer from pursuing the acquisition and (2) to provide the acquirer with insights into the day-to-day operations of the target firm so that an appropriate transaction can take place. Due diligence requires a uniform, disciplined approach to the merger analysis, which presumably will minimize the risk of overlooking issues that are key to the acquisition.[3]

Due diligence analysis normally takes place after a letter of intent has been signed between the acquiring and target firms, but before the terms of the transaction have been completed. It is normally carried out by a team that has been specially assembled for the task. Typically, the team will include one or two top executives, plus specialists from applicable staffs such as finance, legal, medical, nursing, personnel, risk management, and engineering. The team may consist entirely of personnel from the acquiring firm or it may contain consultants in addition to the in-house members.

The due diligence team will gather and analyze information about the acquisition. The end result is a report that summarizes the team's findings and makes recommendations on whether or not to proceed with the acquisition and how the deal, if recommended, should be structured. The time required to conduct a due diligence analysis varies depending on the number of individuals on the team, the nature of the acquisition, and the accessibility of information. Generally, however, due diligence analyses take about 60 to 90 days, so acquirers must allow sufficient time for due diligence analysis when developing merger time tables.

Conducting a thorough due diligence analysis is a necessary component of the acquisition process. In addition to protecting the acquirer against a poor acquisition, it can establish a relationship between acquiring and target firms' managements that not only facilitates successful negotiations but, more importantly, can help lead to a successful merger.

Self-Test Questions:

What is due diligence analysis?

Why is due diligence analysis so important to the merger process?

The Role of Investment Bankers

The investment banking community is involved with mergers in a number of ways: (1) helping to arrange mergers, (2) helping target companies develop and implement defensive tactics, (3) helping in due diligence analysis, especially valuing target companies, (4) helping to finance mergers, and (5) speculating in the stocks of potential merger candidates.

Arranging mergers

The major investment banking firms have merger and acquisition groups that operate within their corporate finance departments. (Corporate finance departments offer advice, as opposed to underwriting or brokerage services, to business firms.) Members of these groups strive to identify firms with excess cash that might want to buy other firms, companies that might be willing to be bought, and firms that might, for a number of reasons, be attractive to others. Similarly, dissident stockholders of firms with poor track records might work with investment bankers to oust management by helping to arrange a merger.

Developing defensive tactics

Target firms that do not want to be acquired generally enlist the help of an investment banking firm, along with a law firm that specializes in helping to block mergers. Defenses include such tactics as (1) changing the bylaws so that only one-third of the directors are elected each year or that a 75 percent approval (a super majority) versus a simple majority is required to approve a merger, or both; (2) trying to convince the target firm's stockholders that the price being offered is too low; (3) raising antitrust issues in the hope that the Federal Trade Commission or the Justice Department will intervene; (4) repurchasing stock in the open market in an effort to push the price above that being offered by the potential acquirer; (5) getting a white knight who is more acceptable to the target firm's management to compete with the potential acquirer; (6) getting a white squire who is friendly to current management to buy some of the target firm's shares, and (7) taking a poison pill, as described next.

Poison pills—which occasionally really do amount to committing economic suicide to avoid a takeover—are such tactics as borrowing on terms that require immediate repayment of all loans if the firm is acquired, selling off at bargain prices the assets that originally made the firm a desirable target, granting such lucrative golden parachutes to their executives that the cash drain from these payments would render the merger infeasible, and planning defensive mergers that would leave the firm with new assets of questionable value and a huge debt load to service.

Currently, the most popular poison pill is for a company to give its stockholders stock purchase rights that allow them to buy at half price the stock of an acquiring firm should the firm be acquired. The blatant use of poison pills is constrained by directors' awareness that excessive use could trigger personal suits by stockholders against directors who voted for them, and, perhaps in the near future, by laws that would further limit management's use of such poison pills. Still, investment bankers and anti-takeover lawyers are busy thinking up new poison pill formulas, and others are just as actively trying to come up with antidotes.

Establishing a fair value

If a friendly merger is being worked out between two firms' managements, it is important to be able to document that the agreed-upon price is a fair one; otherwise, the stockholders of either company may sue to block the merger. Therefore, in many large mergers, each side will hire an investment banking firm to evaluate the target company and to help establish the fair price. Even if the merger is not friendly, investment bankers may still be asked to help establish a price. If a surprise tender offer is to be made, the acquiring firm will want to know the lowest price at which it might be able to acquire the stock, while the target firm may seek help in "proving" that the price being offered is too low.

Arranging financing

Many mergers are financed with the acquiring company's excess cash. At other times, however, the acquiring company has no excess cash; hence, it requires a source of funds to pay for the target company. Perhaps the single most important factor behind the 1980s merger wave was the widespread use of junk bonds, and the system that was developed to market these bonds.

To be a successful investment banker in the mergers and acquisitions (M&A) business, a banker must be able to offer a financing
package to clients, whether they are acquirers that need capital to take
over companies or target companies that need capital to finance stock
repurchase plans or other defenses against takeovers.

Risk arbitrage

Arbitrage generally means simultaneously buying and selling the same
commodity or security in two different markets at different prices, and
pocketing a risk-free return. However, the major brokerage houses, as
well as some wealthy private investors, are engaged in a different type of
arbitrage called *risk arbitrage*. The arbitragers, or "arbs" as they are called,
speculate in the stocks of companies that are likely takeover targets.
Vast amounts of capital are required to speculate in a large number
of securities and thus reduce risk, and also to make money on narrow
spreads, but many institutional investors have the wherewithal to play the
game. To be successful, arbs need to be able to sniff out likely targets,
assess the probability of offers reaching fruition, and move in and out
of the market quickly and with low transaction costs.

Self-Test Questions:

What are some roles that investment bankers play in mergers?

What are some defensive tactics that firms can use to resist hostile
takeover attempts?

What is the difference between pure arbitrage and risk arbitrage?

Who Wins: The Empirical Evidence

The most recent merger waves have been notable not only for the great
number of firms that have combined, but also for the high percentage
of hostile takeovers. With all of this activity, the following questions have
emerged: Do corporate acquisitions create value and, if so, how is the
value shared between the parties involved?

Financial researchers have classified corporate acquisitions as part
of "the market for corporate control." Under this concept, management
teams are viewed as facing constant competition from other management teams. If the team that currently controls a firm is not maximizing
the value of the firm's assets, then an acquisition will likely occur and
increase the value of the firm by replacing its poor managers with good

managers. Furthermore, under this model, intense competition will cause managers to combine or divest assets whenever such steps would increase the value of the firm.

Most researchers agree that mergers increase the wealth of the shareholders of target firms, for otherwise they would not agree to the offer. However, there is a debate about whether or not mergers benefit the acquiring firm's shareholders. In particular, managements of acquiring firms may be motivated by factors other than shareholder wealth maximization; for example, they may want to merge merely to increase the size of the corporations they manage, since increased size usually brings larger salaries and more job security, perquisites, power, and prestige.

The validity of the competing views on who gains from corporate mergers can be tested by examining the stock price changes that occur around a merger announcement. Such changes in the stock prices of the acquiring and target firms represent market participants' beliefs about the value created by the merger, and about how this value will be divided between the target and acquiring firms' shareholders. As long as market participants are neither systematically wrong nor biased in their perceptions of the effects of mergers, examining a large sample of stock price movements will shed light on the issue of who gains from mergers.

One cannot simply examine stock prices around merger announcement dates, because other factors influence stock prices. For example, if a merger was announced on a day when the entire market advanced, the fact that the stock price of a firm involved in a merger rose would not necessarily signify that the merger created value. Hence, studies examine the *abnormal returns* associated with merger announcements, where abnormal returns are defined as that part of a stock price change caused by factors other than changes in the general stock market.

Many studies have examined both acquiring and target firms' stock price responses to mergers and tender offers. Jointly, these studies have covered nearly every acquisition involving publicly traded firms from the early 1960s to the present, and they are remarkably consistent in their results: On average, the stock price of target firms increases by about 30 percent in hostile tender offers, while in friendly mergers the average increase is about 20 percent. However, for both hostile and friendly deals, the stock prices of acquiring firms, on average, remain constant. Thus, the evidence strongly indicates (1) that acquisitions do create value, but (2) that shareholders of target firms reap virtually all of the benefits.

In hindsight, these results are not too surprising. First, target firms' shareholders can always say no, so they are in the driver's seat. Second, takeovers are a competitive game, so if one potential acquirer does not offer full value for a target company, then another potential acquirer will generally jump in with a higher bid. Finally, managements of acquiring firms might well be willing to give up all of the value created by the merger, because the merger would enhance the acquiring managers' personal positions with no explicit cost to their shareholders.

It has also been argued that acquisitions increase shareholder wealth at the expense of bondholders. Specific instances can be cited where bonds were downgraded and bondholders did suffer losses as a direct result of an acquisition, but most of the studies find no evidence to support the contention that bondholders generally lose in corporate mergers.

Self-Test Questions:

Explain how researchers can investigate the effects of mergers on shareholder wealth.

Do mergers create value? If so, who profits from this value?

Does the research result discussed in this section seem logical? Explain.

Corporate Alliances

Mergers are one way for two companies to join forces, but many companies are striking cooperative deals, called *corporate alliances,* that fall short of merging. Whereas mergers combine all of the assets of the firms involved, as well as managerial and technical expertise, alliances allow firms to create combinations that focus on specific business lines that have the most potential for synergies. These alliances take many forms, from straightforward marketing agreements to joint ownership of world-scale operations.

A common form of corporate alliance is the *joint venture,* in which parts of companies are joined together to achieve specific, limited objectives. A joint venture is controlled by a management team consisting of representatives of the two (or more) parent companies. Joint ventures are becoming more prevalent in the health care industry as it strives to consolidate both insurance and provider services. For example, both state officials and the Justice Department blocked the merger of two not-for-profit hospitals—Morton Plant and Mease—because the combined entity would dominate acute care delivery in an area near St. Petersburg, Florida. However, the hospitals were allowed to form a joint venture to consolidate billing and record keeping and to offer expensive high-tech services such as open-heart surgery, magnetic resonance imaging, and neonatal care. By forming a joint venture, the hospitals were able to gain at least some benefits of merging, yet satisfy antitrust laws.

A joint venture analysis is similar to a merger analysis, except that there are multiple classes of equity investors. Thus, in such analyses, the venture's cash flows must be broken down into distributions to each of the joint venture partners, and each partner must analyze its flows on the basis of their riskiness to determine if the venture is in its best interest.

Self-Test Questions:

What is the difference between a merger and a corporate alliance?

What is a joint venture? Give some reasons why joint ventures may be advantageous to the parties involved.

Mergers Involving Not-for-Profit Firms

One of the unique aspects of the health care industry is the large proportion of not-for-profit firms. Although the general principles discussed up to this point apply to all businesses, there are some problems that arise when not-for-profit firms are involved in mergers. In general, the merger of two not-for-profit firms does not require special consideration, but the acquisition of a not-for-profit firm by an investor-owned acquirer presents two significant problems.

The first problem involves the *charitable trust doctrine.* This doctrine, which was first developed in English common law and has been adopted by most states, holds that assets used for charitable purposes must be held in trust. This doctrine shaped the state incorporation laws for not-for-profit firms, which require that assets being used for charitable purposes must be used for such purposes in perpetuity (forever). The result is that the proceeds from the sale of a not-for-profit corporation to an investor-owned business must be held in trust and continue to be used for charitable purposes. These laws place two requirements on the board of trustees of a not-for-profit firm about to be acquired by an investor-owned firm. First, the trustees must ensure that the acquisition price reflects the full fair market value of the assets being acquired. This assurance is normally obtained by getting the opinion of an investment banker or professional appraiser. Second, the trustees must establish a charitable foundation to administer the proceeds from the sale for a charitable purpose. The usual vehicle for continuing the charitable purpose of the not-for-profit corporation is the tax-exempt *foundation.*

By the end of 1995, over 30 foundations had been spawned by the sales of not-for-profit businesses to investor-owned companies, primarily in the hospital industry and primarily as a result of acquisitions by Columbia/HCA Healthcare. Note, however, that foundations have also been created by sales of HMOs and other not-for-profit health care companies. To illustrate the foundation concept, Presbyterian Health Foundation was created in 1985 when Presbyterian Hospital in Oklahoma City was acquired by Hospital Corporation of America (HCA). The foundation began with $60 million in assets, but now has over $110 million. By law, at least 5 percent of assets of charitable foundations must be distributed each year, and Presbyterian Health Foundation has given a total of $30 million alone for rural outreach programs at the University of Oklahoma Health Science Center.

Although merger-related foundations are clearly doing a lot of good work with their vast amount of assets, they are not without criticism. Most of the criticism stems from the close relationships that many foundations have with the for-profit providers that created them. Indeed, some foundations, instead of being funded entirely with cash, have ownership interests in the newly created for-profit entity, and it is easy for conflicts of interest to occur. One not-for-profit foundation has even lost its tax-exempt status because it squandered millions of dollars on overpriced clinics, excessive compensation, and extravagant spending on personal items for managers and employees. At least not-for-profit hospitals are constrained somewhat by competitive markets, whereas the burden of oversight at charitable foundations falls completely on the board of trustees.

The second major problem in the acquisition of a not-for-profit provider by an investor-owned company involves the tax-exempt, or municipal, debt that is often outstanding. Typically, such debt is issued for the sole purpose of funding plant and equipment owned by not-for-profit corporations. Furthermore, such debt usually has covenants that constrain the provider from merger activity that would lower the creditworthiness of the bonds or negatively affect the bonds' tax-exempt status. However, the issuer normally has the right to refund that debt when transactions of this nature occur. The result is that, in most situations, the entire amount of outstanding tax-exempt debt has to be refunded coincident with the acquisition of a not-for-profit provider by a for-profit firm.

Clearly, the restrictions on mergers involving not-for-profit firms and for-profit firms make such activities much more complicated than mergers involving only for-profits or only not-for-profits. Nevertheless, as evidenced by the amount of merger activity, these kinds of mergers do occur, and their volume is likely to increase, not decrease, in the future.

Summary

This chapter has focused on mergers in the health care industry, with emphasis on merger analysis. The key concepts covered are listed below:

- A *merger* occurs when two firms combine to form a single company.

- In most mergers, one company (the *acquirer*) initiates action to take over another (the *target*).

- There have been five prominent *merger waves* in the United States. The current wave includes a great deal of activity in the health care industry, which, for the most part, involves mergers to better position firms to respond to the changing health care marketplace.

- The primary *motives* for mergers are (1) synergy, (2) excess cash, (3) purchase of assets below replacement cost, (4) diversification, and (5) personal incentives.

- A *horizontal* merger occurs when two firms in the same line of business combine. A *vertical* merger is the combination of a firm with one of its customers or suppliers. A *congeneric* merger involves firms in related industries, but for which no customer-supplier relationship exists. A *conglomerate* merger occurs when firms in totally different industries combine.

- In a *friendly merger* the managements of both firms approve the merger, whereas in a *hostile merger* the target firm's management opposes the merger.

- Merger regulation falls into two broad categories: *bid procedure regulation* and *antitrust regulation*.

- *Merger analysis* consists of three tasks: (1) valuing the target firm, (2) setting the bid price, and (3) structuring the bid.

- Two methodologies are most commonly used to value firms: *discounted cash flow analysis* and *market multiple analysis*.

- Potential acquirers undertake *due diligence analysis* (1) to uncover issues that would prevent the acquirer from pursuing the acquisition and (2) to provide the acquirer with insights into the day-to-day operations of the target firm so that an appropriate transaction can take place.

- *Investment bankers* are involved in mergers in a number of ways: (1) they help arrange mergers, (2) they help target companies develop and implement defensive tactics, (3) they help value target companies, (4) they help finance mergers, and (5) they speculate in the stocks of potential merger candidates.

- Many studies have been conducted to determine who wins in mergers. These studies indicate that mergers do create value, but that most of this value goes to the shareholders of target companies.

- Mergers are one way for two companies to join forces, but many companies are striking cooperative deals, called *corporate alliances,* that fall short of merging. A *joint venture* is a corporate alliance in which two or more companies combine some of their resources to achieve a specific, limited objective.

- Some unique problems arise when not-for-profit firms are involved in mergers with for-profit firms. The two largest are that (1) a *charitable foundation* must be created from the merger proceeds, and (2) all *tax-exempt debt* must be refunded.

Notes

1. See E. W. Walker, and J. W. Petty II, *Financial Management of the Small Firm* (Englewood Cliffs, NJ: Prentice-Hall, 1986), chap. 13.
2. For more information on due diligence analysis, see P. Louiselle, "Conducting Financial Due Diligence Analysis of Medical Practices," *Healthcare Financial Management* (December 1995): 29–33.
3. For an example of a due diligence checklist, see HFMA Principles and Practices Board, "Practice Acquisition: A Due Diligence Checklist," *Healthcare Financial Management* (December 1995): 36–39.

Selected Additional References

Baumann, B. H., and M. R. Oxaal. 1993. "Estimating the Value of Group Medical Practices." *Healthcare Financial Management* (December): 58–65.
Becker, S., and R. J. Pristave. 1995. "Physician-Based Transactions: The Sale of Medical Practices, Ambulatory Surgery Centers, and Dialysis Facilities." *Journal of Health Care Finance* (Winter): 13–26.
Boo, M., and P. Louiselle. 1994. "Structuring Medical Practice Acquisitions." *Healthcare Financial Management* (December): 23–27.
Bryant, L. E., Jr. 1993. "Avoiding Antitrust Compliance Difficulties in Mergers and Acquisitions." *Healthcare Financial Management* (August): 48–58.

Collins, H., and G. Simpson. 1995. "Avoiding Pitfalls in Medical Practice Valuation." *Healthcare Financial Management* (March): 20–22.

Federa, R. D., and J. S. Ketcham. 1993. "The Valuation of Medical Practices." *Topics in Health Care Financing* (Spring): 67–75.

Hahn, W. 1994. "Determining a Healthcare Organization's Value." *Healthcare Financial Management* (August): 40–44.

Hill, J. E., and J. Wild. 1995. "Survey Provides Data on Practice Acquisition Activity." *Healthcare Financial Management* (September): 54–72.

Meiling, T. M. (ed.). 1989. "Mergers and Acquisitions." *Topics in Health Care Financing* (Summer issue).

Peregrine, M. W., and D. L. Glaser. 1995. "Legal Issues in Medical Practice Acquisitions." *Healthcare Financial Management* (February): 70–76.

Reilly, R. F. 1990. "The Valuation of a Medical Practice." *Health Care Management Review* (Summer): 25–34.

Rimmer, T. B. 1995. "Physician Practice Acquisitions: Valuation Issues and Concerns." *Hospital & Health Services Administration* (Fall): 415–425.

Unland, J. J. 1989. *Valuation of Hospitals and Medical Centers.* Chicago: Health Management Research Institute.

Ward, M. E., and S. E. Krentz. 1988. "Diversification: Myths versus Realities." *Topics in Health Care Financing* (Fall): 32–39.

Williams, L. 1995. "Structuring Managed Care Joint Ventures." *Healthcare Financial Management* (August): 32–36.

Case 17A

Ocean View General Hospital: Merger Analysis

Ocean View General Hospital is a 400-bed, not-for-profit, acute care hospital that was established in 1928 in Ocean View, Florida. For 50 years it was operated as a county hospital, and hence developed a reputation for providing quality health care services to the poor. After many years of operating losses, the county concluded that it could no longer afford to operate the hospital. So, in 1978, the county sold the hospital for one dollar to Citrus Healthcare Company, a not-for-profit managed care organization and provider, which by 1996 had become the state's largest integrated health care company.

Citrus Healthcare's major business line is managed care. Its numerous plans, including HMO, PPO, POS, Medicare, and Medicaid, serve 250,000 members in 31 Florida counties, encompassing all of the major metropolitan areas. In addition to the managed care plans, Citrus Healthcare owns nine different providers: two acute care hospitals, including Ocean View General, two primary care hospitals, one rehabilitation hospital, one mental health hospital, one hospice, one home health care provider, and one retirement facility.

Ocean View General Hospital is the flagship of Citrus Healthcare's provider network. In recent years, Ocean View has built a new, state-of-the art HeartCare Center and a modern MaternityCare Center. Furthermore, it operates a full-service emergency department. In spite of its solid reputation and recent additions, the hospital faces a very difficult competitive environment. It is one of three hospitals in Ocean View, which has a service area population of about 200,000. The two competing hospitals are Logan Teaching Hospital, a not-for-profit university-affiliated hospital with 525 beds, and Palm Shores Regional Medical Center, an investor-owned hospital with 200 beds. Thus, the service area has a total of 1,125 licensed beds for 200,000 people, or over 5.6 beds per 1,000 population, which is higher than the national average and much greater than the roughly 2 beds per 1,000 population needed under the moderately aggressive case management techniques used by HMOs. Of course, as a tertiary care academic health center, Logan receives patients from throughout the state, but the bulk of its patients still come from the local area.

With such excess capacity of hospital beds, it is doubtful that all three hospitals will survive the changing health care environment. Indeed, Ocean View has had some tough years recently, as evidenced by its number of discharges, which have fallen to 11,412 in 1996 from 12,055 in 1995 and 12,824 in 1994. Another factor that has forced local health care leaders to reevaluate the future of the area's three hospitals is the fact that Palm Shores Regional Medical Center is part of Columbia/HCA Healthcare Corporation, a for-profit chain that has been very aggressive in building market share by acquisition in the areas that it serves. With this background, it is clear that some consolidation in the local hospital market will have to take place, and the most likely result will be the acquisition of Ocean View General by either Logan Teaching Hospital or Columbia/HCA.

In response to the current situation, Logan Teaching Hospital has formed a special committee to consider the feasibility of making an acquisition offer for Ocean View General Hospital. The committee's primary goals are as follows:

1. To place a dollar value on Ocean View General's equity (fund) capital, assuming that the hospital will be acquired and operated by Logan Teaching Hospital

2. To develop a financing plan for the acquisition.

In addition, the committee has been asked to consider two other issues related to the potential acquisition:

1. What is the best organizational structure for the combined enterprise? Currently, both Ocean View General and Logan Teaching Hospital have separate boards of directors and management staffs. Of course, the senior members of the board of Ocean View General currently are Citrus Healthcare officers.

2. Should the medical staffs of the two hospitals be integrated and, if so, in what way? The medical staff of Ocean View General consists of local physicians, including many family practice physicians, while the medical staff at Logan Teaching Hospital is made

up almost entirely of specialists, all of whom are members of the university's college of medicine with responsibilities beyond clinical practice.

A new committee will be formed to address the above issues should Logan's management agree to move forward with the acquisition offer, but some preliminary judgments are sought at this time.

As a starting point in the valuation analysis, the committee has obtained historical income statement and balance sheet data on both hospitals. Table 1 contains the data for Ocean View General Hospital, while Table 2 provides the data for Logan Teaching Hospital. Note that both sets of statements focus on operating data, which are considered to be most relevant to the analysis. In addition, some relevant comparative data are presented in Table 3. Finally, relevant market data are contained in Table 4. (Note that these data are assumed to reflect early 1997 conditions. Use the Table 4 data in your analysis regardless of actual market conditions.)

One of the toughest tasks that the committee faces is the development of Ocean View General's pro forma cash flow statements. Two basic questions must be answered before any numbers can be generated. First, what synergies, if any can be realized from the merger, and how long will it take for any synergies to be realized? For example, can duplications be eliminated? Both hospitals have "mercy flight" helicopters and both offer full emergency department services, even though the two hospitals are less than two miles apart. And what is the impact of such operational changes on revenues and costs, and hence on the net cash flows that Ocean View General's assets can produce? Second, once the consolidation takes place and all synergies have been realized, what are the long-term growth prospects for Ocean View General's revenues? The answers to these questions, and others, are the basis for the pro forma cash flow statements.

Assume that you chair the special committee formed at Logan Teaching Hospital to evaluate the potential acquisition. You must present your findings and recommendations to Logan's board of trustees. Note that it is recognized that Tables 1 through 4 contain far less data than normally available to parties involved in merger analyses, especially when the potential merger is friendly. In effect, the case discussion and accompanying data raise many more questions than they answer. You will be required to make a myriad of difficult assumptions to complete the analysis. Although you do not know much about Ocean View General's local market, you do know the current trends in health care delivery.

Table 1   Ocean View General Hospital: Historical Financial
Statements (millions of dollars)

	1992	*1993*	*1994*	*1995*	*1996*
Income Statements					
Inpatient revenue	$ 81.624	$ 88.249	$ 99.010	$105.332	$110.384
Outpatient revenue	22.861	27.067	34.628	43.616	50.810
Gross patient revenue	$104.485	$115.316	$133.638	$148.948	$161.194
Allowances and discounts	33.699	38.626	44.622	51.198	62.006
Net patient revenue	$ 70.786	$ 76.690	$ 89.016	$ 97.750	$ 99.188
Other operating revenue	1.922	1.515	1.367	1.725	1.048
Total operating revenue	$ 72.708	$ 78.205	$ 90.383	$ 99.475	$100.236
Patient services expenses	$ 60.245	$ 73.858	$ 81.525	$ 90.645	$ 89.505
Interest expense	3.045	3.147	3.093	3.002	2.980
Depreciation	3.466	3.689	4.395	4.258	6.031
Total operating expense	$ 66.756	$ 80.694	$ 89.013	$ 97.905	$ 98.516
Net income	$ 5.952	($ 2.489)	$ 1.370	$ 1.570	$ 1.720
Balance Sheets					
Cash and investments	$ 2.388	$ 1.538	$ 0.162	$ 0.185	$ 0.198
Accounts receivable	18.860	20.581	20.821	21.570	16.732
Other current assets	4.539	8.475	4.669	2.585	2.898
Total current assets	$ 25.787	$ 30.594	$ 25.652	$ 24.340	$ 19.828
Gross plant and equipment	$102.596	$116.694	$122.611	$133.499	$146.130
Accumulated depreciation	27.243	30.505	34.900	39.158	45.189
Net plant and equipment	$ 75.353	$ 86.189	$ 87.711	$ 94.341	$100.941
Total assets	$101.140	$116.783	$113.363	$118.681	$120.769
Current liabilities	$ 9.182	$ 13.584	$ 5.771	$ 10.689	$ 11.431
Long-term debt	33.572	47.302	50.325	49.155	48.781
Total liabilities	$ 42.754	$ 60.886	$ 56.096	$ 59.844	$ 60.212
Fund balance	58.386	55.897	57.267	58.837	60.557
Total claims	$101.140	$116.783	$113.363	$118.681	$120.769

Use this knowledge to help make judgments about the case. It is a fact
of life that the quality of many, if not most, real world financial analyses
depends more on the validity of the underlying assumptions than on
the theoretical "correctness" of the analytical techniques. There is no
"correct" answer to this case, so your case analysis will be judged as much

Table 2   Logan Teaching Hospital: Historical Financial
Statements (millions of dollars)

	1992	1993	1994	1995	1996
Income Statements					
Inpatient revenue	$238.510	$287.559	$328.047	$363.236	$398.997
Outpatient revenue	47.963	57.351	69.252	89.992	103.746
Gross patient revenue	$286.473	$344.910	$397.299	$453.228	$502.743
Allowances and discounts	82.053	107.256	128.645	170.058	185.301
Net patient revenue	$204.420	$237.654	$268.654	$283.170	$317.442
Other operating revenue	5.587	8.899	12.193	22.672	9.979
Total operating revenue	$210.007	$246.553	$280.847	$305.842	$327.421
Patient services expenses	$178.788	$207.596	$231.673	$254.704	$277.938
Interest expense	9.232	10.468	11.983	10.691	9.997
Depreciation	12.289	16.637	19.621	23.286	26.489
Total operating expense	$201.309	$234.701	$263.277	$288.681	$314.424
Net income	$ 8.698	$ 11.852	$ 17.570	$ 17.161	$ 12.997
Balance Sheets					
Cash and investments	$ 17.918	$ 19.862	$ 24.660	$ 27.726	$ 25.220
Accounts receivable	66.212	72.989	99.867	100.297	97.494
Other current assets	12.315	16.771	20.741	20.542	22.757
Total current assets	$ 96.445	$109.622	$145.268	$148.565	$145.471
Gross plant and equipment	$348.288	$341.064	$335.313	$362.152	$400.546
Accumulated depreciation	75.139	76.575	90.056	109.468	123.567
Net plant and equipment	$273.149	$246.489	$245.257	$252.684	$276.979
Total assets	$369.594	$374.111	$390.525	$401.249	$422.450
Current liabilities	$ 42.437	$ 35.061	$ 39.511	$ 37.733	$ 39.817
Long-term debt	146.997	147.038	141.432	136.773	142.893
Total liabilities	$189.434	$182.099	$180.943	$174.506	$182.710
Fund balance	180.160	192.012	209.582	226.743	239.740
Total claims	$369.594	$374.111	$390.525	$401.249	$422.450

on the assumptions used in the analysis as on the analysis itself. Finally,
remember that there are numerous risk analysis techniques available
that can be used to give decision makers some feel for the risks involved.

Samson, Sara Beth
HEA

03/14/2011

OSU Libraries - Circulation Desk
1858 Neil Avenue
Columbus OH 43210-1286

Samson, Sara Beth
1303 King Ave.

Columbus, OH 43212

PAGE SLIP: retrieve item & CHECK IN to holdshelf. See exceptions below.
Remember that items on holdshelf are not yet CHECKED OUT to patron! If
pick up location is MY OFFICE: CHECK OUT to patron and send to
CAMPUS OFFICE. If pick up location is another library: Put IN TRANSIT
and send to pickup location.

CALL #: NUMBER: **RA971.3 .G37 1996**

VOL #: NUMBE   CPY #: NUMBE   **1**

(AUTHOR: Gapenski, Louis C

TITLE: Understanding health care financial management : text, cases, and models

BARCODE: 31055216

LOCATION: LIM Stacks

PICKUP LOCATION: HEA-Health Sciences Lib.

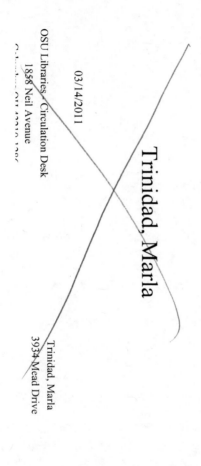

03/14/2011

Trinidad, Marla

OSU Libraries - Circulation Desk
1858 Neil Avenue

Trinidad, Marla
3934 Mead Drive

Table 3 Selected Comparative Data for 1996

	Ocean View	*Logan*
Average age of plant	6.8 years	8.5 years
Licensed beds	400	525
Occupancy rate	52.7%	64.2%
Average length of stay	5.5 days	6.6 days
Number of discharges	11,412	19,748
Medicare percent	57.2%	29.7%
Medicaid percent	10.3%	13.0%
Medicare case mix index	1.51	2.13
Gross price per discharge	$11,688	$20,204
Net price per discharge	$5,850	$12,757
Cost per discharge	$5,703	$12,144

Table 4 Selected Market Data for January 1997

U.S. Treasury Yield Curve

Maturity	*Interest Rate*
6 months	5.50%
1 year	6.00
5 years	6.25
10 years	6.50
20 years	6.75
30 years	7.00

Market Risk Premium

Historical, as reported by Ibbotson Associates	7.4%.
Average ex ante premium as reported by three investment banking firms	6.0%.

Market Betas, Capitalization, and Tax Rates of Two Publicly Traded Hospital Companies

Company	*Beta*	*Debt/Asset Ratio*	*Tax rate*
Columbia/HCA	1.1	48%	40%
Tenet Healthcare	1.2	65%	43%

Ratio of Stock Price to EBITDA per Share

Columbia/HCA	5.3
Tenet Healthcare	4.7

Note: Most of the above data reflect assumptions to ease the case analysis, as opposed to actual data.

Case 17B

West Florida Memorial Hospital: Joint Venture Analysis

West Florida Memorial Hospital (WFMH) is a 320-bed, acute care, not-for-profit hospital located in Tallahassee. The hospital is well known as a leader in new technology, and hence draws patients from as far away as Pensacola to the west and Lake City to the east. The hospital contracts with the Tallahassee Radiology Group (the Group) to provide radiology services for its patients. Basically, the hospital furnishes the radiology equipment and technicians, and performs the tests, while the physicians in the Group agree to "read" the results. Since the Group bills the patients separately for the readings, there is no direct payment from the hospital to the Group.

At the end of one of the monthly medical staff meetings, Dr. Vincent Medina, head of the Tallahassee Radiology Group, presents a proposal to Philip Mikelson, WFMH's CEO. The Group wants the hospital to purchase a biliary lithotripter, a device that uses shock waves to crush gallstones. The machine, which costs about $1.1 million, is expected to be a major technological advance in the treatment of gallstones, since it permits most patients to avoid major surgery. A similar machine is approved for use on kidney stones, but the biliary lithotripter has not yet received FDA approval, and hence it does not qualify for Medicare/Medicaid reimbursement. The Group would be involved in lithotripter usage because radiologists must read the ultrasound images that are used to locate the stones and confirm that the treatment has been effective.

Mikelson recently read an article on biliary lithotripters, and he is supportive of the idea. Furthermore, Medina has mentioned that he talked to the president of Medical Equipment International (MEI), the manufacturer of the equipment, and that MEI promised to give WFMH exclusive purchase rights in the Florida panhandle while the equipment is pending FDA approval, a process expected to take about two years. The idea of being an exclusive provider of gallstone lithotripsy appeals to Mikelson, even if it only lasts for two years. First, by offering this procedure, WFMH is reinforcing its position as the regional leader in new technology. Second, an early start would position WFMH as the leading provider once the equipment becomes available to competing hospitals. Mikelson does not believe that WFMH's board of trustees will be willing to bear the entire risk of the purchase, but he thinks that they might be willing to go along with a joint venture. Thus, Mikelson suggests that Medina look into the matter further and develop a specific joint venture proposal.

Two months later, when Mikelson had just about forgotten the matter, Medina appears with the following proposal: (Table 1 contains a summary of the proposed financing.)

1. A separate business entity, the Tallahassee Lithotripsy Partnership (the Partnership), would be formed.

2. The Partnership would have two general partners: the Group and WFMH. The Group would put up $150,000 in capital and retain 60 percent management control, while WFMH would furnish $100,000 in capital and obtain 40 percent control. (The Group is incorporated, but it files federal income taxes as an S corporation. It would incorporate a subsidiary S corporation for the sole purpose of investing in the Partnership. S corporations pay no federal income taxes—like a partnership, the income is constructively prorated among the owners and taxed as ordinary income.)

3. Thirty-five limited partnerships would be offered to local physicians for $10,000 each. The limited partners would have no liability beyond their $10,000 investments but, on the other hand, they would have no control rights. (The Partnership is purposely restricted to 35 limited partners, because a larger number would require registration with the State of Florida Corporation Commission.)

4. An additional $600,000 would be obtained from the Tallahassee National Bank in the form of a five-year term (amortized) loan carrying an interest rate of 12 percent. The bank would require that the Partnership pledge the equipment as collateral for the loan. In the event of default by the Partnership, the market value of the equipment would first be used to offset the principal

balance; then the Group would be liable for 60 percent and WFMH for 40 percent of any remaining balance.

The $1.2 million initial capital infusion would be just sufficient to purchase and install the equipment, and to pay the consulting, legal, and accounting costs associated with forming the Partnership. WFMH would lease the Partnership the space for the lithotripter, furnish the technical support required to operate the equipment, and handle billing and collections. Of course, all services provided to the Partnership by WFMH would be handled at "arm's length," and hence the Partnership would pay WFMH prevailing market rates for the services provided.

The Partnership itself would not be taxed, but its distributions represent income, and hence would be taxed on the basis of each partner's tax status. The distributions to WFMH would be nontaxable, since the joint venture is consistent with the hospital's not-for-profit mission. The distributions to the Group and to the limited partners would be taxed as ordinary income. However, about 50 percent of the distributions would represent a return of capital (depreciation cash flow), which is not taxed, and hence taxable investors would pay taxes at an effective rate of only about 15 percent. The cash flows from the Partnership would be distributed in the following way:

1. The Partnership would distribute all earned net cash flow to the partners at the end of each year.

2. In the first year, the limited partners would receive 70 percent of the cash flow and the general partners 30 percent. Following the distribution at the end of each year, the total accumulated dollar return provided to the limited partners would be calculated. If this amount was less than the limited partners' total contribution, they would continue to receive 70 percent of the

Table 1   Partnership Financing Summary

Capital Contribution	General Partners	Limited Partners	Debt Financing
$ 150,000	Group		
100,000	WFMH		
350,000		35 @ $10,000 each	
600,000			Tallahassee NB
$1,200,000			

cash flow in the next year, and the general partners would receive 30 percent.

3. In the years following the year in which the limited partners recover their initial contribution, 50 percent of the cash flow would be distributed to the general partners, while 50 percent would go to the limited partners.

4. The cash flow allocated to the general partners would be distributed proportionally to the Group and to WFMH on the basis of each partner's relative contribution; that is, 60 percent would go to the Group and 40 percent to WFMH.

Of course, the key to a sound financial analysis is good cash flow estimates. Medina and Mikelson devoted an entire day to the cash flow estimation process, and many other individuals provided inputs. If the joint venture gets off the ground, the lithotripter would be in operation by the end of the year (Year 0). The equipment would be available for 50 weeks each year, and the best estimate is that two procedures would be performed per week during the first year (Year 1). It is expected that, on average, the Partnership would receive $4,500 per procedure, net of allowances and bad debt losses. Thus, the net revenue in Year 1 is forecasted to be 2(50)($4,500) = $450,000. Physician and public awareness would be increased significantly after the first year, and hence usage is projected to increase to four procedures per week during Year 2. Although FDA approval would mean additional usage by Medicare/Medicaid patients in Year 3, it is likely that at least one competing hospital would have its own lithotripter at this time. Thus, usage would be expected to fall off to three procedures per week in Year 3, and to two procedures per week in Years 4 and 5.

It is difficult to project the trend for net revenue per procedure. On the one hand, it may be possible to build inflation increases into the charges. On the other hand, more and more patients are joining managed care plans, and these plans often negotiate discounts, sometimes quite large. Furthermore, FDA approval would mean that Medicare and Medicaid patients would join the patient mix, but these payments could be set below the standard charge; indeed, such payments could be below costs. To be conservative, no inflation adjustments are applied to charge estimates.

Technology is moving quickly in this area, so it is very difficult to assess whether the lithotripter would have an economic life of more than five years. For the same reason, it is difficult to estimate the machine's salvage value at the end of five years. Because of the uncertainties involved, Mikelson and Medina decided to take a very conservative approach regarding the life of the Partnership. Thus, for planning purposes, they agreed to assume a five-year life for the Partnership and a zero salvage value for the equipment.

Table 2 contains the pro forma cash flow statements for the Partnership for Years 1 and 2. Note the following points:

1. Technician payments are estimated at $40 per procedure, so total technician support for Year 1 is $(2)(50)\$40 = \$4,000$.

2. Clerical payments are estimated at $15 per procedure, so total clerical expense for Year 1 is $(2)(50)\$15 = \$1,500$.

3. Technician and clerical salaries, and hence payments per procedure, are expected to increase at an annual rate of 5 percent.

4. Rent, insurance, and marketing expenses are forecasted to be $15,000, $10,000, and $5,000, respectively, in Year 1. These costs are expected to increase at the projected inflation rate, 5 percent.

5. Expendable supplies are estimated to cost $10 per procedure, and hence the Year 1 total supplies cost is $(2)(50)\$10 = \$1,000$. Further, the cost of expendables is expected to increase at the 5 percent inflation rate.

6. The service contract on the lithotripter is expected to cost $50,000 in Years 1 and 2, $75,000 in Years 3 and 4, and $100,000 in Year 5. These costs will increase over time because cumulative usage increases the need for equipment maintenance and parts replacement.

7. The Partnership will have to pay property taxes on the equipment, and these taxes are estimated to be $23,000 in Year 1, $24,000 in Year 2, $25,000 in Year 3, $26,000 in Year 4, and $27,000 in Year 5.

8. The Partnership's administrative expenses are estimated to be $30,000 per year. These expenses consist of accounting and legal fees, as well as reimbursement for management time spent on Partnership business. These costs are expected to increase at the 5 percent inflation rate.

9. Principal and interest expenses are based on annual amortization of a 12 percent, five-year loan of $600,000.

10. Miscellaneous expenses, which consist of the costs involved in the semiannual partners meeting, forms printing, expendable

clerical supplies, and so on, are expected to be a constant $20,000 over the next five years.

Medina and Mikelson are most concerned about the estimates for weekly usage and net revenue per visit, and hence they spent a great deal of time developing the following data:

			Weekly Usage		
Case	Year 1	Year 2	Year 3	Year 4	Year 5
Worst	1	3	2	1	1
Most likely	2	4	3	2	2
Best	3	5	4	3	3

They consider $3,500 to be the worst, $4,500 to be the most likely, and $5,500 to be the best case net revenue per visit. Also, they believe that usage and per case revenues are highly positively correlated, so low usage means low revenue per visit, and so on. Finally, they believe that the

Table 2   Pro Forma Cash Flow Statements

	Year 1	Year 2
Net revenues	$450,000	$900,000
Cash operating costs:		
Technician support	$ 4,000	$ 8,400
Clerical support	1,500	3,150
Rent	15,000	15,750
Insurance	10,000	10,500
Marketing expenses	5,000	5,250
Expendable supplies	1,000	2,100
Service contract	50,000	50,000
Property taxes	23,000	24,000
Administrative expense	30,000	31,500
Principal repayment	94,446	105,779
Interest expense	72,000	60,666
Miscellaneous expenses	20,000	20,000
Total expenses	$325,946	$337,096
Partnership net cash flow	$124,054	$562,904

probability of the worst case scenario is 25 percent, the probability of the most likely case is 50 percent, and the probability of the best case is 25 percent.

The current yield on five-year T-bonds is 6 percent, while the rate on 20-year T-bonds is 8 percent. A local brokerage firm estimates the market risk premium to be 7 percentage points. Thus, according to the Capital Asset Pricing Model (CAPM), the current required rate of return on an average risk equity investment is 15 percent.

All parties have previously expressed concern over two issues. First, are there any indirect costs or benefits (that is, costs or benefits that do not appear in the cash flows) to any of the parties to the merger? Second, does the merger raise any legal or ethical issues?

Assume that you have been hired as a consultant to examine the feasibility of the proposed joint venture. You must assess the situation and prepare a report for WFMH and the Group. Medina and Mikelson know that the joint venture will never be successful unless all parties are satisfied with the terms. Thus, they believe that an impartial analysis should be conducted to assess the risk/return potential for each party. Furthermore, if any of the parties do not appear to be treated fairly under the initial proposal, they seek recommendations concerning possible changes that might increase overall fairness, and hence give the proposal a better chance of success.

18

Capitation and Risk Sharing

$\mathbf{T}$hus far in the book, we have focused on making financial management decisions in what might be termed a *conventional reimbursement* environment. In such an environment, providers are reimbursed on the basis of each patient encounter. Thus, each hospital stay in an inpatient setting and each patient visit in an outpatient setting will generate additional revenue. The basis for payment may be charges, discounted charges, prospective payment, per diem, or some other methodology, but the key feature of conventional reimbursement is that higher patient volume leads to increased revenues. Also, in most conventional payment methodologies, the greater the intensity of service provided, and hence the higher the costs, the greater the reimbursement amount.

In recent years, a new reimbursement methodology called *capitation* has been introduced that completely changes providers' financial incentives. Under capitation, providers receive a fixed fee for each member (patient) enrolled, regardless of the amount or intensity of services provided. Clearly, capitation represents a reimbursement methodology that requires a different approach to financial management decision making than that used under conventional reimbursement. The basic cornerstones of finance, such as discounted cash flow analysis, risk and return, and opportunity costs, remain unchanged, but the manner in which these concepts are applied must recognize the unique features of capitation.

This chapter was coauthored by Deborah S. Kolb and J. Bruce Ryan of Jennings Ryan & Kolb, and Peter F. Straley of Baycare Health Partners.

In this chapter, we first present some background information about capitation and why some people believe it will be the dominant reimbursement methodology of the future. Then we discuss the mechanics of capitation and its implications for health care financial management.

An Overview of Capitation

Formally defined, *capitation* is a flat periodic payment per enrollee to a health care provider that is the sole reimbursement for providing services to a defined population. The word "capitation" is derived from the term "per capita," which means per person. Generally, capitation payments are expressed as some dollar amount *per member per month (PMPM)*, where the word "member" typically means enrollee in some managed care plan, usually a health maintenance organization (HMO). For example, a primary care physician may receive a capitated payment of $15 PMPM for attending to the health care needs of 250 members of BetterCare, a regional HMO. Under this contract, the physician would receive $15(250)(12) = $45,000 in total capitation payments over the year, and this amount must cover all of the primary care services offered to the patient population that are specified in the contract. Usually, capitated payments are adjusted for age and gender, but no other adjustments are typically made.

The primary impetus for capitation is health care reform. However, by health care reform, we do not mean political reform, but rather the reform in the health care system mandated by purchasers who are convinced that the current system costs too much and provides too little in return. In essence, the U.S. health care system accomplishes miraculous feats in curing disease and saving the lives of individuals with life-threatening injuries, yet it falls far short in the areas of prevention and health promotion. Also, delivery of health care has become so expensive that employers, who are the primary purchasers of health insurance, are seeking lower-cost alternatives to the current system.

In an attempt to control costs, employers are forming coalitions to gain more bargaining clout when purchasing health care services. To illustrate, in 1995 ten major employers, including American Express, IBM, Merrill Lynch, and Sears, banded together to purchase $1 billion of health care services for 600,000 employees from HMOs in 27 locations across the United States. The coalition gives the companies more leverage in controlling costs and quality than they would have on their own, especially at locations where each employer doesn't have a sufficient number of employees to wield much influence. Merrill's 1994 experience with a smaller coalition indicated that HMO premium rates dropped 7 percent in coalition cities but only 1 percent in other markets. These results are preliminary evidence that market forces are affecting, and even deflating, costs to health care purchasers. Furthermore, Merrill estimated that buyer coalitions result in health care costs that are about 8 percent lower than when companies contract individually. The coalition is inviting bids from 200 HMOs, and it plans to select two to four plans in each market, on the basis of both quality and costs, to help foster competition.

It appears, at least for now, that the health care reform movement is dictating the increased use of managed care as a potential means of both controlling costs to employers and increasing the emphasis on disease prevention. Within managed care plans, the preferred choice of employers is the HMO, and within HMOs, capitation is a commonly used payment mechanism. Figure 18.1 presents a comparison of the conventional and capitation payment systems. In the conventional system, as illustrated here by fee-for-service (FFS), the financial risk of providing health care is shared between purchasers and insurers. Hospitals, physicians, and other providers bear negligible risk because they are paid on the basis of services provided. Insurers bear short-term risk in that in any year payments to providers can exceed the amount of premiums collected. However, poor profitability by insurers in one year usually can be offset by price increases to purchasers the next year, so the long-term risk of financing the health care system is borne by purchasers.

Under capitation, fixed payments to providers are made that are independent of the volume of services rendered, so risk sharing occurs among all three parties. Providers bear the short-term risk that the costs of providing service, including opportunity costs (profits), might exceed the capitation payment. Insurers/networks bear a longer-term risk, in that provider costs can increase when contracts are renewed, but purchasers still bear the ultimate risk of having to support the cost of the health care system.

Self-Test Questions:

What is capitation?

What are the primary differences between a conventional payment system and capitation?

The Growth of Capitated Payment Plans

To many providers, capitation is viewed currently as a payment system that is used elsewhere but will never be used at their organization. Well,

Figure 18.1   Comparison of Conventional and Capitation
Payment Systems

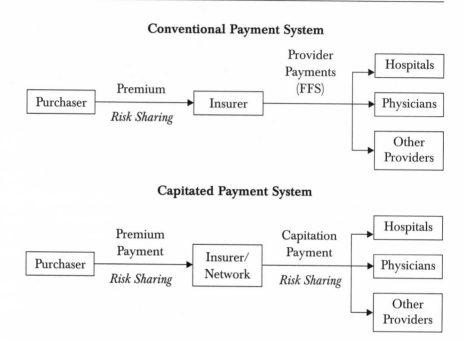

Conventional Payment System

Purchaser — Premium / *Risk Sharing* → Insurer — Provider Payments (FFS) → Hospitals, Physicians, Other Providers

Capitated Payment System

Purchaser — Premium Payment / *Risk Sharing* → Insurer/ Network — Capitation Payment / *Risk Sharing* → Hospitals, Physicians, Other Providers

that may seem to be the case, but don't count on it! Health care buyers prefer capitation because it best meets their goal of controlling health care costs by creating incentives (1) to limit access to only those services that are medically necessary and (2) to provide those services in the most cost-effective setting. Of course, it is possible to become overzealous in limiting services, so it is very important that capitated providers ensure that all services that are medically required be rendered when they are needed. The provision of necessary services when they are needed should actually lower costs in the long run because early intervention and treatment often reduces the need for more intensive services down the road.

For the reasons just mentioned, the march to capitation is being led by the managed care band. Thus, the movement to capitated payment systems can be traced by the movement to managed care plans, particularly HMOs. In 1995, about 55 million Americans (almost 20 percent of the population) were members of HMOs, and this number is expected to increase to about 85 million by 1998. In the health plans of the *Fortune*

1,000 firms, only 34 percent of employees elected managed care plans in 1990, while today over 60 percent are enrolled in these plans.

The increasing size and strength of managed care plans means that more and more providers will be paid under capitation in the future. What types of services can be capitated? Although capitation payment was first used with primary care physicians, virtually any type of health care service can be reimbursed by capitation. Thus, acute care and specialty hospitals can be capitated, as can physician specialists and allied health professionals. Even companies that sell medical supplies can be paid on a capitated basis. In 1994, about 70 percent of all HMOs capitated primary care physicians, 50 percent capitated some or all specialists, and 25 percent capitated some or all hospital services. Fitch Investors Service, a New York credit-rating agency, estimates that 70 percent of hospitals' revenues will be capitated before the turn of the century. Fitch also predicts that Medicare will eventually establish a capitated system for both hospitals and physicians, because capitation offers the only hope for controlling Medicare's massive drain on federal revenues.

Note that capitation can also be applied to total disease management. To illustrate, in the first contract of its kind, Salick Health Care in 1994 agreed to provide comprehensive cancer care—including hospital, outpatient, and home health care—at a fixed price to nearly 100,000 members of Physicians Corporation of America, a Miami-based HMO. Prior to the contract, Salick had spent over two years preparing detailed oncology practice guidelines, in part to control costs, but also to assuage critics who argue that capitation induces providers to withhold needed care.

The Salick illustration gives you some idea of the use of capitation, but it represents only one of thousands of such contracts in use today. There is every indication that capitation payment systems will spread, and perhaps some day will dominate the reimbursement scene.

Self-Test Questions:

What is the driving force behind the growth of capitated payment systems?

What services can be reimbursed by capitation?

Capitation, Provider Incentives, and Behavior

Capitation has a dramatic impact on provider incentives, and hence on provider behavior. To begin our discussion of these issues, we will first discuss the impact of capitation on provider incentives. Then, we present some evidence on what has occurred in markets that are dominated by capitated payment systems.

Incentives under capitation

Consider Figure 18.2, which depicts revenues and costs to a provider under both fee-for-service and capitated payment. Regardless of the payment system, total costs (TC), which are merely the sum of fixed costs (FC) and variable costs (VC), are tied directly to volume, so the greater the volume of services delivered, the greater the amount of total costs. The difference between the two graphs is the revenue line, and the ways in which profits and losses are realized. Under fee-for-service, the revenue line (Rev) is upward sloping, and it starts at the origin. At zero volume, the provider receives zero revenue, and the greater the volume, the higher the revenue. Under capitation, assuming a fixed number of enrollees, revenues are fixed independently of volume, and hence the revenue line is horizontal. On each graph, breakeven (BE) is shown at that volume where revenues equal total costs.

Although the graphs are somewhat similar in general appearance, there is a profound difference in how profits and losses occur. First, consider fee-for-service. All volumes to the left of breakeven produce a

Figure 18.2   Revenue and Cost Structures Under Fee-for-Service
and Capitation

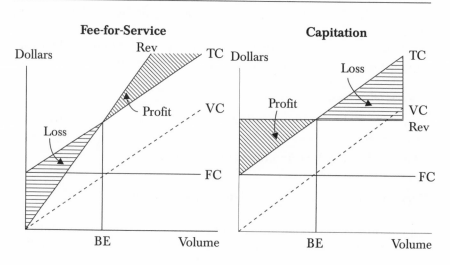

loss for the provider, while all volumes to the right of breakeven produce a profit. Thus, the incentive for providers is to increase utilization because increased volume leads to increased profits. Now look at the capitation graph. Here, all volumes to the left of breakeven produce a profit, whereas all volumes to the right of breakeven result in a loss. Under capitation, providers have the incentive to decrease utilization, because decreased volume leads to increased profits. The only way to increase revenues is to increase the number of covered lives (enrollees).

Capitation completely reverses the actions that providers must take to assure financial success, and many providers will find it difficult to adjust to the new, perverse (by conventional reimbursement standards) incentive system. Under fee-for-service, the keys to success are to work harder, increase volume, and hence increase profits, while under capitation, the keys to profitability are to work smarter and decrease volume. Since the primary means to profitability with fee-for-service is increased volume, increased reimbursement rates, or both, the primary task of managers is to maximize utilization and reimbursement rates. Furthermore, any deficiencies in cost control often can be overcome by higher volume. Under capitation, the primary path to profitability is through cost control, so the key to success is lower volume and cost-effective treatment plans.

Although much has been written about the negatives of capitation, particularly the incentive to withhold needed services, it must also be recognized that there are positive aspects to capitation. Here are some potential benefits associated with capitation:

- Providers receive a fixed payment regardless of whether services are actually rendered. Capitation revenues are predictable and timely, and thus are less risky than revenues from conventional payment methodologies, which are tied to volume.

- Capitation payments are received before services are rendered, so, in effect, payers are extending credit to providers rather than vice versa, as under conventional reimbursement.

- Capitation supports national health care goals, primarily increased emphasis on cost control as well as on wellness and prevention.

- Capitation may ease the reimbursement paperwork burden and hence reduce expenditures on administrative costs.

- Capitation aligns the economic interests of physicians and hospitals because risk-sharing systems are typically established that allow all of the providers in a capitated system to benefit from reducing costs.

- Similarly, capitation encourages utilization of lower-cost treatments, such as outpatient surgery and home health care, as opposed to higher-cost inpatient alternatives. Thus, capitation creates incentives to use those services that are typically preferred by patients when such alternatives are clinically appropriate.

Behavior under capitation

In attempting to predict the future, it is interesting to examine the impact of capitation on provider behavior in those markets where HMOs have the strongest presence. Several markets, such as Rochester, New York, and Madison, Wisconsin, now have HMOs controlling more than 50 percent of the health care market, but the HMOs in southern California have been particularly aggressive in gobbling up market share. For example, in Los Angeles, seven large integrated networks control 75 percent of the city's commercial health care market. Thus, southern California in general, and Los Angeles in particular, are often cited as examples where providers have already responded to the pressures of capitation, and hence represent a view of what the entire country would resemble if capitation becomes the predominant reimbursement system.

Table 18.1 illustrates the impact of capitation on hospital utilization. Whereas current hospital utilization averages over 700 inpatient days annually per 1,000 patient population, capitated systems that aggressively control inpatient stays have reduced utilization to only 238 inpatient days. When these data are converted to daily census, and allowing for 85 percent occupancy as full capacity, only about 0.8 beds are required per 1,000 population versus a current need of about 2.3 beds per 1,000 based on national average usage rates. The implication for hospitals is clear: if the capitated targets are realistic, and if the bulk of the U.S. population becomes covered by HMO plans, then the hospital industry has significant overcapacity and continued shrinkage is likely to occur. Even if the most aggressive utilization targets are not met, HMO penetration and capitation will surely increase the pace of hospital closings, consolidation, and downsizing already taking place.

Table 18.2 focuses on the impact of capitation on selected physician utilization. The key feature here is that managed care, with its emphasis on wellness and prevention as opposed to treatment, requires a different mix and fewer physicians than currently exist. Furthermore, managed care plans use more physician extenders, such as nurse practitioners and physician assistants, than are currently utilized.

Of course, not all predictions come true, and the structure of the

Table 18.1   Impact of Capitation on Annual Hospital Utilization

Age	Number of Inpatient Days per 1,000 Covered Population		
	National Average	*HMO Average*	*Capitated Target*
Under 65	433	297	155
Over 65	2,676	1,691	850
Overall*	702	465	238

*Based on an age mix of 12 percent over age 65.

Source: Estimated by Jennings Ryan & Kolb on the basis of 1994 data from the National Center for Health Statistics; 1994. *Managed Care Digest.* Marion Merrill Dow; and the Advisory Board Government Committee.

Table 18.2   Impact of Capitation on Physician and Physician Extender Utilization

Specialty	FTEs per 100,000 Covered Population		Percent of Current Supply Needed Under Capitation
	1992 Supply	*HMO Needs*	
Family practice/General medicine	29.3	11.7	39.9%
Internal medicine	23.3	23.8	102.1
Pediatrics	13.1	11.9	90.8
Total primary care	65.7	47.4	72.1%
Obstetrics/Gynecology	11.4	10.1	86.0%
Medical specialties	17.8	12.7	71.3
Surgical specialties	32.5	21.2	65.2
Total specialists	61.7	44.0	71.3%
Total physicians	127.4	91.4	71.7%
Physician extenders	19.6	25.0	127.6%

Source: Adapted from Jonathan P. Weiner. 1994. "Forecasting the Effects of Health Care Reform on U.S. Physician Workforce Requirements: Evidence from HMO Staffing Patterns." *Journal of the American Medical Association* (20 July).

health care industry may not change as drastically as these forecasts indicate. However, as we are writing this chapter, the handwriting on the wall suggests two powerful trends: fewer hospital beds and a physician mix that contains a greater proportion of primary care physicians. Most importantly, the data tell us that historical utilization rates based on conventional reimbursement methodologies are not good predictors of future utilization when the payment system is capitation.

Self-Test Questions:

What are the differences in provider incentives under conventional reimbursement and capitation?

What are the advantages of a capitated payment system?

What does the California experience tell us about the look of the future health care delivery system?

Financial Risk under Capitation

One of the key issues facing providers is the impact of capitation on financial risk. To examine this issue, we will first present a descriptive picture of financial risk, then examine the nature of financial risk, and finally present the results of an analysis that examined the financial risk inherent in capitation contracts.

Descriptive risk

One way to assess the risk inherent in capitation versus other reimbursement contracts is to describe in words the nature of the risks incurred. Table 18.3 lists the most common provider reimbursement methodologies and describes the financial risks inherent in each system. *Fee-for-service* is the least risky because the only risk facing providers is the risk that volume will be too low to cover total costs, including both variable and fixed costs. Note that regardless of the reimbursement method, providers bear the cost of service risk, in that costs can exceed revenues. However, a primary difference among the reimbursement types is the ability of the provider to influence the revenue-to-cost ratio. If providers set fees for each type of service provided, they can most easily ensure that revenues exceed costs. Furthermore, if providers have the power to set rates above those that would exist in a truly competitive market, fee-for-service becomes even less risky. Finally, providers can increase usage by *churning*—creating more visits, ordering more tests, extending inpatient stays, and so on—which in turn increases revenues and reduces risks. *Discounted fee-for-service* may lower the profit potential of providers, but it does not alter the risks borne by providers.

Prospective payment, in which a fixed payment is made on the basis of each patient's diagnosis, adds a second dimension of risk to reimbursement contracts because the bundle of services needed to treat a particular patient may be more costly than that assumed in the payment. If, on average, patients require more intensive treatments and, for hospitals, a longer length of stay than assumed in the prospective payment amount, the provider must bear the added costs.

Per diem reimbursement, whereby providers are paid a preset amount per patient day, is often used for hospitals and long-term care facilities. In addition to a single all-inclusive per diem rate, *stratified per diems* are sometimes used whereby different rates are paid for dissimilar categories of care, such as general acute inpatient, obstetrical, and intensive care. Even under stratified per diems, one rate usually covers a large number of diagnoses, and providers bear case-mix risk along

Table 18.3   Descriptive Risk Under Various Reimbursement Methodologies

Contract Type	Provider Risks
Fee-for-service (charges)	Volume too low to cover total costs
Discounted fee-for-service (discounted charges)	Volume too low to cover total costs
Prospective payment	Volume too low to cover fixed costs Case intensity Length of stay
Per diem	Volume too low to cover fixed costs Case intensity Case mix Payer-limited length of stay
Global pricing	Volume too low to cover fixed costs Case intensity Pre- and post-operative care Physician services
Capitation	Volume too high for payment amount Case intensity Case mix Utilization Actuarial accuracy

with intensity risk. In addition, providers bear the risk that the payer, through utilization reviews, will constrain lengths of stay, and hence increase intensity during the days that a patient is hospitalized. Thus, under per diem, the "compression" of services and shortened lengths of stay can put significant pressure on providers' profitability.

Under *global pricing*, payers pay a single prospective payment that covers all services delivered in a single episode, whether the services are rendered by a single or by multiple providers. For example, a global fee may be set for all obstetric services associated with a pregnancy provided by a single physician, including all prenatal and postnatal visits, as well as the delivery itself. Or a global price may be paid for all physician and hospital services associated with a cardiac bypass operation. From a payer's perspective, global pricing eliminates the potential for problems associated with unbundling and upcoding. *Unbundling* involves pricing the individual components of a service separately, rather than as a package. For example, a physician's treatment of a fracture could be bundled and hence billed as one episode, or it could be unbundled, with separate bills submitted for diagnosis, x-rays, setting the fracture, removing the cast, and so on. The rationale for unbundling is usually to provide more detailed records of treatments rendered, but often the result is higher total charges for the parts than would be charged for the entire package. *Upcoding* is the practice of billing for a procedure that yields a higher prospective payment than the one actually performed. Clearly, the more services that must be rendered for a single payment, the more providers are at risk for intensity of services.

Finally, under *capitation*, providers receive a fixed payment per member per month to provide all covered services to some defined population. Now, providers assume utilization and actuarial risks along with the risks assumed under the other reimbursement methods.

When the risks under different reimbursement systems are outlined in this descriptive fashion, it is easy to jump to the conclusion that capitation is by far the riskiest to providers, while fee-for-service is the least risky. However, before finalizing our conclusions regarding the risk to providers under capitation contracts, we need to examine the issue a little more closely. We begin our more detailed examination with a discussion of the nature of financial risk.

The nature of financial risk

As discussed in Chapters 5 and 11, financial risk stems from uncertainties inherent in expected cash flows. If all forecasted cash flows were known with certainty, there would be no financial risk. However, because of uncertainties, there is some probability that a reimbursement contract will be less profitable than expected, and the greater the probability of a realized profitability far below that expected, the greater the financial risk.

Financial risk can be classified along several dimensions, but two dimensions are of particular relevance to our discussion of financial risk under capitation. *Objective risk* occurs when the risk inherent in a uncertain outcome is known with certainty. For example, the flip of a coin has only objective risk. It is uncertain whether the flip will result in a head or a tail, so the flip is risky, but the probability of flipping a head or tail, 50 percent, is known with certainty. *Subjective risk* occurs when the probability distribution itself is uncertain. For example, a particular weather forecaster may predict that the chance of rain is 20 percent, but different forecasters may attach different probabilities to the event. Here there are two dimensions to risk: the risk inherent in the probability distribution (20 percent rain/80 percent no rain) and the risk that the probability distribution itself (the weather forecast) is wrong.[1]

We will see that the objective financial risk inherent in capitation contracts is not as high as many people suspect. However, their subjective financial risk is often very high, so the overall impact of capitation on the financial risk of most providers is much higher than indicated by an objective risk analysis because, by definition, subjective risk cannot be measured.

It is important to make one other point concerning financial risk. Under most types of reimbursement, rates can be set too low to cover costs. In such contracts, providers will lose money, but they do not necessarily bear a great deal of financial risk, as defined here, because such risk is a function of uncertainty, not profitability. If you loan $1,000 to your brother-in-law with every expectation that the loan will never be repaid, the loan is not very risky at all, even though its expected rate of return is −100 percent. Similarly, a hospital's reimbursement contract with a certain loss of, say, $100,000, has no financial risk because there is no uncertainty regarding the contract's profitability. The point here is that many payers offering capitated contracts have a great deal of bargaining power that can be used to negotiate very tough terms with providers. These tough terms, and the resulting potential for losses on the contract, are not a result of the financial risk inherent in the capitation contracts, but rather a result of the negotiating power of the payer. That same payer could negotiate a low-profitability contract regardless of the reimbursement method specified.

A quantitative analysis

The financial risk associated with provider contracts stems from uncertainty in profitability, so both revenues and costs must be considered. We will use hospitals to analyze the financial risk inherent in prospective payment and capitation contracts, but the results also apply to physicians and other health care providers.[2]

Under prospective payment, there is significant revenue risk since the amount of reimbursement depends on the number of admissions, with higher volume yielding greater revenues. However, under capitation, and assuming a fixed number of enrollees, there is virtually no revenue risk. The hospital will receive the contractually fixed amount per member per month regardless of patient volume.

On the cost side, the financial risks are identical under the two contracts. There are fixed costs inherent in providing the service that must be met regardless of volume, and variable costs that are incurred for each patient admission. Thus, total costs, the sum of fixed and variable components, are dependent on volume. If we assume, at least initially, that the number and nature of admissions are unaffected by the reimbursement contract, then realized total costs are the same for a given population whether the payment method is prospective payment or capitation.

The financial risk facing hospitals is tied to uncertainty in profitability, and hence stems from both uncertainties in the revenue stream and uncertainties in total costs. To examine the impact of these uncertainties, we will consider two hospitals: Hospital F, whose costs are all fixed, and Hospital V, whose costs are all variable. Clearly, no real world hospital has all fixed or all variable costs, but by looking at these extremes we can gain a better appreciation of the factors that influence financial risk under prospective payment and capitation.

To keep the analysis manageable, assume a hypothetical situation in which the contract involves 1,000 members; the annual capitation payment is $300 per member per year (PMPY); the expected number of inpatient stays is 0.1 PMPY, or 100 admissions per year; and the prospective payment per admission is $3,000. On the cost side, assume that Hospital F has fixed costs of $300,000, and no variable costs, to treat the population served, while Hospital V has variable costs of $3,000 per inpatient stay, and no fixed costs.

Table 18.4 contains the annual cash flows to each hospital associated with the two contracts. Note that the initial values were chosen so that the revenues are the same under each contract type and total costs are the same at both hospitals. Also, for ease, the values were chosen so that the net income under both contracts is zero.

Now, let's introduce risk into the analysis. Again, to keep the example manageable, assume that the only uncertainty in the contracts is patient volume. That is, the capitation payment, prospective payment per admission, fixed costs, and variable costs per inpatient stay are known with certainty at the beginning of the year (beginning of the contract period). What would happen to profitability if realized volume differed from expected volume? Table 18.5 answers this question.

Uncertain volume has no effect on Hospital F under capitation or on Hospital V under prospective payment. In each instance, revenues and costs move in step with one another. Hospital F has all fixed costs, and under capitation its revenues are fixed, so changes in volume have no impact on profitability. Under prospective payment, revenues vary

Table 18.4   Annual Cash Flows

	Hospital F		Hospital V	
	Prospective Payment	Capitation	Prospective Payment	Capitation
Total revenues	$300,000	$300,000	$300,000	$300,000
Fixed costs	300,000	300,000	0	0
Variable costs	0	0	300,000	300,000
Net income	$ 0	$ 0	$ 0	$ 0

Table 18.5   Net Income at Different Volume Levels

Number of Inpatient Stays	Hospital F		Hospital V	
	Prospective Payment	Capitation	Prospective Payment	Capitation
80	($60,000)	$0	$0	$60,000
85	(45,000)	0	0	45,000
90	(30,000)	0	0	30,000
95	(15,000)	0	0	15,000
100	0	0	0	0
105	15,000	0	0	(15,000)
110	30,000	0	0	(30,000)
115	45,000	0	0	(45,000)
120	60,000	0	0	(60,000)

with volume, while costs are fixed, so higher volume leads to higher profitability. Thus, with prospective payment contracts, Hospital F has a financial incentive to increase volume, because increased volume leads to higher profits.

The situation is reversed at Hospital V. When all costs are variable, profits are constant under prospective payment, but variable under capitation. Increased volume leads to increased revenue under prospective payment, but the revenue increase is offset exactly by higher costs. Hospital V receives $3,000 for each admission, but its variable costs also equal $3,000 per admission, so additional admissions add nothing to the bottom line. Lower volume means lower costs regardless of the reimbursement method, but under capitation the revenue stream is fixed, so Hospital V has a financial incentive with capitation to decrease volume because lower volume leads to higher profits.

The analysis could be extended to include uncertainty in variable costs and prospective payment per admission, but the general results would remain the same. If all costs are fixed, there is less objective financial risk to capitation contracts than to prospective payment contracts. If all costs are variable, there is less objective financial risk to prospective payment contracts than to capitation contracts.

When assessing the relative objective financial risk of capitation contracts, the key question to providers is this: "Are the costs at my organization predominantly fixed or predominantly variable?" If the costs are mostly fixed, then objective financial risk is actually reduced when moving from prospective payment to capitation because the fixed revenue stream better matches the fixed cost structure. On the other hand, if the cost structure is predominantly variable, moving to capitation will increase objective financial risk since the fixed revenue stream is a poor match for a cost structure that is highly correlated to volume.

Most health care providers, and hospitals in particular, have relatively high fixed-to-total-cost ratios. Thus, for most providers, capitation contracts actually have less objective financial risk than prospective payment contracts because financial risk is reduced by matching the uncertainties inherent in the revenue and cost streams. When organizations have a high percentage of fixed costs, a fixed revenue stream stabilizes profits, and hence reduces financial risk.

If objective financial risk is reduced under capitation contracts, why did our earlier descriptive analysis conclude that capitation is more risky than prospective payment? One reason, of course, is that the descriptive assessment did not consider in any systematic way the relationships between revenues and costs. More importantly, the numerical analysis ignored the subjective risk inherent in capitation contracts. The numerical analysis focused solely on objective financial risk—we assumed that providers know their cost structures and population characteristics well enough to be confident of the revenue and cost estimates. Under these conditions, capitation contracts are clearly less risky to providers with a high percentage of fixed costs.

However, to limit the overall financial risk of capitation contracts to objective risk, it is necessary that providers be able to forecast accurately costs and volumes for a large number of diagnoses. For example, assume a hospital signs a capitation contract to provide all common inpatient services to a patient population of 100,000. If the hospital is to bear only objective financial risk, it must know with some confidence the expected volume by diagnosis, as well as the costs for treating those diagnoses. Thus, the hospital needs relatively sophisticated actuarial and cost data.

Even if a contract has substantial underlying financial risk, whether objective or subjective, its effective riskiness is lessened if management can take actions to counter unexpected adverse trends as they develop. Suppose a hospital enters into a capitation contract without good estimates of volume and costs. If six months into the contract realized total costs exceed estimates, the contract will likely be less profitable than expected, and if the volume and cost estimates were very inaccurate, the results could prove disastrous. The only two means available to turn the bad contract into a good one are to decrease volume, lower costs, or both. In the past, hospitals with profitability problems solved such problems by raising charges and increasing volume. Under capitation, however, the prescription for increased profit requires actions—decreasing volume or lowering costs and increasing enrollment—with which providers have limited experience, and hence are more difficult to implement than previous prescriptions. Furthermore, when a high proportion of costs is fixed, cost reduction efforts are extremely challenging because they can be achieved only by selling off plant and equipment and shrinking the labor force. Under capitation contracts, providers are less able to influence the profitability of a contract once it goes into force, so they are less able to cope with the given amount of financial risk faced.

Another risk that providers face under capitation is the impact of outliers. The costs associated with a single patient, especially to a hospital, can fall well beyond normal bounds, and hence one or just a few outliers can result in financial losses well beyond those estimated at the time a contract is signed. In general, prospective payment contracts have outlier provisions, so providers are somewhat protected against the risks associated with high-cost outliers. If capitation contracts do not contain such provisions, the risk of outliers increases the financial risk inherent in such contracts.[3] Furthermore, to increase the probability that realized volume, and hence cash flows, will be close to that forecasted, providers must have a relatively large number of covered lives under capitation contracts.

Our quantitative analysis leads to two primary conclusions about the relative risk of capitation contracts. First, the objective financial risk inherent in capitation contracts is not as high as most people think. Providers with a high percentage of fixed costs can actually stabilize earnings under capitation, and hence reduce financial risk. Second, the overall financial risk of capitation contracts, including both objective and subjective risk, can be very high if providers (1) do not have the actuarial and cost data available to make sound capitation pricing decisions, and (2) do not have the capability to reduce volume and cut costs, if necessary, to react to any adverse trends that might develop.

Taken together, these conclusions have several implications for health care providers. To prosper in a health care system moving rapidly toward capitation, providers must be able to estimate accurately not only their own costs, but also the diagnoses and patient volumes that would result from a particular contract. This means that many providers will need better costing systems than they currently have, and also that providers will need to acquire actuarial expertise, a domain historically left to insurers. Without these data, it will be impossible to enter into capitation contracts without bearing a high degree of subjective financial risk. One efficient way for providers to acquire actuarial data is to enter into integrated networks that possess such data, so the trend toward networks can reduce subjective financial risk.

Also, providers will have to break with traditional paradigms. Financial problems can no longer be solved by raising charges and increasing volume. Under capitation, raising charges (having a high bid on a contract proposal) will mean fewer patients for the provider, which will have an adverse effect both on revenues and on achieving a capitated population sufficiently large to realize actuarial predictions. Furthermore, the key to success once the contract has been signed is to lower costs and volume. This requires nontraditional strategies, so today's health care managers must exhibit flexibility and adaptability to successfully manage the transition to capitation.

Finally, providers that are less efficient than their local counterparts confront very difficult issues when negotiating managed care contracts. Capitation contracts are usually set at rates that assume the efficient delivery of services in order to control unnecessary services and costs. Less efficient providers will experience more challenges under capitation since they must choose between accepting rates that, at least in the short run, may not cover costs, or losing market share that they may not be able to regain. The difficulties inefficient providers face do not result from financial risk differentials, but rather from prior management practices that did not sufficiently stress the efficient delivery of services.

Self-Test Questions:

Briefly describe the following reimbursement systems and, using the descriptive approach, analyze the risks to providers under each system:

1. Fee-for-service
2. Discounted fee-for-service
3. Prospective payment
4. Per diem
5. Global pricing
6. Capitation.

What is the basic source of financial risk?

Distinguish between objective and subjective financial risk.

What lessons can be learned from the quantitative risk assessment of prospective payment and capitation contracts?

Development of Premium Rates

One of the primary financial management functions within managed care plans and integrated delivery systems is the development of premium rates for health care buyers, which involves estimating the total costs of providing health care services. In this section, we discuss several methodologies for estimating provider payments, which are then aggregated to estimate total costs, the basis for the premium rate.

Allocation of premium dollars

HMOs and other managed care organizations collect premium dollars from employers and other purchasers of health care, and then use those dollars to pay providers, cover administrative expenses, and earn profits. To help better understand how HMOs set their premium rates, first consider Table 18.6, which shows how a typical premium dollar is spent. First, HMOs have the same types of management and marketing expenses as any other business, and the premium dollar must cover such costs. Also, it is necessary for HMOs to earn profits, both to create reserves for contingencies and for distribution to stockholders if investor owned. About 16 percent of the premium dollar goes for administration and profit, while the remaining 84 percent is paid out to providers. The biggest provider expense typically is for physicians, with approximately 12 percent of the premium dollar going to primary care physicians and 32 percent to specialists who are part of the HMO's provider panel.

The next major item is payments for hospital and other institutional care provided within the system (within the HMO's provider panel), which totals 36 percent of the premium dollar. Finally, HMO members sometimes require services from providers that are out of the HMO's system, either because there are no in-system providers for that service or the services are required outside the geographic area served by the HMO. Payments to out-of-system providers, including both physicians and hospitals/institutions, average 4 percent of the premium dollar.

Note that the Table 18.6 percentages are averages, that there are wide variations among HMOs on how the premium dollar is allocated. Health care purchasers want a high percentage of the premium dollar to go to providers, to encourage them to provide needed services in a timely manner. Conversely, HMOs have an incentive to lower the amount paid to providers, both to increase profits and to ensure competitive pricing to buyers in an increasingly hostile marketplace.

Developing premium rates: an illustration

There are many ways to develop the premium rates that managed care plans charge health care purchasers. In this section, we illustrate several

Table 18.6   Typical Allocation of the HMO Premium Dollar

Total premium dollar	100%
Administration and profit	16%
Paid to within-system physicians:	
Primary care	12%
Specialists	32
Total to within-system physicians	44%
Paid to within-system hospitals/institutions	36%
Paid to out-of-system providers	4%

Source: Jennings Ryan & Kolb.

methods that an HMO or integrated delivery system can use to estimate the payments it must make to its providers to cover a defined population, and which it can then aggregate and combine with its own costs to estimate a premium rate.[4] Rates are developed as if all providers were capitated, because the final premium rate will be quoted on a per member per month basis. However, actual reimbursement could be by capitation, discounted fee-for-service, or by any other method.

Assume that BetterCare, Inc., an aggressively managed HMO, must develop a premium bid to submit to Big Business, a major employer in BetterCare's service area. To keep the illustration manageable, assume that all medically necessary in-area services can be provided by a single hospital that offers both inpatient and outpatient services, including emergency room services, a single nursing home, a panel of primary care physicians, and a panel of specialist physicians. In addition, BetterCare must budget for covered care to be delivered out of area when its members are traveling. Thus, to develop its bid, BetterCare has to estimate the amount of payments to this set of providers for the covered population, in addition to allowing for administrative expenses and profits.

Hospital inpatient rate

The *fee-for-service equivalent method* is often used to set the within-system hospital inpatient capitation rate. This method is based on expected usage and negotiated charges, rather than underlying costs, although there clearly should be a link between charges and costs. To illustrate, assume that BetterCare targets 350 inpatient days for each 1,000 members, or 0.350 inpatient days per member. Furthermore, BetterCare believes that a fair fee-for-service charge in a competitive environment would be $938 per inpatient day. Note that the values chosen both for utilization and payment are not based on conventional reimbursement experience. Rather, the number of inpatient days reflects a highly managed working-age population, and the fee-for-service charge is designed to cover all hospital costs, including profits, in an efficiently run hospital operating in a highly competitive environment. The inpatient cost per member per month (PMPM) is found as follows:

Inpatient cost PMPM

$$= \frac{\text{Per member utilization rate} \times \text{Fee-for-service rate}}{12}$$

$$= \frac{0.350 \times \$938}{12} = \$27.35 \text{ PMPM.}$$

Thus, using the fee-for-service method, BetterCare estimates that inpatient costs for Big Business's HMO enrollees is $27.35 *PMPM.*

Other institutional rates

The rate for out-of-area hospital usage and hospital outpatient visits, as well as for skilled nursing home stays, is developed using the fee-for-service equivalent method discussed above. Here is a summary of BetterCare's estimates for these services:

Service	Annual Usage per 1,000 Members	Fee-for-Service Rate	Capitation Rate PMPM
Out-of-area inpatient days	25	$1,495	$3.11
Outpatient surgeries	50	1,082	4.51
Emergency room visits	125	138	1.44
Skilled nursing home days	5	150	0.06
			$9.12

Here, each PMPM capitation rate was calculated by multiplying annual usage times the fee-for-service rate, and then dividing the resulting product first by 1,000 to obtain a per member amount, and then by 12 to get the PMPM rate. The end result is a capitation estimate of $9.12 PMPM for the services listed above. Of course, actual payments to these providers typically would be made on a discounted fee-for-service basis.

Primary care rate

We will use the *budgetary,* or *cost, approach* to estimate primary physicians' costs for Big Business's enrollees. This method is the most common for setting physicians' payments, and it is based on usage and underlying costs, as opposed to charges. The starting point is expected patient demand, by specialty, for physicians' services. This demand is then translated into the number of full-time equivalent (FTE) physicians required per 1,000 members (enrollees), which depends on physician productivity. Finally, the cost for physician services is estimated by multiplying staffing requirements by the average cost per FTE, including base compensation, fringe benefits, and malpractice premiums. In addition, an amount is added for clinical and administrative support for physicians, usually some dollar amount per 1,000 members.

In developing its capitation rate for primary care physicians, BetterCare made the following assumptions:

- On average, since each enrollee makes 3.0 visits to a primary care physician per year, each 1,000 enrollees will make 3,000 visits per year.
- Each primary care physician is able to handle 4,000 patient visits per year.
- Total yearly compensation per primary care physician is $175,000.

Under these assumptions, each 1,000 enrollees will require 3,000/4,000 = 0.75 primary care physicians, and hence each 1,000 enrollees will require 0.75($175,000) = $131,250 in primary care physicians' services. Finally, the annual cost per member is $131,250/1,000 = $131.25, and the cost PMPM = $131.25/12 = $10.94. Thus, the rate that BetterCare will propose to Big Business will include a capitation payment of $10.94 PMPM for primary care physician compensation.

Specialty care rate

The capitation rate for specialists' care is developed using the cost approach in a manner similar to that for primary care. Here are BetterCare's assumptions:

- On average, each enrollee is referred for 1.2 visits to specialists per year, so each 1,000 enrollees makes 1,200 visits per year.
- Each specialty physician can handle 2,000 patient visits per year.
- Total compensation per specialist is $284,000 per year.

Under these assumptions, each 1,000 enrollees will require 1,200/2,000 = 0.60 specialists, and hence each 1,000 enrollees will require 0.60($284,000) = $170,400 in specialists' services. Finally, the annual cost per member is $170,400/1,000 = $170.40, so the cost PMPM = $170.40/12 = $14.20. Thus, the rate that BetterCare will propose to Big Business will include a capitation payment of $14.20 PMPM for specialist physician compensation.

Other physician-related costs rate

Thus far, we have estimated the capitation rate for physicians' compensation, but we have not accounted for the other costs associated with physicians' practices. First, physicians require, on average, 1.7 FTEs for clinical and administrative support, and each supporting staff member receives an average of $35,000 per year in total compensation. Since the physician requirement to support 1,000 members is 0.75 primary care plus 0.60 specialists, for a total of 1.35 physicians, each 1,000 members will require $1.35(1.7)(\$35,000) \approx \$80,000$ of physician's support, or $\$80,000/1,000/12 = \$6.67$ PMPM.

Next, expenditures on supplies, including administrative, medical, and diagnostic supplies, average $10 per visit, and members are expected to make 4.2 visits per year to both primary and specialty care physicians. Thus, the annual cost per member is $42, and the cost PMPM is estimated to be $42/12 = \$3.50$ PMPM. Finally, overhead expenses, including depreciation, rent, utilities, and so on, are estimated at $6.00 PMPM.

Total physician rate

BetterCare has estimated numerous categories of costs related solely to physicians. For ease, assume now that BetterCare plans to contract with a single medical group practice to provide all physicians' service and to pay the group a capitated rate. Then the total capitation rate for the medical group would be as follows:

Primary care	$10.94 PMPM
Specialist care	14.20
Support staff	6.67
Supplies	3.50
Overhead	6.00
Subtotal	$41.31 PMPM
Profit (10%)	4.13
In-area total	$45.44 PMPM
Outside referrals	3.40
Total	$48.84 PMPM

The $48.84 PMPM total capitation rate for the medical group is merely the aggregate of the rates previously developed for physicians' services, plus two additional elements. First, BetterCare believes that a fair profit margin on group practice businesses is 10 percent, so $4.13 PMPM is allowed for profit on the in-area physician subtotal of $41.31 PMPM. Second, $3.40 PMPM is allocated to cover referrals outside the group practice when needed either because a particular specialty is not available within the group or the member is outside the service area. Finally, note that the group might not capitate all of its physicians even though it receives a capitated rate from BetterCare.

An alternative method for physician's rates

In general, the rates obtained from the first two methods would include adjustments for age and sex. An alternative method would be to start with utilization data broken down by age and sex. The *demographic-based approach* focuses on the age/sex distribution of the population being served, which is then coupled with cost or fee-for-service data to estimate the capitation rate. Table 18.7 illustrates the demographic-based approach by applying it to the population that would be served if BetterCare wins the contract to provide an HMO plan for Big Business.

The male/female costs were calculated by multiplying the population percentages for each sex times the applicable costs per member per month. The total cost for each service is merely the sum of the male and female costs.

Note that the total cost for physicians, $16.17 + $29.27 = $45.44 PMPM, is the same as BetterCare estimated using the budgetary approach. If the data are consistent, both methods should lead to the same capitation rate. Also, the hospital/other institutional capitation rate of $36.47 PMPM is the same as the rate obtained earlier for these services: $27.35 + $9.12 = $36.47. Clearly, we "fudged" the data so our results would be consistent. In most cases, capitation rates developed

Table 18.7 Demographic-Based Rates for the Medical Group

			Cost per Member per Month					
	Demographics		Primary Care		Specialist/Referral		Hospital/Other	
Age Band	Male	Female	Male	Female	Male	Female	Male	Female
0–1	1.9%	1.9%	$47.00	$47.00	$31.42	$31.42	$ 29.93	$29.93
2–4	2.8	2.8	20.25	20.25	11.19	11.19	16.29	16.29
5–19	12.4	12.4	11.04	11.04	11.19	11.19	15.35	15.35
20–29	11.4	15.4	10.53	15.92	18.44	49.30	11.58	55.65
30–39	9.6	10.0	13.04	17.56	23.26	44.51	24.95	58.97
40–49	5.3	5.7	16.40	19.56	32.64	41.05	53.74	52.31
50–59	3.6	3.6	20.74	22.74	47.13	47.74	80.60	66.91
60+	0.7	0.5	24.93	25.60	73.43	58.91	121.54	87.60
Total	47.7%	52.3%						
Male/female cost			$ 7.07	$ 9.10	$10.58	$18.69	$ 13.24	$23.23
Service average			$16.17		$29.26		$36.46	

using different methodologies will be different, and hence a great deal of judgment will have to applied in the rate-setting process.

Setting the final rate

Remember that our goal here is to set a premium rate that BetterCare can use to make a bid to cover Big Business's employees. So far, we have estimated the capitation rates required to pay all of the providers needed to serve the population, both in area and out of area. In addition, we are assuming that pharmacy benefits will be handled separately, or *carved out*, and that the cost of these benefits would be $7.00 PMPM. After all costs have been considered, BetterCare concludes that it can submit a bid of $108.21 PMPM.

Hospital inpatient	$ 27.35	PMPM
Other institutional	9.12	
Outpatient prescription drugs	7.00	
Physician care	48.84	
Total medical care	$ 92.31	PMPM
HMO costs:		
Administration	$ 13.85	PMPM
Contribution to reserves/profits	2.05	
Total HMO costs	$ 15.90	PMPM
Total premium	$108.21	PMPM

Note that if BetterCare wins the contract from Big Business, the monthly revenue to providers will be somewhat higher (usually about 5 percent) than the embedded capitated rates, because enrollees will be required to make copayments for selected services.

In closing, note that BetterCare's bid most likely will be subject to market forces. That is, there will be multiple bidders for Big Business's health contract. If BetterCare's bid is to be accepted, it must offer the right combination of price and quality. If BetterCare's costs, and hence bid, is too high, or its quality too low, it will not get the contract, and it must reassess its cost and quality structure to ensure that it is competitive on future bids.

Self-Test Questions:

Roughly, what is the allocation of an HMO premium dollar?

Briefly describe these three methods for developing capitation rates:

1. Fee-for-service equivalent method
2. Budgetary, or cost, approach
3. Demographic-based approach.

Of the three approaches, which one do you think would be the most accurate? The easiest to apply in practice?

Risk-Sharing Arrangements

In an integrated delivery system, or within the provider panel of a managed care plan, different providers are brought together in some type of formal or informal arrangement to provide health care services to a defined population. Often, system participants are paid under different reimbursement methods, and different reimbursement systems clearly create different incentives. To illustrate, assume that an integrated delivery system uses capitation for primary care physicians, discounted fee-for-service for specialists, and per diem for institutional providers— hospitals and long-term care providers. In such a system, primary care physicians have the incentive to shift care to specialists and institutions because primary care physicians are capitated, and hence not rewarded for higher utilization. On the other hand, specialists and institutions would welcome the added volume, because they are being paid on the basis of the amount of services provided. Overall, this differential in reimbursement creates incentives that increase total system costs, and hence costs to insurers and purchasers.

If both primary care and specialist physicians are capitated, primary care physicians will still have the incentive to make unnecessary referrals, but such referrals will no longer be welcome by specialists. If the institutions also are capitated, no provider wants increased volume, so conflicts are bound to occur between primary care physicians and specialists and between physicians and institutions.

In such situations, *risk-sharing* arrangements are often implemented to create incentives that encourage providers to act in the best interest of the system, rather than in their own self-interest. Generally, proper incentives are created within integrated systems by establishing *withholds*, or *risk pools*, which are pools of money that are initially withheld, and then distributed to providers only if preestablished goals are met.

Risk-sharing basics

Risk pools can be used with any type of reimbursement system, such as the use of withholds in a per diem system, whereby the hospital is rewarded if utilization is less than expected and, in effect, penalized by not getting some portion or all of the amount withheld if utilization exceeds targets. In effect, risk pools are designed to reward those providers that are most able to control costs through better utilization management, better cost control, or both. Risk-sharing arrangements can occur among physicians only, among physicians and institutions, or among all providers. Furthermore, risk pools can be established to promote only financial goals or some combination of financial and nonfinancial goals.

Note that if a system is fully integrated and all subsidiary providers are owned by, and hence directly responsible to, the same parent, there is only one bottom line and no need for risk-sharing arrangements. Proper incentives are created by managerial control. However, in most systems today, providers are loosely affiliated in some way rather than part of the same corporation, and hence risk-sharing arrangements are needed to align the incentives of the diverse parties involved.

Typically, risk-sharing arrangements allocate 10–20 percent of each reimbursement dollar to one or more risk pools, often for primary care, specialty (referral) care, and institutional. Then, throughout the year, expenses are charged against the applicable pools, and at year end, each pool's expenses are reconciled, that is, compared with those budgeted. Any surpluses are distributed to the participating providers on the basis of a prearranged formula. Any deficits are typically funded from network reserves, which, as we will discuss later, are established specifically to cover system cost overruns.

Primary care withhold: an illustration of a single risk pool

The best way to grasp the basics of risk sharing is through examples. In this section, we illustrate a withhold system for primary care physicians only. In the next section, we will illustrate a risk-sharing system that encompasses primary care physicians, specialists, and a hospital.

Here is the risk pool arrangement for primary care physicians (PCPs) used by one HMO. The HMO pays its PCPs by capitation, but a percentage of the total capitated amount is held in reserve and distributed to individual physicians if certain financial goals are met. In general, PCP goals are based on specialty care and hospital costs. Of course, the goal is to lower the overall cost of providing care, but cost reduction goals should not reduce the quality of care afforded to patients.

Assume that the HMO's capitation payment to PCPs is $15 PMPM, but that 20 percent of this amount is placed into the PCP risk pool. The budgeted amount for specialty and hospital costs is $45 PMPM. Of course, the purpose of the pool is to encourage PCPs to take actions that result in realized specialty and hospital costs that are less than those budgeted. For simplicity, assume that there are only three PCPs in the plan: Physician L (for low-cost), Physician M (for medium-cost), and Physician H (for high-cost). Furthermore, assume that each physician has 1,000 patients under the plan, so there are 3,000 patients in total.

Table 18.8 contains the risk pool distributions under two different outcome scenarios. Line 1 gives each PCP's initial annual capitation payment: $15 PMPM(12 months)(1,000 members) = $180,000. Thus, 3($180,000) = $540,000 in total is allocated for PCP payments. However, 20 percent of the capitated amount is placed into the risk pool, so each PCP's annual capitated payment is reduced by 0.20($180,000) = $36,000. This reduction and the resulting $144,000 actual payment are shown on Lines 2 and 3. Note that each of the members served by the three PCPs is allocated $45 for specialty and hospital costs, so the budgeted goal for these costs is 1,000($45)(12) = $540,000 per PCP, or $1,620,000 in total, as shown on Line 4. Also, note that the total amount in the PCP risk pool is 3($36,000) = $108,000.

Now consider Scenario 1, contained in Lines 4 through 8. Here, the assumption is made that no PCP will receive any funds from the pool if it is empty at year end. The actual referral costs for each PCP are the amounts shown on Line 5. The referral gain (loss) for each PCP is shown on Line 6, while the total gain (loss) for all three PCPs is $40,000 − $20,000 − $140,000 = −$120,000. This exceeds the $108,000 in the risk pool, so no funds remain for distribution. In fact, BetterCare will have to fund the $108,000 − $120,000 = −$12,000 shortfall from its own reserves. Since no funds remain in the pool for distribution, each PCP's realized compensation would be his or her initial capitation payment, $144,000.

Clearly, there is a problem with the way that the risk pool is allocated. Since no funds remained in the pool, all three PCPs were equally penalized, even though Physician L did an excellent job of controlling costs and Physician M came in only $20,000 over budget. The real cause of the failure to meet the overall referral budget was Physician H, who was a whopping $140,000 over budget. Is it fair to penalize L and M because of H's actions? If, over time, it appears to Physicians L and M that the risk pool will always be exhausted due to actions beyond their control, they will have no motivation to continue to practice as efficiently as they do now. Also, it is important to know whether Physician H's failure to meet the risk pool budget is a result of practice patterns, or did H have an extraordinary number of high-cost patients? If the patient mix is not

Table 18.8   Primary Care Physician (PCP) Risk Pool (annual amounts)

	Physician L	Physician M	Physician H
1. Allocated amount	$180,000	$180,000	$180,000
2. Withhold (20 percent)	(36,000)	(36,000)	(36,000)
3. Initial payment	$144,000	$144,000	$144,000
Scenario 1: Distribution Based on Aggregate PCP Performance			
4. Budgeted referral costs	$540,000	$540,000	$540,000
5. Actual referral costs	500,000	560,000	680,000
6. Referral gain (loss)	$ 40,000	($ 20,000)	($140,000)
7. Withhold returned	0	0	0
8. Total compensation	$144,000	$144,000	$144,000
Scenario 2: Distribution Based on Individual PCP Performance			
9. Budgeted referral costs	$540,000	$540,000	$540,000
10. Actual referral costs	500,000	560,000	600,000
11. Referral gain (loss)	$ 40,000	($ 20,000)	($140,000)
12. Withhold returned	36,000	16,000	0
13. Total compensation	$180,000	$160,000	$144,000

equal across PCPs, obvious problems will arise, so the HMO must be careful in assigning patients to ensure (to the extent possible) that the usage and intensity mix is evenly spread across PCPs or that adjustments are made to account for such differences.

Scenario 2 in Table 18.8 is similar to Scenario 1, except that payments are made from the withhold to individual physicians regardless of the aggregate position of the pool. In this situation, the aggregate pool is really an artificiality, because the HMO will reward individual PCPs that come in at or under budget regardless of aggregate performance. In this situation, each PCP has his or her own individual risk pool. Thus, as shown on Line 12, Physician L, because he or she came in below budget, received the entire withhold amount from his or her pool, which resulted in total compensation of $144,000 + $36,000 = $180,000. Physician M received $36,000 − $20,000 = $16,000 from his or her pool, for total compensation of $160,000, while Physician H received nothing from his or her pool, for a total compensation of $144,000. This type of arrangement creates better incentives for PCPs, but the HMO had to bear the total cost of the pool payments, $52,000, because the actions of Physician H depleted the pool. The key here is to modify the behavior of Physician H so that funds remain in the pool to make the incentive payments. Perhaps, after one year, Physician H will be motivated to follow lower-cost practice patterns because of the potential monetary rewards.

Note that there is an almost infinite number of ways in which a PCP risk pool can be distributed. Another alternative to Scenario 2 would be this: if the aggregate risk pool is depleted, payments to individual physicians will be cut in half. If this were the situation in Scenario 2 in Table 18.8, Physician L would get only $18,000 from the pool on Line 12, while Physician M would be paid $8,000. Now, the actions of Physician H have a direct bearing on the payments to L and M, so it is in the best interests of L, M, and the system to encourage H to lower costs. Also, with this distribution system, the HMO does not replace the full amount of the pool if it is depleted.

Primary care and referral withholds: an illustration of two risk pools

The previous risk pool illustration placed only one set of providers at risk, the primary care physicians. In this section, we illustrate the use of two risk pools.

Assume that HealthyHMO, with 10,000 covered lives in a given service area, reimburses its primary care physicians under a capitated system, its specialty care physicians under a discounted fee-for-service system, and the hospital under a per diem system. To create proper incentives, HealthyHMO establishes two risk pools: a professional services risk pool for the physicians only and an inpatient services risk pool that is shared equally by the HMO, physicians, and hospital.

Professional services risk pool (PSRP)

Ten percent of the funds budgeted for specialty services are withheld in the professional services risk pool (PSRP). The total amount budgeted for professional services, including both primary and specialty care physicians, is $37 PMPM. With 10,000 members, the HMO's annual budget for professional services is $37(10,000)(12) = $4,440,000.

The capitated payment for primary care physicians is $12 PMPM, for a total of $12(10,000)(12) = $1,440,000. The difference between the total allocated for professional services and the capitated total for primary care services is $4,440,000 − $1,440,000 = $3,000,000, which is the amount allocated for specialty services. Since 10 percent of the specialists' budget is placed in the PSRP, it is funded at a level of $300,000, and the budget for specialist payments, after withhold, is $2,700,000.

When the budget year is over, a year-end reconciliation process adjusts for under- and overutilization, and allocates the pool among the primary care and specialist physicians. If actual costs exceed the $3,000,000 total specialty care budget, no distributions are made from the PSRP, and HealthyHMO must cover the shortfall. Table 18.9 illustrates end-of-year reconciliation under four different scenarios. In Scenario 1, actual payments for specialty services are assumed to be $3,000,000, as shown on Line 2. This results in a −$300,000 variance from the after-withhold budget, and the risk pool is depleted. Primary care physicians gain no additional income because the specialists have taken the entire amount in the pool in their fee-for-service payments.

Scenario 2 assumes specialist payments of $3,100,000, resulting in a −$400,000 budget variance. Like Scenario 1, nothing is left for the primary care physicians. In fact, the specialists have not only exhausted the pool, but receive $100,000 in additional payments from HealthyHMO, which must bear all losses exceeding the amount placed into the pool.

Scenario 3, which begins on Line 13 in Table 18.9, presents a lower-cost situation, assuming specialty care payments of only $2,800,000. Now the budget variance is −$100,000, leaving $200,000 in the pool for distribution. There are many methodologies that could be used to make the distribution. The $200,000 could be evenly split among all physicians. Or, the pool could be distributed to physicians on a basis proportional to the amount of effort that they expend on HealthyHMO's patients, say, as measured by the number of patient visits or the dollar amount paid to each physician. Alternatively, the distribution could be based on the number of referrals made by primary care physicians and the number received by specialty physicians. In this situation, primary care physicians with fewer referrals would get a larger share of the pool, while specialists with a higher number of referrals would receive a larger share of the pool.

Scenario 4 is similar to Scenario 3, except that with only $2,600,000 paid to specialists over the year, the pool is left with $400,000. Now, $300,000 is available for distribution to physicians and $100,000 is reclaimed by HealthyHMO.

Inpatient services risk pool (ISRP)

HealthyHMO budgets for the inpatient services risk pool (ISRP) based on 350 inpatient days per 1,000 members, which is the rate experienced by the HMO last year for its entire membership. The negotiated per diem

Table 18.9   Professional Services Risk Pool (PSRP)
(annual amounts)

Scenario 1: Specialty Payments of $3,000,000	
1. Budgeted payments for specialty services	$2,700,000
2. Actual payments for specialty services	3,000,000
3. Variance from budget	($ 300,000)
4. Risk pool starting amount	300,000
5. Remainder in pool	$ 0
6. Risk pool allocation	$ 0
Scenario 2: Specialty Payments of $3,100,000	
7. Budgeted payments for specialty services	$2,700,000
8. Actual payments for specialty services	3,100,000
9. Variance from budget	($ 400,000)
10. Risk pool starting amount	300,000
11. Remainder in pool	($ 100,000)
12. Risk pool allocation	$ 0
Scenario 3: Specialty Payments of $2,800,000	
13. Budgeted payments for specialty services	$2,700,000
14. Actual payments for specialty services	2,800,000
15. Variance from budget	($ 100,000)
16. Risk pool starting amount	300,000
17. Remainder in pool	$ 200,000
18. Risk pool allocation	$ 200,000
Scenario 4: Specialty Payments of $2,600,000	
19. Budgeted payments for specialty services	$2,700,000
20. Actual payments for specialty services	2,600,000
21. Variance from budget	$ 100,000
22. Risk pool starting amount	300,000
23. Remainder in pool	$ 400,000
24. Risk pool allocation	
a. Physicians	$ 300,000
b. HMO	100,000

rate is $750. Thus, its 10,000 members are expected to use 10(350) = 3,500 inpatient days, giving a before-withhold amount of 3,500($750) = $2,625,000. HealthyHMO withholds 10 percent of the inpatient budget for the ISRP, or $262,500. Thus, the adjusted per diem rate is 0.90($750) = $675, resulting in a total budgeted payment for inpatient services of 3,500($675) = $2,362,500.

For reconciliation, suppose that actual utilization was 385 inpatient days versus the 350 forecast (10 percent variance higher than forecasted). The resulting ISRP distribution is contained in Table 18.10. With overutilization (as compared to the budget), realized payments total 3,850($675) = $2,598,750, as shown on Line 2, resulting in a dollar variance of −$236,250, as shown on Line 3. Since the pool was initially funded with $262,500, the amount left in the pool after reconciliation is $262,500 − $236,250 = $26,250, which is shown on Line 5. This amount, according to distribution guidelines, is split evenly among primary care physicians, specialty care physicians, and the hospital, as shown in Lines 6a through 6c.

Note that the hospital's per diem payment before withhold was $750. After reconciliation, the hospital's total payment is $2,598,750 + $8,750 = $2,607,500. Since this total resulted from 3,850 inpatient days, the realized per diem payment was $2,607,500/3,850 = $677. This amount is less than the starting $750 amount, because more than the budgeted amount was spent on inpatient care. However, since some funds remained in the pool, the final per diem amount is slightly more than the $675 after-withhold amount. Note that even if less than the budgeted amount is spent on inpatient care, the hospital will still receive less than the initial $750 per diem amount because any savings is split three ways.

The intent of the ISRP is to encourage the parties that have some control over hospital utilization to limit the number of inpatient days to those that are absolutely essential to patients' welfare. Of course, since the hospital is being reimbursed on a per diem basis, it has the incentive

Table 18.10   Inpatient Services Risk Pool (ISRP)
                   (annual amounts)

1. Budgeted payments for inpatient services	$2,362,500
2. Actual payments for inpatient services	2,598,750
3. Variance from budget	($ 236,250)
4. Risk pool starting amount	262,500
5. Remainder in pool	$ 26,250
6. Risk pool allocation	
a. Hospital (⅓)	$ 8,750
b. Primary care physicians (⅓)	8,750
c. Specialty care physicians (⅓)	8,750
7. Total allocated	$ 26,250

to maximize the number of inpatient days. Any gain from additional per diem payments will be three times as profitable as pool distributions, because per diem payments are not shared with physicians. Therefore, the ISRP is really set up to motivate physicians, who actually control hospital admissions and discharges. Under per diem, the hospital does have the incentive to lower costs, because lower costs lead to higher profits. However, the best way to motivate the hospital to control utilization would be to put it under capitation payments.

Performance-based pools

In our discussion of risk pools thus far, we have focused exclusively on risk pools designed to control utilization and costs, but such pools can be structured to influence other types of behavior. To illustrate, primary care as well as specialty physicians may participate in a *performance-based pool*, wherein the pool is distributed on the basis of both financial and nonfinancial performance.

Here is how a performance-based pool might work for primary care physicians. As before, some percentage, say, 20, of the total capitation payment is withheld. At the end of the year, the pool is distributed to physicians based on performance in four areas: (1) quality of care, (2) quality of service, (3) cost control, and (4) organizational participation. Thirty percent of the pool is allocated to each of the first three areas, and ten percent is allocated to organizational participation. Physicians are "graded" in each area. For example, quality of care could be based on chart reviews, continuing medical education hours, and number of liability claims; quality of service could be based on patient satisfaction surveys, as well as the ease with which patients can make appointments and the time spent waiting during visits; cost control could depend on cost of referrals and other resource utilization; and organizational participation could be based on number of staff meetings attended and committee posts held.

At the end of the year, the pool distribution would reward those physicians who scored highest in each area and penalize those physicians who did worst. For example, assume that $10,000 remained in a pool for three physicians, so $0.30(\$10,000) = \$3,000$ is available for distribution based on quality of care performance. Furthermore, the physicians' quality of care performance scores are 55 for Physician X, 44 for Physician Y, and 33 for Physician Z. Note that these scores have no absolute meaning, but they do tell us how well the physicians have performed relative to one another on the quality of care dimension.

Since the scores total 132, Physician X would receive 55/132 = 0.42 of the $3,000 pool, or $1,260; Physician Y would receive 44/132 = 0.33 of the pool, or $990; and Physician Z would receive the remaining $750. Of course, some minimum score could be established, so that physicians would receive nothing from the pool if the minimum level of performance was not met. It is clear that the type of risk pool described in this section creates incentives for physicians to perform well along both financial and nonfinancial dimensions.

Self-Test Questions:

What is the purpose of a risk pool?

Describe how a typical risk pool works.

Can a delivery system with multiple providers have more than one risk pool? Explain.

What is a performance-based risk pool?

Financial Risk Management

As discussed earlier, capitated payments expose providers to financial risks that differ from those associated with conventional reimbursement systems. As with all financial risks, there are actions that can be taken to reduce the impact of capitation-induced risks. We discuss two in this section: (1) the establishment of reserves and (2) stop-loss provisions (reinsurance).

Reserves

The first line of defense against financial risk by any organization is the maintenance of adequate *reserves*. Any provider—including physicians and hospitals—that assumes the financial risk for covered lives without having adequate reserves could easily end up, so to speak, as roadkill along the capitation highway. When health care providers accept capitated rates, they agree to provide whatever services are required for a fixed monthly fee. If all goes well, that is, if utilization and costs are controlled, the provider will end the year with a profit. But, if realized utilization and costs exceed estimates, the losses have to be covered in some way, and hence the need for reserves becomes apparent. There are several classifications of reserves. We will cover the two most important types: required reserves and reserves for incurred but not reported costs.

Required reserves

Required reserves are those reserves necessary to cover costs that exceed capitation revenues. The term "required reserves" stems from the fact that insurance companies—and HMOs are considered to be insurance companies in most states—are required by state regulators to maintain reserves. Typically, such regulations specify a minimum fixed dollar amount of reserves, some percentage of premium income, or even some dollar amount per individual insured. It is interesting to note that some state insurance regulators are now examining the risk positions of providers to ascertain whether it would be appropriate to require licensure and reserves.

At the provider level, where reserves are not currently required by law, it makes good business sense to have sufficient cash and marketable securities on hand (in reserve) to cover losses that have a reasonable likelihood of occurring. In Chapter 14, we discussed the use of Monte Carlo simulation to set a firm's target cash balance. Here we noted that firms' cash inflows and outflows are not known with certainty, so in any period, say, a month, cash outflows could exceed inflows, and a reserve cash balance should be established to cover the potential shortfall. The concept is exactly the same for capitation reserves, but here it is applied to a particular contract. By applying Monte Carlo simulation to utilization and costs, it is possible to estimate the sizes and probabilities of occurrence of potential contract losses. Then, based on the risk aversion of the organization's managers, a reserve can be established to cover all but the most unlikely loss scenarios.

To illustrate the concept, consider a capitation contract that Westside Memorial Hospital has with a local HMO to serve 50,000 enrollees. The capitation rate is $27.50 PMPM, resulting in $16.50 million in total revenue. Table 18.11 contains Westside's best estimate for the cost distribution of enrollees along with the resulting profit distribution. These distributions were developed on the basis of estimates of enrollees' admission rates, average length of stay, and average per diem cost. The expected total contract cost is $15.78 million, resulting in an expected profit of $720,000, which gives Westside a profit margin of 4.4 percent.

Focusing solely on this one contract, it is clear that Westside's profit is not guaranteed. There is a 60 percent chance that the profit realized will be greater than the $720,000 estimate. That's the good news! The bad news is that there is a 40 percent chance that the profit will be less than expected, and a 10 percent chance that the contract will lose money. How can Westside protect itself against the possibility

Table 18.11   Westside Memorial Hospital: Contract Cost and
Profit Distribution (millions of dollars)

Probability	Contract Cost	Contract Profit or Loss
0.10	$14.00	$2.50
0.20	15.00	1.50
0.30	15.50	1.00
0.20	16.00	0.50
0.10	16.50	0.00
0.05	17.50	(1.00)
0.03	19.00	(2.50)
0.02	21.50	(5.00)
1.00 Expected value =	$15.78	$0.72

Note: Contract revenues total $16.50 million.

that losses on this contract will push the hospital into financial distress? Of course, the answer is to have sufficient reserves. On the basis of the Table 18.11 distributions, Westside could fund a $5 million reserve that would totally protect the hospital (assuming that the probability distribution itself is correct). But this very conservative approach to reserves would, assuming an opportunity cost rate of 10 percent, cost Westside $500,000 in carrying costs, and hence almost wipe out the contract's expected profit.

As an alternative, Westside might conclude that a 2 percent probability of occurrence represents a very unlikely event, and hence does not warrant reserve protection. If this were the case, Westside would set a reserve for the contract of less than $5,000,000, say, $1,000,000 or $2,500,000. The choice is a risk/return trade-off, with more risk protection requiring a larger reserve, which in turn leads to lower contract profits. In general, the larger the contract, and the greater the uncertainty in contract costs, the higher the reserve must be to offer realistic protection against negative outcomes.

In most situations, the reserve requirement is not as clear-cut as discussed here. First, it is not easy to estimate utilization and cost distributions, so it is very difficult to have much confidence in the Table 18.11 values. Second, most providers have a large number of contracts with numerous payers, and what is most relevant is the chance of an overall loss rather than the probability of a loss on a particular contract. If the loss distributions on the individual contracts are not perfectly positively correlated, then portfolio effects will mitigate somewhat the risks inherent in each contract.

Note that financial withholds are, in effect, a type of reserve. If certain financial goals are met, the withhold is distributed to providers. However, if goals are not met, the withhold is used to cover the excess costs incurred. Also, note that of all the providers, physicians are particularly vulnerable when entering capitation contracts because historically they have not used reserves. In most cases, physician group practices do everything they can to clear their books at year end. Instead of posting profits that would be taxable, the tendency has been to spend any surplus on salaries and equipment. With this type of behavior as the norm, it is especially difficult to think in terms of establishing reserves.

Reserves for incurred but not reported (IBNR) costs

Another type of reserve is that held to cover *incurred but not reported (IBNR) costs*. To illustrate these reserves, consider HealthyHMO. At the end of every accounting period—for purposes here, assume a year—it must close its books and reconcile its established risk pools. Healthy-HMO uses capitation to pay for primary care services, but it uses fee-for-service reimbursement to pay for specialist services. When it closes its books at the end of the year, HealthyHMO might not realize that there are specialist referrals that have been made by its primary care physicians that have not yet been billed. Indeed, some required specialist services may not have even been performed.

If a provider is capitated, yet has referral responsibility for services that it does not provide, there is a strong likelihood that at the end of the year there will be payment obligations for costs that have been incurred but not reported. Obviously, such costs must be planned for and covered, and the impact of such costs on risk pool distributions must be taken into account. There are relatively sophisticated methods available for establishing IBNR reserves, as well as some rather ad hoc methods such as setting two or three months worth of historical IBNR dollar claims aside as a reserve. It is not important for you to know the details of setting up IBNR reserves—we will leave that to the accountants—but it is important for you to recognize that providers bear extra risk whenever they are responsible for payments for services that they do not provide.

Stop-loss provisions (reinsurance)

Rather than establishing reserves to cover every conceivable cost situation, many providers elect to "reinsure" the risk. Such insurance, which is now offered by dozens of insurance companies, is called *reinsurance* or medical *stop-loss insurance.*[5] Providers have several options for handling stop-loss insurance. One option is to have the HMO withhold a portion of the capitation rate for the sole purpose of buying insurance. However, if the HMO elects to self-insure, and then fails to establish adequate reserves, the provider remains at risk. Another option is for the provider to receive the full capitation payment, and then purchase stop-loss insurance directly from a company that specializes in such insurance. Of course, the option always exists for the provider to self-insure.

Stop-loss insurance is written to protect providers from losses on individual patients, rather than from aggregate losses on a contract. The idea is to insure the provider against catastrophic "budget buster" patients, not to guarantee a certain level of overall profitability. For example, a hospital might purchase stop-loss insurance with a deductible or *threshold,* of $100,000. For any patient with charges over $100,000, the insurer might agree to pay 80 percent of billed charges in excess of this threshold amount. Of course, the lower the threshold and the higher the percentage of any excess paid by the insurer, the higher the stop-loss insurance premium.

Self-Test Questions:

Why is it important that capitated providers establish reserves?

What are the two primary types of reserves?

What is stop-loss insurance, and when should it be taken?

Summary

- *Capitation* is a flat periodic payment to a physician or other health care provider that is the sole reimbursement for providing services to a defined population.

- Capitation payments are generally expressed as some dollar amount *per member per month (PMPM),* where the word "member" typically means enrollee in some managed care plan, usually a *health maintenance organization (HMO).*

- The impetus behind capitation is *health care reform,* which is being mandated by purchasers that can no longer bear the high costs of the current system.

- The increasing size and strength of HMOs means that more and more providers will be *paid under capitation* in the future.

- Although capitation payment was first used with *primary care physicians*, virtually any type of health care service can be reimbursed by capitation.

- Under *fee-for-service*, all volumes less than breakeven produce a loss for the provider, while all volumes greater than breakeven produce a profit. Under *capitation*, all volumes less than breakeven produce a profit, whereas all volumes greater than breakeven result in a loss. Thus, *provider incentives* under capitation are opposite those under conventional reimbursement.

- In markets where capitation has made inroads, the trend is toward *fewer hospital beds* and a physician mix that contains a *greater proportion of primary care physicians*. Most importantly, as capitation gains in importance, historical utilization rates based on conventional reimbursement methodologies are not good predictors of future utilization.

- *Objective risk* occurs when the risk inherent in an uncertain outcome can be specified with confidence. *Subjective risk* occurs when the probability distribution itself is uncertain. Although the objective risk in capitation contracts is no greater, and potentially less, than that under conventional reimbursement, the subjective risk can be high.

- Several methods are used to set capitation rates for providers, including (1) the *fee-for-service equivalent method*, (2) the *budgetary*, or *cost, approach*, and (3) the *demographic-based approach*.

- In *integrated delivery systems*, it is important to establish incentives that encourage providers to act in the best interest of the system, rather than in their own self-interest. One way to create proper incentives is to establish *withholds*, or *risk pools*, which are pools of money that are initially withheld, and then distributed to providers only if preestablished goals are met.

- The two primary actions taken to reduce the impact of capitation-induced risks are (1) the establishment of *reserves* and (2) *stop-loss provisions (reinsurance)*.

Notes

1. Decision scientists classify risk in a more rigorous fashion as follows: *Ignorance* is the condition when decision makers can't even estimate the probable outcomes, say, the cash flows associated with a research and development project; *uncertainty* is present when outcomes can be predicted, but no

probabilities can be attached; and *risk* occurs when both outcomes and probabilities can be forecasted. These classifications are not commonly used by real world decision makers, so we will stick to the simpler objective and subjective risk classifications discussed in this paragraph.

2. This section summarizes results reported in the following two articles by L. C. Gapenski and B. Langland-Orban: "Predicting Financial Risk under Capitation," *Healthcare Financial Management* (November 1995); and "The Impact of Capitation Contracts on Financial Risk," *Health Services Management Review* (forthcoming).

3. Providers that have capitation contracts can limit outlier risk by purchasing *stop-loss* insurance. However, such insurance reduces the profitability of the capitation contract. Stop-loss insurance is discussed in more detail in a later section.

4. Note that the utilization, charge, and cost data used in this section to develop capitation rates are for illustration only, and do not necessarily reflect actual values being used today.

5. The term "reinsurance" has traditionally been used to mean insurance bought by insurance companies from other insurance companies to limit the risk assumed by the first insurer in covering a potential loss. However, the term is now being used in the health care industry when a provider seeks insurance to limit capitation risk.

Selected Additional References

Baker, J. J. 1995. "Activity-Based Costing for Integrated Delivery Systems." *Journal of Health Care Finance,* (Winter): 57–61.

Bond, M. T., and B. Stevenson Marshall. 1994. "Offsetting Unexpected Healthcare Costs with Futures Contracts." *Healthcare Financial Management* (December): 54–58.

———. 1995. "Managing Financial Risk with Options on Futures." *Healthcare Financial Management* (May): 50–56.

Cave, D. G. 1995. "Vertical Integration Models to Prepare Health Systems for Capitation." *Health Care Management Review* (Winter): 26–39.

Coyne, J. S., and S. D. Simon. 1994. "Is Your Organization Ready to Share Financial Risk with HMOs?" *Healthcare Financial Management* (August): 30–34.

Davidson, D. M., and J. Wester. 1995. "Addressing Integrated Systems' Tax-Exemption Problems." *Healthcare Financial Management* (January): 46–30.

Finkler, S. A. 1995. "Capitated Hospital Contracts." *Health Care Management Review* (Summer): 88–91.

Keegan, A. J. 1994. "Hospitals Become Cost Centers in Managed Care Scenario." *Healthcare Financial Management* (August): 36–39.

Kolb, D. S., and J. L. Horowitz. 1995. "Managing the Transition to Capitation." *Healthcare Financial Management* (February): 65–69.

Herrle, G. N., and W. M. Pollock. 1995. "Multispecialty Medical Groups: Adapting to Capitation." *Journal of Health Care Finance* (Spring): 37–43.

Pallarito, K. 1994. "Gatekeepers of Capitation." *Modern Healthcare* (27 June): 93–100.

Peregrine, M. W., and D. L. Glaser. 1995. "Choosing Medical Practice Acquisition Models." *Healthcare Financial Management* (March): 58–64.

Ryan, J. B., and S. B. Clay. 1995. "How to Determine Financial Reserves for Capitated Contracts." *Healthcare Financial Management* (March): 18.

Schultz, D. V. 1995. "The Importance of Primary Care Providers in Integrated Systems." *Healthcare Financial Management* (January): 58–63.

Seaver, D. J., and S. H. Kramer. 1994. "Direct Contracting: The Future of Managed Care." *Healthcare Financial Management* (August): 21–27.

Shortell, S. M. 1995. "The Future of Integrated Systems." *Healthcare Financial Management* (January): 24–30.

Teske, J. M. 1995. "Second-Generation Legal Issues in Integrated Delivery Systems," *Healthcare Financial Management* (January): 54–57.

Toso, M. E., and A. Farmer. 1994. "Using Cost Accounting Data to Develop Capitation Rates." *Topics in Health Care Financing* (Fall): 1–12.

Witek, J. E., and H. Davidson. 1994. "Assessing Organizational Readiness for Capitation and Risk Sharing." *Healthcare Financial Management* (August): 18–19.

Case 18

Frazier Health System: Capitation and Risk Sharing

Frazier Health System (the System) is a physician-hospital organization (PHO) formed by Frazier Memorial Hospital and its affiliated physicians. Over the past five years, the System has had an annual contract to provide exclusive local health care services to enrollees in Capital City Health Plan (the Plan), the local Blue Cross/Blue Shield HMO. In last year's contract with the System, the Plan paid primary care physicians on a capitated basis, but paid specialists and the hospital on a negotiated (discounted) fee-for-service basis. Now, the Plan wants to fully capitate the System, and has proposed a capitation rate that would result in System revenues that are roughly equal to those received last year. The System's executive director, Dr. George O'Donnell, a cardiologist and recent graduate of the University of Wisconsin's Nonresident Program in Administrative Medicine, initially took the position of "no way." However, the Plan has indicated that it will take its 50,000 members (covered lives) to the System's primary competitor if negotiations do not work out.

As detailed in Table 1, the System's medical panel currently consists of 249 physicians. To better assess physician needs, the System recently hired a health care consulting firm to estimate the number of physicians, by specialty, required to support a patient population of 50,000 under aggressive case management. The results of this study are also contained in Table 1. Note, however, that the System serves patients other than those in the Capital City HMO, so the total number of physicians required to treat all of the System's patients far exceeds the Table 1 amount of 59.

An analysis of recent physician data has shown that there is significant variation among physicians' practice patterns, both in their offices and in the hospital. For example, Table 2 contains summary data on hospital charges for three common DRGs. Consider DRG 127, heart failure, for which Frazier Memorial Hospital had 59 admissions. The System physician with the lowest hospital charges for this DRG averaged $9,241 in hospital charges per patient, the highest-charge physician averaged $11,394, and the average charge for all physicians was $10,319. On average, the Plan indicated that its enrollees are hospitalized at a rate of 380 patient-days per 1,000 enrollees.

To help in analyzing the Plan's proposal to capitate the system, Dr. O'Donnell has requested data from the Plan concerning last year's actual payments to the System. Payments to the System last year were

Table 1 System Physician Mix and Estimated Needs per 50,000 Enrollees

Specialty	Number in System	Estimated Need per 50,000 Enrollees
General medicine	42	20.9
Pediatrics	15	4.1
Total primary care	57	25.0
Anesthesiology	9	2.5
Cardiology	12	1.4
Emergency medicine	10	2.5
General surgery	13	2.7
Neurosurgery	3	0.3
Obstetrics/gynecology	27	5.4
Orthopedics	11	2.5
Psychiatry	19	1.9
Radiology	8	3.0
Thoracic surgery	0	0.4
Urology	5	1.3
Other specialties	75	10.1
Total specialists	192	34.0
Grand total	249	59.0

Table 2 Average Hospital Charges for Three Common DRGs by Physician

DRG	Minimum	Average	Maximum
98: Bronchitis/Asthma	$2,872	$ 4,018	$ 4,638
127: Heart failure	9,271	10,319	11,394
373: Vaginal delivery without complications	6,498	7,568	8,015

approximately $100 per member per month (PMPM), for a total annual payment of $100(50,000 members)(12 months) = $60 million. Of this $60 million, 42 percent went to the hospital, 12 percent was paid to primary care physicians, 38 percent went to specialty physicians, and 8 percent went for miscellaneous "other services," such as medical equipment, nursing home care, and home health care. The system would be responsible for providing these services under the proposed contract, but outpatient pharmacy and out-of-area services would be funded by the Plan separately.

As part of normal operations, the System has a standing committee to identify and resolve differences among its disparate elements. When Dr. O'Donnell asked the committee for a short report on current problem areas, including the possibility of a capitated contract with the Plan, he was provided the following information:

Frazier Memorial Hospital

Hospital managers are worried about profitability. In total, the hospital barely broke even last year when the Plan paid 75 percent of charges. Although no one knows for sure, the best guess is that the hospital lost 1 percent on last year's Plan contract. They believe that the only way to control hospital costs is to create a subpanel of physicians for participation in the capitation contract. When asked how the subpanel should be chosen, their reply was to choose the physicians who have done the best job of containing hospital costs.

Primary Care Physicians

Most of the primary care physicians believe that they have been the losers under past contracts with the Plan. On average, primary care physicians received only about 60 percent of what charges would have been for treating the Plan's enrollees. Primary care physicians are the only ones bearing the risk of capitated payments, they get the lowest compensation, and they believe that they have to work much harder than the specialists. Furthermore, primary care physicians believe that the specialists supplement their own incomes by overusing in-office tests and procedures. Some primary care physicians are even talking about dropping out of the PHO, forming their own contracting group, and "taking the whole capitation payment from the Plan and contracting themselves for specialist and hospital services."

Specialist Care Physicians

The specialists believe that the primary care physicians refer too many patients to them. The specialists don't mind as long as they are being paid charges—they received between 80 and 90 percent of charges under last year's contract with the Plan—but if they are capitated they want the primary care physicians to handle more of the problems themselves. Also, whenever the subject of subpanels is raised, many of the specialists become incensed. "After all," they say, "the whole idea behind the System is to protect the specialists." Both sets of physicians—primary care and specialists—agree that the hospital is hopelessly inefficient. Says one specialist, "The hospital is getting the lion's share of the contract monies and they still don't seem to be able to make a profit."

In order to respond to the Plan's initiative, the System must grapple with the following issues:

1. How should the $100 PMPM capitation payment from the Plan be allocated to each component (hospital, primary care physicians, specialists, and other)?

2. What payment methodology should the system use for each component?

3. What risk pools or other incentives should be put in place?

4. Should all of the System's physicians participate in the contract, or should subpanels be formed? If subpanels should be formed, how will they be constituted?

5. What other actions must the System undertake to increase the chances of successfully managing a capitation contract?

In pondering these questions, Dr. O'Donnell and the System's executive committee are forced to face up to the fact that the hospital really needs this contract. If the Plan takes its business elsewhere, the hospital will lose 52 patients per day. A blow of this magnitude to the hospital's occupancy rate would force it into a major restructuring. Furthermore, all physicians would be hurt, to a greater or lesser extent, if the contract goes to a competing delivery system.

Assume that you have been hired to advise Dr. O'Donnell and the board of directors of Frazier Health System regarding its response to the Capital City Health Plan. At a minimum, your report should address all of the issues listed above, as well as the concerns raised by the physicians and the hospital.

Index

About the Author

Louis C. Gapenski, Ph.D., is an associate professor in both health services administration and finance at the University of Florida. He is the author or coauthor of twenty textbooks on corporate and health care finance. Dr. Gapenski's books are used world wide, with Canadian and international editions as well as translations into Russian, Bulgarian, Chinese, Indonesian, and Spanish. In addition, he has published over 25 journal articles related to corporate and health care finance.

Dr. Gapenski received a B.S. degree from the Virginia Military Institute, an M.S. degree from the U.S. Naval Postgraduate School, and M.B.A. and Ph.D. degrees from the University of Florida.

Dr. Gapenski is an active member of the Association of University Programs in Health Administration, the American College of Healthcare Executives, and the Healthcare Financial Management Association. He has acted as academic advisor, chaired sessions, and presented papers at numerous national meetings, and has been a reviewer for eleven academic and professional journals.